Handbook of Inflammatory Bowel Disease

Handbook of Inflammatory Bowel Disease

Edited by Charlotte Ramirez

hayle
medical

New York

Hayle Medical,
750 Third Avenue, 9th Floor,
New York, NY 10017, USA

Visit us on the World Wide Web at:
www.haylemedical.com

ISBN: 978-1-63241-914-9

Cataloging-in-Publication Data

Handbook of inflammatory bowel disease / edited by Charlotte Ramirez.
    p. cm.
Includes bibliographical references and index.
ISBN 978-1-63241-914-9
1. Inflammatory bowel diseases. 2. Gastroenteritis. I. Ramirez, Charlotte.
RC862.I53 H36 2020
616.344--dc23

Table of Contents

Preface

Inflammatory bowel disease (IBD) comprises of two conditions- ulcerative colitis and Crohn's disease. These involve chronic inflammation of the colon and small intestine. IBD is caused by a combination of genetic and environmental factors interacting with the body's defense system. IBD can exhibit intestinal complications such as toxic megacolon, ulcers, strictures and fistulas. Extraintestinal complications such as skin rashes, eye problems, liver disease and arthritis are also common. IBD is rarely a fatal disease. Fatalities may however arise due to bowel perforation, toxic megacolon and surgical complications. The goal of IBD treatment is achieving total remission. Often an acute resurgence of symptoms may occur, which may again require medication. Some of the research dimensions in the management of IBD explore the healing effects of helminthic therapy, prebiotics and probiotics, and cannabis. This book is a valuable compilation of topics, ranging from the basic to the most complex advancements in the diagnosis and therapy for inflammatory bowel disease. From theories to research to practical applications, case studies related to all contemporary topics of relevance to this condition have been included herein. It will help new researchers by foregrounding their knowledge in inflammatory bowel disease.

The information shared in this book is based on empirical researches made by veterans in this field of study. The elaborative information provided in this book will help the readers further their scope of knowledge leading to advancements in this field.

Finally, I would like to thank my fellow researchers who gave constructive feedback and my family members who supported me at every step of my research.

Editor

The Vitamin D Status in Inflammatory Bowel Disease

Lauren Elizabeth Veit[1], Louise Maranda[2], Jay Fong[1], Benjamin Udoka Nwosu[1]*

1 Department of Pediatrics, University of Massachusetts Medical School, Worcester, Massachusetts, United States of America, 2 Department of Quantitative Health Sciences, University of Massachusetts Medical School, Worcester, Massachusetts, United States of America

Abstract

Context: There is no consensus on the vitamin D status of children and adolescents with inflammatory bowel disease (IBD).

Aim: To determine the vitamin D status of patients with IBD by comparing their serum 25(OH)D concentration to that of healthy controls.

Hypothesis: Serum 25(OH)D concentration will be lower in patients with IBD compared to controls.

Subjects and Methods: A case-controlled retrospective study of subjects with IBD (n = 58) of 2–20 years (male n = 31, age 16.38±2.21 years; female n = 27, age16.56±2.08 years) and healthy controls (n = 116; male n = 49, age 13.90±4.59 years; female n = 67, age 15.04±4.12years). Study subject inclusion criteria: diagnosis of Crohn's disease (CD) or ulcerative colitis (UC). Vitamin D deficiency was defined as 25(OH)D of (<20 ng/mL) (<50 nmol/L), overweight as BMI of ≥85th but <95th percentile, and obesity as BMI ≥95th percentile. Data were expressed as mean ± SD.

Results: Patients with CD, UC, and their controls had mean serum 25(OH)D concentrations of 61.69±24.43 nmol/L, 53.26±25.51, and 65.32±27.97 respectively (ANOVA, p = 0.196). The overweight/obese controls had significantly lower 25(OH)D concentration compared to the normal-weight controls (p = 0.031); whereas 25(OH)D concentration was similar between the normal-weight and overweight/obese IBD patients (p = 0.883). There was no difference in 25(OH)D between patients with UC and CD, or between subjects with active IBD and controls. However, IBD subjects with elevated ESR had significantly lower 25(OH)D than IBD subjects with normal ESR (p = 0.025), as well as controls (65.3±28.0 nmol/L vs. 49.5±25.23, p = 0.045).

Conclusion: There is no difference in mean serum 25(OH)D concentration between children and adolescents with IBD and controls. However, IBD subjects with elevated ESR have significantly lower 25(OH)D than controls. Therefore, IBD subjects with elevated ESR should be monitored for vitamin D deficiency.

Editor: Andrzej T. Slominski, University of Tennessee, United States of America

Funding: This work was funded in part by the Faculty Diversity Scholars Program, and the Department of Pediatrics, University of Massachusetts Medical School, Worcester, Massachusetts, USA. The funders had no role in study design, data collection and analysis, decision to publish, or preparation of the manuscript.

Competing Interests: The authors have declared that no competing interests exist.

* Email: Benjamin.Nwosu@umassmemorial.org

Introduction

There is no consensus on the vitamin D status of children and adolescents with inflammatory bowel disease (IBD). The composite term IBD refers to two diseases, Crohn's disease (CD) and ulcerative colitis (UC), which are characterized by chronic inflammation of the gastrointestinal tract, marked by recurrent periods of remission and exacerbation [1]. Pediatric CD is characterized by discontinuous, transmural inflammation of the gastrointestinal tract with preferential involvement of the ileo-colonic segment, while UC is characterized by a more superficial, continuous inflammation that extends proximally from the rectum to variable areas of the large intestine [1].

Prolonged vitamin D deficiency could lead to poor health, as strong associations between vitamin D deficiency and increased risk for several diseases such as type 1 and type 2 diabetes, cardiovascular diseases, rheumatoid arthritis, infectious diseases, depression, and cancers of the breast, prostate, colon, and pancreas, have been reported [2–4]. Though there is an ongoing debate on the significance of these extra-skeletal functions of vitamin D in humans [5,6], there is a universal consensus on its skeletal functions, as vitamin D has been demonstrated to be vital for bone mineralization, maintenance of bone strength, and the prevention of fractures and consequent immobilization [6,7].

The lack of consensus on the vitamin D status of children and adolescents with IBD stems from two primary reasons: first, the studies that investigated the vitamin D status of children and adolescents with IBD [8–12] focused primarily on determining the prevalence of vitamin D deficiency in IBD, and secondarily on comparing the vitamin D status of patients with the subtypes of

IBD, i.e., UC and CD, but failed to compare their results directly to a local control group of healthy children and adolescents.

Secondly, only one study has directly compared the vitamin D status of children and adolescents with IBD to the vitamin D status of age- and gender-matched peers [13]. This cross-sectional study of 60 children with newly-diagnosed IBD and 56 controls found that 25(OH)D level was significantly lower in children with IBD compared to the controls. However, no subsequent studies have been performed to confirm these findings. Furthermore, to our knowledge, there has been no case-controlled study examining the vitamin D status of patients with established IBD of more than one year duration. This lack of clarity on the vitamin D status of children and adolescents with IBD compared to their peers has made it difficult to propose a coherent recommendation for vitamin D supplementation in patients with IBD [9,14].

We designed this study to explore the hypothesis that serum 25(OH)D concentration is significantly lower in patients with IBD compared to controls. The primary aim of this study was to characterize the vitamin D status of patients with IBD by directly comparing their mean serum 25(OH)D concentration to that of a local group of healthy children.

Materials and Methods

Ethics statement

The study protocol was approved by the University of Massachusetts Institutional Review Board. All patient records and information were anonymized and de-identified prior to analysis.

Subjects

All data were sourced from the Children's Medical Center Database of the UMassMemorial Medical Center, Worcester, Massachusetts, USA. The medical records of children and adolescents of ages 2–20 years with a confirmed diagnosis of Crohn's disease or ulcerative colitis from January 1, 2007 through June 30, 2013, were reviewed. Study subjects (n = 58; 31 males) were included if they had a diagnosis of Crohn's disease or ulcerative colitis. Subjects' height, weight, gender, race, IBD diagnosis, date of endoscopic IBD diagnosis, and any history of vitamin D supplementation were recorded.

A group of healthy peers served as controls. The controls were identified from the same database as the subjects. Subjects were included in the control group (n = 116; 49 males) if they carried no diagnosis of Crohn's disease or ulcerative colitis. Subjects' height, weight, gender, race, and history of vitamin D supplementation were similarly recorded.

Patients were excluded from this study if they carried a concurrent diagnosis of any disease that affects calcium or vitamin D metabolism. Subjects with a malabsorption syndrome, other than IBD, were excluded. Further exclusion criteria included patients with a history of vitamin D or calcium supplementation prior to the date of 25(OH)D measurement, subjects on continuous doses of oral corticosteroids for the management of any disease other than IBD, pregnant or lactating subjects, and patients with chronic liver disease.

We identified 76 children and adolescents of ages 2–20 years with a diagnosis of IBD. Eighteen subjects were excluded based on the above exclusion criteria. Fifty-eight subjects were included in the study. The control group consisted of 116 non-IBD peers who were randomly drawn from the same database using a systematic sampling scheme. For this method, we alphabetized the list of control patients then selected every 5th patient for inclusion in our control group, thereby preserving randomization.

The ages of both the study subjects and their controls were determined by the date of 25(OH)D measurement. The duration of disease was designated as the interval from the date of endoscopic diagnosis of IBD to the date of 25(OH)D measurement. The percentages of subjects from the various ethnic/racial groups for the control group were as follows: Non-Hispanic 75%, African American 8%, White Hispanic 5%, Multi-ethnicity 5%, Unknown 4%. Similarly, the percentages from the various ethnic/racial groups for the IBD groups were: Non-Hispanic white 85%, African American 3%, White Hispanic 3%, Multi-ethnicity 3%, Unknown 5%.

Because vitamin D status varies with sunlight exposure and the seasons, we categorized each subject's date of vitamin D draw according to the seasons as follows: fall (September 22–December 21), winter (December 22–March 21), spring (March 22–June 21), and summer (June 22–September 21)[15].

Anthropometry

Height was measured to the nearest 0.1 cm using a wall-mounted stadiometer (Holtain Ltd, Crymych, Dyfed, UK) that was calibrated daily. Weight was measured to the nearest 0.1 kg using an upright scale. BMI was derived using the formula weight/height^2 (kg/m^2), and expressed as standard deviation score (SDS) for age and gender based on National Center for Health Statistics (NCHS) data [16]. Overweight was defined as BMI of $\geq$85th but <95th percentile, while obesity was defined as a BMI of $\geq$95th percentile for age and gender.

Assay

Serum 25(OH)D concentration was analyzed using 25-hydroxy chemiluminescent immunoassay (DiaSorin Liaison; Stillwater, Minnesota), which has a 100% cross-reactivity with both metabolites of 25(OH)D namely, 25(OH)D$_2$ and 25(OH)D$_3$ and thus measures total serum 25(OH)D content. Its functional sensitivity is 10 nmol/L, and its intra- and inter-assay coefficients of variation are 5% and 8.2%, respectively. Vitamin D status was defined using 25(OH)D values based on criteria by The Endocrine Society Clinical Practice Guideline as follows: vitamin D deficiency<20 ng/mL (50 nmol/L), insufficiency 20–29.9 ng/mL (50–74.5 nmol/L), and sufficiency$\geq$30 ng/mL (75 nmol/L)[5], which is similar to the classification of vitamin D status by the American Academy of Pediatrics and the Institutes of Medicine criteria which denote vitamin D deficiency as 25(OH)D <50 nmol/L; and sufficiency as 25(OH)D >50 nmol/L [6,17].

Statistical analyses

Statistical analyses were performed using the SPSS Predictive Analytics SoftWare v.21 (IBM Corporation, Armonk, NY) and Microsoft Excel (2007). Means and standard deviations were calculated for descriptive summary statistics and 25(OH)D measurements. Multivariate and univariate comparisons on anthropometrics, 25(OH)D, and other variables were conducted using ANOVA and two-tailed student's t-test respectively. Specifically, ANOVA was used to compare the differences in the parameters of interests between the controls, UC, and CD subjects. Height, weight, and BMI data were expressed as z-scores. Race, gender proportionality, and seasons of blood draw were compared using Fisher's exact test. Data were expressed as mean $\pm$ standard deviation (SD).

Table 1. A Comparative Analysis of the Characteristics of Subjects with Ulcerative Colitis, Crohn's Disease, and Healthy Controls.

Parameter	CD	95% CI	UC	95% CI	Controls	95% CI	p
Total	40	-	18	-	116	-	-
Age (years)	16.61±2.20	(15.91, 17.32)	16.13±1.99	(15.14, 17.12)	14.56±4.35	(13.76, 15.36)	0.008
Height z-score	-0.63±1.18	(-1.01, -0.25)	0.00±0.98	(-0.49, 0.49)	-0.02±1.42	(-0.28, 0.24)	0.040
Weight z-score	-0.31±1.45	(-0.77, 0.16)	0.30±1.11	(-0.26, 0.85)	0.40±1.60	(0.11, 0.70)	0.041
BMI z-score	-0.08±1.35	(-0.51, 0.35)	0.28±0.99	(-0.21, 0.78)	0.48±1.38	(0.23, 0.74)	0.076
Sex (% males)	24/40 (60.0%)	-	7/18 (38.9%)	-	49/116 (42.2%)	-	0.124
Race (% white)	36/40 (90.0%)	-	15/18 (83.3%)	-	87/116 (75.0%)	-	0.118
Season (%Winter-Spring)	17/40 (42.5%)	-	8/18 (44.4%)	-	51/116 (44.0%)	-	0.985
BMI status (% overweight/obese)	11/40 (27.5%)	-	2/18 (11.1%)	-	45/116 (38.8%)	-	0.046
Disease duration (years)	2.61±2.76	(1.68, 3.54)	2.76±2.54	(1.49, 4.02)	-	-	0.854
Mean serum 25(OH)D (nmol/L)	61.69±24.43	(53.88, 69.50)	53.26±25.51	(40.57, 65.94)	65.32±27.97	(60.18, 70.46)	0.196
25(OH)D ≤15 ng/mL (%)	6/40 (15.0%)	-	5/18 (27.8%)	-	12/116 (10.3%)	-	0.118
25(OH)D ≤20 ng/mL (%)	16/40 (40.0%)	-	9/18 (50.0%)	-	31/116 (26.7%)	-	0.070
25(OH)D ≤30 ng/mL (%)	29/40 (72.5%)	-	15/18 (83.3%)	-	87/116 (75%)	-	0.671

SDS standard deviation score; 25(OH)D 25-hydroxyvitamin D.

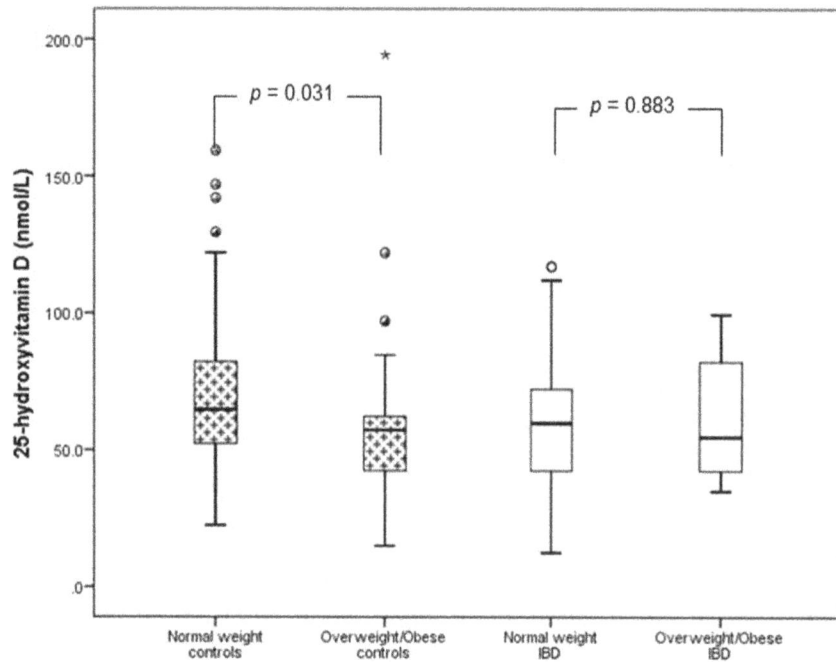

Figure 1. Box plots of the comparison of 25-hydroxyvitamin D concentration of patients with inflammatory bowel disease (IBD) and normal controls stratified by body mass index. This figure shows that the overweight/obese controls had significantly lower value for 25(OH)D than the normal weight controls (58.32±27.63 vs. 69.76±27.45, p = 0.031), while there was no significant difference in 25(OH)D value between the normal weight and overweight/obese IBD patients (59.71±26.44 vs. 60.91±23.26, p = 0.883). Note: 50 nmol/L = 20 ng/mL.

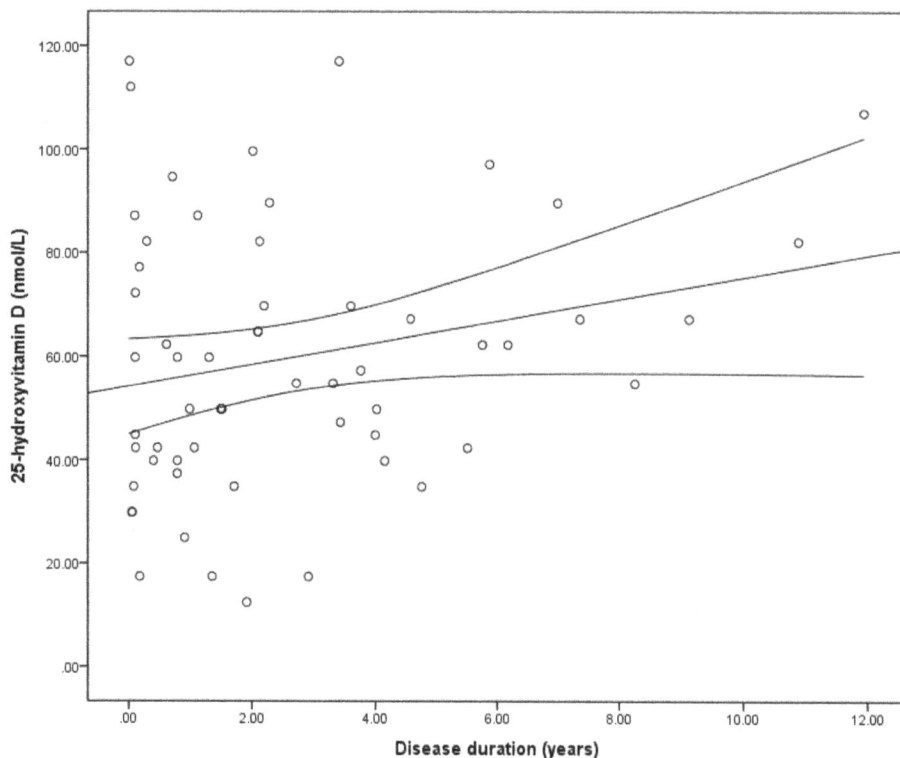

Figure 2. Scatterplot of the comparison of the 25-hydroxyvitamin D concentration and the duration of disease in inflammatory bowel disease. This figure shows a non-significant positive relationship between serum 25(OH)D concentration and the duration of disease ($r^2 = 0.054$, $\beta = 0.23$, p = 0.08).

Results

Comparative analysis of the characteristics of subjects with UC, CD, and their controls

Table 1 shows the analysis of the characteristics of the subjects with UC, CD, and controls using a one-way ANOVA. The controls were younger, had higher value for weight SDS, and a higher prevalence of overweight/obese status compared to the UC and CD groups. There was no difference in mean serum 25(OH)D concentration (p = 0.196) between the groups. There was a non-significantly higher prevalence of vitamin D deficiency as defined by a 25(OH)D value of <50 nmol/L (20 ng/mL) in both the UC and CD compared to controls (p = 0.070).

Comparison of the characteristics of the subjects with UC vs. CD

When the IBD cohort was stratified by IBD sub-types, UC vs. CD, there were no significant differences in age, gender, weight, BMI, disease duration, or season of vitamin D measurement. Subjects with CD were non-significantly shorter than the UC patients (p = 0.05). There was no difference in mean serum 25(OH)D concentration between groups (53.3±25.4 vs. 61.8±24.4, p = 0.24). Subjects with UC had a non-significantly higher prevalence of vitamin D deficiency compared to the CD subjects (50% vs. 40%, p = 0.53).

The effect of adiposity on serum 25(OH)D in IBD vs. controls

To investigate the effect of adiposity on 25(OH)D concentration in IBD vs. controls, the subjects were stratified into normal-weight vs. overweight/obese groups (Figure 1). The overweight/obese controls had significantly lower 25(OH)D concentration compared to the normal-weight controls (p = 0.031), whereas 25(OH)D concentration was similar between the normal-weight and overweight/obese IBD patients (p = 0.883). Further stratification of the IBD cohort into UC and CD showed no difference in 25(OH)D concentration between the normal-weight and overweight/obese groups for CD (p = 0.98) or UC (p = 0.70). These data suggest that adiposity has no effect on serum 25(OH)D concentration of patients with IBD.

The relationship between the duration of IBD and serum 25(OH)D concentration

We first compared the mean 25(OH)D concentration of the control group to 13 patients with IBD who had serum 25(OH)D estimation at the time of diagnosis of IBD, i.e. during active disease, and found no significant difference in their mean 25(OH)D concentration (65.3±28.0 vs. 63.8±30.1 nmol/L, p = 0.86). Next, we investigated the relationship between the duration of disease and serum concentration of 25(OH)D (Figure 2). There was a non-significant, positive relationship between serum 25(OH)D concentration and the duration of disease ($r^2 = 0.054$, $\beta = 0.23$, p = 0.08).

The relationship between the severity of IBD and serum 25(OH)D concentration

Using the Pediatric Crohn's Disease Activity Index (PCDAI)[18] and Lichtiger Colitis Activity Index (LCAI)[19], to quantify the severity of IBD, we investigated the differences in serum 25(OH)D concentration in the three groups: controls, n = 116; quiescent IBD cases n = 22; active IBD cases n = 8. There was no difference in serum 25(OH)D concentration between three groups: [controls, 65.3±27.7 nmol/L; quiescent IBD cases

61.3±28.3; active IBD cases 54.5±22.5, ANOVA p = 0.498. Post hoc comparisons detected no significant difference in 25(OH)D levels between the groups.

We then stratified the IBD cohort using ESR as a marker of inflammation and compared their serum 25(OH)D level to the controls. Within the IBD cohort, serum 25(OH)D concentration was significantly lower in patients with elevated ESR levels (ESR of >21 mm/hr) compared to those with normal ESR values (49.5±25.2 nmol/L vs. 65.6±22.1, p = 0.025).

Subsequent analysis of the mean serum 25(OH)D concentrations of the 3 groups: controls (n = 116), IBD with elevated ESR (n = 19), and IBD with normal ESR (n = 37), showed a near-significant difference in 25(OH)D between the groups (ANOVA p = 0.052). Post hoc comparisons showed a significant difference in 25(OH)D concentration between the controls and IBD subjects with elevated ESR (65.3±28.0 nmol/L vs. 49.54±25.23, p = 0.045), but not between the controls and the IBD subjects with normal ESR (65.3±28.0 vs. 65.6±22.1, p = 0.998).

Discussion

This study found no significant difference in the serum concentration of 25(OH)D in children and adolescents with IBD compared to normal controls. The normal-weight controls had significantly higher 25(OH)D concentration compared to the overweight/obese controls as well as the normal-weight IBD subjects. There was no difference in 25(OH)D between the normal-weight IBD and the overweight/obese IBD subjects. In contrast, subjects with IBD and elevated ESR had significantly lower serum 25(OH)D concentration compared to the healthy controls, and subjects with IBD and normal ESR level.

This is the second study to directly compare the vitamin D status of children and adolescents with IBD to healthy controls. Our finding, however, is contrary to the report by El-Matary et al [13] who described lower 25(OH)D concentration in a cross-sectional study of children with newly-diagnosed IBD compared to controls. Our report differed from the above-referenced study in that our study included subjects with more established IBD, with mean disease duration of thirty-two months. However, our sub-analysis found no difference in the mean 25(OH)D concentration measure at the time of IBD diagnosis compared to the mean 25(OH)D of the controls. Thus, this study found no evidence for subnormal vitamin D status in patients with newly-diagnosed IBD compared to controls in our cohort.

This study's findings on the 25(OH)D levels of established IBD are consistent with the report of a case-controlled study that reported no significant difference in serum 25(OH)D in adult patients with established IBD [20].

The effect of disease duration on vitamin D deficiency is unclear, as some studies report longer disease duration as a risk factor for vitamin D deficiency [20], while others found a positive correlation between disease duration and serum 25(OH)D concentration [8]. This study's findings are in agreement with the above report of a positive relationship between disease duration in IBD and 25(OH)D concentration (Figure 2). One explanation for this association is that the initiation of treatment in patients with IBD results in some degree of healing of the mucosal damage and consequent improvement in the absorption of vitamin D. It is also possible that the phenomenon of compensation which has been described in celiac disease, also occurs in IBD and leads to increased vitamin D absorptive capacity by the unaffected mucosal surfaces [21].

Additional case-controlled studies are warranted to accurately characterize the vitamin D status of patients with IBD at various phases of the disease. This is necessary because the other studies that have examined the vitamin D status of patients with IBD lacked control groups, focused primarily on either the prevalence rate of vitamin D deficiency in IBD, or limited their comparison of vitamin D status to patients with the subtypes of IBD, i.e., UC and CD. For example, one study found normal 25(OH)D concentration in children with CD [12], while another study reported lower 25(OH)D concentration in children with CD compared to those with UC, even though the mean 25(OH)D concentration was normal for the two IBD sub-types [11]. Two studies that defined vitamin D deficiency using a cut-off value of 37.4 nmol/L (15 ng/mL) reported prevalence rates of 16% for children with CD [10] and 10.8% for children and adolescents with IBD [8]. Three studies have investigated the vitamin D status of children and adolescents using a 25(OH)D cut-off value of 50 nmol/L (20 ng/mL), similar to the current study. The first of these studies which was conducted in Australia [22] reported a 19% prevalence of vitamin D deficiency while the other two studies from the same center in New England, USA, reported prevalence rates of 34.6% [8] and 14.3%[9]. A similar study in healthy adolescents in New England that used a cut-off value of 50 nmol/L to define vitamin D deficiency reported a prevalence of 42.0% [23]. An analysis of the prevalence of vitamin D deficiency in the subtypes of IBD detected no significant differences between UC and CD at 25(OH)D cut-off values of 38 nmol/L or 50 nmol/L [8]. Thus, the results of studies investigating the vitamin D status of children and adolescents with IBD are limited and discordant.

Though the studies that characterized the prevalence of vitamin D deficiency in IBD have provided important information in this field, they have not proven that vitamin D deficiency is a feature of IBD as they did not compare their vitamin D data to those of healthy children and adolescents in a case-controlled research design. This is expressed in a recent call for more studies comparing the vitamin D status of patients with IBD to those of healthy controls [9].

The lack of a demonstration of subnormal vitamin D status in IBD compared to controls may be explained by the fact that in addition to oral intake, this prohormone is synthesized in the skin through exposure to ultra-violet radiation. Hence, dietary intake of vitamin D is not necessarily required to maintain normal vitamin D status in individuals who maintain adequate exposure to sunlight.

There was neither a significant difference in serum 25(OH)D concentration between IBD subjects and controls, nor between IBD subjects with active vs. quiescent disease.

In contrast, IBD subjects with elevated ESR had significantly lower 25(OH)D concentration than IBD subjects with normal ESR values. When compared to controls, subjects with IBD and normal ESR level had similar 25(OH)D concentration as controls, whereas subjects with IBD and elevated ESR had significantly lower 25(OH)D than controls (65.3±28.0 nmol/L vs. 49.54±25.23, p = 0.045). This finding supports previous reports of an independent association between ESR and lower 25(OH)D concentration in IBD [8,14]. However, to the best of our knowledge, this is the first study to report significantly lower 25(OH)D concentration in patients with IBD and elevated ESR compared to healthy controls.

Adiposity and 25-hydroxyvitamin D

Obesity occurs in IBD despite the strong association between IBD and growth retardation [24]. A recent study of nearly 1600 children reported an obesity rate of 20% in children with IBD; and a rate for overweight status that is similar to that of the general population at nearly 30% [25]. The control group in this study

had a non-significantly higher BMI z-score than the subjects with IBD. To determine the effect of adiposity on 25(OH)D concentration, we stratified the subjects and controls into normal-weight and overweight/obese groups based on BMI criteria(Figure 1). Even though there was no difference in mean serum 25(OH)D between the IBD patients and controls (Table 1), upon stratification into BMI sub-groups, the normal-weight controls had significantly higher 25(OH)D concentration compared to the overweight/obese IBD patients (p = 0.031). In contrast, serum 25(OH)D concentration was similar between the normal-weight IBD and the overweight/obese IBD patients (p = 0.883). The normal-weight controls had significantly higher 25(OH)D concentration compared to the normal-weight IBD subjects (p = 0.023), but there was neither a difference in serum 25(OH)D concentration between the overweight/obese controls vs. the overweight/obese IBD subjects, nor between normal-weight IBD vs. overweight/obese IBD.

We and others have shown that increased adiposity is associated with vitamin D deficiency [26,27]. The mechanism of this association is unclear, however, proposed causative factors include poor nutrition, inadequate exposure to sunlight, and the sequestration of vitamin D in fat stores in overweight/obese individuals [28]. Interestingly, adiposity had no effect on the vitamin D status of our IBD cohort. More research is needed to determine the adiposity threshold necessary to induce significant reduction in serum 25(OH)D concentration [9] through processes such as the sequestration of vitamin D in fat stores in patients with IBD [28].

Strengths and limitations

This study has some limitations. First, the cross-sectional study design limits causal inference on the effects of seasons, race, and adiposity on vitamin D status. Second, we did not administer a food-recall to accurately determine dietary vitamin D intake. Third, we did not exhaustively evaluate the components of the complex vitamin D metabolic pathway, such as parathyroid hormone (PTH), 1,25-dihydroxyvitamin D, 24,25-dihydroxyvitamin D, and vitamin D receptor activity. This is important because PTH could be elevated in states of vitamin D deficiency and hypocalcemia, while 24,25-dihyroxyvitamin D could be elevated in states on increased vitamin D degradation. However, 25(OH)D is the major circulation form of vitamin D and its stability in plasma, and a long half-life of >15 days makes it a highly sensitive and specific marker of vitamin D status [29]. Fourth, our control group was younger than the IBD cohort: such a difference could potentially influence our results, however, earlier studies found no relationship between age and 25(OH)D concentration in children and adolescents with IBD [8,13]. Fifth, we did not adjust for the effect of pubertal maturation on 25(OH)D concentration, however, others have shown that pubertal maturation does not influence vitamin D concentration in IBD [30]. Finally, our results were derived from a single tertiary care center in the northern United States located at latitude 42°N. Therefore, we are uncertain that our results are generalizable to other centers, countries, and geographical latitudes.

The unique strength of this study is its case-controlled design which enabled us to evaluate a large cohort of patients with IBD and compare their results to a control group. This large sample size enabled us to detect subtle differences between the groups of interest. Our sample contained a fair representation of the fractional composition of each of the major racial groups in Central Massachusetts, thus enabling us to analyze the effects of differential insolation on racial groups. The control group was randomly selected using a structured randomization scheme. This study was conducted exclusively amongst subjects living in the same geographical latitude (42°N), thus ensuring uniformity of exposure to solar radiation. Phlebotomy was performed at different seasons of the year, thus ensuring that seasonality did not confound our results. Furthermore, the relationship between duration of IBD and 25(OH)D was analyzed, and effect of disease severity on 25(OH)D concentration in IBD was analyzed and compared to controls. All anthropometric data were expressed as z-score, and the analyses were adjusted for covariates.

Conclusions

There was no difference in mean serum 25(OH)D concentration between children and adolescents with IBD and controls. IBD subjects with elevated ESR had significantly lower serum 25(OH)D concentration compared to the healthy controls, and subjects with IBD and normal ESR level. This finding of vitamin D deficiency in subjects with IBD and elevated ESR suggests that inflammation is a risk factor for vitamin D deficiency in IBD. Therefore, it may be prudent to closely monitor patients with IBD and elevated ESR for vitamin D deficiency.

Acknowledgments

We thank Francis M. Wanjau for his assistance with data management, and Jessica L. Kowaleski for her clerical assistance.

Author Contributions

Conceived and designed the experiments: BUN. Performed the experiments: LV BUN LM JF. Analyzed the data: LM LV BUN. Contributed reagents/materials/analysis tools: LM JF. Contributed to the writing of the manuscript: BUN LV LM JF.

References

1. Day AS, Ledder O, Leach ST, Lemberg DA (2012) Crohn's and colitis in children and adolescents. World J Gastroenterol 18: 5862–5869.
2. Stewart R, Hirani V (2010) Relationship between vitamin D levels and depressive symptoms in older residents from a national survey population. Psychosom Med 72: 608–612.
3. Holick MF (2007) Vitamin D deficiency. N Engl J Med 357: 266–281.
4. Bikle D (2009) Nonclassic actions of vitamin D. J Clin Endocrinol Metab 94: 26–34.
5. Holick MF, Binkley NC, Bischoff-Ferrari HA, Gordon CM, Hanley DA, et al. (2011) Evaluation, treatment, and prevention of vitamin D deficiency: an Endocrine Society clinical practice guideline. J Clin Endocrinol Metab 96: 1911–1930.
6. Ross AC, Manson JE, Abrams SA, Aloia JF, Brannon PM, et al. (2011) The 2011 report on dietary reference intakes for calcium and vitamin D from the Institute of Medicine: what clinicians need to know. J Clin Endocrinol Metab 96: 53–58.
7. Cranney A, Horsley T, O'Donnell S, Weiler H, Puil L, et al. (2007) Effectiveness and safety of vitamin D in relation to bone health. Evid Rep Technol Assess (Full Rep): 1–235.
8. Pappa HM, Gordon CM, Saslowsky TM, Zholudev A, Horr B, et al. (2006) Vitamin D status in children and young adults with inflammatory bowel disease. Pediatrics 118: 1950–1961.
9. Pappa HM, Langereis EJ, Grand RJ, Gordon CM (2011) Prevalence and risk factors for hypovitaminosis D in young patients with inflammatory bowel disease. J Pediatr Gastroenterol Nutr 53: 361–364.
10. Sentongo TA, Semaeo EJ, Stettler N, Piccoli DA, Stallings VA, et al. (2002) Vitamin D status in children, adolescents, and young adults with Crohn disease. Am J Clin Nutr 76: 1077–1081.
11. Gokhale R, Favus MJ, Karrison T, Sutton MM, Rich B, et al. (1998) Bone mineral density assessment in children with inflammatory bowel disease. Gastroenterology 114: 902–911.
12. Issenman RM, Atkinson SA, Radoja C, Fraher L (1993) Longitudinal assessment of growth, mineral metabolism, and bone mass in pediatric Crohn's disease. J Pediatr Gastroenterol Nutr 17: 401–406.
13. El-Matary W, Sikora S, Spady D (2011) Bone mineral density, vitamin D, and disease activity in children newly diagnosed with inflammatory bowel disease. Dig Dis Sci 56: 825–829.
14. Pappa HM, Mitchell PD, Jiang H, Kassiff S, Filip-Dhima R, et al. (2012) Treatment of vitamin D insufficiency in children and adolescents with inflammatory bowel disease: a randomized clinical trial comparing three regimens. J Clin Endocrinol Metab 97: 2134–2142.
15. Svoren BM, Volkening LK, Wood JR, Laffel LM (2009) Significant vitamin D deficiency in youth with type 1 diabetes mellitus. J Pediatr 154: 132–134.
16. Kuczmarski RJ, Ogden CL, Guo SS, Grummer-Strawn LM, Flegal KM, et al. (2002) 2000 CDC Growth Charts for the United States: methods and development. Vital Health Stat 11: 1–190.
17. Sacheck J, Goodman E, Chui K, Chomitz V, Must A, et al. (2011) Vitamin D deficiency, adiposity, and cardiometabolic risk in urban schoolchildren. J Pediatr 159: 945–950.
18. Hyams JS, Ferry GD, Mandel FS, Gryboski JD, Kibort PM, et al. (1991) Development and validation of a pediatric Crohn's disease activity index. J Pediatr Gastroenterol Nutr 12: 439–447.
19. Lichtiger S, Present DH, Kornbluth A, Gelernt I, Bauer J, et al. (1994) Cyclosporine in severe ulcerative colitis refractory to steroid therapy. N Engl J Med 330: 1841–1845.
20. Suibhne TN, Cox G, Healy M, O'Morain C, O'Sullivan M (2012) Vitamin D deficiency in Crohn's disease: prevalence, risk factors and supplement use in an outpatient setting. J Crohns Colitis 6: 182–188.
21. Semeraro LA, Barwick KW, Gryboski JD (1986) Obesity in celiac sprue. J Clin Gastroenterol 8: 177–180.
22. Levin AD, Wadhera V, Leach ST, Woodhead HJ, Lemberg DA, et al. (2011) Vitamin D deficiency in children with inflammatory bowel disease. Dig Dis Sci 56: 830–836.
23. Gordon CM, DePeter KC, Feldman HA, Grace E, Emans SJ (2004) Prevalence of vitamin D deficiency among healthy adolescents. Arch Pediatr Adolesc Med 158: 531–537.
24. Zwintscher NP, Horton JD, Steele SR (2014) Obesity has minimal impact on clinical outcomes in children with inflammatory bowel disease. J Pediatr Surg 49: 265–268; discussion 268.
25. Long MD, Crandall WV, Leibowitz IH, Duffy L, del Rosario F, et al. (2011) Prevalence and epidemiology of overweight and obesity in children with inflammatory bowel disease. Inflamm Bowel Dis 17: 2162–2168.
26. Vimaleswaran KS, Berry DJ, Lu C, Tikkanen E, Pilz S, et al. (2013) Causal relationship between obesity and vitamin D status: bi-directional Mendelian randomization analysis of multiple cohorts. PLoS Med 10: e1001383.
27. Setty-Shah N, Maranda L, Candela N, Fong J, Dahod I, et al. (2013) Lactose intolerance: lack of evidence for short stature or vitamin D deficiency in prepubertal children. PLoS One 8: e78653.
28. Liel Y, Ulmer E, Shary J, Hollis BW, Bell NH (1988) Low circulating vitamin D in obesity. Calcif Tissue Int 43: 199–201.
29. Jones G (2008) Pharmacokinetics of vitamin D toxicity. Am J Clin Nutr 88: 582S–586S.
30. Pappa HM, Grand RJ, Gordon CM (2006) Report on the vitamin D status of adult and pediatric patients with inflammatory bowel disease and its significance for bone health and disease. Inflamm Bowel Dis 12: 1162–1174.

2

The Fecal Microbiome in Dogs with Acute Diarrhea and Idiopathic Inflammatory Bowel Disease

Jan S. Suchodolski[1]*, Melissa E. Markel[1], Jose F. Garcia-Mazcorro[2], Stefan Unterer[3], Romy M. Heilmann[1], Scot E. Dowd[4], Priyanka Kachroo[5], Ivan Ivanov[5], Yasushi Minamoto[1], Enricka M. Dillman[5], Jörg M. Steiner[1], Audrey K. Cook[5], Linda Toresson[6]

1 Gastrointestinal Laboratory, Small Animal Clinical Sciences, College of Veterinary Medicine and Biomedical Sciences, Texas A&M University, College Station, Texas, United States of America, 2 Facultad de Medicina Veterinaria, Universidad Autónoma de Nuevo León. Gral. Escobedo, Nuevo León, México, 3 Clinic of Small Animal Medicine, Ludwig-Maximillians-University, Munich, Germany, 4 Molecular Research DNA Laboratory, Shallowater, Texas, United States of America, 5 College of Veterinary Medicine and Biomedical Sciences, Texas A&M University, College Station, Texas, United States of America, 6 Helsingborg Referral Animal Hospital, Helsingborg, Sweden

Abstract

Background: Recent molecular studies have revealed a highly complex bacterial assembly in the canine intestinal tract. There is mounting evidence that microbes play an important role in the pathogenesis of acute and chronic enteropathies of dogs, including idiopathic inflammatory bowel disease (IBD). The aim of this study was to characterize the bacterial microbiota in dogs with various gastrointestinal disorders.

Methodology/Principal Findings: Fecal samples from healthy dogs (n = 32), dogs with acute non-hemorrhagic diarrhea (NHD; n = 12), dogs with acute hemorrhagic diarrhea (AHD; n = 13), and dogs with active (n = 9) and therapeutically controlled idiopathic IBD (n = 10) were analyzed by 454-pyrosequencing of the 16S rRNA gene and qPCR assays. Dogs with acute diarrhea, especially those with AHD, had the most profound alterations in their microbiome, as significant separations were observed on PCoA plots of unweighted Unifrac distances. Dogs with AHD had significant decreases in Blautia, Ruminococcaceae including *Faecalibacterium*, and *Turicibacter* spp., and significant increases in genus *Sutterella* and *Clostridium perfringens* when compared to healthy dogs. No significant separation on PCoA plots was observed for the dogs with IBD. *Faecalibacterium* spp. and Fusobacteria were, however, decreased in the dogs with clinically active IBD, but increased during time periods of clinically insignificant IBD, as defined by a clinical IBD activity index (CIBDAI).

Conclusions: Results of this study revealed a bacterial dysbiosis in fecal samples of dogs with various GI disorders. The observed changes in the microbiome differed between acute and chronic disease states. The bacterial groups that were commonly decreased during diarrhea are considered to be important short-chain fatty acid producers and may be important for canine intestinal health. Future studies should correlate these observed phylogenetic differences with functional changes in the intestinal microbiome of dogs with defined disease phenotypes.

Editor: Markus M. Heimesaat, Charité, Campus Benjamin Franklin, Germany

Funding: These authors have no support or funding to report.

Competing Interests: The authors have read the journal's policy and have the following conflict. Author Scot E. Dowd is an employee of MR DNA (Molecular Research), Shallowater. There are no patents, products in development or marketed products to declare.

* E-mail: jsuchodolski@cvm.tamu.edu

Introduction

Recent molecular-phylogenetic studies have revealed a complex assembly of bacteria in the mammalian gastrointestinal (GI) tract [1–3]. Intestinal microbes play a crucial role in the maintenance of host health. They act as a defending barrier against transient pathogens, support the host in digestion and energy harvest from the diet, stimulate the immune system, and provide nutritional support for enterocytes [4].

The intestinal microbiota has also been implicated in the pathogenesis of various canine GI disorders, either associated with the presence of specific pathogens (e.g., enterotoxigenic *C. perfringens*, *Salmonella*, viruses, and parasites) in acute episodes of diarrhea [5,6], or a non-specific dysbiosis such as that described in dogs with idiopathic inflammatory bowel disease [7–10]. Canine

idiopathic IBD is one of the most common causes of chronic GI disease in dogs and encompasses a group of chronic enteropathies of unknown cause, which are characterized by infiltration of the intestinal mucosa with inflammatory cells [11]. Although histopathologic changes may be found in any segment of the GI tract, the small intestine is typically the most frequently affected segment. The diagnosis of idiopathic IBD is made after known causes of GI inflammation have been ruled out, the animal has not shown a favorable response to a dietary and antibiotic therapeutic trial, and typically requires immunosuppressive or anti-inflammatory therapy [11].

Molecular-phylogenetic studies have revealed a bacterial and/or fungal dysbiosis in the duodenum of dogs with idiopathic IBD. Most commonly, a decrease in the proportions of Clostridiales and

Table 1. Summary of basic characteristics and alpha diversity measures.

	Healthy	NHD	AHD	A_IBD	S_IBD	p-value
Age (years; median, range)	4.6, 0.3–15.0	5.3, 0.5–15.0	5.0, 2.0–16.0	3.5, 0.6–7.6	5.7, 3.7–8.7	0.496
Weight (lbs; median, range)	47.0, 5.8–81.5	47.1, 5.5–75.0	19.8, 4.0–68.3	55.0, 9.0–130.0	56.1, 18.5–91.7	0.574
CIBDAI (median, range)	N/A	N/A	N/A	7, 5–9	1.5, 1–2	<0.001
gender (female/male)	14/18	8/4	7/6	3/5	3/7	0.449
Country	Sweden n = 8; USA n = 24	USA	Germany	Sweden	Sweden	n/a
OTU$_{97}$ (mean ± SD)	242±93	188±95	175±57	163±91	119±85	0.111
Shannon index (mean ± SD)	3.3±0.8	2.4±1.4	2.6±0.9	2.3±1.1	1.9±1.0	0.104
Chao1 (mean ± SD)	504±181	390±232	327±126	357±212	251±203	0.053

IBD = inflammatory bowel disease.
CIBDAI = canine IBD disease activity index.
NHD = acute non-hemorrhagic diarrhea, AHD = acute hemorrhagic diarrhea, A_IBD = active IBD, S_IBD = clinically insignificant IBD.

an increase in Proteobacteria is observed [7,9,10,12]. Only few molecular studies have described the fecal microbiota of dogs with acute and chronic GI disorders. One study, using fluorescent *in situ* hybridization (FISH) probes, found *Bacteroides* counts to be significantly increased in Beagle dogs with chronic diarrhea [13]. In contrast, using 454-pyrosequencing of the cpn60 gene, significantly decreased proportions of Bacteroidetes were observed in dogs with unspecified diarrhea [14]. Using terminal restriction fragment length polymorphism (T-RFLP) analysis and quantitative PCR (qPCR), an increased abundance of *Clostridium perfringens*, *Enterococcus faecalis*, and *E. faecium* was observed in dogs during diarrheic episodes [15]. While these studies suggest a dysbiosis present in fecal samples of dogs with diarrhea, additional studies using high-throughput sequencing technologies in dogs with well-

Table 2. Oligonucleotides primers/probes used in this study.

qPCR primers/probe	Sequence (5'-3')	Target	Annealing (°C)	Reference
CFB555f	CCGGAWTYATTGGGTTTAAAGGG	Bacteroidetes	60	[38]
CFB968r	GGTAAGGTTCCTCGCGTA			
BifF	TCGCGTCYGGTGTGAAAG	*Bifidobacterium*	60	[39]
BifR	CCACATCCAGCRTCCAC			
FaecaF	GAAGGCGGCCTACTGGGCAC	*Faecalibacterium*	60	[22]
FaecaR	GTGCAGGCGAGTTGCAGCCT			
RumiF	ACTGAGAGGTTGAACGGCCA	Family Ruminococcaceae	59	[22]
RumiR	CCTTTACACCCAGTAAWTCCGGA			
CPerf165F	CGCATAACGTTGAAAGATGG			
CPerf269R	CCTTGGTAGGCCGTTACCC	*C. perfringens* 16S	58	[40]
CPerf187F (probe)	TCATCATTCAACCAAAGGAGCAATCC			
TM-cpe-F	AACTATAGGAGAACAAAATACAATAG			
TM-cpe-R	TGCATAAACCTTATAATATACATATTC	*C. perfringens* enterotoxin	55	[41]
TM-cpe-pr	TCTGTATCTACAACTGCTGGTCCA			
tcdB-F	GGTATTACCTAATGCTCCAAATAG			
tcdB-R	TTTGTGCCATCATTTTCTAAGC	*C. difficile* toxin B gene	58	[42]
tcdB-P (probe)	ACCTGGTGTCCATCCTGTTTCCCA			
Fuso-F	KGGGCTCAACMCMGTATTGCGT	Fusobacterium	51	This study
Fuso-R	TCGCGTTAGCTTGGGCGCTG			
Blaut-F	TCTGATGTGAAAGGCTGGGGCTTA	*Blautia spp.*	56	This study
Blaut-R	GGCTTAGCCACCCGACACCTA			
341-F	CCTACGGGAGGCAGCAGT	Universal Bacteria	59	[43]
518-R	ATTACCGCGGCTGCTGG			
TuriciF	CAGACGGGGACAACGATTGGA	*Turicibacter*	63	This study
TuricR	TACGCATCGTCGCCTTGGTA			

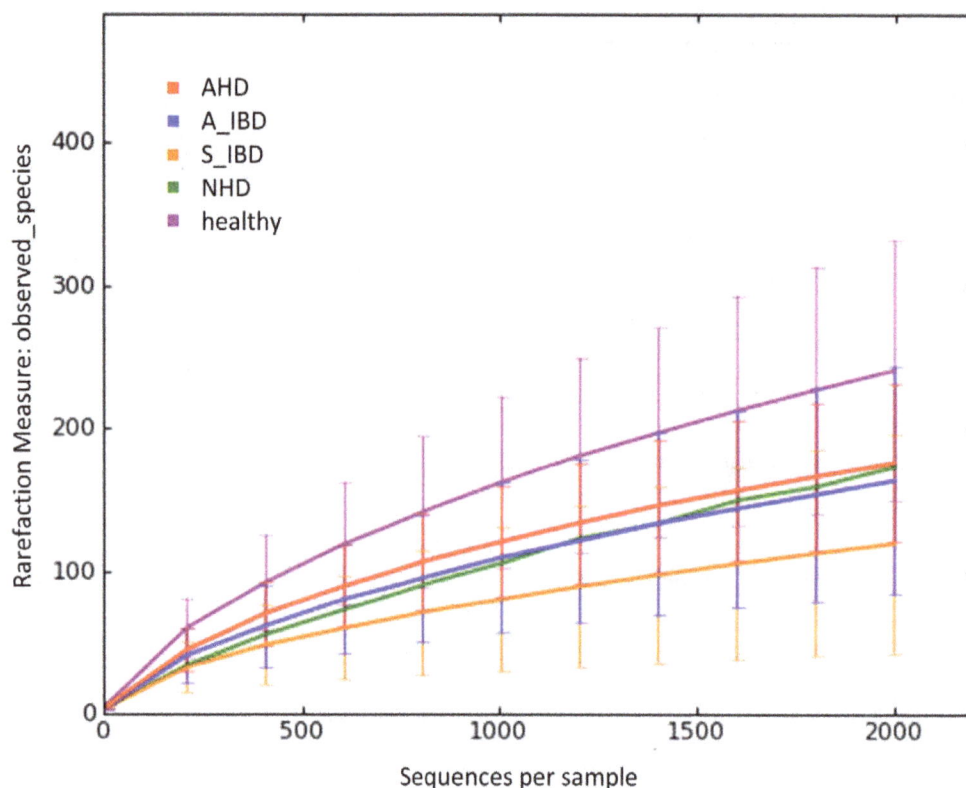

Figure 1. Rarefaction analysis of 16 S rRNA gene sequences obtained from canine fecal samples. Lines represent the average of each group, while the error bars represent the standard deviations. The analysis was performed on a randomly selected subset of 2,000 sequences per sample. A_IBD = active IBD; S_IBD = therapeutically controlled IBD; NHD = acute non-hemorrhagic diarrhea; AHD = acute hemorrhagic diarrhea.

defined acute and chronic disease phenotypes are needed to further characterize changes in the fecal microbiome. In addition, comparison of fecal findings in dogs with IBD with those previously observed in duodenal biopsies is of interest [7], as collection of fecal samples is more practical. Furthermore, it is unclear if the pattern of dysbiosis observed in dogs with IBD is specific for this disorder, or if similar patterns are present in acute GI diseases.

This study compared the fecal microbiome of healthy dogs, dogs with acute non-hemorrhagic diarrhea (NHD), dogs with acute hemorrhagic diarrhea (AHD), and dogs with active and therapeutically controlled clinically insignificant IBD. The results indicate differences in the fecal microbiome among the dogs with various GI diseases. Dogs with acute diarrhea had the most pronounced changes, with several bacterial groups altered when compared to healthy dogs. Only *Faecalibacterium* spp. and Fusobacteria were decreased in dogs with clinically active IBD, but increased during time periods of clinically insignificant IBD.

Materials and Methods

Ethics Statement

The collection and analysis of fecal samples was approved by the institutional Clinical Research Review Committee of the College of Veterinary Medicine, Texas A&M University (CRRC#09-06).

Animals and Sample Collection

Fecal samples from a total of 76 dogs were analyzed. These dogs were either healthy (n = 32), or had signs of either acute non-

hemorrhagic diarrhea (NHD; n = 12), acute hemorrhagic diarrhea (AHD, n = 13), active inflammatory bowel disease (A-IBD; n = 9), or therapeutically controlled clinically insignificant IBD (S-IBD; n = 10), as scored by a published canine clinical IBD activity index (CIBDAI) [16]. Left-over naturally-passed feces collected for routine fecal examination were frozen within a few hours of collection at either $-20°C$ or $-80°C$, and were stored frozen until processing of samples for DNA extraction. The summary of the baseline characteristics for each animal group is listed in Table 1, and detailed descriptions of each enrolled dog are listed in supplementary Tables S1–S3.

Healthy controls. Fecal samples from a total of 32 pet dogs were analyzed by 454-pyrosequencing and quantitative PCR assays (qPCR). All dogs were privately owned and lived in diverse home environments, were on a variety of commercial diets, and none of the dogs had a history of gastrointestinal signs or administration of antibiotics for at least the past 3 months (Table S1). Eight healthy dogs lived in Sweden, while the remaining 24 healthy dogs lived in Texas, USA.

Dogs with acute non-hemorrhagic diarrhea (NHD). Fecal samples from a total of 12 pet dogs that presented to a first-opinion practice (Austin, TX) with acute, uncomplicated, non-hemorrhagic diarrhea were evaluated (duration of diarrhea <3 days). Of those, 7 samples were analyzed by 454-pyrosequencing, while all 12 samples were analyzed by qPCR assays. None of the dogs had a previous history of GI signs or had received antibiotics within the previous 3 months (Table S2). Diagnostic evaluation included complete blood count (CBC), serum chemistry profiles, and partial fecal analysis for enteric pathogens by fecal flotation and fecal cytology. *Clostridium*

Table 3. Relative percentages of the most abundant bacterial groups at the various phylogenetic levels (phylum, class, order, family, genus) based on pyrosequencing.

	Medians % (min-max%)*					
	Healthy	NHD	AHD	Active IBD	Controlled IBD	Kruskal-Wallis P-value**
Firmicutes	96.6 (81–100)	95.6 (83–100)	56 (13–100)	98.7 (95–100)	98.6 (24–100)	0.0985
Clostridia	78.1 (21–97)	86.8 (46–99)	55.6 (12–99)	45.5 (1–94)	47 1–91)	1
Clostridiales	78.1 (21–97)	86.8 (46–99)	55.6 (12–99)	45.5 (1–94)	47 (1–91)	1
Clostridiaceae	36.2 (6–84)	81.5 (32–99)	46.4 (7–99)	26.4 (1–82)	18.2 (1–75)	0.302
Clostridium	33.7[a] (5–84)	81.5[b] (32–99)	44.0[a,b] (6–99)	13.7[a] (0–82)	14.2[a] (0–82)	**0.03**
Ruminococcaceae	16.0[a] (0–46)	4.7[b] (0–21)	0.8[b] (0–18)	5.6[a,b] (0–54)	7.9[a,b] (0–53)	**0.004**
Faecalibacterium	0.1 (0–16)	0 (0–5)	0 (0–3)	0 (0–0)	0.3 (0–3)	1
Ruminococcus	15.4[a] (0–46)	4.7[b] (0–16)	0.7[b] (0–18)	5.6[a,b] (0–54)	6.8[a,b] (0–53)	**0.008**
Lachnospiraceae	0.4 (0–2)	0.1 (0–3)	0 (0–1)	0.3 (0–1)	0.3 (0–3)	0.114
Blautia	9.9[a] (0–28)	0.2[b] (0–17)	0.2[b] (0–4)	5.9[a,b] (0–9)	3.6[b] (0–16)	**0.002**
Roseburia	0.2 (0–1)	0.1 (0–3)	0 (0–1)	0.1 (0–0)	0.1 (0–1)	0.642
Coprococcus	0 (0–1)	0 (0–0)	0 (0–0)	0.1 (0–0)	0.1 (0–1)	1
Veillonellaceae	0 (0–4)	0 (0–0)	0 (0–1)	0 (0–0)	0 (0–0)	1
Eubacteriaceae	0.2 (0–2)	0.1 (0–13)	0.1 (0–17)	0.2 (0–0)	0.5 (0–4)	1
Eubacterium	0.8 (0–27)	0.1 (0–13)	0.1 (0–17)	0.3 (0–1)	1 (0–5)	0.564
Erysipelotrichi	7.8[a] (0–45)	0.7[a,b] (0–9)	0.1[b] (0–2)	0.8[a,b] (0–99)	0.8[b] (0–8)	**0.0009**
Erysipelotrichales	7.8[a] (0–45)	0.7[a,b] (0–9)	0.1[b] (0–2)	0.8[a,b] (0–99)	0.8[b] (0–8)	**0.0009**
Erysipelotrichaceae	7.8[a] (0–45)	0.7[a,b] (0–9)	0.1[b] (0–2)	0.8[a,b] (0–99)	0.8[b] (0–8)	**0.0009**
Turicibacter	0.5 (0–39)	0.1 (0–4)	0 (0–0)	0 (0–0)	0.1 (0–1)	0.138
Allobaculum	0.3 (0–14)	0.4 (0–8)	0 (0–1)	0 (0–3)	0 (0–2)	1
Bacilli	0 (0–15)	0.2 (0–16)	0 (0–3)	0 (0–1)	0 (0–1)	0.2169
Lactobacillales	0.2 (0–74)	1.7 (0–29)	0.4 (0–5)	18.2 (0–60)	7.9 (0–98)	1
Streptococcaceae	0.1 (0–74)	0.3 (0–19)	0.1 (0–4)	6 (0–60)	2.7 (0–95)	1
Streptococcus	0 (0–74)	0.3 (0–19)	0.1 (0–4)	3.4 (0–60)	2.5 (0–95)	1
Lactobacillaceae	0 (0–61)	0 (0–2)	0 (0–0)	0 (0–11)	0.2 (0–98)	0.86
Enterococcaceae	0 (0–3)	0 (0–2)	0 (0–3)	0 (0–1)	0 (0–1)	1
Proteobacteria	0.30[a] (0–3)	1.3[a,b] (0–16)	4.3[b] (0–17)	0.1[a] (0–1)	0.1[a] (0–46)	**0.016**
Betaproteobacteria	0.0[a] (0–0)	0.0[a,b] (0–3)	2.1[b] (0–14)	0.0[a,b] (0–0)	0.0[a] (0–8)	**0.0099**
Sutterella	0.0[a] (0–0)	0.0[a] (0–0)	1.6[b] (0–14)	0.0[a] (0–0)	0.0[a] (0–1)	**0.008**
Gammaproteobacteria	0 (0–3)	1 (0–16)	0.6 (0–15)	0 (0–0)	0 (0–29)	0.0648
Enterobacteriales	0 (0–3)	0.2 (0–16)	0.1 (0–13)	0 (0–0)	0 (0–19)	1
Enterobacteriaceae	0 (0–0)	0.2 (0–16)	0.1 (0–13)	0 (0–0)	0 (0–19)	1
Alphaproteobacteria	0.1 (0–0.9)	0.1 (0–1.2)	0 (0–0.2)	0.1 (0–0.3)	0 (0–2)	0.063
Rickettsiales	0.1[a] (0–0.9)	0.0[a,b] (0–0.2)	0.0[b] (0–0.2)	0.1[a,b] (0–0.3)	0.0[b] (0–0.4)	**0.0072**
Anaplasmataceae	0.1[a] (0–0.9)	0.0[a,b] (0–0.2)	0.0[b] (0–0.2)	0.1[a,b] (0–0.3)	0.0[b] (0–0.4)	**0.016**
Anaplasma	0.1[a] (0–0.9)	0.0[a,b] (0–0.2)	0.0[b] (0–0.2)	0.1[a,b] (0–0.3)	0.0[b] (0–0.4)	**0.016**
Bacteroidetes	0 (0–18)	0 (0–3)	0.5 (0–17)	0 (0–0)	0 (0–12)	0.0685
Bacteroidia	0 (0–18)	0 (0–0)	0.5 (0–17)	0 (0–0)	0 (0–11)	0.1683
Bacteroidales	0 (0–18)	0 (0–0)	0.5 (0–17)	0 (0–0)	0 (0–11)	0.1683
Bacteroidaceae	0 (0–4)	0 (0–0)	0.5 (0–10)	0 (0–0)	0 (0–3)	0.524
Bacteroides	0 (0–3)	0 (0–0)	0.5 (0–10)	0 (0–0)	0 (0–3)	0.696
Actinobacteria	1.8[a] (0–13)	1.4[a,b] (0–6)	0.2[b] (0–3)	0.8[a,b] (0–5)	1.0[a,b] (0–15)	**0.019**
Actinobacteria (class)	1.8[a] (0–13)	1.4[a,b] (0–6)	0.2[b] (0–3)	0.8[a,b] (0–5)	1.0[a,b] (0–15)	**0.0342**
Coriobacteriales	1.8[a] (0–13)	1.0[a,b] (0–6)	0.1[b] (0–2)	0.8[a,b] (0–5)	0.7[a,b] (0–15)	**0.0162**
Coriobacteriaceae	1.8[a] (0–13)	1.0[a,b] (0–6)	0.1[b] (0–2)	0.8[a,b] (0–5)	0.7[a,b] (0–15)	**0.036**
Collinsella	1.5[a] (0–13)	1.0[a,b] (0–4)	0.0[b] (0–2)	0.7[a,b] (0–5)	0.5[a,b] (0–13)	**0.018**
Fusobacteria	0.1 (0–4)	0 (0–2)	23.5 (0–75)	0 (0–0)	0 (0–17)	0.0865

Table 3. Cont.

	Medians % (min-max%)*					
	Healthy	**NHD**	**AHD**	**Active IBD**	**Controlled IBD**	**Kruskal-Wallis P-value****
Fusobacteriales	0 (0–4)	0 (0–2)	23.4 (0–0)	0 (0–0)	0 (0–14)	0.1647
Fusobacteriaceae	0 (0–4)	0 (0–2)	23.4 (0–0)	0 (0–0)	0 (0–14)	0.366
Fusobacterium	0 (0–4)	0 (0–2)	23.2 (0–0)	0 (0–0)	0 (0–6)	0.5

Taxa present in at least 50% of dogs (either healthy or diseased) included in analysis.
**p-values adjusted based on the Benjamini and Hochberg False discovery rate.
*Medians not sharing a common superscript are significantly different (p<0.05 based on a Dunn's multiple comparisons test).
NHD = acute hemorrhagic diarrhea; AHD = acute hemorrhagic diarrhea; IBD = inflammatory bowel disease.

perfringens enterotoxin and *C. difficile* toxin A/B were analyzed using commercially available ELISA kits (*C. perfringens* Enterotoxin Test™ and *C. difficile* Tox A/B II™, TechLab, Blacksburg, VA). Based on review of the medical records, all dogs in this group recovered after non-specific symptomatic therapy (e.g., fluid supplementation, gastric acid blockers) within a few days.

Dogs with acute hemorrhagic diarrhea (AHD). Fecal samples were analyzed from a total of 13 pet dogs that presented to the Clinic of Small Animal Medicine, LMU University of Munich, Germany, with acute hemorrhagic diarrhea (duration of <3 days). None of the dogs had a previous history of GI signs or had received antibiotics within the previous 3 months (Table S2). Diagnostic evaluation included CBC, serum chemistry profiles, and partial fecal analysis for enteric pathogens (*C. perfringens* enterotoxin ELISA, *C. difficile* toxin A/B ELISA, and fecal culture).

Dogs with idiopathic IBD. Fecal samples were analyzed from pet dogs that had been presented to the Helsingborg Referral Animal Hospital, Helsingborg, Sweden with signs of chronic GI disease. Dogs underwent clinical evaluation by a veterinary internist (LT). Diagnostic tests that were performed included a CBC, serum chemistry profiles, fecal flotation, serum concentrations of cobalamin and folate, and depending on the clinical signs, serum concentrations of trypsin-like immunoreactivity (cTLI) and pancreatic lipase-immunoreactivity (cPLI). During the months of diagnostic work-ups, dogs underwent various forms of antibiotic

and/or dietary trials. All dogs failed the trials and subsequently underwent endoscopy with collection of intestinal biopsies. All dogs then received and responded to immunosuppressive therapy, leading to a diagnosis of idiopathic IBD (Table S3).

The disease activity of these dogs was scored using the published clinical canine IBD activity index (CIBDAI) [16]. The CIBDAI is based on 6 criteria, each scored on a scale from 0–3: attitude/activity, appetite, vomiting, stool consistency, stool frequency, and weight loss. The total composite score is determined to be clinically insignificant (score 0–3), mild (score 4–5), moderate (score 6–8), or severe (score 9 or greater). We analyzed a total of 19 dogs (Table S3). Of those 19 dogs, 9 were newly diagnosed with active IBD (A_IBD) as judged by their CIBDAI score (median 7, range 5–9), and fecal samples collected at the time of diagnosis were analyzed (5 samples were analyzed by pyrosequencing; all 9 samples were analyzed by qPCR). The other 10 dogs had been on medical treatment (Table S3) for their idiopathic IBD for several months to years (therapeutically controlled stable IBD; S_IBD) and had clinically insignificant or no signs of IBD as scored by the CIBDAI (median 1.5, range 1–2) at the time of sample collection. From the latter group of dogs all 10 samples were analyzed by pyrosequencing and qPCR assays. None of these 19 dogs received antibiotics for at least 2 months before sample collection.

In addition, paired samples were obtained from 8 dogs, representing time points when, based on CIBDAI scoring, the dogs showed either a clinically significant CIBDAI (median 5,

Table 4. Summary statistics for qPCR results.

	Medians (min-max)* log DNA					
	Healthy	**NHD**	**AHD**	**Active IBD**	**Controlled IBD**	**Kruskal-Wallis P-value**
Bacteroidetes	6.4ᵃ (0.0–12.1)	4.5ᵇ (0.0–6.1)	6.7ᵃ (4.7–9.9)	7.3ᵃ (0.0–9.3)	5.3ᵃ,ᵇ (0.0–7.5)	0.0009
Bifidobacterium	2.9 (0.0–7.3)	3.1 (0.0–6.2)	0 (0.0–3.9)	2.2 (0.0–6.6)	3.8 (0.0–7.5)	0.0959
Blautia	9.7ᵃ (8.2–10.7)	6.3ᵇ (5.7–10.2)	8.2ᵇ (6.9–10.2)	9.2ᵃ,ᵇ (7.3–9.9)	9.5ᵃ,ᵇ (5.9–9.9)	0.0003
C. perfringens	2.0ᵃ (0.0–6.1)	4.0ᵃ,ᵇ (0.0–7.4)	6.2ᵇ (0.6–7.6)	3.0ᵃ,ᵇ (0.0–6.7)	2.4ᵃ,ᵇ (0.6–5.7)	0.0002
Faecalibacterium	5.8ᵃ (4.1–7.9)	0.0ᵇ (0.0–7.7)	4.7ᵇ (0.0–7.8)	4.2ᵇ (0.0–6.3)	5.5ᵃ,ᵇ (0.0–7.3)	0.0002
Fusobacteria	7.3ᵃ,ᵇ (5.5–8.8)	6.9ᵃ,ᶜ (3.9–8.6)	8.2ᵇ (6.0–10.3)	6.4ᶜ (4.7–6.7)	7.1ᵃ,ᵇ,ᶜ (3.0–7.9)	0.0014
Ruminococcaceae	7.6ᵃ (2.4–8.9)	5.7ᵇ (2.7–7.1)	5.6ᵇ (0.0–7.5)	7.3ᵃ,ᵇ (0.0–8.6)	7.9ᵃ (6.5–8.6)	<0.0001
Turicibacter	2.9ᵃ (0.0–7.7)	0.0ᵇ (0.0–4.8)	0.0ᵇ (0.0–0.0)	1.5ᵃ,ᵇ (0.0–6.6)	3.8ᵃ (0.0–5.9)	0.0003
Universal	12.0 (10.9–13.2)	10.8 (8.3–12.7)	11.6 (10.7–12.4)	12.0 (9.7–12.2)	12.3 (8.2–12.8)	0.0935

*Medians not sharing a common superscript are significantly different (p<0.05 based on a Dunn's multiple comparisons test).
NHD = acute non-hemorrhagic diarrhea; AHD = acute hemorrhagic diarrhea; IBD = inflammatory bowel disease

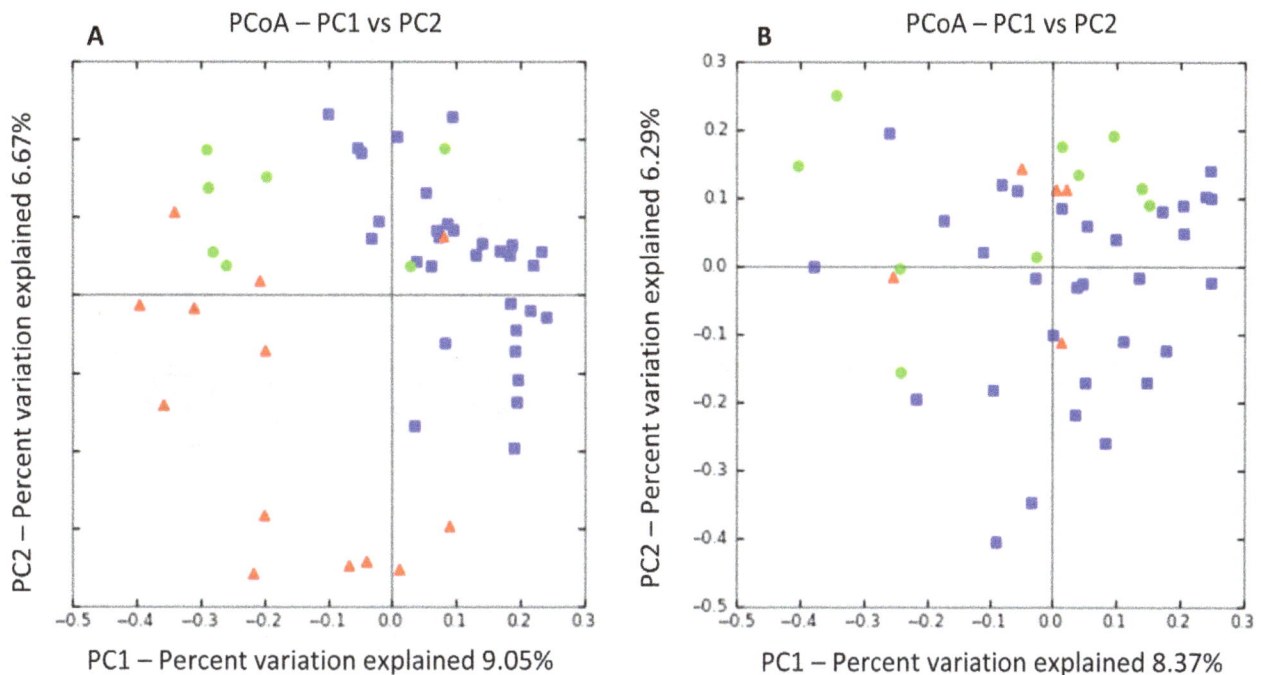

Figure 2. Principal Coordinates Analysis (PCoA) of unweighted UniFrac distances of 16 S rRNA genes. (A) Analysis for healthy dogs (blue), dogs with acute non-hemorrhagic diarrhea (NHD; green), and dogs with acute hemorrhagic diarrhea (AHD; red). These results indicate that fecal microbial communities differ in dogs with acute forms of diarrhea compared to healthy control dogs. Statistical analysis revealed a significant separation between samples obtained from NHD and AHD (ANOSIM; p = 0.004) and both groups were also significantly different from the healthy dogs (ANOSIM; NHD vs. healthy dogs, p = 0.003; AHD vs. healthy dogs, p = 0.001). (B) Analysis for healthy dogs (blue), dogs with active IBD (red), and dogs with therapeutically controlled IBD (green). In contrast to the dogs with acute diarrhea, fecal communities in dogs with chronic forms of diarrhea (active idiopathic IBD) were not significantly different from healthy dogs in this study.

range 4–9) or a clinically insignificant CIBDAI (median 1.5, range 1–3). The time period between the collections of repeated samples ranged from 2–8 months (median 5.5 months). These paired samples were analyzed separately by qPCR assays, as these follow up samples were obtained after the pyrosequencing analysis had been completed.

DNA Extraction

An aliquot of 100 mg (wet weight) of each fecal sample was extracted by a bead-beating method using a commercial DNA extraction kit (ZR Fecal DNA Kit™, Zymo Research Corporation) following the manufacturer's instructions. The bead beating step was performed on a homogenizer (FastPrep-24, MP Biomedicals) for 60 s at a speed of 4 m/s.

454-pyrosequencing

Bacterial tag-encoded FLX-titanium amplicon pyrosequencing (bTEFAP) based on the V1–V3 region (*E. coli* position 27–519) of the 16 S rRNA gene was performed on 67 of the 77 samples as described previously with primers forward 28F: GAGTTT-GATCNTGGCTCAG and reverse 519R: GTNTTACNGCGGCKGCTG [3,17]. Raw sequence data were screened, trimmed, denoised, and filtered with the QIIME pipeline version 1.4.0 (http://qiime.sourceforge.net) [18] with the following settings: minimum read length of 300 bp; no ambiguous base calls; no homopolymeric runs longer than 8 bp; average quality value>q25 within a sliding window of 50 bp. Chimeras were excluded using the software B2C2 (http://www.researchandtesting.com/B2C2.html) [7,19]. Operational taxonomic units (OTUs) were defined as sequences with at least

97% similarity using QIIME. For classification of sequences on a genus level the naïve Bayesian classifier within the Ribosomal Database Project (RDP, v10.28) was used. The confidence threshold in RDP was set to 80% [7].

Quantitative PCR (qPCR)

For validation of pyrosequencing results and/or to evaluate bacterial groups that are typically present at very low abundance or typically not detected in sequence data based on the authors' experience from previous studies (i.e., *Bifidobacterium* spp.; *Faecalibacterium* spp.) [3,20,21], qPCR assays for selected bacterial groups were performed: total bacteria, Bacteroidetes, Fusobacteria, *Blautia*, Ruminococcaceae, *Faecalibacterium* spp., *Turicibacter* spp., *Bifidobacterium* spp., and *Clostridium perfringens*. PCR was also used to detect the genes encoding *C. perfringens* enterotoxin (*cpe*) and *C. difficile* toxin B (*tcd* B). Real-time PCR conditions were performed as described previously [22]. The oligonucleotide sequences of primers and probes, and respective annealing temperatures are summarized in Table 2. The qPCR data was expressed as log amount of DNA (fg) for each particular bacterial group per 10 ng of isolated total DNA.

Statistical Analysis

To account for unequal sequencing depth across samples, and to avoid exclusion of samples with lower number of sequence reads, the subsequent analysis was performed on a randomly selected subset of 2,000 sequences per sample. Differences in microbial communities between disease groups were investigated using the phylogeny-based unweighted UniFrac distance metric, and PCoA plots and rarefaction curves were plotted using QIIME.

Blautia

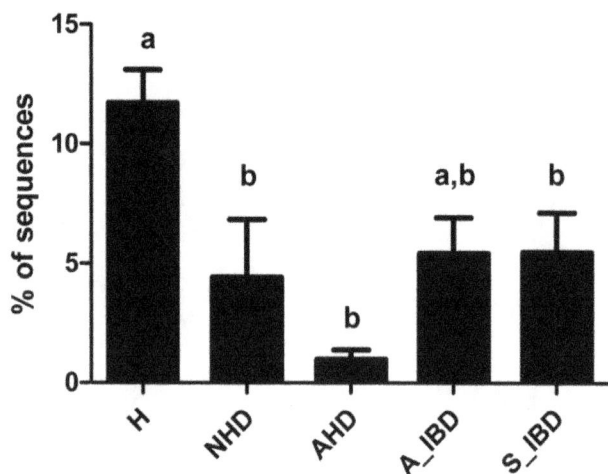

Ruminococcaceae

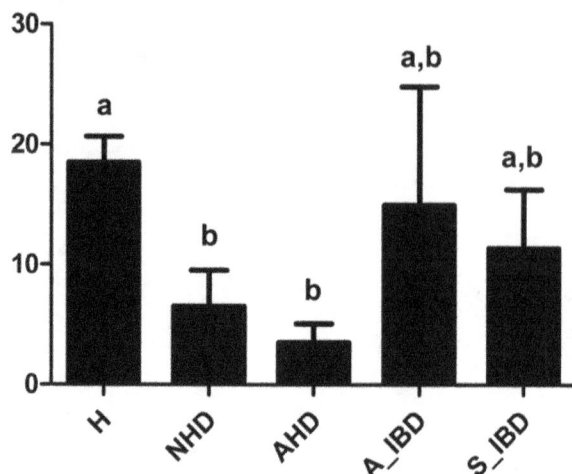

Actinobacteria

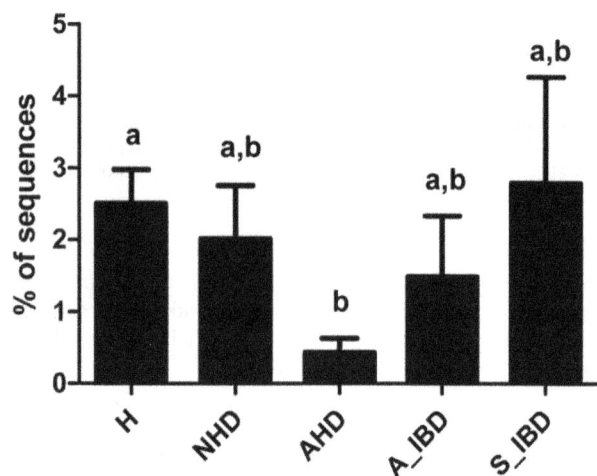

Lactobacillales

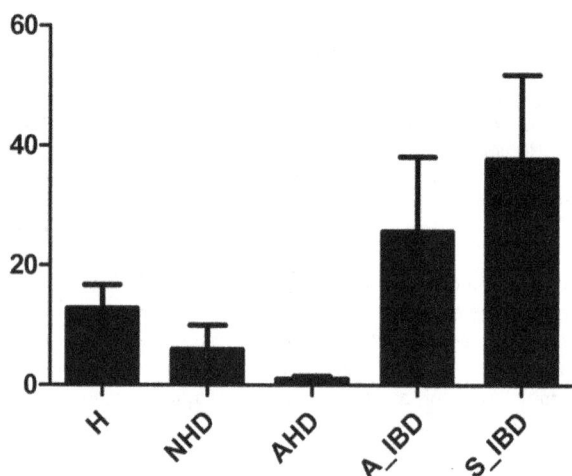

Fusobacteria

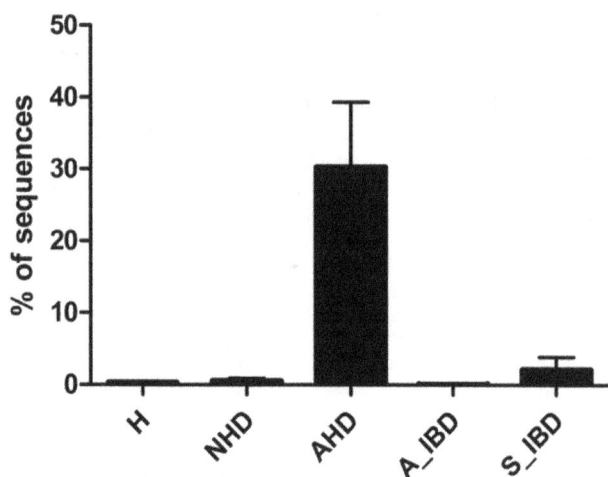

Sutterella

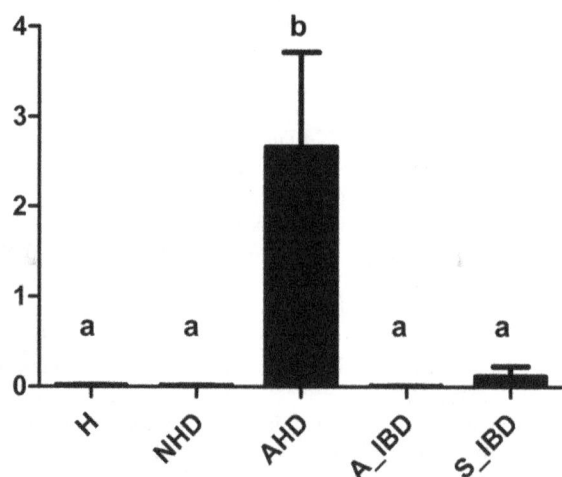

Figure 3. Results of sequence analysis for selected bacterial groups. H = healthy, NHD = acute non-hemorrhagic diarrhea, AHD = acute hemorrhagic diarrhea, A_IBD = active IBD, S_IBD = therapeutically controlled, clinically insignificant IBD. Columns not sharing a common superscript are significantly different (P<0.05).

To determine differences in microbiota composition between the animal groups, the analysis of similarities (ANOSIM) function in the statistical software package PRIMER 6 (PRIMER-E Ltd., Lutton, UK) was used on the unweighted UniFrac distance matrixes. To visualize the relative abundance of bacterial families for individual fecal samples, heat maps were generated in NCSS 2007 (NCSS, Kaysville, Utah).

For all datasets, assumption of normality was tested using the D'Agostino and Pearson normality test (Prism 5.00, GraphPad Software Inc.). Only bacterial taxa that were present in at least 50% of dogs (either healthy or diseased) were included in the analysis. Because most datasets did not meet the assumptions of normal distribution, the differences in the proportions of bacterial taxa (defined as percentage of total sequences) or qPCR results between healthy and disease groups were determined using non-parametric Kruskal-Wallis tests (Prism v5.00, GraphPad Software Inc.). The resulting p-values of the Kruskal-Wallis tests were corrected for multiple comparisons on each phylogenetic level using the Benjamini & Hochberg's False Discovery Rate, and a $p<0.05$ was considered statistically significant [23]. For those bacterial groups that were still significant after p-value adjustment, a Dunns' post-test was used to determine which disease categories were significantly different. A Fisher's exact test was used to determine the proportions of dogs that harbored specific bacterial taxa or toxins.

Paired samples were available for 8 dogs with IBD, representing samples at time of clinically active and therapeutically controlled IBD (i.e., clinically insignificant IBD), respectively. The qPCR assays for these paired samples were performed as batch in the same assay run, and the obtained data for the paired time points were compared using a Wilcoxon signed rank test.

Linear Discriminant Analysis (LDA) was used to achieve dimensionality reduction and thereby to identify combinations of bacterial groups that would discriminate between healthy dogs and all diseased dogs (independent of disease phenotype) [24]. Using the OTUs as features for the classification, the single, two, or three feature LDA classifiers were constructed and ranked based on their error estimates [25,26]. More detailed descriptions of LDA classification are provided as supplementary Method S1.

Results

Animals and Disease Characteristics

No significant differences in age, gender, or body weight were found among the various animal groups (Table 1).

Sequence Analysis

The 454- pyrosequencing pipeline yielded 189,138 quality sequences for the 67 samples analyzed. Across all disease groups, sequences were classified into nine bacterial phyla (Table 3). Figure 1 illustrates the rarefaction curves for all disease groups. No significant differences in the number of OTUs, the Shannon index, and the Chao1 metric were observed (Table 1).

Microbial Communities in Controls and in Dogs with Acute and Chronic Gastrointestinal Diseases

No significant differences were observed in total bacterial abundance among the groups based on qPCR analysis (Table 4;

p = 0.09). Significant differences in microbial communities were, however, observed among the various groups. According to the linear discriminant analysis (LDA; Method S1), the triple combination of *Blautia* spp., *Faecalibacterium* spp., and *Turicibacter* spp. had the highest discriminatory power when healthy dogs were compared to all the dogs with gastrointestinal disease (independent of disease phenotype).

PCoA plots (Fig. 2) were constructed to compare the individual groups of dogs, and showed notable differences between healthy dogs and dogs with acute GI disorders (ANOSIM; NHD vs. healthy dogs, p = 0.003; AHD vs. healthy dogs, p = 0.001). Furthermore, both acute disease groups differed significantly from each other (Fig. 2) (ANOSIM; NHD vs. AHD, p = 0.004).

In contrast, neither the A_IBD nor the S_IBD group were significantly different from the healthy group or different from each other based on PCoA plots (ANOSIM; A_IBD vs. S-_IBD, p = 0.91; A_IBD vs. controls, p = 0.75; S_IBD vs. controls, p = 0.07). However, sequence analysis and qPCR results revealed that *Faecalibacterium* spp. and Fusobacteria were significantly lower in dogs with clinically active IBD when compared to healthy dogs (see below).

Dogs with acute hemorrhagic diarrhea (AHD). Based on PCoA plots, dogs with AHD had profound microbiome changes. Several bacterial groups were altered in dogs with AHD compared to the healthy dogs, but also to dogs with other forms of GI disease (Table 3). Increases in proportions were observed for the genus *Sutterella* (class β-Proteobacteria) and *Clostridium perfringens*--like sequences (Table 3, Fig. 3). The phylum Fusobacteria was also increased in dogs with AHD (Fig. 3), but this difference did not reach significant differences when p-values were adjusted for multiple comparisons (p = 0.08). Decreases in proportions were observed for Actinobacteria (i.e., Coriobacteriaceaea) and several members within the Firmicutes, most notably Ruminococcaceae, *Blautia* spp. (Lachnospiraceae), and *Turicibacter* spp. (Erysipelotrichaceae) (Table 3, Fig. 3).

Results of qPCR assays confirmed significant decreases in Blautia, Ruminococcaceae including *Faecalibacterium*, and *Turicibacter* spp. (Fig. 4). *Clostridium perfringens* was significantly increased only in the dogs with AHD when compared to healthy dogs.

Dogs with acute non-hemorrhagic diarrhea (NHD). PCoA plots also revealed shifts in the fecal microbiome of dogs with NHD (ANOSIM; NHD vs. healthy dogs, p = 0.003). While several bacterial taxa showed similar trends as observed for dogs with AHD, only few groups reached significance (Table 3). Sequence analysis revealed decreased proportions of *Blautia* spp. and Ruminococcaceae. Analysis by qPCR confirmed these decreases and also revealed decreases in *Turicibacter* spp., *Faecalibacterium* spp., and Bacteroidetes (Table 4).

Dogs with idiopathic IBD. PCoA plots did not indicate a significant separation between dogs with idiopathic IBD and control dogs (Fig. 2.). However, trends were observed for decreases in proportions of *Faecalibacterium* spp. and *Turicibacter* spp. (p = 0.06) in active IBD when compared to the healthy dogs, and the proportions of these groups tended to be similar to control dogs in the samples of dogs with controlled IBD. One reason for lack of significance in the sequencing results was most likely due to the low percentage of sequencing tags for *Faecalibacterium*, with medians of 0.1% in healthy dogs and 0.0%

Bifidobacterium

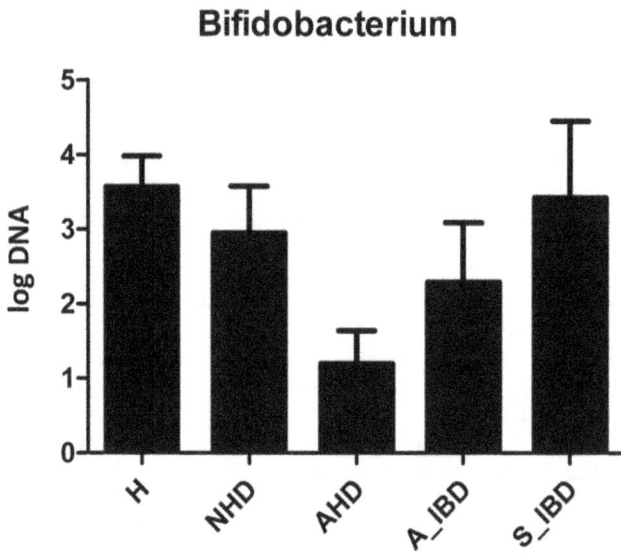

C. perfringens

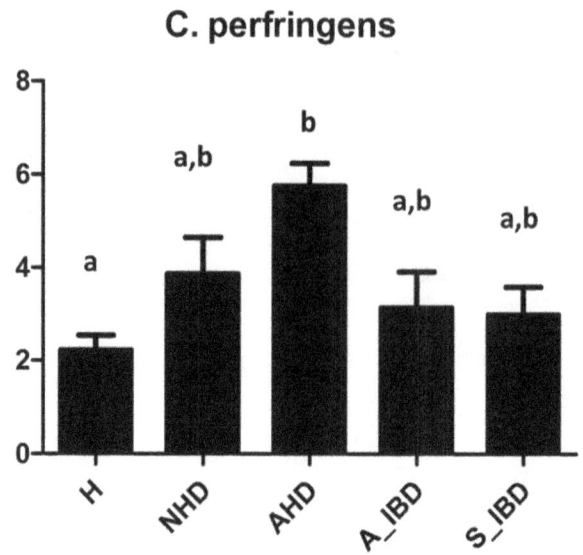

Turicibacter

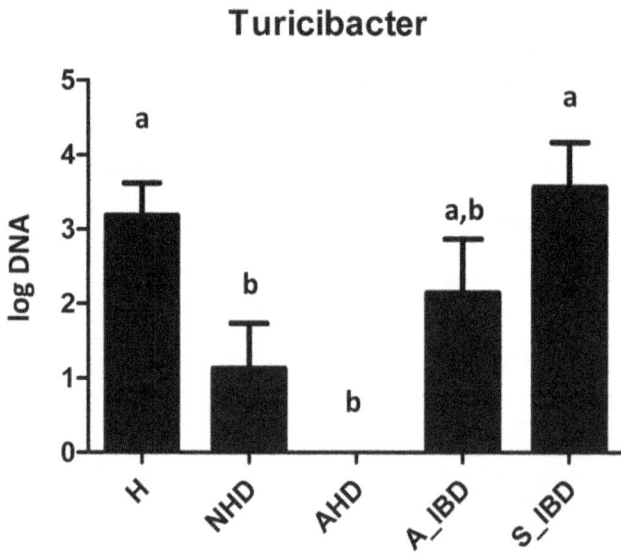

Bacteroidetes

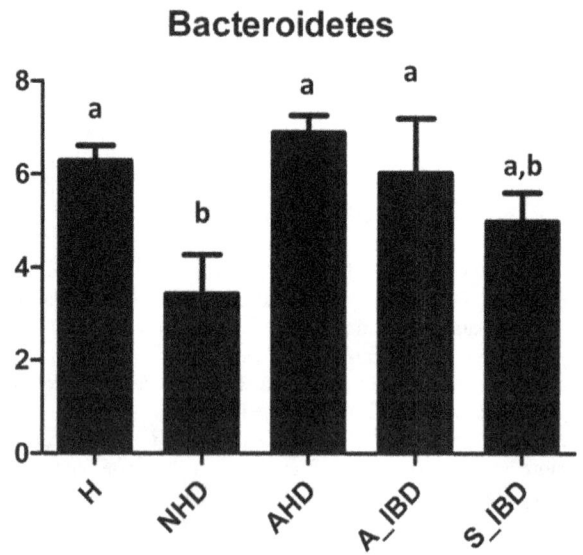

Faecalibacterium

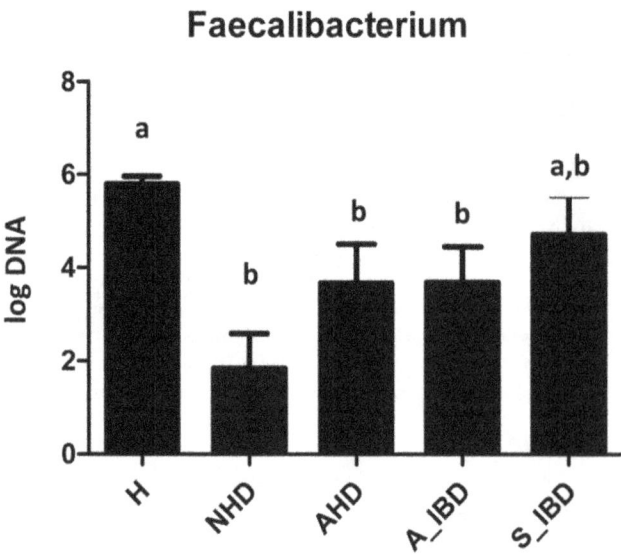

Universal

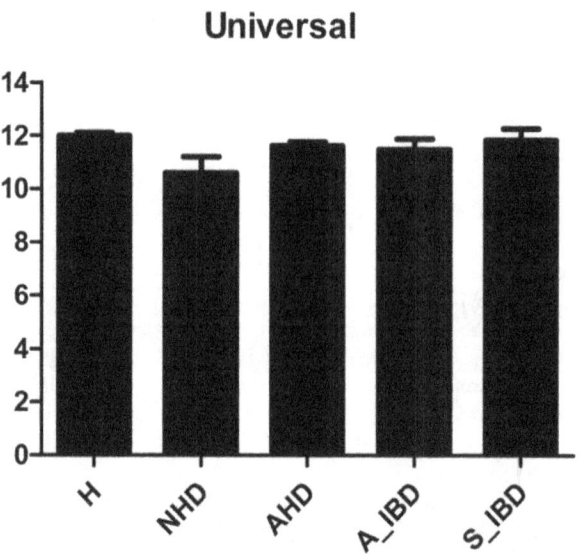

Figure 4. Results of quantitative PCR assays for selected bacterial groups. H = healthy, NHD = acute non-hemorrhagic diarrhea, AHD = acute hemorrhagic diarrhea, A_IBD = active IBD, S_IBD = therapeutically controlled, clinically insignificant IBD. Columns not sharing a common superscript are significantly different (P<0.05).

in diseased animals. However, *Faecalibacterium* was detectable in 23/32 healthy dogs, 6/10 dogs with controlled IBD, but only 1/5 with active IBD (p = 0.04 vs. healthy dogs). Results of qPCR analysis for *Faecalibacterium* spp. confirmed the trend observed for the pyrosequencing results and showed a significant decrease in dogs with active IBD, but no significant difference between the healthy dogs and dogs with clinically insignificant IBD. Furthermore, when paired samples were analyzed from dogs (n = 8) at time periods of active and clinically insignificant IBD, the abundance of *Faecalibacterium* was significantly higher in samples collected during time periods of clinically insignificant IBD (Fig. 5, p = 0.0313).

Based on qPCR analysis, also Fusobacteria were significantly decreased in dogs with active IBD compared to the healthy dogs. Fusobacteria were also significantly increased in samples collected during time periods of clinically insignificant IBD compared to those during active disease when paired samples were analyzed (Fig. 5, p = 0.0148).

None of the other bacterial groups evaluated by qPCR, including total bacteria, revealed significant differences between healthy dogs and those with active IBD, or between time periods of active disease vs. time periods of clinically insignificant IBD.

Discussion

This study evaluated the fecal microbiome of healthy dogs and dogs with acute and chronic GI disorders. Significant differences were observed in microbiome composition among the various disease groups. Dogs with acute diarrhea showed the most profound alterations in their microbiome. *Faecalibacterium* spp. and the phylum Fusobacteria were decreased in active IBD, but not significantly different during time periods of clinically insignificant IBD. Rarefaction curves (Fig. 1.) and alpha diversity measures (Table 1) suggested a trend for lower species richness and microbial diversity in the diseased groups. However, statistical

differences (e.g., p = 0.053 for the Chao1) were not identified, most likely due to the large inter-animal variation and the relative small number of animals analyzed.

Various pathogens, but also other causes such as hypersensitivities, have been associated with causing acute diarrhea [27,28]. In this study only a partial evaluation for bacterial and parasitic enteropathogens was conducted. Potential pathogens identified were *E. coli*, *Isospora*, *Giardia/Cryptosporidium*, enterotoxigenic *C. perfringens*, and toxigenic *C. difficile* (Table S2), but no clear evidence for an association between specific pathogens and acute diarrhea was identified. Patients were, therefore, classified based on clinical signs (i.e., AHD and NHD) rather than the presence of specific pathogens. The results of this study are in general agreement with previous molecular studies examining the fecal microbiota of dogs with diarrhea. In one study, dogs with acute episodes of diarrhea had an increased abundance of *C. perfringens* and *Enterococcus* spp., and a decrease in *Bacteroides* spp. [15]. Decreased proportions of Bacteroidetes were also observed in 9 dogs with unspecified diarrhea when compared to 9 healthy dogs [14]. Similarly, this study observed significant decreases in Bacteroidetes in the dogs with acute non-hemorrhagic diarrhea, but interestingly not in dogs with AHD. We also observed significant increases in *Clostridium* spp. in dogs with NHD and increases in *C. perfringens* in dogs with AHD (Fig. 4). Additionally, dogs with AHD showed increases in Fusobacteria and the genus *Sutterella* (family Alcaligenaceae). We also observed that dogs with acute diarrhea displayed significant decreases in prominent members of the intestinal microbiota, such as Erysipelotrichaceae (i.e., genus *Turicibacter*), Ruminococcaceae (i.e., *Ruminococcus*, *Faecalibacterium*) and Lachnospiraceae (i.e., *Blautia*) (Fig. 6). Some of these groups are believed to be important producers of short-chain fatty acids (SCFA), which are important for intestinal health. For example, butyrate protects against colitis by inducing apoptosis in cells with DNA damage, while acetate beneficially modulates intestinal permeability [29,30]. The mem-

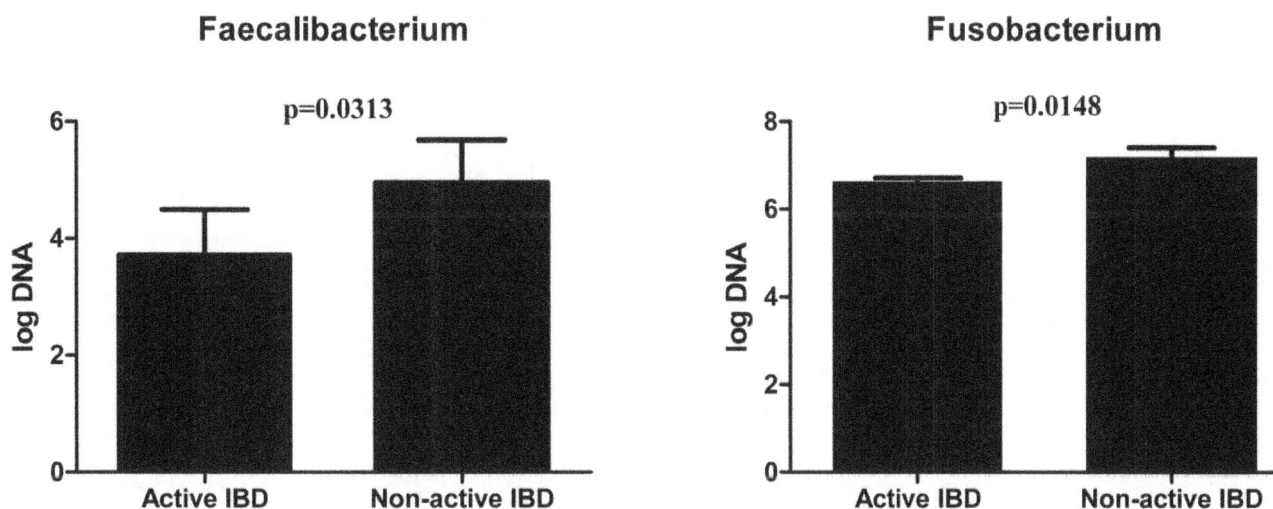

Figure 5. *Faecalibacterium* spp. and the phylum Fusobacteria in active and non-active IBD. Using qPCR, paired fecal samples were analyzed from dogs (n = 8) at time periods of active and clinically insignificant IBD as scored by a clinical IBD disease activity index (CIBDAI). The time period between the collections of repeated samples ranged from 2–8 months (median 5.5 months). None of the other bacterial groups evaluated by qPCR, including total bacteria, revealed significant differences between the paired time periods.

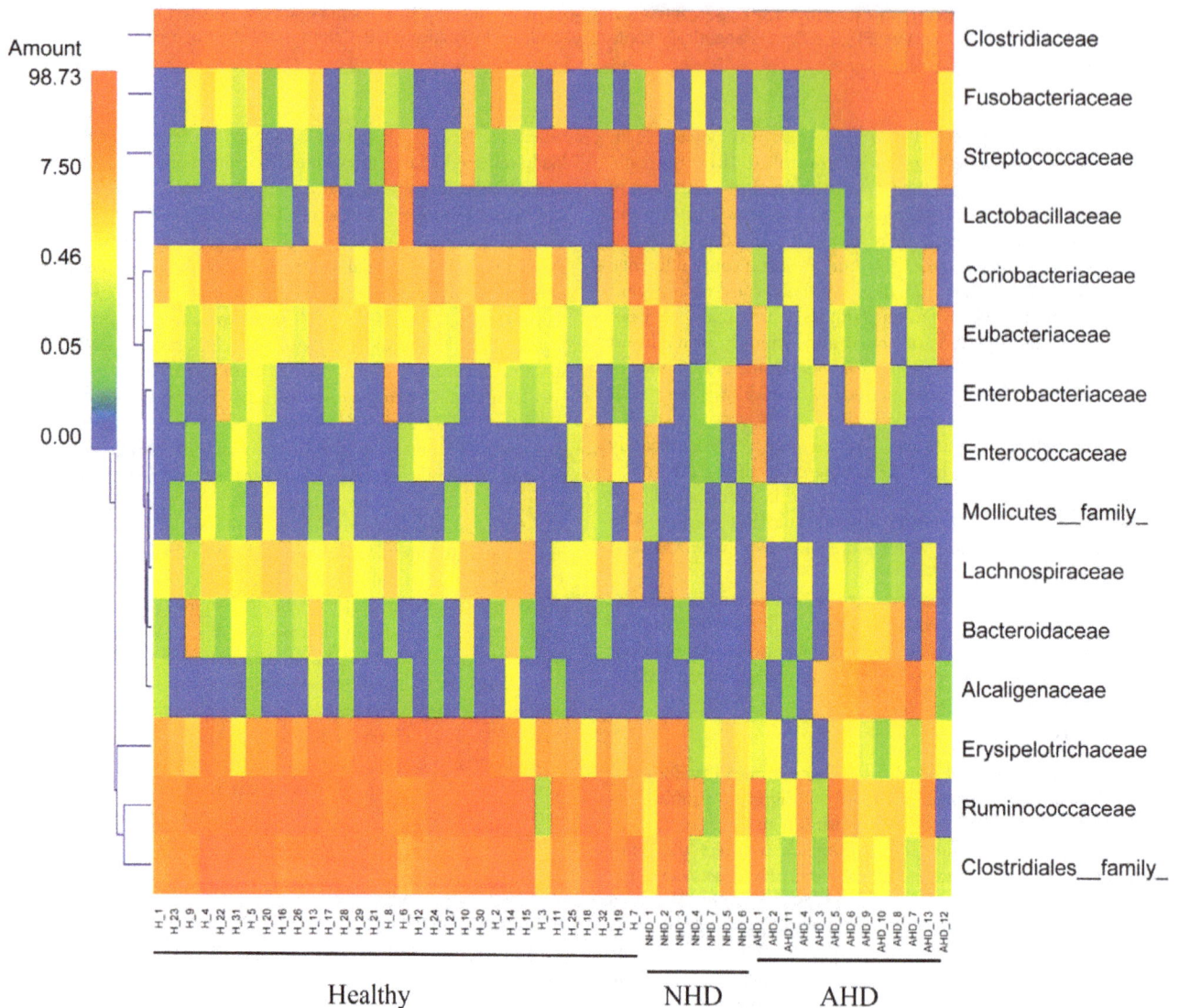

Figure 6. Heatmap illustrating the relative abundance of predominant bacterial families in fecal samples of healthy dogs and dogs with acute diarrhea based on 454-pyrosequencing. Samples from healthy dogs (H), dogs with acute non-hemorrhagic diarrhea (NHD), and dogs with acute hemorrhagic diarrhea (AHD) are shown. The heatmap represents the relative percentage of each family within each sample.

bers of the intestinal microbiota produce various other metabolites (e.g., indole) that have direct immunomodulatory properties [30,31]. Future studies are warranted to evaluate microbiome function (e.g., microbial derived metabolites) in dogs with acute diarrhea.

Idiopathic IBD is a common chronic GI disorder of dogs. As in humans, an interplay between the intestinal microbiota together with an underlying genetic susceptibility of the host and dietary and environmental factors, are implicated in the development of disease [7,32]. While recent studies have reported a dysbiosis in duodenal samples of dogs with IBD, limited data are available describing the fecal microbiota in these dogs [7–10]. In this study, *Faecalibacterium* spp. and Fusobacteria were significantly decreased in dogs with active IBD. Furthermore, when paired fecal samples were analyzed, the abundances of *Faecalibacterium* spp. and Fusobacteria were significantly decreased in samples collected during episodes of clinically active disease vs. periods of clinically insignificant IBD (Fig. 5). In contrast to previous findings in duodenal biopsies of dogs with IBD [7], we did not observe

significant differences in members of Proteobacteria between healthy dogs and dogs with IBD. Proteobacteria were only significantly higher in dogs with acute diarrhea.

Faecalibacterium spp. were found decreased in dogs with acute diarrhea and active IBD. *Faecalibacterium prausnitzii* has garnered attention as it is often observed to be decreased in humans with IBD [33]. Furthermore it has been shown to secrete anti-inflammatory peptides in *in-vitro* studies [34]. Recent studies suggest that *Faecalibacterium* spp. are prominent members of the canine gut microbiota, as FISH analysis of fecal samples of healthy dogs estimated the abundance of the *Faecalibacterium–Subdoligranulum* group as a median 16% of total bacterial counts [21]. It has been suggested that dogs may harbor *Faecalibacterium* spp. other than *F. prausnitzii*, as an initial phylogenetic assessment of a near-full-length 16S rRNA gene clone obtained from the canine colon clustered distinct from a human strain of *F. prausnitzii* (AJ270469) [35]. Therefore, the phylogenetic classification of *Faecalibacterium* spp and their functional properties in the canine intestine deserve further research.

As a limitation to this study, we evaluated only a small number of animals in the various disease groups. We initially evaluated only a subset of animals by 454-pyrosequencing, as these samples were initially available at the time of sequence analysis. Therefore, due to the small sample size we may have missed some bacterial groups that are altered in certain groups of diseased dogs. Our study population was also not homogenous, as some of the dogs lived in different countries. Geographical differences in fecal microbiota have not been well examined in dogs. In this study we evaluated samples from control dogs and diseased dogs from Sweden, and also control and diseased dogs (NHD) from Texas. We did not have matching controls from Germany, the site where samples from dogs with hemorrhagic diarrhea were collected, as these were part of an unrelated study. For initial evaluation for potential differences in the canine fecal microbiome based on country and other variables, we performed clustering based on the Unifrac distance metric on all healthy dogs in this study and did not observe clustering based on country of origin (USA vs. Sweden), weight or gender (data not shown). We also performed a separate Unifrac analysis on all dogs from Sweden (healthy vs. active IBD vs. controlled IBD), and similar to the analysis that contained all dogs regardless of country of origin, we did not observe clustering between healthy dogs and dogs with IBD, but sequence and qPCR analysis revealed similar results as observed when all dogs were included in the analysis. These results would also suggest that dog microbiota could potentially be classified into specific enterotypes [36,37]. In humans, enterotypes are characterized as compositional categories of organisms, most notably *Bacteroides*, *Prevotella*, or *Ruminococcus*, respectively, which are typically independent of nationality, gender, age, or short-term dietary interventions [36,37]. Definition of specific microbial community enterotypes may open up new therapeutic approaches to companion animal health, by designing or prescribing appropriate diets for specific disease phenotypes.

In conclusion, we observed differences in the fecal microbiome composition between dogs with acute and chronic diarrhea compared to healthy dogs. These changes were more profound in dogs with acute diarrhea, and were not identified in dogs with therapeutically controlled IBD. These results form a roadmap for additional studies focused on a more defined population of diseased dogs.

Supporting Information

Table S1   Control dogs enrolled into the study.

Table S2   Dogs with acute hemorrhagic diarrhea (AHD) and acute non-hemorrhagic diarrhea (NHD).

Table S3   Dogs with active IBD and with therapeutically controlled IBD.

Methods S1   Linear discriminant analysis.

Author Contributions

Conceived and designed the experiments: JSS SU JMS AKC LT. Performed the experiments: JSS MEM JFG SU RMH SED YM EMD LT. Analyzed the data: JSS MEM JFG SED PK II YM. Wrote the paper: JSS MEM JFG SU RMH SED PK II YM JMS AKC LT.

References

1. Frank DN, St Amand AL, Feldman RA, Boedeker EC, Harpaz N, et al. (2007) Molecular-phylogenetic characterization of microbial community imbalances in human inflammatory bowel diseases. Proc Natl Acad Sci U S A 104: 13780–13785.
2. Ritchie LE, Steiner JM, Suchodolski JS (2008) Assessment of microbial diversity along the feline intestinal tract using 16S rRNA gene analysis. FEMS Microbiol Ecol 66: 590–598.
3. Handl S, Dowd SE, Garcia-Mazcorro JF, Steiner JM, Suchodolski JS (2011) Massive parallel 16S rRNA gene pyrosequencing reveals highly diverse fecal bacterial and fungal communities in healthy dogs and cats. FEMS Microbiol Ecol 76: 301–310.
4. Suchodolski JS (2011) Companion animals symposium: Microbes and gastrointestinal health of dogs and cats. J Anim Sci 89: 1520–1530.
5. Marks SL, Rankin SC, Byrne BA, Weese JS (2011) Enteropathogenic bacteria in dogs and cats: diagnosis, epidemiology, treatment, and control. J Vet Intern Med 25: 1195–1208.
6. Kempf C, Schulz B, Strauch C, Sauter-Louis C, Tuyen U, et al. (2010) Virusnachweis in Kotproben und klinische sowie labordiagnostische Befunde von Hunden mit akutem haemorrhagischem Durchfall. Tieraerztliche Praxis 38 79–86.
7. Suchodolski JS, Dowd SE, Wilke V, Steiner JM, Jergens AE (2012) 16S rRNA gene pyrosequencing reveals bacterial dysbiosis in the duodenum of dogs with idiopathic inflammatory bowel disease. Plos ONE 7: e39333.
8. Allenspach K, House A, Smith K, McNeill FM, Hendricks A, et al. (2010) Evaluation of mucosal bacteria and histopathology, clinical disease activity and expression of Toll-like receptors in German shepherd dogs with chronic enteropathies. Vet Microbiol 146: 326–335.
9. Suchodolski JS, Xenoulis PG, Paddock CG, Steiner JM, Jergens AE (2010) Molecular analysis of the bacterial microbiota in duodenal biopsies from dogs with idiopathic inflammatory bowel disease. Vet Microbiol 142: 394–400.
10. Xenoulis PG, Palculict B, Allenspach K, Steiner JM, Van House AM, et al. (2008) Molecular-phylogenetic characterization of microbial communities imbalances in the small intestine of dogs with inflammatory bowel disease. FEMS Microbiol Ecol 66: 579–589.
11. Simpson KW, Jergens AE (2011) Pitfalls and progress in the diagnosis and management of canine inflammatory bowel disease. Vet Clin North Am Small Anim Pract 41: 381–398.
12. Suchodolski JS, Morris EK, Allenspach K, Jergens AE, Harmoinen JA, et al. (2008) Prevalence and identification of fungal DNA in the small intestine of healthy dogs and dogs with chronic enteropathies. Vet Microbiol 132: 379–388.
13. Jia J, Frantz N, Khoo C, Gibson GR, Rastall RA, et al. (2010) Investigation of the faecal microbiota associated with canine chronic diarrhoea. FEMS Microbiol Ecol 71: 304–312.
14. Chaban B, Links MG, Hill JE (2012) A Molecular Enrichment Strategy Based on cpn60 for Detection of Epsilon-Proteobacteria in the Dog Fecal Microbiome. Microb Ecol 63: 348–357.
15. Bell JA, Kopper JJ, Turnbull JA, Barbu NI, Murphy AJ, et al. (2008) Ecological characterization of the colonic microbiota of normal and diarrheic dogs. Interdiscip Perspect Infect Dis 2008: 149694.
16. Jergens AE, Schreiner CA, Frank DE, Niyo Y, Ahrens FE, et al. (2003) A scoring index for disease activity in canine inflammatory bowel disease. J Vet Intern Med 17: 291–297.
17. Suchodolski JS, Dowd SE, Westermarck E, Steiner JM, Wolcott RD, et al. (2009) The effect of the macrolide antibiotic tylosin on microbial diversity in the canine small intestine as demonstrated by massive parallel 16S rRNA gene sequencing. BMC Microbiol 9: 210.
18. Caporaso JG, Kuczynski J, Stombaugh J, Bittinger K, Bushman FD, et al. (2010) QIIME allows analysis of high-throughput community sequencing data. Nat Methods 7: 335–336.
19. Gontcharova V, Youn E, Wolcott RD, Hollister EB, Gentry TJ, et al. (2010) Black Box Chimera Check (B2C2): a Windows-Based Software for Batch Depletion of Chimeras from Bacterial 16S rRNA Gene Datasets. Open Microbiol J 4: 47–52.
20. Ritchie LE, Burke KF, Garcia-Mazcorro JF, Steiner JM, Suchodolski JS (2010) Characterization of fecal microbiota in cats using universal 16S rRNA gene and group-specific primers for Lactobacillus and Bifidobacterium spp. Vet Microbiol 144: 140–146.
21. Garcia-Mazcorro JD, Dowd SE, Poulsen J, Steiner JM, Suchodolski JS (2012) Abundance and short-term temporal variability of fecal microbiota in healthy dogs. Microbiology Open 1: 340–347.
22. Garcia-Mazcorro JF, Suchodolski JS, Jones KR, Clark-Price SC, Dowd SE, et al. (2012) Effect of the proton pump inhibitor omeprazole on the gastrointestinal bacterial microbiota of healthy dogs. FEMS Microbiol Ecol 80: 624–636.
23. Benjamini Y, Hochberg Y (1995) Controlling the false discovery rate: a practical and powerful approach to multiple testing. J Roy Stat Soc B 57: 289–300.
24. Kachroo P, Ivanov I, Davidson LA, Chowdhary BP, Lupton JR, et al. (2011) Classification of diet-modulated gene signatures at the colon cancer initiation and progression stages. Dig Dis Sci 56: 2595–2604.
25. Chapkin RS, Zhao C, Ivanov I, Davidson LA, Goldsby JS, et al. (2010) Noninvasive stool-based detection of infant gastrointestinal development using

gene expression profiles from exfoliated epithelial cells. Am J Physiol Gastro-intest Liver Physiol 298: G582–589.

26. Sima C, Braga-Neto UM, Dougherty ER (2011) High-dimensional bolstered error estimation. Bioinformatics 27: 3056–3064.

27. Unterer S, Strohmeyer K, Kruse BD, Sauter-Louis C, Hartmann K (2011) Treatment of aseptic dogs with hemorrhagic gastroenteritis with amoxicillin/clavulanic acid: a prospective blinded study. J Vet Intern Med 25: 973–979.

28. Weese JS (2011) Bacterial enteritis in dogs and cats: diagnosis, therapy, and zoonotic potential. Vet Clin North Am Small Anim Pract 41: 287–309.

29. Pryde SE, Duncan SH, Hold GL, Stewart CS, Flint HJ (2002) The microbiology of butyrate formation in the human colon. FEMS Microbiol Lett 217: 133–139.

30. Fukuda S, Toh H, Taylor TD, Ohno H, Hattori M (2012) Acetate-producing bifidobacteria protect the host from enteropathogenic infection via carbohydrate transporters. Gut Microbes 3: 449–454.

31. Bansal T, Alaniz RC, Wood TK, Jayaraman A (2010) The bacterial signal indole increases epithelial-cell tight-junction resistance and attenuates indicators of inflammation. Proc Natl Acad Sci U S A 107: 228–233.

32. Packey CD, Sartor RB (2009) Commensal bacteria, traditional and opportu-nistic pathogens, dysbiosis and bacterial killing in inflammatory bowel diseases. Curr Opin Infect Dis 22: 292–301.

33. Sokol H, Seksik P, Furet JP, Firmesse O, Nion-Larmurier I, et al. (2009) Low counts of *Faecalibacterium prausnitzii* in colitis microbiota. Inflamm Bowel Dis 15: 1183–1189.

34. Sokol H, Pigneur B, Watterlot L, Lakhdari O, Bermudez-Humaran LG, et al. (2008) *Faecalibacterium prausnitzii* is an anti-inflammatory commensal bacterium identified by gut microbiota analysis of Crohn disease patients. Proc Natl Acad Sci U S A 105: 16731–16736.

35. Suchodolski JS, Camacho J, Steiner JM (2008) Analysis of bacterial diversity in the canine duodenum, jejunum, ileum, and colon by comparative 16S rRNA gene analysis. FEMS Microbiol Ecol 66: 567–578.

36. Wu GD, Chen J, Hoffmann C, Bittinger K, Chen YY, et al. (2011) Linking long-term dietary patterns with gut microbial enterotypes. Science 334: 105–108.

37. Arumugam M, Raes J, Pelletier E, Le Paslier D, Yamada T, et al. (2011) Enterotypes of the human gut microbiome. Nature 473: 174–180.

38. Muhling M, Woolven-Allen J, Murrell JC, Joint I (2008) Improved group-specific PCR primers for denaturing gradient gel electrophoresis analysis of the genetic diversity of complex microbial communities. ISME J 2: 379–392.

39. Malinen E, Rinttila T, Kajander K, Matto J, Kassinen A, et al. (2005) Analysis of the fecal microbiota of irritable bowel syndrome patients and healthy controls with real-time PCR. Am J Gastroenterol 100: 373–382.

40. Wise MG, Siragusa GR (2005) Quantitative detection of *Clostridium perfringens* in the broiler fowl gastrointestinal tract by real-time PCR. Appl Environ Microbiol 71: 3911–3916.

41. Gurjar AA, Hegde NV, Love BC, Jayarao BM (2008) Real-time multiplex PCR assay for rapid detection and toxintyping of *Clostridium perfringens* toxin producing strains in feces of dairy cattle. Mol Cell Probes 22: 90–95.

42. Houser BA, Hattel AL, Jayarao BM (2010) Real-time multiplex polymerase chain reaction assay for rapid detection of *Clostridium difficile* toxin-encoding strains. Foodborne Pathog Dis 7: 719–726.

43. Lubbs DC, Vester BM, Fastinger ND, Swanson KS (2009) Dietary protein concentration affects intestinal microbiota of adult cats: a study using DGGE and qPCR to evaluate differences in microbial populations in the feline gastrointestinal tract. J Anim Physiol Anim Nutr (Berl) 93: 113–121.

3

MIF Participates in *Toxoplasma gondii*-Induced Pathology following Oral Infection

Marta G. Cavalcanti[1,3]*[9], **Jacilene S. Mesquita**[1][9], **Kalil Madi**[5,6], **Daniel F. Feijó**[1], **Iranaia Assunção-Miranda**[2], **Heitor S. P. Souza**[4], **Marcelo T. Bozza**[1,4]*

1 Departamento de Imunologia, Instituto de Microbiologia Professor Paulo de Góes, Universidade Federal do Rio de Janeiro (UFRJ), Rio de Janeiro, Brazil, 2 Departamento de Virologia, Instituto de Microbiologia Professor Paulo de Góes, Universidade Federal do Rio de Janeiro (UFRJ), Rio de Janeiro, Brazil, 3 Serviço de Doenças Infecciosas e Parasitárias, Universidade Federal do Rio de Janeiro (UFRJ), Rio de Janeiro, Brazil, 4 Departamento de Clínica Médica, Laboratório Multidisciplinar de Pesquisa, Universidade Federal do Rio de Janeiro (UFRJ), Rio de Janeiro, Brazil, 5 Departamento de Patologia, Hospital Universitário Clementino Fraga Filho, Universidade Federal do Rio de Janeiro (UFRJ), Rio de Janeiro, Brazil, 6 Laboratório Sérgio Franco, Rio de Janeiro, Brazil

Abstract

Background: Macrophage migration inhibitory factor (MIF) is essential for controlling parasite burden and survival in a model of systemic *Toxoplasma gondii* infection. Peroral *T. gondii* infection induces small intestine necrosis and death in susceptible hosts, and in many aspects resembles inflammatory bowel disease (IBD). Considering the critical role of MIF in the pathogenesis of IBD, we hypothesized that MIF participates in the inflammatory response induced by oral infection with *T. gondii*.

Methodology/Principal Findings: Mif deficient (*Mif⁻/⁻*) and wild-type mice in the C57Bl/6 background were orally infected with *T. gondii* strain ME49. *Mif⁻/⁻* mice had reduced lethality, ileal inflammation and tissue damage despite of an increased intestinal parasite load compared to wt mice. Lack of MIF caused a reduction of TNF-α, IL-12, IFN-γ and IL-23 and an increased expression of IL-22 in ileal mucosa. Moreover, suppressed pro-inflammatory responses at the ileal mucosa observed in *Mif⁻/⁻* mice was not due to upregulation of IL-4, IL-10 or TGF-β. MIF also affected the expression of matrix metalloproteinase-9 (MMP-9) but not MMP-2 in the intestine of infected mice. Signs of systemic inflammation including the increased concentrations of inflammatory cytokines in the plasma and liver damage were less pronounced in *Mif⁻/⁻* mice compared to wild-type mice.

Conclusion/Significance: In conclusion, our data suggested that in susceptible hosts MIF controls *T. gondii* infection with the cost of increasing local and systemic inflammation, tissue damage and death.

Editor: Jörg Hermann Fritz, McGill University, Canada

Funding: This work was supported by CNPq, FAPERJ and Pronex (Programa de Apoio a Núcleos de Excelência – Pronex/FAPERJ (www.faperj.br/interna.phtml?ctx_cod = 1.11)). The funders had no role in study design, data collection and analysis, decision to publish, or preparation of the manuscript.

Competing Interests: The authors have declared that no competing interests exist.

* E-mail: cavalcanti.marta66@gmail.com (MGC); mbozza@micro.ufrj.br (MTB)

[9] These authors contributed equally to this work.

Introduction

The immune/inflammatory response to *Toxoplasma gondii* infection is essential to control parasite replication and tissue spread but also can cause tissue damage, being decisive to pathogenesis. Selective tissue invasion by *T. gondii* causes compartmental immune responses unique to each tissue such as the one present in the placenta, central nervous system and intestinal mucosa, while parasite spreading promotes a systemic response that resembles bacterial sepsis [1–3]. Inhibition or abrogation of TNF-α, IL-12 and/or IFN-γ increase host susceptibility to toxoplasmosis as a result of uncontrolled parasite burden [4–6]. In natural *T. gondii* infection through the oral route, exacerbated inflammatory responses at the small intestine (ileitis) resemble human inflammatory bowel disease (IBD) [1,7]. The inflammatory response coordinate by IL-23/IL-22 is involved in *T. gondii*-induced disruption of intestinal homeostasis and immu-

nopathology, an effect at least in part due to increase expression of matrix metalloproteinase-2 (MMP) [7]. These pro-inflammatory mediators and MMPs are involved in the immune pathogenesis and tissue damage in *T. gondii* peoral infection, increasing host morbidity and mortality despite parasite control [7–9]. Deficient regulation of the inflammatory response observed in the absence of IL-10 results in massive leukocyte infiltration, extensive tissue damage despite control of parasite load, systemic inflammation and increase lethality [2].

MIF is a versatile molecule that comprises hormonal and enzymatic activities in addition to exert pro-inflammatory and chemotactic functions [10–13]. First described as a T-cell-derived factor involved in the inhibition of macrophage migration in delayed–type hypersensitivity response, MIF is also produced by other immune cells such as macrophages, neutrophils and eosinophils but also non immune cells such as endothelial, epithelial, muscle and pituitary cells [10–15]. MIF expression and production are regulated by adrenocorticotrophic hormone which results in counter-regulation of cortisol [11,16]. MIF production is also regulated by TNF and LPS-Toll-like receptor 4 (TLR4) in a positive feedback cascade resulting in enhanced proinflammatory responses [15,17,18]. Furthermore, MIF is an essential regulator of innate and adaptive immune responses with a crucial role in host protection against different pathogens and is involved in the pathogenesis of a broad spectrum of infectious and non infectious inflammatory diseases [10–23].

In parasitic infections MIF is involved both in protective as well as immune pathogenic responses [12,21,24–28]. Upon systemic infection with *T. gondii*, IFN-γ and TNF-α mediated responses are upregulated by MIF, and *Mif⁻/⁻* mice are more susceptible to infection presenting increased parasite burden [27]. A recent study also demonstrated an increased susceptibility, reduced IL-12 production and dendritic cell activation on *Mif⁻/⁻* mice in the Balb/c background to an oral *T. gondii* infection [28]. Balb/c mice are naturally resistant to oral infection with *T. gondii*, while C57BL/6 are highly susceptible and display intestinal inflammation, especially in the ileum [29–31].

Considering the role of MIF on intestinal inflammation, we hypothesize that MIF participates in the pathogenesis of *T. gondii*-induced intestinal tissue damage. Our results indicate that MIF mediates pathogenic responses during *T. gondii* oral infection by exacerbating compartmental and systemic inflammatory responses. The lack of MIF caused an overall reduction of tissue damage despite of an increase in local parasite burden.

Materials and Methods

Mice

C57BL/6 (wild type, wt) and *Mif⁻/⁻* (backcrossed to the C57BL/6 genetic background, n = 8) were obtained from the animal facility at the Universidade Federal do Rio de Janeiro (UFRJ, Rio de Janeiro). Sex and age-matched (8–12 week-old) C57BL/6 were used as controls for *Mif⁻/⁻*. The animals were kept at constant temperature (25°C) with free access to chow and water in a room with a 12 h light/dark cycle. All animal experiments were performed in accordance to Brazilian Government's ethical and animal experiment regulations. The experiments were approved by the Institutional Animal Welfare Committee (approval ID: CEUA/CCS/UFRJ/IMPPG 011).

Parasites and per oral infection

The *T. gondii* strain ME49 was kindly provided by Dr R. Gazzinelli, (UFMG, Minas Gerais, Brazil) and Dr J. Lannes-Vieira (FIOCRUZ, Rio de Janeiro, Brazil). For peroral infection, mice were infected by gavage using 20 and 100 ME49 cysts/animal. Cysts were obtained from C57BL/6 brain homogenates as previously described [2].

Detection of *T. gondii* DNA

Parasites in tissues were quantified by a real-time polymerase chain reaction (RT-PCR) as previously described [7] targeting a repetitive 529-bp DNA fragment of *T. gondii* (GenBank accession no AF487550) [32] which are specific for a cryptic gene as described [33]. Fifty to 100 μg of ileum and liver tissues were crushed in a rotor-stator after frozen in liquid nitrogen and total DNA were isolated with DNAzol reagent (Invitrogen Life Technologies) following the manufactures protocol. Five hundred ng of total DNA extracted from each sample were submitted to real-time PCR using Power SYBR® Green PCR master mix (Applied Biosystems) using each oligonucleotide primer (TOX-9, 5′-AGGAGAGATATCAGGACTGTAG-3′; TOX-10, 5′-

GCGTCGTCTCGTCTAGATCG-3′). The amplification was performed using one cycle at 95°C for 10 min, 45 cycles at 95°C for 30 s, 60°C for 1 min. A standard curve was performed using 5000-5 pg *T. gondii* DNA to quantification of total DNA of samples.

Determination of small intestinal length, histopathology and histological scores

Small intestinal shortening was determined by measuring whole intestinal segment of wt and *Mif⁻/⁻* controls and *T. gondii*-infected mice. It was calculated by dividing the difference of the mean length of the small intestine from control mice minus the length from infected mice at day 8 after infection and then multiplied by 100 over the mean length of mice small intestines [34]. Intestines, liver and brain were fixed in 10% neutral buffered formalin, embedded in paraffin, sectioned at 5 μm, and stained with hematoxylin and eosin using standard techniques. Blinded samples were submitted for semi-quantitative histopathologic analysis. Histological scores were determined in fixed and paraffin-embedded tissue sections taken from the terminal ileum, as previously described [34]. Liver sections were analyzed for the numbers of inflammatory foci at a magnification of ×200 at day 9 after infection in each group. We analyzed the number of inflammatory foci per field (6.5×9 mm, microscope Zeiss, Germany) counting 10 fields of each section.

Determination of cytokine concentrations at the intestinal tissue and plasma

Plasma samples were obtained to measure cytokine concentrations. IFN-γ and TNF-α concentrations were measured by a commercial ELISA from Peprotech (NJ, USA). Concentrations of IL-10 was determined by ELISA using a commercial kit from R&D Systems (MN, USA).

RT-PCR analysis of matrix metalloproteinases and cytokines

Approximately 50–100 μg of ileum tissue were crushed in a rotor–stator after frozen in liquid nitrogen and total RNA were isolated with TRIzol reagent (Invitrogen Life Technologies) following the manufactures protocol. Four micrograms of total RNA extracted were reverse transcribed using a High capacity cDNA reverse transcription kit (Applied Biosystems, Foster City, CA). Each sample was submitted to real-time PCR using Power SYBR® Green PCR master mix (Applied Biosystems). The reactions were carried out using specific primers for the following genes: MMP-2 (forward, 5′-CAATCTTTTCTGG-GAGCTC-3′; reverse, 5′-GCTGATACTGACACTGGTACTG-3′), MMP-9 (forward, 5′-CCTGGAACTCACACGACATCTTC-3′; reverse, 5′-TGGAAACTCACACGCCAGAA-3′), TNF-α (forward, 5′-CCTCACACTCAGATCATCTTCTCA-3′; reverse, 5′-TGGTTGTCTTTGAGATCCATGC-3′), IL-6 (forward, 5′- TCA-TATCTTCAACCAAGAGGTA-3′; reverse, 5′- CAGTGAGGA-ATGTCCACAAACTG-3′), IFN-γ (forward, 5′-AGCAACAGCA-AGGCGAAAA-3′; reverse, 5′- CTGGACCTGTGGGTTGTTGA-3′), IL-17A (forward, 5′-TCCCTCTGTGATCTGGGAAG-3′; reverse, 5′-CTCGACCCTGAAAGTGAAGG-3′), TGF-β (forward, 5′-GACCGCAACAACGCCATCTA-3′; reverse, 5′-AGCCCTG-TATTCCGTCTCCTT-3′), IL-12p35 (forward, 5′-CCACCCTT-GCCCTCCTAAAC-3′; reverse, 5′-GGCAGCTCCCTCTTGTT-GTG-3′), IL-23 (forward, 5′-TGGCATCGAGAAACTGTGAGA-3′; reverse, 5′-TCAGTTCGTATTGGTAGTCCTGTTA-3′), IL-22 (forward, 5′-GACAGGTTCCAGCCCTACAT-3′; reverse, 5′-GTCGTCACCGCTGATGTG-3′), IL-10 (forward, 5′-TAAGG-GTTACTTGGGTTGCCAAG-3′; reverse, 5′-CAAATGCTCCT-

TGATTTCTGGGC-3′). The samples were subjected to 45 amplification cycles consisting in 95°C for 30 s, 60°C for 1 min. The expression of the hypoxanthine guanine phosphoribosyl transferase 1 (Hprt1) gene (forward, 5′-GCTGGTGAAAAG-GACCTCT-3′; reverse 5′-CAC AGG ACT AGA ACA CCT GC-3′) was used to normalize the results, which were presented as fold induction of mRNA expression relative to control samples. Moreover, mouse TaqMan pre-developed assay reagents (Applied Biosystems) were used for IL-4 and Hprt amplification. The analyses of relative gene expression data were performed by $2^{-\Delta\Delta C_T}$ method [35].

Statistical analysis

Data are expressed as means ± SEM. The statistical significance of differences in mean values was determined by using Student's t test or ANOVA. Survival data are presented as a Kaplan-Meier survival curve and analyzed with Log-rank test by software Prism 5 (USA). Differences of at least p≤0.05 are considered significant.

Results

Reduced mortality and morbidity of Mif$^{-/-}$ mice after T. gondii oral infection

It has been recently demonstrated that MIF determines host susceptibility to *T. gondii* infection by peritoneal route [27]. *Mif / ⁻* mice presente increased parasite load and systemic inflammatory response when compared to wt mice. However, *T. gondii* infection through the oral route might determine a different outcome depending on the inflammatory response within the intestinal mucosa [36,37]. To define the role of MIF during natural *T. gondii*

infection in susceptible hosts, wt and *Mif / ⁻* mice were orally infected with 100 or 20 cysts per animal. Wt mice infected with 100 cysts were all dead after 10–12 days post infection while *Mif / ⁻* mice had a significant increase of survival (Fig. 1A). The increase survival of *Mif / ⁻* compared to wt mice was even more pronounced upon infection with 20 cysts/animal (Fig. 1B). To assess morbidity during acute *T. gondii* infection, we used weight loss and hematocrit measurement, considered good markers of morbidity in acute acquired toxoplasmosis [38]. Although both wt and *Mif / ⁻* mice presented weight loss, it was more severe in wt than on *Mif / ⁻* mice (Fig. 1C). Similarly, hematocrit was significantly reduced in infected wt when compared to *Mif / ⁻* mice (Fig. 1D). Thus, *Mif / ⁻* mice displayed increased resistance to acute infection and reduced morbidity following per oral *T. gondii* infection.

Reduced ileal damage despite of increased parasite loads in the absence of MIF

To determine the cause of reduced mortality of *Mif / ⁻* mice, we initially performed macroscopical and histopathological analysis of the small intestine of control and infected animals. At day 9 post infection, wt mice presented significant intestinal shortening compared to *Mif / ⁻* mice (Fig. 2A). This intestinal shrinkage observed in wt mice was associated with histological changes at the terminal ileum, including blunting of the villi, extensive necrosis and full thickness inflammatory infiltration of the lamina propria (Fig. 2B). Infected *Mif / ⁻* mice presented reduced necrosis and decreased loss of mucosal integrity, lamina propria and intestinal wall and more preserved areas of intestine. Tissue damage was determined by histopathological scores of the terminal ileum of infected mice, and most samples from wt mice

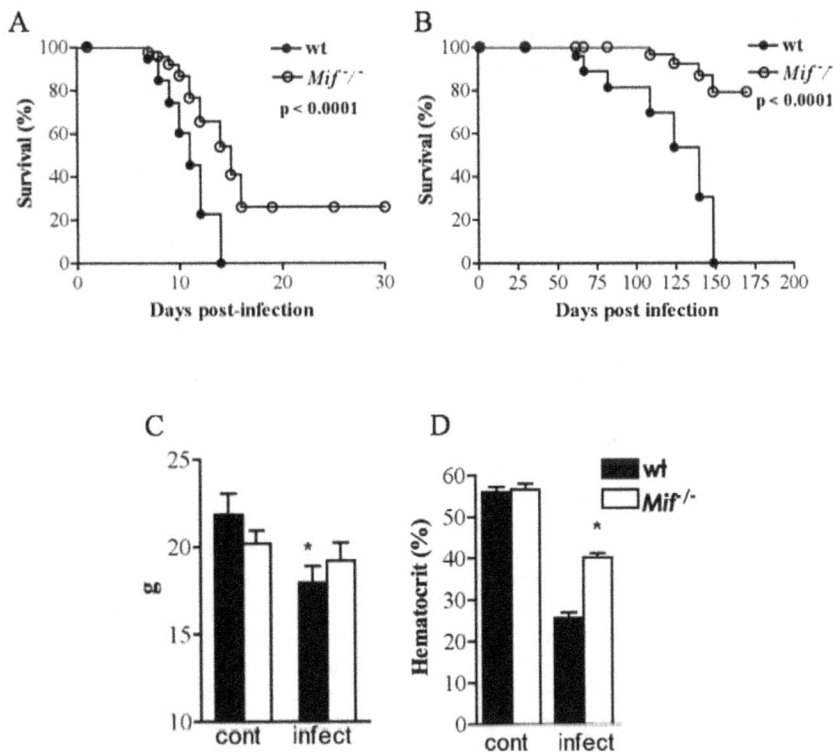

Figure 1. MIF increases morbidity and mortality during peroral *T. gondii* infection. Survival curves of *Mif / ⁻* (C57BL/6) mice (6–8 weeks old) and age and sex-matched wild type controls orally infected with 100 (A) and 20 cysts (B) of ME-49 strain of *T. gondii*. Morbidity was evaluated by determining animal (C) relative weight loss and (D) hematocrit. One representative experiment out of three performed. Data from 8 to 10 animals per group are given as mean ± SEM, and p values were determined by t-test (* p≤0.05) or by Log-rank test (A, B). Cont, control not infected.

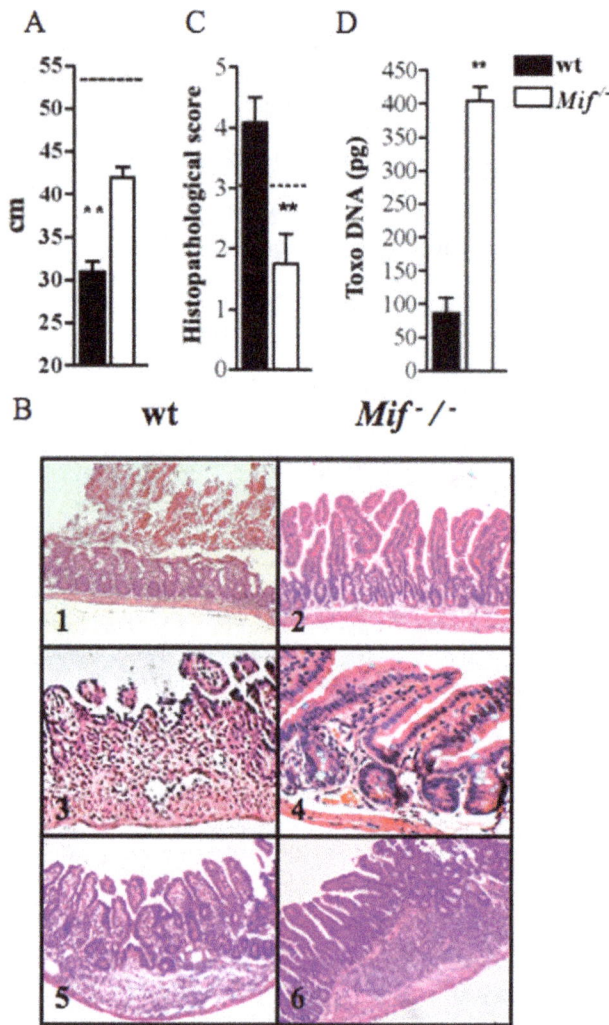

Figure 2. _T. gondii_-induced ileitis is mediated by MIF that induces severe tissue damage despite efficient parasite control. (A) Shortening of small intestine of wt and _Mif⁻/⁻_ mice (n = 6) at 9 days post-infection (dpi). (B) Histopathologycal analysis by hematoxilin and eosin (HE) of terminal ileum was performed at 9 dpi in wt and _Mif⁻/⁻_. Magnification are ×200 (B1, 2, 5 and 6) and ×400 (B3 and 4). In (C) Histologycal scores of ileal biopsies of wt and _Mif⁻/⁻_ mice at 9 dpi. The horizontal line limits absence of inflammatory response (0 to 3) and necrosis (above 3). (D) Toxo DNA concentration was determined in ileal biopsies of wt and _Mif⁻/⁻_ mice. One representative experiment out of three independent experiments. Data from 3 to 6 mice per group is represented by means ± SEM and p values determined by t-test (* p≤0.05, ** p≤0.01). Length of intestinal segments of control not infected wt and _Mif⁻/⁻_ mice are represented by a dotted line in A. Cont, control not infected.

presented higher scores when compared to _Mif⁻/⁻_ mice (Fig. 2C). In fact, _Mif⁻/⁻_ mice displayed less tissue damage in contrast to a significant increase in tissue parasitism (Fig. 2D). These findings indicate that MIF-mediated inflammatory response promotes tissue damage, contributing to morbidity and mortality, but also participates on _T. gondii_ control at the intestinal mucosa.

MIF regulates inflammatory cytokines in _T. gondii_-induced ileitis

To investigate the mechanism by which MIF regulates the inflammatory response at the intestinal mucosa, we examined mRNA expression and the concentrations of inflammatory cytokines in the supernatants of ileal mucosal explants from wt and _Mif⁻/⁻_ infected mice. TNF-α, IL-12, IFN-γ and IL-23 expression were decreased in infected _Mif⁻/⁻_ mice when compared to wt mice (Fig. 3A–C, E). The mRNA expression of IL-6 and IL-17A were also similar in wt and _Mif⁻/⁻_ mice (Fig. 3D, F). Surprisingly, IL-22 expression was significantly increased in infected _Mif⁻/⁻_ compared to wt mice (Fig. 3G). To determine if IL-4, IL-10 and TGF-β could be implicated in the suppression of immunopathology and increased parasite burdens of _Mif⁻/⁻_, we examined the mRNA expression of these regulatory cytokines in the ileal mucosa explants of control and infected wt and _Mif⁻/⁻_ mice. While IL-4 mRNA expression was similar in wt and _Mif⁻/⁻_ mice at 9 days post infection (Fig. 4A), IL-10 mRNA expression and protein in ileal mucosa were reduced in _Mif⁻/⁻_ compared to wt mice (Fig. 4B, data not shown). Similarly, _T. gondii_ infected _Mif⁻/⁻_ mice presented significant decrease of TGF-β expression when compared to infected wt mice (Fig. 4C). These results indicate that the reduced inflammatory response in the ileun of _Mif⁻/⁻_ compared to wt mice is not due to up regulation of IL-4, IL-10 or TGF-β.

T. gondii peroral infection induces decreased expression of MMP-9, but not MMP2, in the intestinal mucosa of _Mif⁻/⁻_ mice

Matrix metalloproteinases have been implicated in the pathogenesis of IBD and most recently in _T. gondii_-induced ileitis [7]. Given that MIF regulates the expression of MMPs during pathological inflammatory responses such as arthritis [39,40], we investigated the possible involvement of MMP-2 and MMP-9 in _T. gondii_-induced MIF-mediated ileitis. We determined the mRNA expression of MMP-2 and MMP-9 in the ileum of control and infected wt and _Mif⁻/⁻_ mice. At day 9 post-infection, both control and infected wt and _Mif⁻/⁻_ mice presented similar MMP-2 expression (Fig. 5A). However, MMP-9 was significantly reduced in the ileum of _Mif⁻/⁻_ infected mice (Fig. 5B). These results suggest that MIF might contribute to pathological responses to _T. gondii_ infection at the intestinal compartment via MMP-9 pathway.

Systemic inflammatory responses are regulated by MIF and enhance _T. gondii_-induced pathology

The systemic inflammation during _T. gondii_ infection resembles bacterial sepsis. Considering the critical role of MIF in the pathogenesis of experimental sepsis, we investigated several markers of systemic inflammation in _T. gondii_-infected wt and _Mif⁻/⁻_ mice. Leukocyte counts were higher in wt mice at day 4 and 7 post-infection when compared to _Mif⁻/⁻_ mice (Fig. 6A). Given that systemic inflammation during per oral infection are induced by pro-inflammatory mediators such as IFN-γ and TNF-α, we investigated the concentrations of these cytokines in the plasma of infected wt and _Mif⁻/⁻_ mice. The concentrations of both cytikones were higher in wt compared to _Mif⁻/⁻_ mice (Fig. 6B, C). Thrombosis was often associated with vascular inflammatory infiltration in the livers of wt and _Mif⁻/⁻_ mice (Fig. 6D). Wt mice had increased numbers of mononuclear cell infiltrates in perivascular areas and scattered at the hepatic parenquima (Fig. 6D, E). In contrast, infected _Mif⁻/⁻_ mice had preserved liver parenquima and reduced mononuclear cell infiltration (Fig. 6D, E). Wt mice presented higher alanine aminotransferase and aspartate aminotransferase plasma concentrations compared to _Mif⁻/⁻_ mice, an indication of liver damage and dysfunction (Fig. 6F, G). Moreover, _T. gondii_ DNA levels were similar in wt and _Mif⁻/⁻_ mice (Fig. 6H). The findings suggest that

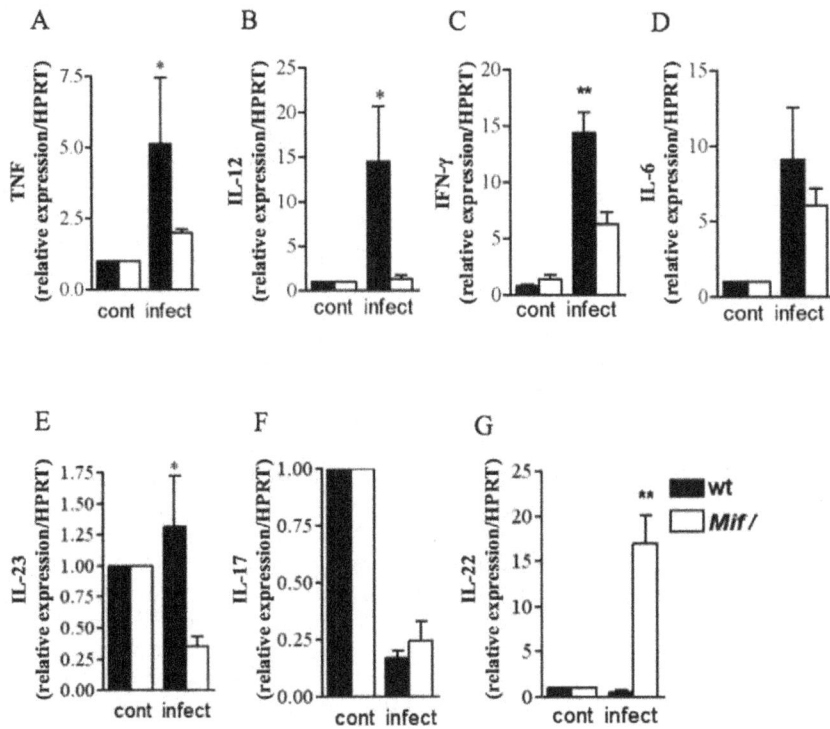

Figure 3. MIF upregulates proinflammatory responses in toxoplasmic ileitis. Real-time PCR of (A) TNF-α, (B) IL-12, (C) IFN-γ, (D) IL-6, (E) IL-23, (F) IL-17 and (G) IL-22 expression in ileal explants from control and infected wt and $Mif^{-/-}$ mice. Results are expressed as fold changes relative to HPRT mRNA expression. Data from 3 to 6 mice per group is represented by means ± SEM and p values determined by t-test (* p≤0.05, ** p≤0.01). Cont, control not infected.

T.gondii-induced systemic response is in part dependent on MIF, while parasite replication and dissemination is not affected by MIF.

Discussion

In the present study we demonstrated that MIF increases the inflammatory response and tissue damage due to *T. gondii* oral infection in susceptible C57BL/6 mice. $Mif^{-/-}$ mice had reduced intestinal and systemic inflammation surviving more compared to wt mice, despite of an increase in intestinal parasite burden. This reduced inflammatory response in the intestine of $Mif^{-/-}$ mice was associated with decreased expression of inflammatory

cytokines and MMP-9 comapared to wt mice. Despite of the lower expression of IL-23 compared to wt mice in ileal explants, IL-22 expression was siginificantly increased in $Mif^{-/-}$ mice. The originally local inflammatory response in the small intestine of *T. gondii*-infected wt mice had systemic repercussions similar to sepsis, including increased plasma concentrations of inflammatory cytokines, leukocytosis and liver damage, all less pronounced in $Mif^{-/-}$ mice. Together, these results indicate that MIF is involved in the response to *T. gondii* infection of the small intestine, increasing the ileitis and the systemic inflammatory response.

The peroral infection with *T. gondii* caused a severe ileitis characterized by intestinal shortening, extensive necrosis, blunting of the villi, loss of Peyer's patches and leukocyte infiltration in the

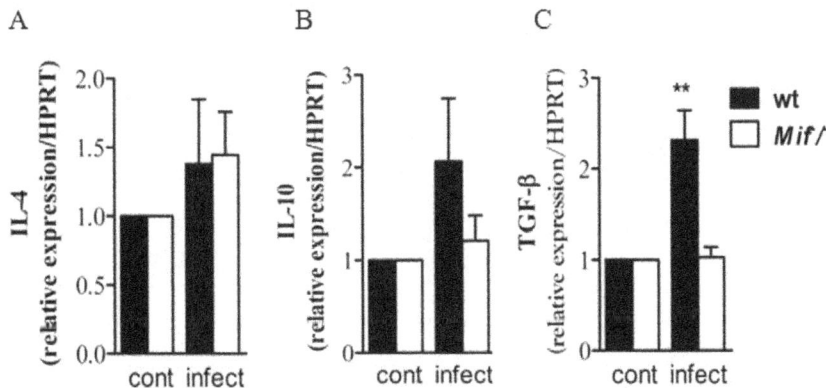

Figure 4. Reduced intestinal expression of IL-10 and TGF-β in $Mif^{-/-}$ mice. Quantitative RT-PCR of of (A) IL-4, (B) IL-10 and (C) TGF-β mRNA expression in ileal explants of control and infected wt and $Mif^{-/-}$ mice. Results are expressed as fold changes relative to HPRT mRNA expression. Data from 3 to 6 mice per group is represented by means ± SEM and p values determined by t-test (*p≤0.05). Cont, control not infected.

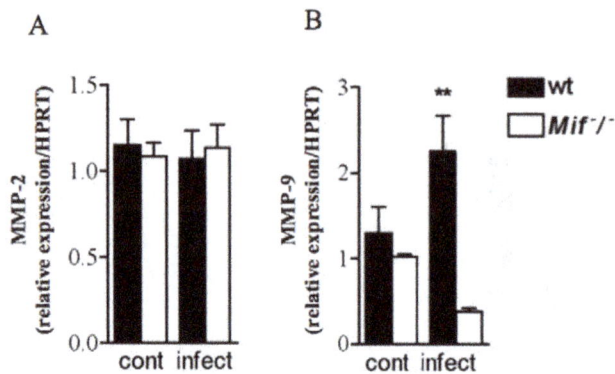

Figure 5. MIF upregulates MMP-9 but not MMP-2 in the terminal ileum of *T. gondii* infected mice. Quantitative real-time PCR of (A) MMP-2 and (B) MMP-9 mRNAs in ileal biopsies of control and infected (9 dpi) wt and *Mif⁻/⁻* mice. Results are expressed as fold changes to HPRT mRNA expression. One representative experiment out of two experiments is shown. Data of three to five mice per group are given as means ± SEM and p values were determined by Mann-Whitney (**p≤0.01). Cont, control not infected.

model of IBD [1,7,41]. An essential role of MIF in experimental colonic inflammation has been demonstrated [20]. It has been also shown that MIF controls the production of inflammatory cytokines including TNF-α and IFN-γ involved in the pathogenesis of intestinal inflammation [42] In the present study, using a model of *T. gondii*-induced ileal inflammation, we demonstrated a critical role of MIF promoting the intestinal inflammatory response and the expression of TNF-α, IL-12 and IFN-γ.

A recent study showed that during peoral *T. gondii* infection IL-23 regulates the ileal inflammatory response independent of IL-17 [7]. We also observed that upon *T. gondii* infection IL-23 expression was upregulated in the intestine while IL-17 was reduced. The inflammatory role of IL-23 was dependent of increased IL-22 production that in turn promoted the ileal inflammation and tissue damage [7]. IL-22, a member of the IL-10 family, is important in epithelial cell homeostasis, in infection and inflammation [43]. In toxoplasmic ileitis, the inflammatory response is a result of IL-22 upregulation induced by IL-23 [7]. In fact, *T. gondii*-infected *IL-22⁻/⁻* mice have reduced intestinal inflammation and are more resistant than wt. Unexpectaly, we observed a significant increased of IL-22 expression in *Mif⁻/⁻* mice with reduction of IL-23 and TGF-β. Others have previously shown increased IL-22 production by T CD4+ lymphocytes in the absence of IL-23 [44,45]. Thus our results suggest a previously unrecognized role of MIF inducing IL-23 and inhibiting IL-22 expression. Our results also implies a MIF-dependent pathogenic role of IL-22 in *T. gondii*-induced ileitis. Interestingly, an anti-

lamina propria [1,7,41]. All these pathological parameters were significantly reduced on *Mif⁻/⁻* compared to wt mice. In natural *T. gondii* infection, gut-associated inflammatory response resembles that observed in Crohn's ileitis and it has been proposed as a

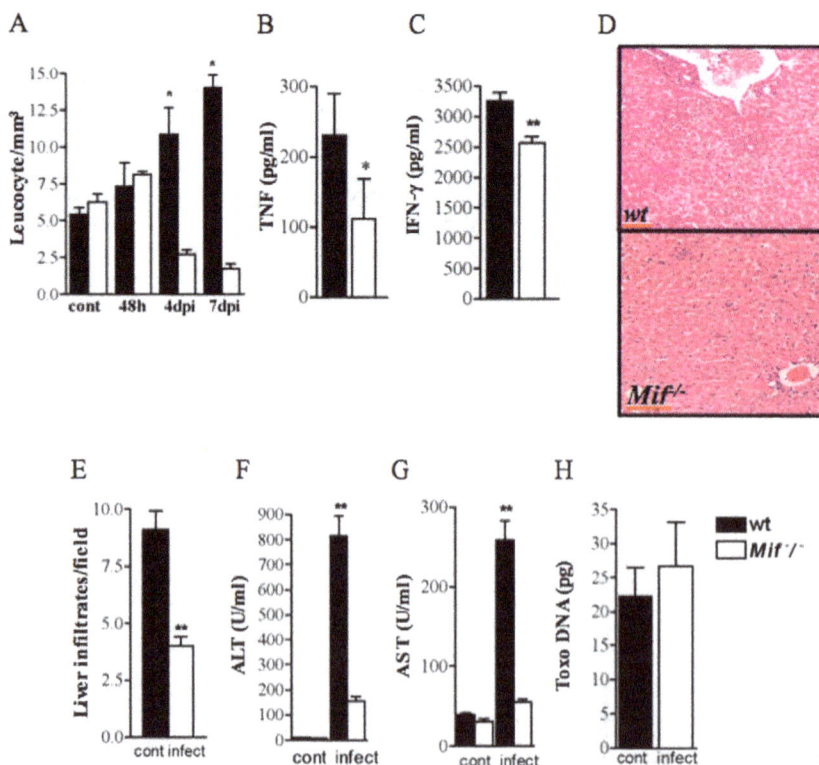

Figure 6. *T. gondii*-induced sepsis-like response is partially dependent of MIF. (A) Leukocyte counts were determined in peripheral blood at indicated times. (B) TNF-α and (C) IFN-γ concetrations in the plasma of wt and *Mif⁻/⁻* mice (n = 3–5) 9 dpi were measured by ELISA. (D) Histopathologycal analysis of the liver at 9 dpi from wt and *Mif⁻/⁻* mice. (E) Quantitative analysis of liver sections (3 slides/animal) of infected wt and *Mif⁻/⁻* mice mice was performed. Liver damage was also determined by quantifying serum concentrations of biochemical marker as (F) alanine aminotransferase (ALT), and (G) aspartate aminotransferase (AST). (H) Toxo DNA concentration was determined in the liver of wt and *Mif⁻/⁻* mice. One representative experiment out of six experiments is shown. Data of three to five mice/group are given as as means ± SEM and p values were determined by t-test (* p≤0.05, ** p≤0.01). Cont, control not infected.

inflammatory role of IL-22 in different models of colitis has been previously demonstrated [46]. Future studies will be importat to define the mechanism by which MIF controls IL-23 and IL-22 expression, and how MIF participates in the pathogenic role of IL-22 on *T. gondii*-induced intestinal inflammation.

We observed that MIF was essential to *T. gondii*-induced expression of MMP-9, suggesting that MIF could be involved in tissue remodeling/repair at the small intestine during *T. gondii* peroral infection by over expressing gelatinase B. Several studies have shown that MIF affects tissue remodeling and the expression of different metalloproteinases [40]. Previous studies demonstrated an increased expression and enzymatic activity of metalloproteinases in humans and mice with intestinal inflammation [7,47]. MMP-2 and MMP-9 are elevated in the intestine of *T. gondii*-infected animals, however in these model, C57BL/6 mice lacking MMP-2 but not MMP-9 have reduced immunopathology of the small intestine [7]. Thus the exact role of the reduced expression of MMP-9 observed on *Mif⁻/⁻* upon *T. gondii* infection requires further investigations.

During intestinal parasitic infection, reduced anti-inflammatory responses could decrease parasite burden but intensify tissue damage, causing loss of epithelial barrier integrity and increased bacterial translocation [34]. Our results showed that MIF mediated *T. gondii*-induced ileitis does not affect IL-4 and increase IL-10 and TGF-β expression. The intestinal inflammatory response induced by *T. gondii* is complex and intestinal homeostasis requires reciprocal control of both Th1 and TGF-β mediated responses. Consequently, MIF exacerbation of intestinal inflammatory responses might involve not only increased pro-inflammatory responses but also TGF-β-mediated responses. MIF and TGF-β are involved in fibrotic responses in several conditions due to regulation of MMPs [48,49]. Since both cytokines upregulate MMP-9 expression, it is possible that MIF regulates tissue remodeling in *T. gondii*-induced ileitis through a TGF-β/MMP-9 pathway.

The reduced inflammatory response and pathological damage in the small intestine of *Mif⁻/⁻* occurred in the context of higher *T. gondii* burden. It has been recently shown in a model of toxoplasmosis induced by intraperitoneal route that MIF is essentially protective [27]. In this model of systemic infection, *Mif⁻/⁻* had higher numbers of cysts in the brain. The increased susceptibility of *Mif⁻/⁻* mice systemically infected was related with reduced production of inflammatory cytokines, however these animals, in opposition to our findings, developed increased liver damage compared to wt mice [27]. *Mif⁻/⁻* mice of the Balb/c background are also more susceptible to *T. gondii* when infected by the oral route, presenting increased lethality and parasite burden in the brain and liver [28]. Compared to susceptible hosts such as C57BL/6, the infection of Balb/c mice with *T. gondii* by the oral route causes a less severe intestinal inflammatory response and a disease that tends to become chronic. These findings suggest that MIF-mediated *T. gondii*-induced pathological responses might be differently regulated depending on the route and site of infection, and the genetic background of the host.

We observed that *Mif⁻/⁻* mice had reduced signs of systemic inflammation compared to wt mice when infected by the oral route. The reduced systemic inflammation of *Mif⁻/⁻* mice was characterized by lower plasma concentrations of TNF-α and IFN-γ, reduced biochemical and histological parameters of liver damage and lower leukocytosis when compared to wt mice. Considering the pathogenic roles of TNF-α and IFN-γ in *T. gondii* oral infection, we postulate that enhancement of systemic

inflammatory response is mediated by MIF acting in concert with TNF-α and IFN-γ [2,4,5]. A deleterious role of MIF was recently observed in a mouse model of lethal dengue virus infection, with reduced systemic inflammatory response in *Mif⁻/⁻* mice compare to wt mice [50]. Although the molecular mechanisms involved in toxoplasmic ileitis are not completely understood, new evidence indicates that co-factors such as Gram-negative intestinal microflora play a role in *T. gondii*-induced acute ileitis and systemic inflammation through LPS-induced TLR-4 signaling [51]. Since MIF up-regulates the expression of TLR-4 [17], it is possible that the reduced inflammatory response observed in *Mif⁻/⁻* mice upon *T. gondii* might be a result of reduced TLR-4 activation. Considering that MIF contributes to IBD even in the absence of TLR-4, it is possible that the effect of MIF on *T. gondii* pathogenesis occurs independently of its effects on TLR-4 expression. Interestingly, MIF also regulates the expression of TLR-11 [28], considered important in the recognition and response to *T. gondii* [52]. It has been suggest that the reduced expression of TLR-11 in the absence of MIF affects the maturation and activation of dendritic cells consequently hampering a protective immune response to *T. gondii* [28]. It will be important to characterize the role of TLR-4 and TLR-11 in the MIF-dependent small bowel injury caused by *T. gondii* in susceptible hosts.

In conclusion, we demonstrated that MIF participates in the pathogenesis of natural *T. gondii* infection in C57BL/6 mice, promoting an intense ileitis and a robust systemic inflammatory response that resulted in poor outcome during the acute phase. Similar to previous studies, we confirmed a central role of MIF in the control of parasite burden in different models of experimental toxoplasmosis [27,28]. Although MIF has been regarded as essential in host protection during *T. gondii* infection, our findings demonstrated a pathogenic role of MIF in natural *T. gondii* infection in susceptible hosts by exacerbating IL-12, IFN-γ, TNF-α and IL-23 dependent responses. MIF also plays a role in tissue remodeling possibly by regulating TGF-β induced MMP-9. Thus, we propose that MIF actually exerts a bidirectional role in toxoplasmosis. This dichotomy is dependent on the route of infection and the genetic background of the host, and has been also observed with other pro-inflammatory cytokines [2]. In this scenario, MIF seems to compromise host protection by exacerbating intestinal tissue damage and by inducing a sepsis-like response. Previous studies demonstrating a participation of MIF on human *T. gondii* infection [27,53,54] enphasize the importance to understand the diffrential role of MIF on immunity and pathogenesis triggered by *T. gondii* in distinct tissues.

Acknowledgments

We thank Dr. Claudia Paiva (IMPPG, UFRJ, Brazil), Dr. Claudia Benjamin (Department of Pharmacy, UFRJ, Brazil), Steffi CH Hanschke and Dr. João P. Viola (Instituto Nacional do Câncer, RJ, Brazil) for their gifts of reagents and Rosa Arras and Letícia Alves for technical assistance.

Author Contributions

Conceived and designed the experiments: MGC MTB. Performed the experiments: MGC JSM DFF IMA. Analyzed the data: MGC MTB. Contributed reagents/materials/analysis tools: KM HSPS. Wrote the paper: MGC MTB.

References

1. Liesenfeld O (2002) Oral infection of C57BL/6 mice with *Toxoplasma gondii*: a new model of inflammatory bowel disease? J Infect Dis 185: S96–101.

2. Gazzinelli RT, Wysocka M, Hieny S, Scharton-Kersten T, Cheever A, et al. (1996) In the absence of endogenous IL-10, mice acutely infected with

Toxoplasma gondii succumb to a lethal immune response dependent on CD4+T cells and accompanied by overproduction of IL-12, IFN-γ, and TNF-α. J Immunol 157: 798–805.

3. Buzoni-Gatel D, Schulthess J, Menard LC, Kasper LH (2006) Mucosal defenses against orally acquired protozoan parasites, emphasis on *Toxoplasma gondii* infections. Cell Microbiol 8: 535–544.

4. Denkers EY, Gazzinelli RT (1998) Regulation and function of T-cell-mediated immunity during *Toxoplasma gondii* infection. Clin Microbiol Rev 11: 569–588.

5. Yap GS, Sher A (1999) Effector cells of both nonhemopoietic and hemopoietic origin are required for interferon (IFN)-gamma and tumor necrosis factor (TNF)-alpha-dependent host resistance to the intracellular pathogen, *Toxoplasma gondii*. J Exp Med 189: 1083–1092.

6. Tait ED, Hunter CA (2009) Advances in understanding immunity to *Toxoplasma gondii*. Mem Inst Oswaldo Cruz 104: 201–210.

7. Muñoz M, Heimesaat MM, Danker K, Struck D, Lohmann U, et al. (2009) Interleukin (IL)-23 mediates *Toxoplasma gondii*-induced immunopathology in the gut via matrixmetalloproteinase-2 and IL-22 but independent of IL-17. J Exp Med 206: 3047–3059.

8. Mordue DG, Monroy F, La Regina M, Dinarello CA, Sibley LD (2001) Acute toxoplasmosis leads to lethal overproduction of Th1 cytokines. J Immunol 167: 4574–4584.

9. Mennechet FJD, Kasper LH, Rachinel N, Li W, Vandewalle A, et al. (2002) Lamina propria CD4+T lymphocytes synergize with murine intestinal epithelial cells to enhance proinflammatory responses against intracellular pathogen. J Immunol 168: 2988–2996.

10. Bernhagen J, Calandra T, Mitchell RA, Martin SB, Tracey KJ, et al. (1993) MIF is a pituitary-derived cytokine that potentiates lethal endotoxaemia. Nature 365: 756–759.

11. Bucala R (1996) MIF rediscovered cytokine, pituitary hormone, and glucocorticoid-induced regulator of the immune response. FASEB J 10: 1607–1613.

12. Calandra TJ, Roger T (2003) Macrophage migration inhibitory factor: a regulator of innate immunity. Nature Rev Immunol 3: 791–800.

13. Weber C, Kraemer S, Drechsler M, Lue H, Koenen RR, et al. (2008) Structural determinants of MIF functions in CXCR2-mediated inflammatory and atherogenic leukocyte recruitment. Proc Natl Acad Sci U S A 105: 16278–16283.

14. Calandra T, Bernhagen J, Metz CN, Spiegel LA, Bacher M, et al. (1995) MIF as a glucocorticoid-induced modulator of cytokine production. Nature 377: 68–71.

15. Calandra T, Bernhagen J, Mitchell RA, Bucala R (1994) The macrophage is an important and previously unrecognized source of macrophage migration inhibitory factor. J Exp Med 179: 1895–1902.

16. Lue H, Kleemann R, Calandra T, Roger T, Bernhagen J (2002) Macrophage migration inhibitory factor (MIF): mechanism of action and role in disease. Microbes Infect 4: 449–460.

17. Roger T, David J, Glauser MP, Calandra T (2001) MIF regulates innate immune responses through modulation of Toll-like receptor 4. Nature 4414: 920–924.

18. Dunne DW, Shaw A, Bockenstedt LK, Allore HG, Chen S (2010) Increased TLR4 expression and downstream cytokine production in immunosuppressed adults compared to non-immunosuppressed adults. PLoS One 5: e11343.

19. Bozza M, Satoskar AR, Lin G, Lu B, Humbles AA, et al. (1999) Target disruption of Migration Inhibitory Factor gene reveals its critical role in sepsis. J Exp Med 189: 341–346.

20. De Jong YP, Abadia-Molina AC, Satoskar AR, Clarke K, Rietdijk ST, et al. (2001) Development of chronic colitis is dependent on the cytokine MIF. Nature Immunol 2: 1061–1066.

21. Satoskar AR, Bozza M, Rodriguez-Sosa M, Lin G, David JR (2001) Migration-Inhibitory gene deficient mice are susceptible to cutaneous *Leishmania major* infection. Infect Immun 69: 1247–1254.

22. Magalhães ES, Mourao-Sa DS, Vieira-de-Abreu A, Figueiredo RT, Pires AL, et al. (2007) Macrophage migration inhibitory factor is essential for allergic asthma but not for Th2 differentiation. Eur J Immunol 37: 1097–1106.

23. Paiva CN, Arras RH, Magalhães ES, Alves LS, Lessa LP, et al. (2009) Migration inhibitory factor (MIF) released by macrophages upon recognition of immune complexes is critical to inflammation in Arthus reaction. J Leukoc Biol 85: 855–861.

24. McDevitt MA, Xie J, Shanmugasundaram G, Griffith J, Liu A, et al. (2006) Critical role for the host mediator macrophage migration inhibitory factor in the pathogenesis of malarial anemia. J Exp Med 193: 1–12.

25. Magalhães ES, Paiva CN, Souza HS, Pyrrho AS, Mourão-Sá D, et al. (2009) Macrophage migration inhibitory factor is critical to interleukin-5-driven eosinophilopoiesis and tissue eosinophilia triggered by *Schistosoma mansoni* infection. FASEB J 23: 1262–1271.

26. Reyes JL, Terrazas LI, Espinoza B, Cruz-Robles D, Soto V, et al. (2006) Macrophage migration inhibitory factor contributes to host defense against acute *Trypanosoma cruzi* infection. Infect Immun 72: 3571–3576.

27. Flores M, Saavedra R, Bautista R, Viedma R, Tenorio EP, et al. (2008) Macrophage migration inhibitory factor (MIF) is critical for the host resistance against *Toxoplasma gondii*. FASEB J 22: 3661–3671.

28. Terrazas CA, Juarez I, Terrazas LI, Saavedra R, Calleja EA, et al. (2010) *Toxoplasma gondii*: Impaired maturation and pro-inflammatory response of dendritic cells in MIF deficient mice favors susceptibility to infection. Exp Parasitol 126: 348–358.

29. Liesenfeld O, Kosek J, Remington JS, Suzuki Y (1996) Association of CD4+ Tcell-dependent interferon γ mediated necrosis of the small intestine with genetic susceptibility of mice to per oral infection with *Toxoplasma gondii*. J Exp Med 184: 597–607.

30. Liesenfeld O, Kang H, Park D, Nguyen TA, Parkhe C, et al. (1999) TNF-α, nitric oxide and IFN-γ are all critical for development of necrosis in small intestine and early mortality in genetically susceptible mice infected per orally with *Toxoplasma gondii*. Parasite Immun 21: 365–376.

31. Suzuki Y, Sher A, Yap G, Park D, Neyer LE, et al. (2000) IL-10 is required for prevention of necrosis in the small intestine and mortality in both genetically resistant BALB/c and susceptible C57BL/6 mice following per oral infection with *Toxoplasma gondii*. J Immunol 164: 5375–5382.

32. Reischl U, Bretagne S, Kruger D, Ernault P, Costa JM (2003) Comparison of two DNA targets for the diagnosis of Toxoplasmosis by real-time PCR using fluorescence resonance energy transfer hybridization probes. BMC Infect Dis 3: 7.

33. Kompalic-Cristo A, Frotta C, Suárez-Mutis M, Fernandes O, Britto C (2007) Evaluation of a real-time PCR assay based on the repetitive B1 gene for the detection of *Toxoplasma gondii* in human peripheral blood. Parasitol Res 101: 619–625.

34. Heimesaat MM, Bereswill S, Fischer A, Niebergall J, Freudenberg M, et al. (2006) Gram-negative bacteria aggravate murine small intestinal Th-1 type immunopathology following oral infection with *Toxoplasma gondii*. J Immunol 177: 8785–8795.

35. Livak KJ, Schmittgen TD (2001) Analysis of relative gene expression data using real-time quantitative PCR and the 2(-Delta Delta C (T)). Method Methods 25: 402–408.

36. Roberts CW, Ferguson DJ, Jebbari H, Satoskar A, Bluethmann H, Alexander J (1996) Different roles for interleukin-4 during the course of *Toxoplasma gondii* infection. Infect Immun 64: 897–904.

37. Nickdel MB, Lyons RE, Roberts F, Brombacher F, Hunter CA, et al. (2004) Intestinal pathology during acute toxoplasmosis is IL-4 dependent and unrelated to parasite burden. Parasite Immunol 26: 75–82.

38. Neves ES, Bicudo LN, Curi AL, Carregal E, Bueno WF, et al. (2009) Acute acquired toxoplasmosis: clinical-laboratorial aspects and ophthalmologic evaluation in a cohort of immunocompetent patients. Mem Inst Oswaldo Cruz 104(2): 393–6.

39. Pakozdi A, Amin MA, Haas CS, Martinez RJ, Haines GK, 3rd, et al. (2006) Macrophage migration inhibitory factor: a mediator of matrix metalloproteinase-2 production in rheumatoid arthritis. Arthritis Res Ther 8: 1–14.

40. Assunção-Miranda I, Bozza MT, Da Poian AT (2010) Pro-inflammatory response resulting from sindbis virus infection of human macrophages: implications for the pathogenesis of viral arthritis. J Med Virol 82: 164–174.

41. Munoz M, Liesenfeld O, Heimesaat MM (2011) Immunology of *Toxoplasma gondii*. Immunol Rev 240: 269–285.

42. Ohkawara T, Nishihira J, Ishiguro Y (2006) Resistance to experimental colitis depends on cytoprotective heat shock proteins in macrophage migration inhibitory factor null mice. Immunol Lett 107: 148–154.

43. Aujla SJ, Kolls JK (2009) IL-22: a critical mediator in mucosal host defense. J Mol Med 87: 451–454.

44. Ramirez JM, Brembilla NC, Sorg O, Chicheportiche R, Matthes T, et al. (2010) Activation of the aryl hydrocarbon receptor reveals distinct requirements for IL-22 and IL-17 production by human T helper cells. Eur J Immunol 40: 2450–2459.

45. Brembilla NC, Ramirez JM, Chicheportiche R, Sorg O, Saurat JH, et al. (2011) In vivo dioxin favors interleukin-22 production by human CD4+ T cells in an aryl hydrocarbon receptor (AhR)-dependent manner. PLoS One 6: e18741.

46. Monteleone I, Rizzo A, Sarra M, Sica G, Sileri P, et al. (2011) Aryl Hydrocarbon Receptor-Induced Signals Up-regulate IL-22 Production and Inhibit Inflammation in the Gastrointestinal Tract. Gastroenterology 141: 237–248.

47. Garg P, Vijay-Kumar M, Wang L, Gewirtz AT, Merlin D, et al. (2009) Matrix metalloproteinase-9-mediated tissue injury overrides the protective effect of matrix metalloproteinase-2 during colitis. Am J Physiol Gastrointest Liver Physiol 296: G175–184.

48. Chou YT, Wang H, Chen Y, Danielpour D, Yang YC (2006) Cited2 modulates TGF-beta-mediated upregulation of MMP9. Oncogene 25: 5547–5560.

49. He XX, Chen K, Yang J, Li XY, Gan HY (2009) Macrophage migration inhibitory factor promotes colorectal cancer. Mol Med 15: 1–10.

50. Assunção-Miranda I, Amaral FA, Bozza FA, Fagundes CT, Sousa LP, et al. (2010) Contribution of macrophage migration inhibitory factor to the pathogenesis of dengue virus infection. FASEB J 24: 218–228.

51. Heimesaat MM, Fischer A, Jahn HK, Niebergall J, Freudenberg M, et al. (2007) Exacerbation of murine ileitis by Toll-like receptor 4 mediated sensing of lipopolysaccharide from commensal *Escherichia coli*. Gut 56: 941–948.

52. Yarovinsky F, Zhang D, Andersen JF, Bannenberg GL, Serhan CN, et al. (2005) TLR-11 activation of dendritic cells by a protozoan profilin-like protein. Science 308: 1626–1629.

53. Ferro EA, Mineo JR, Ietta F, Bechi N, Romagnoli R, et al. (2008) Macrophage migration inhibitory factor is up-regulated in human first-trimester placenta stimulated by soluble antigen of *Toxoplasma gondii*, resulting in increased monocyte adhesion on villous explants. Am J Pathol 172: 50–58.

54. de Oliveira Gomes A, de Oliveira Silva DA, Silva NM, de Freitas Barbosa B, Franco PS, et al. (2011) Effect of macrophage migration inhibitory factor (MIF) in human placental explants infected with *Toxoplasma gondii* depends on gestational age. Am J Pathol 178: 2792–2801.

4

Non-Invasive Mapping of the Gastrointestinal Microbiota Identifies Children with Inflammatory Bowel Disease

Eliseo Papa[1], Michael Docktor[2], Christopher Smillie[3], Sarah Weber[2], Sarah P. Preheim[4], Dirk Gevers[5], Georgia Giannoukos[5], Dawn Ciulla[5], Diana Tabbaa[5], Jay Ingram[2], David B. Schauer[6,7†], Doyle V. Ward[5], Joshua R. Korzenik[8], Ramnik J. Xavier[5,8,9], Athos Bousvaros[2*◐], Eric J. Alm[4,5,6*◐]

1 Harvard/MIT Health Science and Technology Institute, Cambridge, Massachusetts, United States of America, 2 Inflammatory Bowel Disease Center, Children's Hospital Boston, Boston, Massachusetts, United States of America, 3 Computational and Systems Biology Initiative, Massachusetts Institute of Technology, Cambridge, Massachusetts, United States of America, 4 Department of Civil and Environmental Engineering, Massachusetts Institute of Technology, Cambridge, Massachusetts, United States of America, 5 The Broad Institute, 7 Cambridge Center, Cambridge, Massachusetts, United States of America, 6 Department of Biological Engineering, Massachusetts Institute of Technology, Cambridge, Massachusetts, United States of America, 7 Division of Comparative Medicine, Massachusetts Institute of Technology, Cambridge, Massachusetts, United States of America, 8 Gastrointestinal Unit, Center for Inflammatory Bowel Disease, Massachusetts General Hospital, Harvard Medical School, Boston, Massachusetts, United States of America, 9 Center for Computational and Integrative Biology, Harvard Medical School, Massachusetts General Hospital, Boston, Massachusetts, United States of America

Abstract

Background: Pediatric inflammatory bowel disease (IBD) is challenging to diagnose because of the non-specificity of symptoms; an unequivocal diagnosis can only be made using colonoscopy, which clinicians are reluctant to recommend for children. Diagnosis of pediatric IBD is therefore frequently delayed, leading to inappropriate treatment plans and poor outcomes. We investigated the use of 16S rRNA sequencing of fecal samples and new analytical methods to assess differences in the microbiota of children with IBD and other gastrointestinal disorders.

Methodology/Principal Findings: We applied synthetic learning in microbial ecology (SLiME) analysis to 16S sequencing data obtained from i) published surveys of microbiota diversity in IBD and ii) fecal samples from 91 children and young adults who were treated in the gastroenterology program of Children's Hospital (Boston, USA). The developed method accurately distinguished control samples from those of patients with IBD; the area under the receiver-operating-characteristic curve (AUC) value was 0.83 (corresponding to 80.3% sensitivity and 69.7% specificity at a set threshold). The accuracy was maintained among data sets collected by different sampling and sequencing methods. The method identified taxa associated with disease states and distinguished patients with Crohn's disease from those with ulcerative colitis with reasonable accuracy. The findings were validated using samples from an additional group of 68 patients; the validation test identified patients with IBD with an AUC value of 0.84 (e.g. 92% sensitivity, 58.5% specificity).

Conclusions/Significance: Microbiome-based diagnostics can distinguish pediatric patients with IBD from patients with similar symptoms. Although this test can not replace endoscopy and histological examination as diagnostic tools, classification based on microbial diversity is an effective complementary technique for IBD detection in pediatric patients.

Editor: Jacques Ravel, Institute for Genome Sciences - University of Maryland School of Medicine, United States of America

Funding: This work was supported in part by philantropic donations from the MacInnes Friends and Family Fund and by the Rasmussen Family Fund. EP was supported by a NSERC PGS D award. EJA was supported by the NIH award 1-R21-A1084032-01A1. ALPCO diagnostics/Buhlmann laboratories kindly provided calprotectin kits. The funders had no role in study design, data collection and analysis, decision to publish, or preparation of the manuscript.

Competing Interests: The authors have declared that no competing interests exist.

* E-mail: athos.bousvaros@childrens.harvard.edu (AB); ejalm@mit.edu(EJA)

◐ These authors contributed equally to this work.

†Deceased.

Introduction

Crohn's disease (CD) and ulcerative colitis (UC), collectively termed inflammatory bowel diseases (IBD), are incurable conditions that cause ulceration of the intestinal mucosa. If left untreated, IBD may require repeated surgical intervention to remove affected parts of the gastrointestinal system [1] leading to malabsorption and nutritional complications [2]. Despite its importance, timely diagnosis is difficult because patients often present with non-specific symptoms [3], and the presence of CD or UC can only be confirmed by colonoscopy.

Diagnosis is particularly challenging in children, for whom presenting symptoms may vary widely and may only consist of subtle extra-intestinal manifestations [4]. This in turn leads to a typical delay in the diagnosis of pediatric IBD, ranging from 4 weeks in severe colitis [5] to 6–7 months in milder disease [4]. Reducing this diagnostic delay is important, since a long period of unmanaged symptoms can significantly impact growth [5] and early treatment is essential to preserving long-term quality of life [6]. Thus a sensitive yet non-invasive detection tool, that could identify patients at high risk for IBD, and therefore warranting endoscopic evaluation, would be a valuable diagnostic aid.

Non-invasive tests for IBD already exist, including antibodies [7], imaging-based screens [8,9], and fecal biomarkers [10]. Specificities for existing methods range from 89% to 95% for either CD or UC [11], however,these methods are either limited to active disease, poorly sensitive (~55%), or their outcome can be confounded by diseases other than IBD [11], limiting their clinical utility [12,13].

The design of an accurate test for IBD is challenging, since the precise cause of IBD is unknown. No single genetic, environmental or epidemiological factor alone is diagnostic of IBD [14]. Instead, current evidence about the aetiology of IBD points toward a complex interplay between genetic, environmental, and immunological factors[15–17] and the intestinal microbiota[18–20].

Arguing in favour of the involvement of gut microbes in the pathogenesis of IBD, it is known that colonisation with commensal bacteria is required to elicit colitis in mice [19,21]. Similarly, in IBD patients it is known that antibiotics can treat CD colitis in the short term [22] and probiotics may prevent relapse of UC [23]. We hypothesized that changes in the intestinal microbiota, whether causative of or responsive to disease, may provide a viable diagnostic of disease status.

Previous microbial diversity studies have found characteristic changes in the composition of the gut flora during IBD that could potentially be used to screen patients with non-specific symptoms [18,24]. In one of the most comprehensive studies to date, Frank and colleagues [24] mapped microbiota composition in 124 IBD and non-IBD patients by biopsy sampling coupled with 16S rRNA sequencing. Their work showed that patients with a long-standing history of IBD had decreased levels of Firmicutes and increased level of Proteobacteria, when compared to control individuals. While these results firmly established the relationship between GI microbiota and disease status, the overall approach is unsatisfactory as a diagnostic tool because of low sensitivity (31%) and low overall accuracy (51%, as determined from the third figure in [24]).

More recent studies have been able to accurately distinguish CD and healthy individuals on the basis of pyrosequencing data [25], but the same model was unable to distinguish UC from healthy individuals or to differentiate patients in remission from patients with active disease, raising questions about whether such approaches show clinical potential. Finally, none of these studies examined pediatric cohorts.

Here we demonstrate an approach that is capable of routinely differentiating children with IBD from controls with other gastrointestinal diseases in a case-control study of ninety-one pediatric patients. Our methodology shows high sensitivity and specificity over a range of disease prevalence and it can be used to i) identify key taxa associated with each disease state, ii) discriminate CD and UC and iii) differentiate patients with active disease from those in remission. We confirmed our results by blind validation with an independent cohort of seventy-seven pediatric patients. This method applies next-generation sequencing and robust statistical analysis using machine learning techniques and, significantly, is a test for IBD based on non-invasive fecal sampling.

Results

Supervised Classification Distinguishes IBD and Non-IBD Patients in Existing Tissue-based Studies

The case-control study of Frank and colleagues [24] used an unsupervised clustering approach: principal components analysis (PCA). When the class labels (healthy vs. diseased) are known for a training set of samples, then supervised learning methods can also be applied (e.g. support vector machines, random forests, etc.). These algorithms have been widely and successfully applied to many problems in the biomedical sciences [26,27,28] and their use in a clinical setting is emerging in the analysis of gene expression data [29,30,31,32] and microbiome data [33].

We first investigated whether supervised learning could offer sufficient performance to be employed in a microbiota-based IBD detection tool, by applying it to the published IBD data set of Frank et al [24]. We employed our Synthetic Learning in Microbial Ecology (SLiME) method to classify samples from the existing data set as IBD or control. SLiME is a software pipeline which applies supervised classification algorithm to sequencing data, using associated metadata as the classification label. Demultiplexed sequences are classified into lineages, clustered to select a representative set and used to estimate the abundance of each taxa in each sample. The resulting frequency table is normalized and fed to a supervised classification algorithm. SLiME is based on Random Forests (RFs) [34], which we chose for its accuracy and speed, although we achieved similar results using other supervised learning approaches such as bagging, stacking and support vector machines (see Fig. S1). Applying SLiME to the existing data set yielded accurate classification of patients into IBD or non-IBD groups. Based on repeated ten-fold cross validation, the area under the ROC curve (AUC) – which is a measure of the overall accuracy of the classification algorithm over the range of possible disease incidence [35] – was 0.73 (Fig. 1A). Choosing a cutoff on the curve which gives relatively high sensitivity (ie. 87.6%) yields 47.3% specificity, amply surpassing the accuracy of the clustering method originally employed [24].

Supervised Classification Distinguishes IBD and Non-IBD Pediatric Patients on the Basis of Stool

Although the results obtained using the existing Frank et al. [24] data set were encouraging, there are several reasons why they might not translate to a clinically useful diagnostic test. First, samples were obtained invasively through surgical tissue resection from adult patients with advanced disease, and may not reflect changes observed in fecal samples from patients with less advanced disease. Second, the control specimens in the Frank et al. study were largely composed of tissue from cancer patients, and thus were not typical of patients investigated for IBD in the pediatric setting. We therefore designed a new case-control study to evaluate whether fecal samples from children not undergoing surgery could be utilized to differentiate between patients with and without IBD.

We selected a group of ninety-one children and young adults receiving care in the gastroenterology program of Children's Hospital (Boston, USA), and obtained fecal samples. Of these children, 23 had Crohn's disease, 43 had ulcerative colitis, one had undefined IBD (colitis with elements of CD and UC) and 24 had non-IBD functional disease (patients with gastrointestinal symptoms but no intestinal inflammation). To evaluate the potential of our method to differentiate between children with IBD and children without IBD, we thought it essential to study not completely healthy children, but children with gastrointestinal symptoms. These are the children who would present to the gastroenterologist for evaluation, and for whom IBD is in the differential diagnosis. Demographics of the patient populations are given in Table 1. We isolated DNA from the fecal samples and sequenced a portion of the 16S rRNA gene using high throughput 454 pyrosequencing (see Materials and Methods). We then applied SLiME to the resulting microbial compositional data.

A

B

Table 1. demographics of paediatric (training) cohort.

		Crohn's	UC	Control	IBDU
n		**23**	**43**	**24**	**1**
Gender	Male	13(56%)	21(49%)	10(42.%)	1
	Female	10(44%)	22(51%)	14(58%)	0
Age	Median +/− s.d.	14.13±3.84	13.7±4.25	9.08±4.3	14
	Range	3–20	4–24	3–17	
Montreal class.	L1	1(4%)			
	L2	1(4%)			
	L3	15(65%)			
	L4	6(26%)			
	B1	18(78%)			
	B2	4(17%)			
	B3	1(4%)			
	E1		2(5%)		
	E2		6(14%)		
	E3		35(81%)		
Disease Activity	Control	0	0	24	0
	Inactive	14	11		
	Mild	5	15		1
	Moderate	3	9		
	Severe	1	8		
Medications	Salicylates only	1 (4%)	6(14%)		
	6mp/AZA/MTX	11 (48%)	12(28%)		
	Anti-TNF	7 (30%)	4(9%)		
	Calcineurin inhibitor	0	23(53%)		
	Antibiotics	6 (26%)	14(33%)		1
	(Steroids)	13 (57%)	25(58%)		1

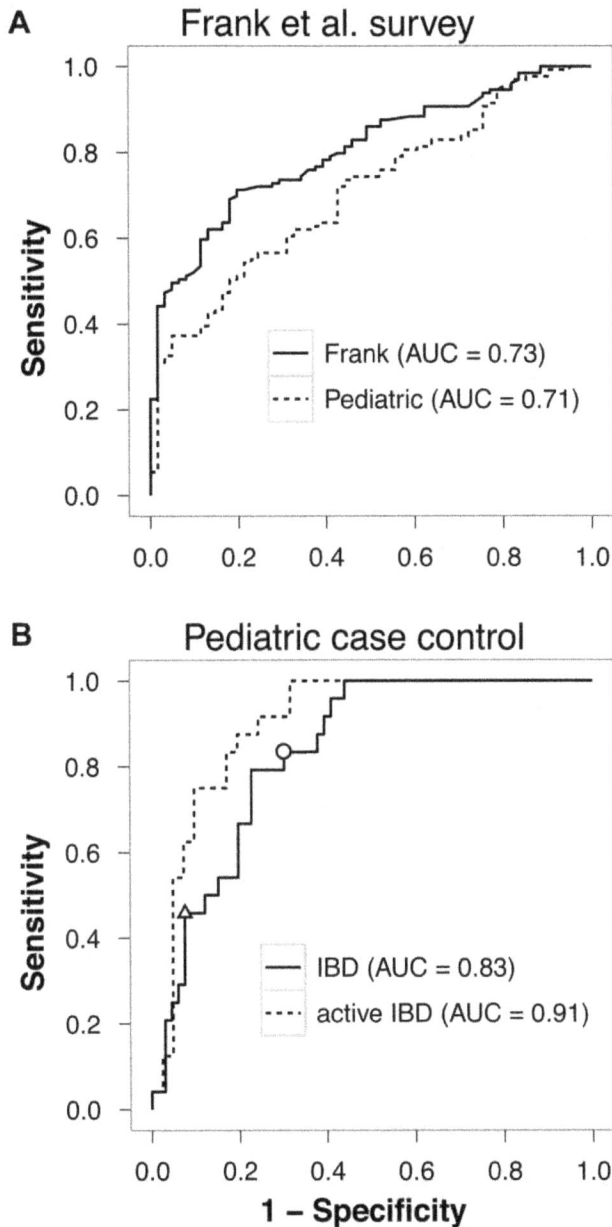

Figure 1. Accuracy of disease classification. (A) SLiME applied to Frank et al. biopsy data set. The black line indicates performance obtained when features were generated by taxonomical binning of the original sequence data (AUC =0.73); dashed line shows performance when features were selected based on their importance in the pediatric case-control data set and then applied to the Frank et al. study (AUC =0.71). (B) ROC curve for SLiME classification of active IBD patients vs controls in the pediatric case-control data set. Two different threshold selections are highlighted: circle, for which SLiME has 80.3% sensitivity and 69.7% specificity; triangle, for which SLiME has 45.8% sensitivity and 92.4% specificity.

Remarkably, performance of our method improved on this data set despite the substitution of mucosal samples with stool samples, yielding a ten-fold cross-validated AUC of 0.83 for distinguishing IBD patients from controls (Fig. 1B). Sensitivity and specificity for the diagnostic test can be obtained by selecting the desired threshold along the curve. For instance, choosing a cutoff on the curve at relatively high sensitivity (Fig. 1B, circle) yields 80.3% sensitivity and 69.7% specificity for the test. The result is particularly remarkable considering that fecal samples may not be truly representative of the total intestinal microbiota. Indeed, bacteria living in association with the intestinal epithelium, and thus capable of interacting with innate immune receptors, are likely not to be present in fecal samples.

The performance of the same classification algorithm was higher when it was applied to distinguish from controls only those IBD patients with clinically active disease, yielding an AUC of 0.91 (Fig. 1B dashed line). Table S6 and S7 show how the classifier performs amongst the three disease groups (CD,UC and control) at one arbitrary threshold. To test if the chosen sequencing technology altered the classification of patients into controls and IBD samples, we repeated sequencing for 10 of the samples using the Sanger sequencing method. Supervised learning results, however, were independent of the sequencing method employed (Fig. S2). We hypothesized that some of the improvement in performance might be due to increased sampling depth if a subset of discriminatory bacteria are present at low abundance. To test this hypothesis, we identified the bacterial taxa most strongly associated with IBD (either positively or negatively), and plotted their abundance. As shown in Fig. S3, many of the most informative taxa are present at a level of less than 1% per sample

– the level at which we would expect to see one count or less at the sequencing depth used in Frank et al [24]. Thus, sequencing depth is an important factor in diagnostic accuracy and may account to a large degree for the lower AUC we obtained in the classification of the Frank et al. data set.

Distinctive Taxonomical Groups are Associated with IBD

We identified a number of bacterial taxa strongly associated with IBD that both confirmed and supplemented previous studies. Fig. 2 shows taxa that are significantly associated with either IBD or control patients (q-value <0.01, Kruskal-Wallis test, FDR adjusted [36], $E(\pi_0) = 0.18$, see Fig. S4). Only a few of these taxa show a distribution consistent with an ideal microbial biomarker – a bacterial group whose presence/absence indicates disease phenotype. For example, the Enterobacteriales are indicators of active IBD (ie. patients with clinically active disease and not in remission), while Rikenellaceae and Porphyromonadaceae are generally found within the control group. By contrast, most of the discriminatory groups in Fig. 2 are more or less abundant in IBD patients, but not exclusive to one population (e.g., the Butyricicoccus and Subdoligranum genera decrease in the IBD patients with clinically active disease, but are still present in some IBD patients with inactive disease). This highlights the need for quantitative global surveys of microbial diversity rather than simple indicators of presence/absence.

Microbial Alterations are Similar in Stool and Tissue Samples

Our finding that classification was similarly accurate in tissue and stool samples led us to ask whether the same alterations in the gut profile were observed in both sample types or whether distinct but similarly predictive changes occurred in each. To test this, we used the bacterial taxa identified in the pediatric case-control (stool-based) study to re-classify the tissue samples in the study by Frank et al. [24] The classification accuracy based on features from the pediatric study was nearly identical to the model using features picked from the tissue-based study: AUC = 0.71 (Fig. 1A), an increase in estimated measurement error of only 3%.

The relative change (upwards or downwards) of taxa in IBD vs. control groups is remarkably concordant between the two studies, with the exception of Lactobacillales (Fig. 3). Unsurprisingly, due to the largely different sequencing depth many of the low-abundance taxa detected in the pediatric case-control (e.g., Alistipes) are of little importance in the classification, when applied to the Frank et al. data (Fig. S5). On the other hand, the Subdoligranulum genus and the Proteobacteria phylum remain two consistently important features across data sets (Fig. 3). These results are encouraging because they suggest stool samples can be used to study changes in other compartments such as the mucosa.

Microbiota Diversity Decreases as Disease Severity Increases

An important clinical question is to establish whether a marker of disease activity exists, and to what extent it can be used to stratify patients according to disease severity. To address this question, we measured disease activity by means of standard clinical indices (PUCAI [37], PCDAI [38]), based on symptoms and blood test results [39], and compared to SLiME predictions. While SLiME could not reliably classify on the basis of activity due to the small number of patients in each distinct level of disease severity, we nevertheless observed that overall microbiota diversity was strongly associated with disease activity. As disease severity

increased, independently of the type of disease (CD or UC), overall bacterial diversity decreased as measured by the Shannon diversity index (Fig. 4). These results further support the view that IBD reflects an overall GI tract dysbiosis rather than the effect of a small number of pathogenic taxa [20,24,40]. Moreover, a number of microbial taxa showed significant association with disease activity levels. Among the most discriminative taxa was the Proteobacteria phylum (Fig. 5, see also Fig. S6). Specifically, the Gammaproteobacteria class was prevalent in all active forms of the disease. Severe disease in particular was associated with the Serratia and Escherichia-Shigella genera as well as the Coryneobacteriacea family.

Gut Microbiota Shows Characteristic Changes from Active Disease to Remission

The factors responsible for triggering episodes of active disease are largely unknown. To identify microbial groups potentially associated with the establishment of active disease, we compared the composition of bacteria in fecal samples taken during active disease and remission periods. Classification with SLiME could distinguish between active and remission samples with an AUC of 0.72. Amongst the taxa which were significantly associated with active disease (Fig. S7) we found Proteobacteria (q-value <0.05, Kruskal-Wallis test, FDR adjusted [36], $E(\pi 0) = 0.35$, see Fig. S8) which was in agreement with previous observations [41]. This finding appears to confirm the hypothesis that before or during active disease Proteobacteria rapidly expand and potentially displace other bacterial groups, such as Actinobacteria. On the other hand, members of the Eubacteriaceae, Incertae Sedis XIV and Bifidobacteriaceae families were associated with remission, which to our knowledge has not been reported previously. The Lachnospiraceae family, Subdoligranulum and Butyricicoccus, a butyrate-producing organism that can ferment dietary polysaccharides, were also associated with remission.

Diversity is Correlated with Antibiotic Therapy

We found that overall microbial diversity, as measured by the Shannon diversity index, was the single most important feature for discriminating between patients undergoing antibiotic therapy or not. Although we could not classify whether samples were obtained from antibiotic-treated patients with high accuracy (AUC <0.6), we did find that Shannon diversity index was significantly and negatively associated with antibiotic therapy in the IBD samples (p-value = 0.0067, Wilcoxon test, see Fig. S9). This observation is consistent with a simple model of antibiotic effect on the gut microbiota: most taxa and bacterial groups are killed by antibiotics, while the few bacterial strains which have resistance survive and increase in relative abundance.

Differential Diagnosis of Ulcerative Colitis and Crohn's Disease is Possible

Ulcerative colitis is generally limited to the colon, while intestinal inflammation in Crohn's disease may occur in any region of the gastrointestinal tract. Classification of pediatric IBD patients into UC or CD at the time of fecal testing is desirable, given the different clinical management of the two diseases. Even though distinguishing UC from CD was not the primary aim of our study design, we found that SLiME applied to the case-control data set could separate UC patients and control patients (Fig. 6A, cross-validated AUC = 0.82 and 0.83 respectively), but was less accurate in distinguishing Crohn's disease patients (AUC = 0.68). When we excluded controls from the data and attempted to distinguish between CD and UC in all IBD patients, we were able

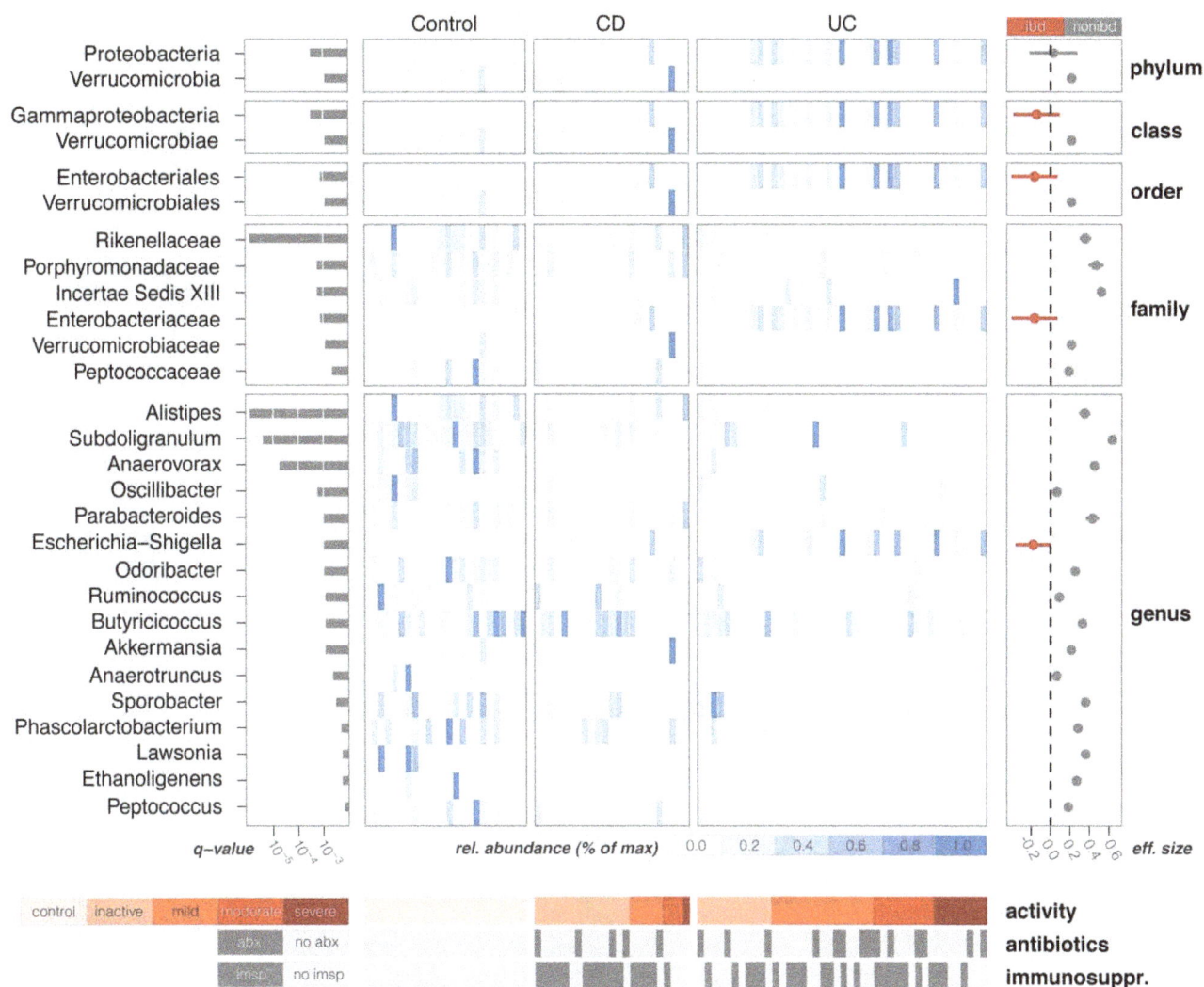

Figure 2. Taxa significantly associated with IBD. Center panel is a compositional heatmap of the selected taxa for each of the samples in the pediatric case-control study. Left panel indicates the significance of the association of each taxa with disease state, as measured by the q-value. Right panel shows a measure of effect size (Cohen's delta), highlighting in red those taxa which are significantly more prevalent in IBD samples. Bottom panels show relevant metadata for each sample, including disease activity as measured by PUCAI [32] and PCDAI indices [33].

to do so with accuracies (AUC = 0.76,ie. a specificity of 49% at 95% sensitivity) superior to current noninvasive clinical methods [13].

The most informative bacterial families in discriminating UC, CD and Control samples as determined by Kruskal-Wallis test were the Eubacteriaceae, Bacteroidaceae, and Verrucomicrobiaceae (Fig. 6B, also see Fig. S10). Verrucomicrobia were consistently employed in the classifier because bacteria of this group were completely absent from UC patients, which tended to be characterized by Lactobacillales or Bacilli and Gammaproteobacteria.

Steroid treatment could potentially affect the composition of the microbiota and in turn the accuracy of the classification between CD and UC. To assess this effect, we limited our analysis to those patients undergoing steroid therapy. However, we found no substantial difference in the accuracy of the classification (AUC = 0.73, 40% specificity at 95% sensitivity, Fig. S11) between CD and UC patients in the steroid subgroup with respect to the totality of all IBD patients.

Classification in CD or UC performed differently depending on whether the patient was experiencing active disease or remission, and surprisingly was more accurate at distinguishing CD and UC patients in remission (AUC = 0.73) than for patients with active disease (AUC = 0.67). This finding suggests that changes in microbiota composition during acute inflammation may be similar in both UC and CD, rendering distinction by microbial diversity more challenging.

Blind Validation with an Independent Patient Sample Confirms the Accuracy of Supervised Classification

To confirm the general validity of our results, we selected an independent patient sample of 68 children and young adults. Following fecal sampling and 16S rRNA sequencing, we applied SLiME – trained on our initial pediatric cohort – to the new dataset. Encouragingly, SLiME maintain good performance in distinguishing IBD patients from controls (AUC = 0.84, Fig. S12). Table S8 illustrates the classification performance of SLiME on the validation cohort at a chosen threshold.

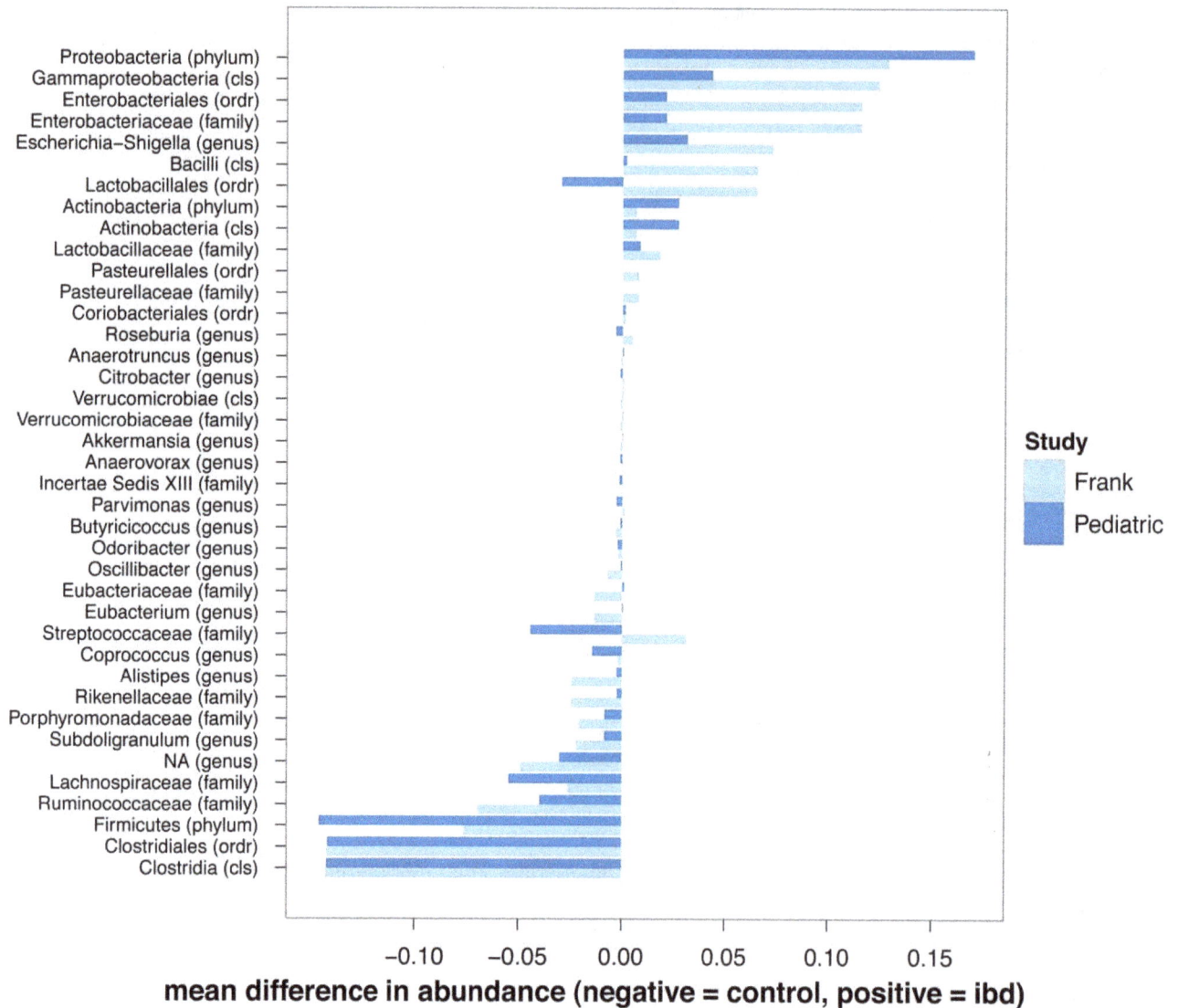

Figure 3. Taxa in the pediatric data set (stool-based) and the Frank et al. data set (tissue-based) agree in their relative abundance. Mean difference in normalized abundance between IBD samples and control samples is plotted for each taxa. Positive values (x-axis) mean the taxa is more prevalent in IBD samples, while negative values are associated with taxa more abundant in control samples. Stool-based and tissue-based data set are differentially colored (dark blue and light blue respectively).

Classification by SLiME is Comparable to Testing by Fecal Calprotectin

We compared the accuracy of SLiME with the outcome of the fecal calprotectin test on a portion of our samples from both the pediatric cohort and the validation cohort, to determine how our method compared to the most clinically accepted non-invasive test for IBD. On those 120 samples where we could obtain calprotectin measurements retrospectively (Table S9), we found that SLiME could classify the samples as IBD with comparable accuracy to calprotectin (AUC = 0.85 compared to calprotectin's AUC of 0.77). Superposing the two ROC curves (Fig. S13) shows that SLiME is slightly more specific, but otherwise comparable to calprotectin. Given that calprotectin levels should be raised in both CD and UC patients, it is not surprising that SLiME could distinguish CD samples from UC samples better than calprotectin (AUC 0.69 compared to AUC 0.50 for calprotectin, Fig. S14).

Discussion

Delay in the diagnosis of pediatric IBD is likely due to the non-specific presentation of the disease. An inexpensive and sensitive diagnostic tool could reduce this delay by rapidly identifying patients at high risk for IBD and, therefore, warranting endoscopic evaluation. In this study, we demonstrated the feasibility of a new approach to detecting pediatric IBD based on analysis of fecal microbiota. The sensitivity and specificity of our approach, as measured by ROC curve analysis, matches or surpasses that of alternative methods proposed for clinical use.

Two key methodological advances are responsible for improved performance compared to previous studies. These include the SLiME software package, which is freely available for public use, and increased sampling depth, which allows low abundance but highly informative groups to be sampled. The advantages of employing machine learning methods to analyze microbiome data have already been discussed [33]. Compared to clustering

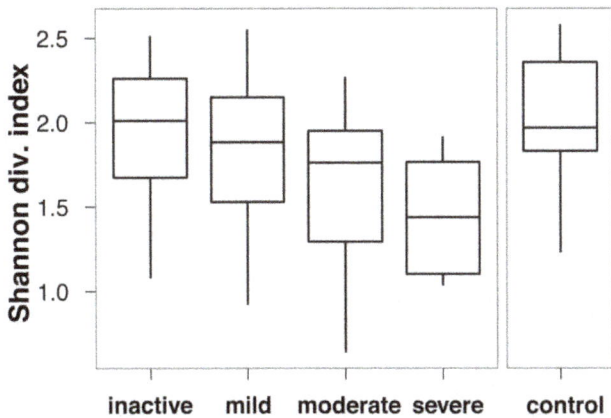

Figure 4. Stratification of patients by activity levels. Overall microbial diversity as measured by the Shannon Diversity Index. Activity was assessed on the basis of patient symptoms using PCDAI and PUCAI clinical indices.

methods, machine learning excels in classifying unlabelled data and extracting pivotal features from large and complex data sets. SLiME is a pipeline which allows the routine application of these algorithms to microbiome data.

Previous surveys of microbial diversity in IBD relied on clustering analyses to differentiate between IBD and non-IBD samples [18,24,41]. As a result, these studies suffered from poor sensitivity and, more importantly, did not generate predictive models that could be employed to distinguish new unlabelled samples. In this study, we employed SLiME to achieve high sensitivity as well as high specificity in differentiating IBD samples from controls. Models generated by SLiME were capable of classifying unlabelled samples with accuracy, as demonstrated by the large AUC obtained both after cross-validation and after blind validation with an independent cohort. Importantly, our approach was effective across disparate data sets using different sample types, and processing and sequencing technologies. Finally, we generated a list of taxa specifically associated with each disease state (active IBD, remission samples, CD and UC) facilitating biological interpretation.

Although we succesfully employed specific taxa as predictive biomarkers, our results indicate that IBD reflects an overall GI tract dysbiosis rather than the effect of a small number of pathogenic taxa. This result is in agreement with previous observations [20,24,40] and suggests that a global community survey rather than a test for bacterial presence/absence is better suited to identifying IBD.

Departing from the traditional clustering analysis, a recent and promising study [25] showed the use of a predictive model in classifying samples as IBD on the basis of microbial diversity. However, the same study arised concerns regarding a) the ability to distinguish UC patients from controls and b) the ability to discriminate between samples from patients with active disease and those in remission. Our study answers these questions, and importantly we report only cross-validated results that should more closely reflect accuracy in a clinical setting.

Some potential limitations in our study stem from its relatively small scale. For instance, while we are able to succesfully distinguish both UC and CD patients, SLiME appears to classify UC patients more succesfully than CD patients. However, we find that this difference in performance disappears after downsampling,

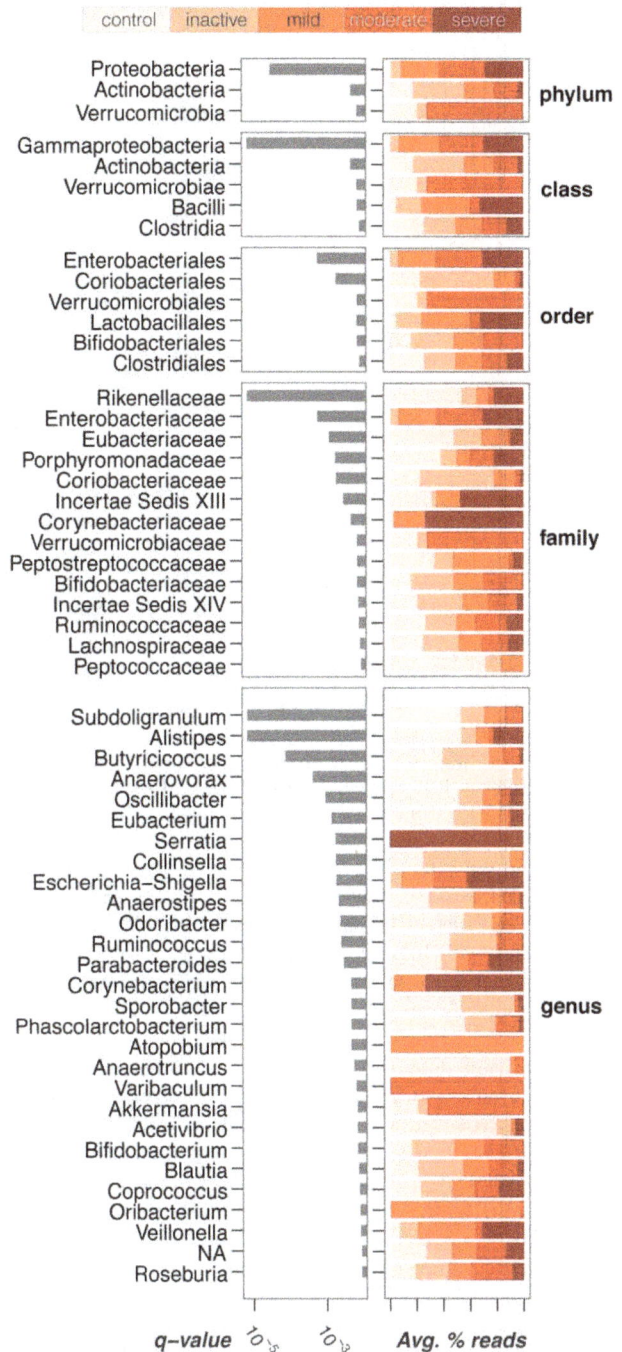

Figure 5. Best features to discriminate by activity levels. Activity levels are considered simultaneously, employing the Kruskal-Wallis test. Grey bar indicate the q-value and thus the strength of the association between the features and the disease state. Color bars indicate the average percentage of reads for each disease activity level.

confirming that it is probably due to the uneven split between CD and UC patients in our training cohort.

We also attempted to find correlations between therapeutic regimens (antibiotics, salicylates, anti-TNF, methotrexate, etc.) and microbial composition. Unfortunately SLiME was not capable to differentiate between subgroups with different therapeutic regimens, most likely due to the broad range of treatments employed in our cohort and the small number of patients in each

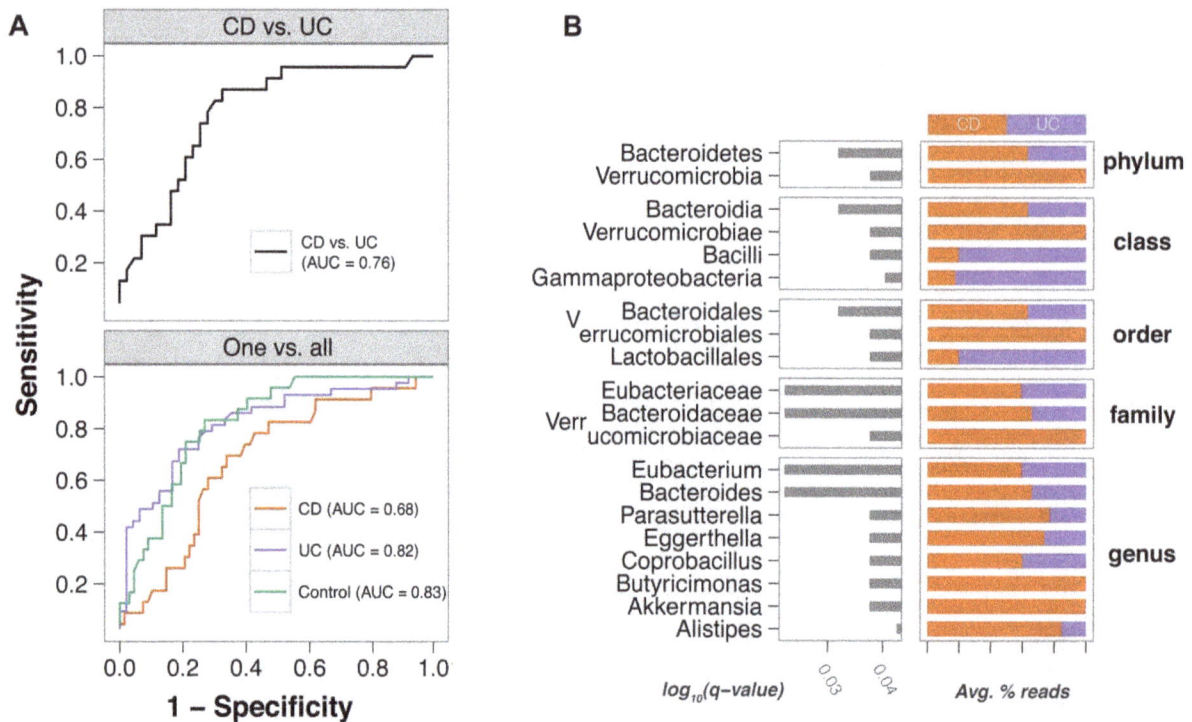

Figure 6. Discrimination of CD and UC. (A) Above, ROC curve for the classification of CD vs UC in samples where diagnosis of IBD is already established. Below, ROC curve for the classification of each disease class against all other classes. (B) Strength of association for the best features (q-value <0.05) [31] which allow discrimination between CD and UC.

subgroup. While these results indicate that SLiME may not be influenced by different therapeutic interventions while differentiating patients with IBD from controls, recruiting a larger number of patients following similar therapeutic regimens would have allowed to identify key microbial changes brought about by the therapy.

It is arguable that both these potential limitations will be addressed by studies with larger patient samples, better suited to compare alternatives in disease behaviour and therapeutic management of IBD. In addition, a cross-sectional study design on fecal samples taken at the time of diagnosis and before the start of any therapy, rather than the case-control study we employed, would allow to estimate more precisely the sensitivity of SLiME when employed in the general population.

Even though our results demonstrate the potential of the gastrointestinal microbiome as a diagnostic tool in IBD, further validation will be necessary before this tool is accepted into clinical practice. Our comparison between SLiME and calprotectin is encouraging, insofar as it shows that the two methods have comparable accuracies on this data set. However, other IBD fecal biomarkers – such as C-reactive protein, fecal lactoferrin, fecal calprotectin [10] – and blood biomarkers [42] have shown high sensitivity in IBD diagnosis. Further comparison of SLiME against these biomarkers in larger patient samples will allow clinicians to gauge the relative benefits of each method.

Despite these limitations, our results demonstrate the considerable potential of microbiome-based diagnostics in the clinic, particularly in the case of pediatric patients where diagnosis is often challenging. Similar approaches could evaluate the efficacy of novel therapies (e.g. probiotics, antibodies), predict the outcome of disease and forecast the timings of flare-ups. While not replacing endoscopy and histological examination as diagnostic tools, we propose that classification based on microbial diversity can be included as an effective complementary technique to aid in the diagnosis of IBD, particularly in pediatric patients.

Materials and Methods

Participants and Ethics

Fecal samples were obtained from 91 children and young adults with Crohn's disease, ulcerative colitis, and a control population composed of children with non-inflammatory conditions of the gastrointestinal tract (such as functional abdominal pain, constipation and diarrhea). The control population was composed of patients with symptomatology suggestive of IBD: constipation (n = 9), abdominal pain (n = 8), gastroesophageal reflux (n = 2), poor weight gain (n = 1), diarrhea (n = 1), blood in stool (n = 2) and oropharyngeal dysphagia (n = 1). Table 1 shows the patient demographics. Recruitment was conducted in the clinic or inpatient hospital wards under a protocol approved by the Children's Hospital Committee on Clinical Investigation. Written informed consent was obtained from patients (if over 18), or from parents or legal guardian (if patients were minors) for participation in the study. Written informed consent was obtained from all participants.

Fecal samples were generally obtained within 4 hours of the bowel movement, and stool was frozen at −80 degrees C on the receipt of the sample from the patient. Clinical data were recorded at the time of sample acquisition including: disease type, disease location, disease duration, disease activity (as determined by the Pediatric Crohn's disease activity index for CD, and the pediatric ulcerative colitis activity index for UC), and current prescribed medications.

An additional independent patient sample of 68 children and young adults was selected for blind validation. Table S1 shows the patient demographics of this additional sample set. Diagnoses for the control populations, data on disease duration and histological evidence for both sample sets are contained in Table S2, S3 and S4 respectively.

DNA Extraction and Sequencing

DNA from stool samples was extracted using the QIAamp DNA Stool Mini Kit (Qiagen, Inc., Valencia, CA) according to manufacturer's instructions. The manufacturer protocol was altered to accommodate larger volumes of stool and to improve homogenization using bead-beating techniques at several steps: a) a minimum of 2 mL of Buffer ASL and 300 mg of stool was used in the protocol; b) a ratio of 700 uL of Buffer ASL per 100 mg of stool weight was used for larger volumes using no more than 1500 mg of stool and 10.5 mL of Buffer ASL; c) following the addition of Buffer ASL to each sample (step #2), 0.70 mm Garnet Beads (MO BIO Laboratories, Inc., Carlsbad, CA) were added to the suspension and vortexed for 10 seconds; d) a second bead-beating was done following the heating of the suspension (step #3) in 0.1 mm Glass Bead Tubes (MO BIO Laboratories, Inc., Carlsbad, CA), and vortexed for 10 minutes.

Extracted DNA was employed for 454 FLX Titaninum pyrosequencing of PCR-amplified windows of the 16S gene.

Variable region V3–V5 amplification primers were designed with FLX Titanium adaptors (A adaptor sequence: 5′ CCATCT-CATCCCTGCGTGTCTCCGACTCAG 3′; B adaptor sequence: 5′ CCTATCCCCTGTGTGCCTTGGCAGTCTCAG 3′) on the 5′ end of the 16S primer sequence: 454B_ 357F (5′ CCTACGGGAGGCAGCAG 3′) and 454A_barcode_926R (5′ CCGTCAATTCMTTTRAGT 3′). See Table S5.

Polymerase chain reaction (PCR) mixtures (25 µl) contained 10 ng of template, 1× Easy A reaction buffer (Stratagene, La Jolla, CA), 200 mM of each dNTP (Stratagene), 200 nM of each primer, and 1.25 U Easy A cloning enzyme (Stratagene). The cycling conditions for the V3–V5 consisted of an initial denaturation of 95°C for 2 min, followed by 25 cycles of denaturation at 95°C for 40 sec, annealing at 50°C for 30 sec, extension at 72°C for 5 min and a final extension at 72°C for 7 min. Amplicons were confirmed on 1.2% Flash Gels (Lonza, Rockland, ME) and purified with AMPure XP DNA purification beads (Beckman Coulter, Danvers, MA) according to the manufacturer and eluted in 25 µL of 1× low TE buffer (pH 8.0). Amplicons were quantified on Agilent Bioanalyzer 2100 DNA 1000 chips (Agilent Technologies, Santa Clara, CA) and pooled in equimolar concentration. Emulsion PCR and sequencing were performed according to the manufacturer's specifications. Sequencing was performed with a target of 5000 raw reads per sample.

Sanger Sequencing

Polymerase chain reaction (PCR) mixtures (25 µl) contained 10 ng of template, 1× Easy A reaction buffer (Stratagene, La Jolla, CA), 200 mM of each dNTP (Stratagene), 200 nM of each primer (63f: 5′ GCCTAACACATGCAAGTC 3′; U1525R: 5′ AAG-GAGGTGWTCCARCC 3′), and 1.25 U Easy A cloning enzyme (Stratagene). The cycling conditions consisted of an initial denaturation of 95°C for 2 min, followed by 30 cycles of denaturation at 95°C for 40 sec, annealing at 50°C for 30 sec, extension at 72°C for 2 min and a final extension at 72°C for 7 min. PCR products were purified with QIAquick PCR purification kit (QIAGEN, Inc, Valencia, CA) according to the manufacturer, and size selected on a 1% agarose gel. The gel bands were purified with QIAquick gel extraction kit (QIAGEN)

according to the manufacturer's instructions with one modification: the gel bands were dissolved at room temperature on a Dynal Bioteck Rotator (Model RKDYNAL, setting 30, Invitrogen, Life Technologies, Carlsbad, CA) for 15 minutes. Cleaned amplicons were cloned (pCR2.1-TOPO vector, TOPO-TA Cloning kit and electrocompetent cells TOP 10; Invitrogen, Carlsbad, CA) and sequenced.

Processing Sequencing Samples

Sequences were processed using a data curation pipeline implemented in MOTHUR [43], which removed sequences from the analysis if they were less than 200 nt or greater than 600 nt, had a low read quality score (<25), contained ambiguous characters, had a non-exact barcode match, or had more than 4 mismatches to the reverse primer sequences (926R). Remaining sequences were assigned to samples based on barcode matches, after which barcode and primer sequences were trimmed. Chimeric sequences were identified using the ChimeraSlayer algorithm [44], and reads were classified with the MSU RDP classifier v2.2 [45] using the taxonomy maintained at the Ribosomal Database Project (RDP 10 database, version 6). After processing, the resulting sequencing depth was 2690±898 (median ± median abs. deviation) reads per sample.

Synthetic Learning in Microbial Ecology (SLiME)

Using a set of training data, supervised learning algorithms can be trained to classify each microbiota sample into distinct classes (eg. IBD/non-IBD) based on a defined set of features (eg. the relative abundance of each OTU). We first assigned each sequence in the data set to a taxonomical group using the RDP Naive Bayesan classifier [46]. For each sample we then calculated the relative abundance of each taxa with respect to the total number of sequences in each sample. We then trained a random forest (RF) classifier (R-project implementation [29,47]) to assign the class (IBD or non-IBD) based on the relative sequence abundances in every taxa. We used ten-fold cross-validation to compute accuracy of the classifier, where training of the classification algorithm employs a random 90% of the available patients and the performance of the generated model is tested on the remaining 10% of patients.

Fecal Calprotectin Test

Calprotectin was assayed using the calprotectin ELISA kit (Bühlmann Laboratories/ALPCO Diagnostics) and followed the manufacter testing protocol. Samples were shaken on an orbital shaker at 600 rpm. ELISA plates were read with the Varioskan (Thermo Scientific). SkanIT software (Thermo Scientific) was used to fit the standard curve using four parameter curve fitting.

Statistical Analyses

Several approaches can be used to identify the features which were most important to the classification task: a) a priori statistical tests, b) statistics intrinsic to the supervised learning algorithm or c) iterative measures of the importance of each variable [48]. To minimize computational complexity and exclusively for the purpose of visualization we selected taxa independently from the classification task and chose to employ an a priori statistical test. Taxa were tested for significant association with disease state by means of non-parametric Kruskal-Wallis test, which does not include an assumption of normality. Multiple p-values were then converted to q-values, by FDR adjustment [36] and a significance threshold was chosen between q-value <0.01 or q-value <0.05 by estimating the π_0

parameter as well as the number of false positives vs. cutoff (see [36] for details). In the case of IBD/control, CD/UC and activity classification, features individuated by Kruskal-Wallis test were largely overlapping with the list of most discriminative features obtained by iterative measures and intrinsic measures (data not shown). No feature selection or other dimensionality reduction was used in the classification task.

Receiver operating characteristic analysis was used to evaluate the classification algorithms across a range of possible disease prevalences. Reported AUC values are median AUC values resulting from 3 repetitions of 10-fold cross validations.

All calculations were performed in R [47] and plots were generated in R using the ggplot library [49].

Supporting Information

Figure S1 Patients are classifiable as IBD and non-IBD with a variety of supervised learning algorithms. ROC curves for SVM, Bagging (decision tree as base classifier), Stacking (decision tree as base classifier) and RFs are shown.

Figure S2 Sequencing technology does not significantly influence classification accuracy. ROC curves for active IBD vs. control classification in ten samples where sequencing was repeated by Sanger methods and yielded the same area under the curve.

Figure S3 Relative abundance of each discriminatory feature compared to the sequencing depth of other IBD microbiota surveys. Two vertical lines indicate the minimum detectable abundance in the Frank et al. study (right) and the Willing et al. study (left). Due to low sequencing depth, the Frank et al. survey could have detected only 13 of the features considered discriminatory for classification (right vertical line).

Figure S4 FDR adjustment of Kruskal-Wallis p-values for those features which best discriminate between IBD samples and control samples. (Top-left) The expected proportion of false positive samples (p_0) is estimated by fitting. (Top-right) A plot of the calculated q-values versus the initial p-values. (Bottom-left) The number of significant tests for every given q-value cut-off. (Bottom-right) The number of expected false positives for a given number of significant tests considered.

Figure S5 Taxa in the pediatric data set (stool-based) and the Frank et al. data set (tissue-based) vary in their importance as features. Best features - as determined by the RandomForest algorithm - applied to the pediatric data set are used to classify the Frank et al. data set. The importance of each feature - calculated as the decrease in accuracy of the algorithm when the feature is not used - is plotted for both studies. Noticeably, feature at the genus level are far more important in the pediatric data set than when used on the Frank et al. data set. This may reflect the greater depth of sequencing (see Figure S2).

Figure S6 FDR adjustment of Kruskal-Wallis p-values for those features which best discriminate between levels of IBD activity. (Top-left) The expected proportion of false positive samples (p_0) is estimated by curve fitting. (Top-right) A plot of the calculated q-values versus the initial p-values.

(Bottom-left) The number of significant tests for every given q-value cut-off. (Bottom-right) The number of expected false positives for a given number of significant tests considered.

Figure S7 Features that show the greatest difference between active and inactive state in the pediatric case-control study. All features with significant association (q-value <0.05, see Figure S12){Storey,2003} to either active disease or remission are shown. Grey bars indicate the q-value of each taxon, heat maps describe the median normalized abundance in each sample. The right panel indicates the effect size and highlights in red the taxa which are prevalent in active samples.

Figure S8 FDR adjustment of Kruskal-Wallis p-values for those features which best discriminate between active IBD samples and inactive IBD samples. (Top-left) The expected proportion of false positive samples (p_0) is estimated by curve fitting. (Top-right) A plot of the calculated q-values versus the initial p-values. (Bottom-left) The number of significant tests for every given q-value cut-off. (Bottom-right) The number of expected false positives for a given number of significant tests considered.

Figure S9 Antibiotic therapy reduces overall microbial diversity. Box plot showing the distribution of Shannon diversity indices for all patients undergoing antibiotic therapy, compared to the patients with IBD and without antibiotics, as well as controls.

Figure S10 FDR adjustment of Kruskal-Wallis p-values for those features which best discriminate between CD samples and UC samples. (Top-left) The expected proportion of false positive samples (p_0) is estimated by curve fitting. (Top-right) A plot of the calculated q-values versus the initial p-values. (Bottom-left) The number of significant tests for every given q-value cut-off. (Bottom-right) The number of expected false positives for a given number of significant tests considered.

Figure S11 ROC curve for the CD vs UC classification in the steroid-treated subgroup. The performance in this subset of the cohort is comparable to the totality of IBD patients.

Figure S12 Blind validation of a SLiME model - previously trained on our pediatric cohort - applied to an independent set of fecal samples from 77 patients. ROC curve shows that high sensitivity and high specificity are maintained across a range of disease prevalences.

Figure S13 Comparison of SLiME and fecal calprotectin assay. The two assays have comparable efficacy in distinguishing IBD patients from control when applied to all samples in the training and validation cohorts for which calprotectin could be measured (n = 120).

Figure S14 Comparison of SLiME and fecal calprotectin assay. SLiME is slightly superior in distinguishing CD from UC samples, when applied to all CD and UC samples (n = 90) in the training and validation cohorts for which calprotectin could be measured.

Table S1 Patient demographics for the validation set

Table S2 Control patients' diagnose

Table S3 Disease Duration at Time of Sample Acquisition

Table S4 Histological evidence of disease at diagnostic colonoscopy

Table S5 454 barcodes and primers

Table S6 Confusion matrix for the SLiME classification of the pediatric training cohort. Sensitivity 87.6%. Specificity 45.8%. Note this is only one possible cutoff value. Different sensitivity and specificity can be obtained by appropriately tuning the cutoff.

Table S7 Confusion matrix for the SLiME classification of the training cohort on the subset of patient with clinically active disease at the time of sampling. Sensitivity 82.5%. Specificity 75%. Note this is only one possible cutoff value. Different sensitivity and specificity can be obtained by appropriately tuning the cutoff.

Table S8 Confusion matrix for the blind validation of the SLiME classifier on an independent validation cohort. Sensitivity for IBD vs controls is 94.5%, while specificity is 46.1%. Note this is only one possible cutoff value. Different sensitivity and specificity can be obtained by appropriately tuning the cutoff.

Table S9 Summary of calprotectin assay results

Acknowledgments

Data availability

Sequencing data is publicly available as a NCBI BioProject, with BioProjectID 82109.

Author Contributions

Conceived and designed the experiments: EP EJA AB DBS JRK DG DJW. Performed the experiments: MD AB DBS DG GG DC DT DJW SPP. Analyzed the data: EP CS DG SW JI. Wrote the paper: EP EJA AB. Critically reviewed the manuscript: RJX.
†Deceased

References

1. Carter MJ, Lobo AJ, Travis SPL (2004) Guidelines for the management of inflammatory bowel disease in adults. Gut 53 Suppl 5: V1–16.
2. Kappelman MD, Bousvaros A (2008) Nutritional concerns in pediatric inflammatory bowel disease patients. Molecular nutrition & food research 52: 867–874.
3. Yantiss RK, Odze RD (2006) Diagnostic difficulties in inflammatory bowel disease pathology. Histopathology 48: 116–132.
4. Heikenen JB, Werlin SL, Brown CW, Balint JP (1999) Presenting symptoms and diagnostic lag in children with inflammatory bowel disease. Inflammatory bowel diseases 5: 158–160.
5. Spray C, Debelle GD, Murphy MS (2001) Current diagnosis, management and morbidity in paediatric inflammatory bowel disease. Acta paediatrica (Oslo, Norway : 1992) 90: 400–405.
6. Devroede GJ, Taylor WF, Sauer WG, Jackman RJ, Stickler GB (1971) Cancer risk and life expectancy of children with ulcerative colitis. The New England journal of medicine 285: 17–21.
7. Peeters M, Joossens S, Vermeire S, Vlietinck R, Bossuyt X, et al. (2001) Diagnostic value of anti-Saccharomyces cerevisiae and antineutrophil cytoplasmic autoantibodies in inflammatory bowel disease. The American journal of gastroenterology 96: 730–734.
8. Andersen K, Vogt C, Blondin D, Beck A, Heinen W, et al. (2006) Multi-detector CT-colonography in inflammatory bowel disease: prospective analysis of CT-findings to high-resolution video colonoscopy. European journal of radiology 58: 140–146.
9. Löffler M, Weckesser M, Franzius C, Schober O, Zimmer K-P (2006) High diagnostic value of 18F-FDG-PET in pediatric patients with chronic inflammatory bowel disease. Annals of the New York Academy of Sciences 1072: 379–385.
10. Lewis JD (2011) The Utility of Biomarkers in the Diagnosis and Therapy of Inflammatory Bowel Disease. Gastroenterology 140: 1817–1826.e2.
11. Ruemmele FM, Targan SR, Levy G, Dubinsky M, Braun J, et al. (1998) Diagnostic accuracy of serological assays in pediatric inflammatory bowel disease. Gastroenterology 115: 822–829.
12. Austin GL, Herfarth HH, Sandler RS (2007) A critical evaluation of serologic markers for inflammatory bowel disease. Clinical gastroenterology and hepatology : the official clinical practice journal of the American Gastroenterological Association 5: 545–547.
13. Dubinsky MC, Ofman JJ, Urman M, Targan SR, Seidman EG (2001) Clinical utility of serodiagnostic testing in suspected pediatric inflammatory bowel disease. The American journal of gastroenterology 96: 758–765.
14. Bernstein CN, Shanahan F (2008) Disorders of a modern lifestyle: reconciling the epidemiology of inflammatory bowel diseases. Gut 57: 1185–1191.
15. Cho JH (2008) The genetics and immunopathogenesis of inflammatory bowel disease. Nature Reviews Immunology 8: 458.
16. Arseneau KO, Tamagawa H, Pizarro TT, Cominelli F (2007) Innate and adaptive immune responses related to IBD pathogenesis. Current gastroenterology reports 9: 508–512.
17. Baumgart DC, Carding SR (2007) Inflammatory bowel disease: cause and immunobiology. Lancet 369: 1627–1640.
18. Dicksved J, Halfvarson J, Rosenquist M, Järnerot G, Tysk C, et al. (2008) Molecular analysis of the gut microbiota of identical twins with Crohn's disease. The ISME journal 2: 716–727.
19. Sartor RB, Muehlbauer M (2007) Microbial host interactions in IBD: implications for pathogenesis and therapy. Curr Gastroenterol Rep 9: 497–507.
20. Sartor RB (2008) Microbial influences in inflammatory bowel diseases. Gastroenterology 134: 577–594.
21. Kim SC, Tonkonogy SL, Albright CA, Tsang J, Balish EJ, et al. (2005) Variable phenotypes of enterocolitis in interleukin 10-deficient mice monoassociated with two different commensal bacteria. Gastroenterology 128: 891–906.
22. Selby W, Pavli P, Crotty B, Florin T, Radford-Smith G, et al. (2007) Two-year combination antibiotic therapy with clarithromycin, rifabutin, and clofazimine for Crohn's disease. Gastroenterology 132: 2313–2319.
23. Böhm SK, Kruis W (2006) Probiotics: do they help to control intestinal inflammation? Annals of the New York Academy of Sciences 1072: 339–350.
24. Frank DN, Amand ALS, Feldman RA, Boedeker EC, Harpaz N, et al. (2007) Molecular-phylogenetic characterization of microbial community imbalances in human inflammatory bowel diseases. Proceedings of the National Academy of Sciences 104: 13780–13785.
25. Willing BP, Dicksved J, Halfvarson J, Andersson AF, Lucio M, et al. (2010) A pyrosequencing study in twins shows that gastrointestinal microbial profiles vary with inflammatory bowel disease phenotypes. Gastroenterology 139: 1844–1854.e1.
26. Baldi P, Brunak S (2001) Bioinformatics: the machine learning approach.
27. Tarca AL, Carey VJ, Chen X-wen, Romero R, Draghici S (2007) Machine learning and its applications to biology. PLoS computational biology 3: e116.
28. Ben-Hur A, Ong CS, Sonnenburg S, Schalkopf B, Ratsch G (2008) Support vector machines and kernels for computational biology. PLoS computational biology 4: e1000173.
29. Shipp MA, Ross KN, Tamayo P, Weng AP, Kutok JL, et al. (2002) Diffuse large B-cell lymphoma outcome prediction by gene-expression profiling and supervised machine learning. Nature medicine 8: 68–74.
30. Parsons DW, Jones S, Zhang X, Lin JC-H, Leary RJ, et al. (2008) An integrated genomic analysis of human glioblastoma multiforme. Science (New York, NY) 321: 1807–1812.
31. Liang Y, Diehn M, Watson N, Bollen AW, Aldape KD, et al. (2005) Gene expression profiling reveals molecularly and clinically distinct subtypes of glioblastoma multiforme. Proceedings of the National Academy of Sciences of the United States of America 102: 5814–5819.
32. Tomaşs G, Tarabichi M, Gacquer D, Habrant A, Dom G, et al. (2012) A general method to derive robust organ-specific gene expression-based differentiation indices: application to thyroid cancer diagnostic. Oncogene.

33. Knights D, Costello EK, Knight R (2010) Supervised classification of human microbiota. FEMS microbiology reviews 1–17.

34. Liaw A, Wiener M (2002) Classification and Regression by randomForest. R News 2: 18–22.

35. Bradley A (1997) The use of the area under the ROC curve in the evaluation of machine learning algorithms. Pattern Recognition 30: 1145–1159.

36. Storey JD, Tibshirani R (2003) Statistical significance for genomewide studies. Proceedings of the National Academy of Sciences of the United States of America 100: 9440–9445.

37. Turner D, Hyams J, Markowitz J, Lerer T, Mack DR, et al. (2009) Appraisal of the pediatric ulcerative colitis activity index (PUCAI). Inflammatory bowel diseases 15: 1218–1223.

38. Turner D, Griffiths AM, Walters TD, Seah T, Markowitz J, et al. (2010) Appraisal of the pediatric Crohn's disease activity index on four prospectively collected datasets: recommended cutoff values and clinimetric properties. The American journal of gastroenterology 105: 2085–2092.

39. Griffiths AM, Otley AR, Hyams J, Quiros AR, Grand RJ, et al. (2005) A review of activity indices and end points for clinical trials in children with Crohn's disease. Inflammatory bowel diseases 11: 185–196.

40. Tamboli CP, Neut C, Desreumaux P, Colombel JF (2004) Dysbiosis in inflammatory bowel disease. Gut 53: 1–4.

41. Sepehri S, Kotlowski R, Bernstein CN, Krause DO (2007) Microbial diversity of inflamed and noninflamed gut biopsy tissues in inflammatory bowel disease. Inflammatory bowel diseases 13: 675–683.

42. Cabrera-Abreu JC, Davies P, Matek Z, Murphy MS (2004) Performance of blood tests in diagnosis of inflammatory bowel disease in a specialist clinic. Arch Dis Child 89: 69–71.

43. Schloss PD (2008) Evaluating different approaches that test whether microbial communities have the same structure. The ISME Journal 2: 265.

44. Haas BJ, Gevers D, Earl A, Feldgarden M, Ward DV, et al. (2011) Chimeric 16S rRNA sequence formation and detection in Sanger and 454-pyrosequenced PCR amplicons. Genome research 21: 494–504.

45. Cole JR, Wang Q, Cardenas E, Fish J, Chai B, et al. (2009) The Ribosomal Database Project: improved alignments and new tools for rRNA analysis. Nucleic acids research 37: D141–5.

46. Wang Q, Garrity GM, Tiedje JM, Cole JR (2007) Naive Bayesian classifier for rapid assignment of rRNA sequences into the new bacterial taxonomy. Applied and environmental microbiology 73: 5261–5267.

47. Team RDC (2011) R: A Language and Environment for Statistical Computing.

48. Saeys Y, Inza I, Larrañaga P (2007) A review of feature selection techniques in bioinformatics. Bioinformatics (Oxford, England) 23: 2507–2517.

49. Wickham H (2009) ggplot2: elegant graphics for data analysis. Springer New York.

5

Association between CD14 Gene C-260T Polymorphism and Inflammatory Bowel Disease

Zhengting Wang[1⑨], **Jiajia Hu**[2⑨], **Rong Fan**[1], **Jie Zhou**[1], **Jie Zhong**[1]*

1 Department of Gastroenterology, Ruijin Hospital, Shanghai Jiaotong University School of Medicine, Shanghai, China, 2 Department of Nuclear Medicine, Ruijin Hospital, Shanghai Jiaotong University School of Medicine, Shanghai, China

Abstract

Background: The gene encoding CD14 has been proposed as an IBD-susceptibility gene with its polymorphism C-260T being widely evaluated, yet with conflicting results. The aim of this study was to investigate the association between this polymorphism and IBD by conducting a meta-analysis.

Methodology/Principal Findings: Seventeen articles met the inclusion criteria, which included a total of 18 case-control studies, including 1900 ulcerative colitis (UC) cases, 2535 Crohn's disease (CD) cases, and 4004 controls. Data were analyzed using STATA software. Overall, association between C-260T polymorphism and increased UC risk was significant in allelic comparison (odds ratio [OR] = 1.21, 95% confidence interval [CI]: 1.02–1.43; P = 0.027), homozygote model (OR = 1.44, 95% CI: 1.03–2.01; P = 0.033), as well as dominant model (OR = 1.36, 95% CI: 1.06–1.75; P = 0.016). However, there was negative association between this polymorphism and CD risk across all genetic models. Subgroup analyses by ethnicity suggested the risk-conferring profiles of -260T allele and -260 TT genotype with UC in Asians, but not in Caucasians. There was a low probability of publication bias.

Conclusions/Significance: Expanding previous results of individual studies, our findings demonstrated that *CD14* gene C-260T polymorphism might be a promising candidate marker in susceptibility to UC, especially in Asians.

Editor: Georgina L. Hold, University of Aberdeen, United Kingdom

Funding: No current external funding sources for this study.

Competing Interests: The authors have declared that no competing interests exist.

* E-mail: Jimmyzj64@medmail.com.cn

⑨ These authors contributed equally to this work.

Introduction

Crohn's disease (CD) and ulcerative colitis (UC) are the two major subtypes of inflammatory bowel disease (IBD), which is a chronic relapsing and remitting inflammatory condition affecting the gastrointestinal tract. Familial aggregation and twin studies reported that patients with IBD carried strong genetic predisposition [1]. Recent genome-wide association studies (GWAS) have identified approximately 100 IBD-susceptibility loci, and thereof more than 70 loci susceptible to CD and 47 to UC have been confirmed in subsequent meta-analyses, especially in the genes encoding microbe recognition, lymphocyte activation, cytokine signaling, and intestinal epithelial defense [2–6]. The results of GWAS provided new insights into the immunopathogenesis of this disease, implicating an important role of the innate and adaptive immune systems in disease occurrence.

Toll-like receptors (TLRs) are a class of proteins that are active in innate and adaptive systems. TLRs are members of a conserved interleukin (IL)-1 superfamily of transmembrane receptors that recognize pathogen-associated molecular patterns (PAMPs) which present on the surface of pathogens. The pathogenesis of IBD, ulcerative colitis and Crohn's disease may be due to increased TLR or decreased TLR signalling respectively [7]. TLR4−/− mice increased susceptibility to bleeding and bacterial trans-

location in DSS (dextran sodium sulfate)-induced colitis model [8,9]. CD14 serves as a receptor for lipopolysaccharides (LPS), and the binding of LPS/CD14 complex to TLR4 could activate NF-κB, and further induce an inflammatory response [10]. Soluble CD14 accompanying with serum LPS-binding protein are markers of disease activity in patients with Crohn's disease [11]. Co-existence of a mutation in either TLR4 or CD14 gene, and in NOD2/CARD15 is associated with an increased susceptibility to developing CD compared to UC, and to developing either CD or UC compared to healthy individuals [12,13]. It is required for the microbe-induced endocytosis of TLR4. In dendritic cells, this CD14-dependent endocytosis pathway is upregulated upon exposure to inflammatory mediators [14]. Meanwhile, human *CD14* gene is mapped on chromosome 5q31.1, adjacent to a region reportedly in linkage with IBD [15,16]. From genetic perspective, the substitution of a promoter polymorphism in *CD14* gene (C-260T, also known as *CD14*. C-159T) results in elevated transcriptional activity and accordingly high serum CD14 levels [17,18]. Therefore, candidacy of *CD14* for IBD is well-defined and its C-260T polymorphism has been reported to be associated with IBD by some but not all studies [19,20]. Generally, studies with insufficient sample sizes account for such inconsistency [21].

To shed some light on this issue, we sought to examine the association of *CD14* gene C-260T polymorphism with the

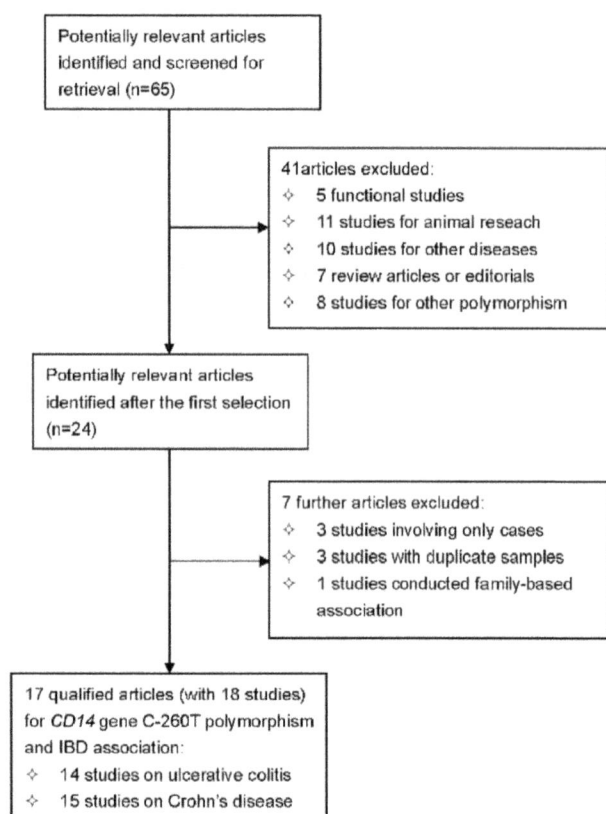

Figure 1. Flow diagram of search strategy and study selection.

occurrence of IBD by a meta-analysis, and simultaneously to identify factors attributed to between-study heterogeneity and publication bias.

Methods

This meta-analysis is reported in accordance with the Preferred Reporting Items for Systematic Reviews and Meta-analyses (PRISMA) guideline (please see supplementary PRISMA checklist) [22].

Search strategy for identification of studies

We searched the PubMed, EMBASE, ISI Web of Knowledge databases and Wanfang databases before July 20, 2012, by using the key subjects "inflammatory bowel disease", "IBD", "Crohn's disease", "CD", "Ulcerative colitis", "UC", in combination with "Cluster of differentiation 14", "CD14 ", "toll like receptor 4", "TLR4" and "TLR-4". We read the full text of the retrieved articles to inspect whether data on the topic of interest were included. Reference lists of the retrieved articles and systematic reviews were also checked for citations of articles that were not initially identified. Special meeting issues of journals (Abstract only) were removed from the searching results. Search results were restricted to human populations and articles written in English or Chinese. If more than one geographic or ethnic heterogeneous group was reported in one report, each was extracted separately. If two or more studies shared the whole or part of study populations, the one with larger sample size was extracted.

Inclusion/exclusion criteria

Identified studies satisfied the following criteria: (1) evaluation of *CD14* gene C-260T polymorphism with the risk for IBD (CD and/or UC); (2) case-control or cross-sectional or nested case-control study in design; (3) availability of genotype or allele counts of studied polymorphisms between patients and controls in order to estimate odds ratio (OR) and its corresponding 95% confidence interval (CI).

Extracted information

The following data were extracted independently and entered into separate databases by two authors (Z. Wang and J. Hu) from each qualified study: first author's last name, publication year, population ethnicity, study design, genotyping methods, baseline characteristics of the study population including age, gender, subtype of the disease, and the genotype or allele distributions in patients and controls. Any encountered discrepancies were adjudicated by a discussion and an 100% consensus was reached.

Statistical analysis

In this meta-analysis, we assessed the association of *CD14* gene C-260T polymorphism with IBD risk under allelic, homozygous and dominant and recessive models, respectively. Crude OR and 95% CI were calculated to compare contrasts of alleles or genotypes between patients and controls.

Deviation from Hardy-Weinberg equilibrium was assessed using Pearson χ^2 test. The random-effects model using DerSimonian & Laird method was employed to bring the individual effect-size estimates together irrespective of between-study heterogeneity [23]. Heterogeneity was evaluated by the I^2 statistic, which was documented for the percentage of the observed between-study variability due to heterogeneity rather than chance with its values ranging 0–100% [$I^2 = 0$–25%, no heterogeneity; $I^2 = 25$–50%, moderate heterogeneity; $I^2 = 50$–75%, large heterogeneity; $I^2 = 75$–100%, extreme heterogeneity [24]. In the case of between-study heterogeneity, we examined the study characteristics that can stratify the studies into subgroups with homogeneous effects. Subgroup analyses were conducted after stratifying studies performed on various ethnic/geographic populations or studies with different study designs (hospital-based and population-based) or studies on different subtype diseases. Here, the design of studies was determined according to the sources of control group, either from hospitals or general populations.

Finally, evidence for publication bias was assessed using Egger's test and visual funnel plot inspection. The Egger's test detects funnel plot asymmetry by determining whether the intercept deviates significantly from zero in a regression of the standardized effect estimates against their precision.

Probability less than 0.05 was judged significant with the exception of the I^2 statistic and publication tests, where a significance level of less than 0.1 was chosen. Statistical analyses were performed using STATA version 11.0 for Windows (StataCorp LP, College Station, Texas, USA).

Results

Search results

The detailed selection process is presented in Figure 1. Based on our search strategy, the primary screening yielded 65 potentially relevant articles. Because the study by Baumgart DC et al included two populations, we treated them separately in this meta-analysis. Therefore, seventeen articles met the inclusion criteria, which included a total of 18 case-control studies. 17 articles met the inclusion criteria, which included a total of 18

Table 1. The baseline characteristics of all eligible studies.

First author	Year	Ethnicity	Study design	Genotyping method	Numbers			T freq. (%)			HWE
					Cases		Controls	Cases		Controls	
					CD	UC		CD	UC		
Klein W et al.	2002	Germany (C)	NA	PCR-RFLP	219	142	410	51.1	43.7	44.5	0.9006
Obana N et al.	2002	Japan (A)	NA	PCR-RFLP	82	101	123	48.2	57.4	44.7	0.5234
Klein W et al.	2003	Germany (C)	HB	PCR-RFLP	253	/	650	51.0	/	44.5	0.993
Torok HP et al.	2004	Germany (C)	PB	PCR-RFLP	102	98	145	48.5	43.4	50.0	0.9983
Arnott IDR et al.	2004	UK (C)	PB	PCR-RFLP	242	233	189	49.0	52.8	51.9	0.6105
Klausz G et al.	2005	Hungary (C)	NA	Probe	133	/	75	48.5	/	46.0	0.9599
Guo QS et al.	2005	Chinese (A)	PB	PCR-RFLP	/	114	160	/	64.0	60.3	0.9989
Gazouli M et al.	2005	Greece (C)	HB	PCR-RFLP	120	85	100	50.4	40.0	37.0	0.6079
Leung E et al.	2005	New Zealand (C)	PB	PCR-RFLP	185	/	187	51.4	/	50.3	0.7974
Peters KE et al.	2005	Australia (C)	PB	PCR-RFLP	235	81	189	49.6	56.8	49.2	0.5584
Ouburg S et al.	2005	Netherlands (C)	HB	PCR-RFLP	112	/	170	44.6	/	47.7	0.9544
XUE H et al.	2007	Chinese (A)	HB	PCR-RFLP	41	43	135	61.0	60.5	59.3	0.6887
Wang F et al.	2007	Japanese (A)	HB	PCR-RFLP	/	97	135	/	66.0	48.5	0.5882
Baumgart DC et al.	2007	Hungary (C)	NA	Probe	144	118	202	42.7	44.1	52.7	0.7091
Baumgart DC et al.	2007	Germany (C)	NA	Probe	235	145	403	45.3	53.8	45.5	0.9415
Petermann I et al.	2009	New Zealand (C)	PB	Taqman	387	405	377	49.6	48.4	49.3	0.984
Sivaram G et al.	2012	India (A)	NA	PCR-RFLP	/	139	176	/	53.2	41.8	0.3855
Kim EJ et al.	2012	Korea (A)	HB	PCR-RFLP	45	99	178	61.1	54.6	36.5	0.8755

Abbreviations: HB = hospital-based design; PB = population-based design; NA = not available; CD = Crohn's disase; UC = ulcerative colitis.

case-control studies in an attempt to examine the association of *CD14* gene C-260T polymorphism with IBD [12,13,19,20,25–37]. A total of 4435 IBD cases (1900 UC and 2535 CD) and 4004 controls were finally analyzed. Of these 18 studies, seventeen [12,13,19,20,25–36] were published in English and one in Chinese [37]. Six studies were conducted in Asians (two in Chinese [20,37], two in Japanese [28,34], and one in India [31] and Korea [13], respectively), whereas 12 [12,13,19,20,25–36] studies were conducted in Caucasians.

Study characteristics

The baseline characteristics of all qualified studies are presented in Table 1. The frequency of -260T allele was 51.71% in UC patients, 49.21% in CD patients and 47.29% in controls, with the higher frequency in average Asians cases than Caucasians cases (65.98% vs 48.47% in UC, 54.76% vs 48.82% in CD), whereas with similar frequency in controls (48.02% in Asians vs 47.08%). Genotyping for C-260T polymorphism across all studies, except three using the probe technology [25,26] and one using TaqMan assay [36], was conducted using polymerase chain reaction-restriction fragment length polymorphism (PCR-RFLP) followed by enzyme ScaI digestion.

Associations between CD14 polymorphism and UC

The pooled OR from all included studies indicated a significant association between *CD14* polymorphism and increased UC risk in allelic comparison (OR = 1.21, 95% CI: 1.02–1.43; P = 0.027) with low possibility of publication bias as reflected by the suggestive asymmetry of funnel plot (Figure 2) and the Egger's test (P = 0.25), although there was strong evidence of between-study heterogeneity (I^2 = 73.5%, P<0.001). The magnitude of OR

in allele comparison was similar to the homozygote (OR = 1.44, 95% CI: 1.03–2.01; P = 0.033) as well as dominant models (OR = 1.36, 95% CI: 1.06–1.75; P = 0.016), while no significant association was found in recessive model (OR = 1.19, 95% CI: 0.96–1.48, P = 0.112).

Considering the fact that study design, the ethnicity difference, as well as the method of genotype might attribute to the sources of heterogeneity, we conducted separate analyses according to these factors.

In view of study design, no obvious association existed in the population-based subgroup and NA group, but significant association between *CD14* C-260T polymorphism and UC risk was observed across all genetic models, in the hospital-based subgroup (Table 2).

Further subgroup analysis by ethnicity suggested heterogeneous associations of C-260T polymorphism with UC, by showing that there was significant association among Asian populations, whereas no substantive changes was observed in Caucasians in any kind of comparisons (Figure 3).

To evaluate the possible effect of genotyping methods on the variability of overall estimates, studies were divided into PCR-based subgroup and Taqman or Probe subgroup, and importantly the magnitude of association in PCR-based studies was reinforced with the -260T allele conferring a significant risk effect on UC (OR = 1.29; 95% CI: 1.06–1.56; P = 0.009), whereas this effect was reversed in Taqman or Probe subgroup studies with no attainable significance (OR = 0.99; 95% CI: 0.70–1.39; P = 0.956).

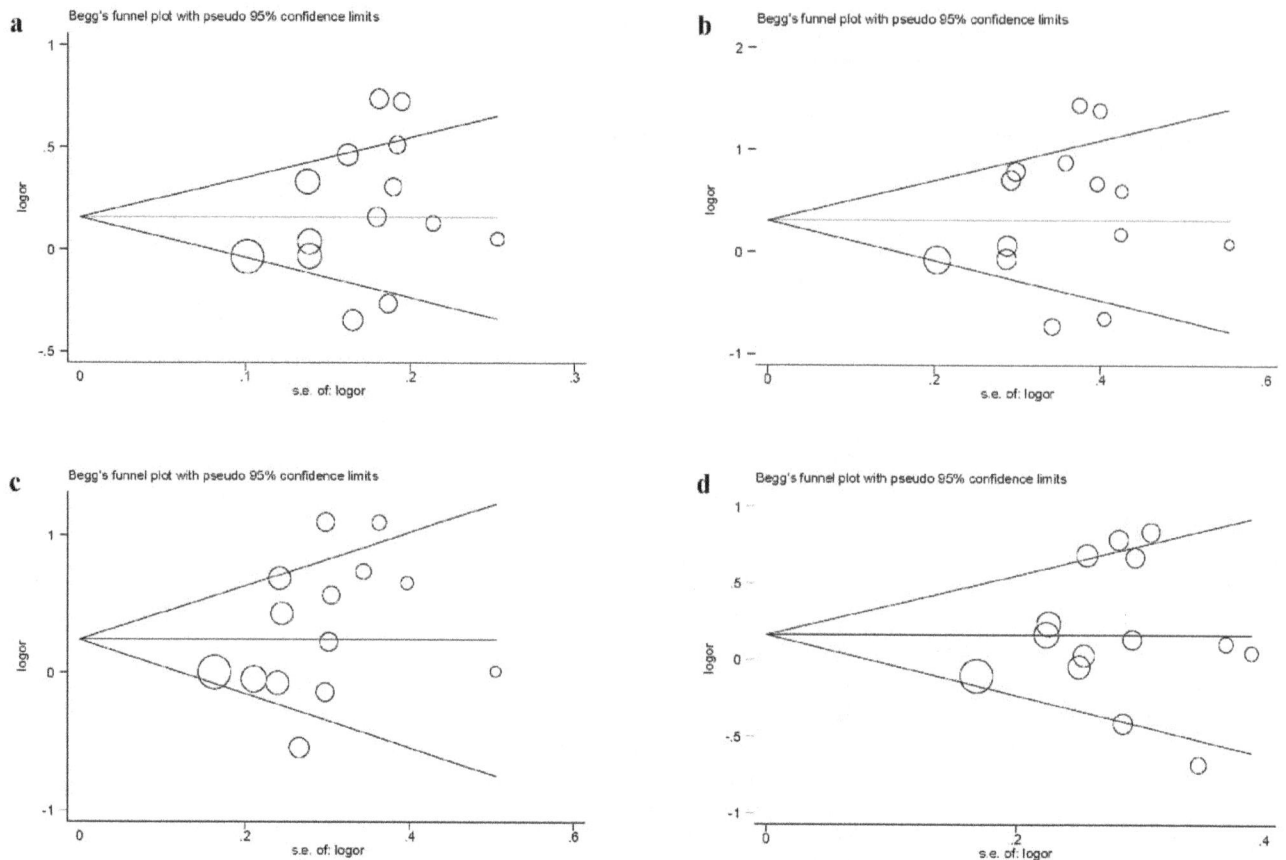

Figure 2. Begg's funnel plots of publication bias test for CD14 C-260T polymorphism with UC (a. -260T vs.-260C allele; b. -260TT vs. -260CC; c. dominant model; d. recessive model). Vertical axis represents the log of OR; horizontal axis represents the SE of log(OR). Funnel plots are drawn with 95% confidence limits. OR, odds ratio; SE, standard error. The graphic symbols represents the data in the plot be sized proportional to the inverse variance.

Associations between CD14 polymorphism and CD

Overall no significant association was found for *CD14* C-260T polymorphism in allele comparison (OR = 1.10, 95% CI: 0.96–1.25; P = 0.167), homozygote (OR = 1.18, 95% CI: 0.92–1.52, P = 0.201), dominant model (OR = 1.05, 95% CI: 0.88–1.23, P = 0.603) and recessive model (OR = 1.20; 95% CI: 0.97–1.49; P = 0.09), even in Asians or Caucasians stratified by ethnicity. However, subgroup analyses by study design detected significance for allele comparison (OR = 1.40; 95% CI: 1.01–1.94; P = 0.046), homozygote model (OR = 1.82; 95% CI: 1.00–3.32; P = 0.05) with increased CD risk, in hospital-based studies, even for the recessive models (OR = 1.67; 95% CI: 1.05–2.65; P = 0.03). When we conducted an stratified analysis by the genotyping methods, there were obvious differences. For example, a increased risk was observed in allele comparison (OR = 1.18, 95% CI: 1.00–1.38; P = 0.045) and homozygote model (OR = 1.35, 95% CI: 1.00–1.81, P = 0.049) for PCR-based subgroup; whereas no materially change in odds was observed in Taqman or Probe subgroup studies (Table 2).

Publication Bias

As reflected by the funnel plots (Figure 2) and the corresponding Egger's test, there was a low probability of publication bias for the *CD14* gene C-260T polymorphisms under study.

Discussion

To the best of our knowledge, the present study involving 8439 subjects represents the first meta-analysis investigating the relationship between *CD14* gene C-260T polymorphism and risk for IBD. Our results demonstrated that -260T allele carriers were at moderate increased risk of developing UC, especially in Asians, although this finding might suffer from the disturbance of significant heterogeneity. Moreover, differences in ethnicity and study design were identified as potential sources of heterogeneity. Furthermore, the relatively large samples examined and low probability of publication bias as reflected by visual inspection of the funnel plots along with Egger's tests indicated the robustness of our results.

It is inevitable to encounter genetic heterogeneity in any disease identification strategy [38]. As exemplified in the present study, frequency of -260T allele in patients differed remarkably between Caucasians and Asians (65.98% vs. 48.47% in UC, 54.76% vs. 48.82% in CD), leaving open the question that divergent genetic backgrounds or linkage disequilibrium patterns may account for this difference. Meanwhile, the possibility of *CD14* gene C-260T being in close linkage with different nearby causal variants in different populations cannot be excluded. Additionally, it is widely believed that genetic markers in predisposition to IBD vary across geographical and racial groups. As evidenced, nucleotide oligo-merization domain (NOD)2/caspase-activation recruitmentdo-mains (CARD)-15 polymorphisms have been strongly associated

Table 2. Subgroup analysis of CD14 C-260T gene polymorphisms and IBD (CD and UC).

Variables	Allele contrast		Homozygote model		Dominant model		Recessive model	
	OR (95% CI)	p	OR (95% CI)	p	OR (95% CI)	p	OR (95% CI)	p
CD14 C-260T gene polymorphism and CD								
Total	1.10(0.96,1.25)	0.167	1.18(0.92,1.52)	0.201	1.05(0.88,1.23)	0.603	1.20(0.97,1.49)	0.090
Descent of populations								
Caucasians	1.05(0.93,1.18)	0.479	1.08(0.85,1.38)	0.510	1.00(0.85,1.18)	0.991	1.12(0.91,1.38)	0.265
Asians	1.49(0.84,2.66)	0.171	2.03(0.70,5.91)	0.193	1.53(0.83,2.82)	0.169	1.77(0.76,4.13)	0.185
Source of controls								
HB	1.40(1.01,1.94)	0.046	1.82(1.00,3.32)	0.050	1.36(0.92,2.01)	0.127	1.67(1.05,2.65)	0.030
PB	0.99(0.88,1.11)	0.808	0.97(0.77,1.23)	0.801	0.96(0.79,1.16)	0.669	1.00(0.83,1.22)	0.970
NA	1.02(0.81,1.29)	0.879	1.03(0.64,1.65)	0.914	0.95(0.69,1.31)	0.761	1.10(0.72,1.69)	0.663
Genotyping methods								
PCR-based	1.18(1.00,1.38)	0.045	1.35(1.00,1.81)	0.049	1.12(0.93,1.36)	0.225	1.33(1.03,1.71)	0.027
Probe or Taqman	0.93(0.77,1.13)	0.459	0.86(0.58,1.26)	0.430	0.87(0.62,1.23)	0.444	0.93(0.69,1.24)	0.607
CD14 C-260T gene polymorphism and UC								
Total	1.21(1.02,1.43)	0.027	1.44(1.03,2.01)	0.033	1.36(1.06,1.75)	0.016	1.19(0.96,1.48)	0.112
Descent of populations								
Caucasians	1.01(0.87,1.19)	0.866	1.01(0.73,1.41)	0.938	1.09(0.83,1.43)	0.538	0.95(0.79,1.15)	0.626
Asians	1.58(1.28,1.95)	0.000	2.51(1.77,3.55)	0.000	1.97(1.46,2.65)	0.000	1.69(1.27,2.25)	0.000
Source of controls								
HB	1.54(1.08,2.20)	0.017	2.27(1.11,4.66)	0.025	1.92(1.12,3.31)	0.018	1.65(1.10,2.48)	0.016
PB	1.03(0.88,1.20)	0.754	1.09(0.73,1.61)	0.679	1.16(0.85,1.58)	0.354	0.95(0.75,1.20)	0.674
NA	1.20(0.88,1.63)	0.251	1.37(0.77,2.45)	0.287	1.24(0.80,1.91)	0.336	1.25(0.85,1.85)	0.258
Genotyping methods								
PCR-based	1.29(1.06,1.56)	0.009	1.63(1.12,2.36)	0.010	1.48(1.13,1.94)	0.005	1.30(1.01,1.68)	0.044
Probe or Taqman	0.99(0.70,1.39)	0.956	0.98(0.48,2.00)	0.954	1.06(0.57,1.95)	0.863	0.93(0.68,1.28)	0.668

Abbreviations: OR = odds ratio; CI = confidence interval; HB = Hospital based; PB = Population based; NA = Not available.

with CD in Caucasians [39,40], but not in individuals of Asian descent [41,42]. Accordingly, in our ethnicity-stratified analyses, *CD14* gene C-260T polymorphism exhibited remarkable heterogeneity with UC across ethnic groups, with significance attained in Asians but not in Caucasians, suggesting that *CD14* C-260T might exert a pleiotropic impact in the pathogenesis of UC or interact with other genetic or environmental factors. Furthermore, CD14 is a monocytic differentiation antigen that regulates innate immune responses to pathogens. *CD14* C-260T polymorphism has been reported to be associated with some immune-related diseases, such as allergic rhinitis [43], pediatric asthma [44] and juvenile idiopathic arthritis [45], most in Asians [46]. These results are similar to ours, and may provide a hint for exploring the complex relationship between CD14 genetic polymorphisms, ethnic difference and susceptibility to human immune-related diseases. To unravel this uncertainty, more and more large, well-designed studies are required to understand the genetic variability of IBD.

Besides the disturbing influence of ethnicity in this meta-analysis, it should still be treated with caution that differences in study design constituted another potential source of heterogeneity. Although positive association of *CD14* gene C-260T polymorphism with UC risk was observed across all genetic models in hospital-based studies, we run the risk of overestimating this association in view of the striking weaknesses of this type of design, such as population stratification and admixture. To obtain

convincing evidence, well-designed studies with less error-prone methods are encouraged.

So far, as two major subtypes of IBD, CD and UC are believed to share overlapping but distinct clinical and pathological features, and have great differences in etiology and genetic backgrounds [47,48]. In this study, we found that carriers of -260T allele were at moderate increased risk of developing UC, but not in CD, indicating the different roles of *CD14* polymorphism in the IBD different subgroups. Given the insufficient study power in each subgroup, much more research within the framework of genetics and biology is warranted.

Despite the clear strengths of our study including relatively large sample sizes and robustness of statistical analyses, interpretation of our current study, however, should be viewed in light of several technical limitations. First, all included studies were cross-sectional in design, which precludes us to make inference on causality. Second, because only published studies were retrieved and articles in languages other than English or Chinese were not included, publication bias might be possible, even though our funnel plots and statistical tests indicated no observable bias. Third, our results were based on unadjusted estimates. It seems likely that the *CD14* gene C-260T polymorphism individually make a moderate contribution to risk prediction in UC patients, but whether the polymorphism integrated with other risk factors will enhance the prediction requires additional research. Thus, a more precise analysis should be conducted with individual data, which would

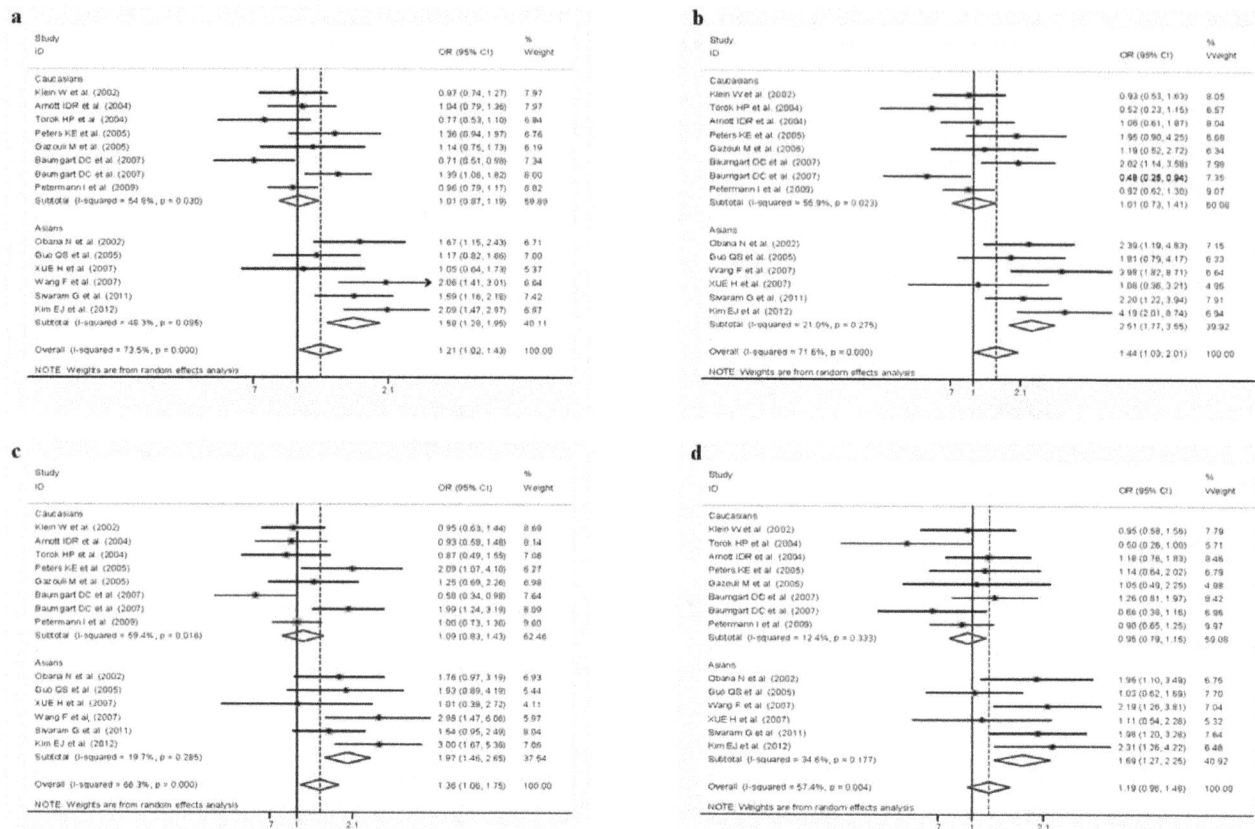

Figure 3. Subgroup analyses of CD14 C-260T polymorphism to UC by ethnicity (a. -260T vs. -260C allele; b. -260TT vs. -260CC; c. dominant model; d. recessive model). There was significant association among Asian populations, whereas no substantive changes was observed in Caucasians in any kind of comparisons.

allow for the adjustment by other co-varieties such as age, gender, lifestyle and other genetic factors.

Taken together, we expand previously individual studies on IBD by suggesting that *CD14* gene C-260T polymorphism might contribute to the occurrence of UC, especially in Asians. Also our observations leave open the question regarding the heterogeneous effect of -260T allele across different ethnic populations. Nonetheless, for practical reasons, we hope that this study will not remain

just another endpoint of research instead of a beginning to establish the background data for further investigation on pathphysiological mechanisms of *CD14* gene on IBD.

Author Contributions

Conceived and designed the experiments: J. Zhong. Performed the experiments: ZW JH RF. Analyzed the data: ZW JH J. Zhou. Contributed reagents/materials/analysis tools: ZW JH. Wrote the paper: ZW JH.

References

1. Vermeire S, Rutgeerts P (2005) Current status of genetics research in inflammatory bowel disease. Genes Immun 6: 637–645.
2. Abraham C, Cho JH (2009) Inflammatory bowel disease. N Engl J Med 361: 2066–2078.
3. Thompson AI, Lees CW (2011) Genetics of ulcerative colitis. Inflamm Bowel Dis 17: 831–848.
4. Franke A, McGovern DP, Barrett JC, Wang K, Radford-Smith GL, et al. (2010) Genome-wide meta-analysis increases to 71 the number of confirmed Crohn's disease susceptibility loci. Nat Genet 42: 1118–1125.
5. Cho JH, Brant SR (2011) Recent insights into the genetics of inflammatory bowel disease. Gastroenterology 140: 1704–1712.
6. Lee JC, Parkes M (2011) Genome-wide association studies and Crohn's disease. Brief Funct Genomics 10: 71–76.
7. Fukata M, Abreu MT (2007) TLR4 signalling in the intestine in health and disease. Biochem Soc Trans 35: 1473–1478.
8. Rakoff-Nahoum S, Paglino J, Eslami-Varzaneh F, Edberg S, et al.(2004) Recognition of commensal microflora by toll-like receptors is required for intestinal homeostasis. Cell 118: 229–241.

9. Fukata M, Michelsen KS, Eri R, Thomas LS, Hu B, et al. (2005) Toll-like receptor-4 is required for intestinal response to epithelial injury and limiting bacterial translocation in a murine model of acute colitis. Am J Physiol Gastrointest Liver Physiol 288: G1055–1065.
10. Wright SD, Ramos RA, Tobias PS, Ulevitch RJ, Mathison JC (1990) CD14, a receptor for complexes of lipopolysaccharide (LPS) and LPS binding protein. Science 249: 1431–1433.
11. Lakatos PL, Kiss LS, Palatka K, Altorjay I, Antal-Szalmas P, et al. (2011) Serum lipopolysaccharide-binding protein and soluble CD14 are markers of disease activity in patients with Crohn's disease. Inflamm Bowel Dis 17: 767–777.
12. Gazouli M, Mantzaris G, Kotsinas A, Zacharatos P, Papalambros E, et al. (2005) Association between polymorphisms in the Toll-like receptor 4, CD14, and CARD15/NOD2 and inflammatory bowel disease in the Greek population. World J Gastroenterol 11: 681–685.
13. Kim EJ, Chung WC, Lee KM, Paik CN, Jung SH, et al. (2012) Association between toll-like receptors/CD14 gene polymorphisms and inflammatory bowel disease in Korean population. J Korean Med Sci 27: 72–77.

14. Zanoni I, Ostuni R, Marek LR, Barresi S, Barbalat R, et al. (2011) CD14 controls the LPS-induced endocytosis of Toll-like receptor 4. Cell 147: 868–880.

15. Rioux JD, Silverberg MS, Daly MJ, Steinhart AH, McLeod RS, et al. (2000) Genomewide search in Canadian families with inflammatory bowel disease reveals two novel susceptibility loci. Am J Hum Genet 66: 1863–1870.

16. Ma Y, Ohmen JD, Li Z, Bentley LG, McElree C, et al. (1999) A genome-wide search identifies potential new susceptibility loci for Crohn's disease. Inflamm Bowel Dis 5: 271–278.

17. Griga T, Wilkens C, Schmiegel W, Folwaczny C, Hagedorn M, et al. (2005) Association between the promoter polymorphism T/C at position -159 of the CD14 gene and anti-inflammatory therapy in patients with inflammatory bowel disease. Eur J Med Res 10: 183–186.

18. Baldini M, Lohman IC, Halonen M, Erickson RP, Holt PG, et al. (1999) A Polymorphism* in the 5' flanking region of the CD14 gene is associated with circulating soluble CD14 levels and with total serum immunoglobulin E. Am J Respir Cell Mol Biol 20: 976–983.

19. Peters KE, O'Callaghan NJ, Cavanaugh JA (2005) Lack of association of the CD14 promoter polymorphism–159C/T with Caucasian inflammatory bowel disease. Scand J Gastroenterol 40: 194–197.

20. Guo QS, Xia B, Jiang Y, Morre SA, Cheng L, et al. (2005) Polymorphisms of CD14 gene and TLR4 gene are not associated with ulcerative colitis in Chinese patients. Postgrad Med J 81: 526–529.

21. van Heel DA, Fisher SA, Kirby A, Daly MJ, Rioux JD, et al. (2004) Inflammatory bowel disease susceptibility loci defined by genome scan meta-analysis of 1952 affected relative pairs. Hum Mol Genet 13: 763–770.

22. Moher D, Liberati A, Tetzlaff J, Altman DG (2009) Preferred reporting items for systematic reviews and meta-analyses: the PRISMA statement. Ann Intern Med 151: 264–269, W264.

23. Cohn LD, Becker BJ (2003) How meta-analysis increases statistical power. Psychol Methods 8: 243–253.

24. Higgins JP, Thompson SG, Deeks JJ, Altman DG (2003) Measuring inconsistency in meta-analyses. BMJ 327: 557–560.

25. Baumgart DC, Buning C, Geerdts L, Schmidt HH, Genschel J, et al. (2007) The c.1-260C>T promoter variant of CD14 but not the c.896A>G (p.D299G) variant of toll-like receptor 4 (TLR4) genes is associated with inflammatory bowel disease. Digestion 76: 196–202.

26. Klausz G, Molnar T, Nagy F, Gyulai Z, Boda K, et al. (2005) Polymorphism of the heat-shock protein gene Hsp70-2, but not polymorphisms of the IL-10 and CD14 genes, is associated with the outcome of Crohn's disease. Scand J Gastroenterol 40: 1197–1204.

27. Arnott ID, Nimmo ER, Drummond HE, Fennell J, Smith BR, et al. (2004) NOD2/CARD15, TLR4 and CD14 mutations in Scottish and Irish Crohn's disease patients: evidence for genetic heterogeneity within Europe? Genes Immun 5: 417–425.

28. Obana N, Takahashi S, Kinouchi Y, Negoro K, Takagi S, et al. (2002) Ulcerative colitis is associated with a promoter polymorphism of lipopolysaccharide receptor gene, CD14. Scand J Gastroenterol 37: 699–704.

29. Ouburg S, Mallant-Hent R, Crusius JB, van Bodegraven AA, Mulder CJ, et al. (2005) The toll-like receptor 4 (TLR4) Asp299Gly polymorphism is associated with colonic localisation of Crohn's disease without a major role for the Saccharomyces cerevisiae mannan-LBP-CD14-TLR4 pathway. Gut 54: 439–440.

30. Torok HP, Glas J, Tonenchi L, Mussack T, Folwaczny C (2004) Polymorphisms of the lipopolysaccharide-signaling complex in inflammatory bowel disease: association of a mutation in the Toll-like receptor 4 gene with ulcerative colitis. Clin Immunol 112: 85–91.

31. Sivaram G, Tiwari SK, Bardia A, Anjum F, Vishnupriya S, et al. (2012) Macrophage migration inhibitory factor, Toll-like receptor 4, and CD14 polymorphisms with altered expression levels in patients with ulcerative colitis. Hum Immunol 73: 201–205.

32. Leung E, Hong J, Fraser AG, Merriman TR, Vishnu P, et al. (2005) Polymorphisms of CARD15/NOD2 and CD14 genes in New Zealand Crohn's disease patients. Immunol Cell Biol 83: 498–503.

33. Klein W, Tromm A, Griga T, Fricke H, Folwaczny C, et al. (2002) A polymorphism in the CD14 gene is associated with Crohn disease. Scand J Gastroenterol 37: 189–191.

34. Wang F, Tahara T, Arisawa T, Shibata T, Nakamura M, et al. (2007) Genetic polymorphisms of CD14 and Toll-like receptor-2 (TLR2) in patients with ulcerative colitis. J Gastroenterol Hepatol 22: 925–929.

35. Klein W, Tromm A, Griga T, Folwaczny C, Hocke M, et al. (2003) Interaction of polymorphisms in the CARD15 and CD14 genes in patients with Crohn disease. Scand J Gastroenterol 38: 834–836.

36. Petermann I, Huebner C, Browning BL, Gearry RB, Barclay ML, et al. (2009) Interactions among genes influencing bacterial recognition increase IBD risk in a population-based New Zealand cohort. Hum Immunol 70: 440–446.

37. Xue H, Ni P, Wu J, Tong J (2007) CD14 gene promoter region -159 polymorphism and its significance in patients with inflammatory bowel disease. Journal of Shanghai Jiaotong University Medical Science 27: 1127–1131.

38. Hemminki K, Lorenzo Bermejo J, Forsti A (2006) The balance between heritable and environmental aetiology of human disease. Nat Rev Genet 7: 958–965.

39. Hugot JP, Chamaillard M, Zouali H, Lesage S, Cezard JP, et al. (2001) Association of NOD2 leucine-rich repeat variants with susceptibility to Crohn's disease. Nature 411: 599–603.

40. Nagy Z, Karadi O, Rumi G, Rumi G Jr, Par A, et al. (2005) Crohn's disease is associated with polymorphism of CARD15/NOD2 gene in a Hungarian population. Ann N Y Acad Sci 1051: 45–51.

41. Yamazaki K, Takazoe M, Tanaka T, Kazumori T, Nakamura Y (2002) Absence of mutation in the NOD2/CARD15 gene among 483 Japanese patients with Crohn's disease. J Hum Genet 47: 469–472.

42. Leong RW, Armuzzi A, Ahmad T, Wong ML, Tse P, et al. (2003) NOD2/CARD15 gene polymorphisms and Crohn's disease in the Chinese population. Aliment Pharmacol Ther 17: 1465–1470.

43. Han D, She W, Zhang L (2010) Association of the CD14 gene polymorphism C-159T with allergic rhinitis. Am J Rhinol Allergy 24: e1–3.

44. Wu X, Li Y, Chen Q, Chen F, Cai P, et al. (2010) Association and gene-gene interactions of eight common single-nucleotide polymorphisms with pediatric asthma in middle china. J Asthma 47: 238–244.

45. Zeng HS, Chen XY, Luo XP (2009) The association with the -159C/T polymorphism in the promoter region of the CD14 gene and juvenile idiopathic arthritis in a Chinese Han population. J Rheumatol 36: 2025–2028.

46. Zhang Y, Tian C, Zhang J, Li X, Wan H, et al. (2011) The -159C/T polymorphism in the CD14 gene and the risk of asthma: a meta-analysis. Immunogenetics 63: 23–32.

47. Marks DJ (2011) Defective innate immunity in inflammatory bowel disease: a Crohn's disease exclusivity? Curr Opin Gastroenterol 27: 328–334.

48. Waterman M, Xu W, Stempak JM, Milgrom R, Bernstein CN, et al. (2011) Distinct and overlapping genetic loci in Crohn's disease and ulcerative colitis: correlations with pathogenesis. Inflamm Bowel Dis 17: 1936–1942.

6

Identification of Restricted Subsets of Mature microRNA Abnormally Expressed in Inactive Colonic Mucosa of Patients with Inflammatory Bowel Disease

Magali Fasseu[1,2☯], **Xavier Tréton**[1,2,3☯], **Cécile Guichard**[1,2], **Eric Pedruzzi**[1,2], **Dominique Cazals-Hatem**[1,2,4], **Christophe Richard**[1,2], **Thomas Aparicio**[1,2,5], **Fanny Daniel**[1,2], **Jean-Claude Soulé**[1,2,5], **Richard Moreau**[1,2], **Yoram Bouhnik**[1,2,3], **Marc Laburthe**[1,2], **André Groyer**[1,2*¶], **Eric Ogier-Denis**[1,2¶]

1 INSERM U773, Centre de Recherche Biomédicale Bichat Beaujon, Paris, France, 2 Université Paris 7 Denis Diderot, Paris, France, 3 Service de Gastroentérologie et d'Assistance Nutritive, Hôpital Beaujon, Clichy, France, 4 Service d'Anatomo-Pathologie, Hôpital Beaujon, Clichy, France, 5 Service de Gastroentérologie, Hôpital Xavier Bichat, Paris, France

Abstract

Background: Ulcerative Colitis (UC) and Crohn's Disease (CD) are two chronic Inflammatory Bowel Diseases (IBD) affecting the intestinal mucosa. Current understanding of IBD pathogenesis points out the interplay of genetic events and environmental cues in the dysregulated immune response. We hypothesized that dysregulated microRNA (miRNA) expression may contribute to IBD pathogenesis. miRNAs are small, non-coding RNAs which prevent protein synthesis through translational suppression or mRNAs degradation, and regulate several physiological processes.

Methodology/Findings: Expression of mature miRNAs was studied by Q-PCR in inactive colonic mucosa of patients with UC (8), CD (8) and expressed relative to that observed in healthy controls (10). Only miRNAs with highly altered expression (>5 or <0.2 -fold relative to control) were considered when Q-PCR data were analyzed. Two subsets of 14 (UC) and 23 (CD) miRNAs with highly altered expression (5.2->100 -fold and 0.05–0.19 -fold for over- and under- expression, respectively; $0.001 < p \leq 0.05$) were identified in quiescent colonic mucosa, 8 being commonly dysregulated in non-inflamed UC and CD (mir-26a,-29a,-29b,-30c,-126*,-127-3p,-196a,-324-3p). Several miRNA genes with dysregulated expression co-localize with acknowledged IBD-susceptibility loci while others, (eg. clustered on 14q32.31), map on chromosomal regions not previously recognized as IBD-susceptibility loci. In addition, *in silico* clustering analysis identified 5 miRNAs (mir-26a,-29b,-126*,-127-3p,-324-3p) that share coordinated dysregulation of expression both in quiescent and in inflamed colonic mucosa of IBD patients. Six miRNAs displayed significantly distinct alteration of expression in non-inflamed colonic biopsies of UC and CD patients (mir-196b,-199a-3p,-199b-5p,-320a,-150,-223).

Conclusions/Significance: Our study supports miRNAs as crucial players in the onset and/or relapse of inflammation from quiescent mucosal tissues in IBD patients. It allows speculating a role for miRNAs as contributors to IBD susceptibility and suggests that some of the miRNA with altered expression in the quiescent mucosa of IBD patients may define miRNA signatures for UC and CD and help develop new diagnostic biomarkers.

Editor: Guillaume Dalmasso, Emory University, United States of America

Funding: Institut National de la Sante et de la Recherche Medicale (Inserm) and in parts by grants from Association Francois Aupetit AFA, Assistance Publique-Hopitaux de Paris, Ferring Laboratories, Ipsen Laboratories, Societe Nationale Francaise de Gastro-enterologie (SNFGE), Association Francaise pour l'etude du foie (AFEF), and Programme National de Recherche en Hepato-Gastroenterologie. The funders had no role in study design, data collection and analysis, decision to publish, or preparation of the manuscript.

Competing Interests: Funding by Ipsen Laboratories was only a small part of the doctoral fellowships dedicated to Xavier Treton.

* E-mail: andre.groyer@inserm.fr

☯ These authors contributed equally to this work.

¶ These authors also contributed equally to this work.

Introduction

Ulcerative Colitis (UC) and Crohn's Disease (CD) are two subphenotypes of inflammatory bowel disease (IBD) affecting the intestinal mucosa. UC and CD share similarities such as a chronic relapsing-remitting course and common extra-intestinal manifestations. However, several differences in localization (any part of the gastrointestinal tract -CD- or restricted to the colon -UC),

endoscopic appearance and histology support differences in underlying physiopathology.

The current understanding of IBD pathogenesis points out the interplay of genetic, epigenetic and environmental factors in the dysregulated immune response of the intestinal mucosa [1–3] where inappropriate control of innate and acquired immunity plays a major role [4].

Long term follow-up stressed that basal colonic lesions extend progressively in more than 50% of UC patients [5]. In CD patients, ileal recurrence involving microscopically quiescent tissues at the time of ileo-colonic resection was reported to reach 73% at one year [6]. These observations suggest that quiescent mucosa of IBD patients display increased susceptibility to inflammation. In this connection, animals models (mice carrying intestinal epithelial cell-specific invalidation of genes involved in the unfolded protein response -XBP1, X-box Protein 1- or essential for embryonic development of the colon -HNF4, Hepatic Nuclear Factor 4) support the notion that epithelial cell dysfunction in the quiescent mucosa can trigger intestinal inflammation [7–8]. However the early epithelial disorders that, in pre-inflammatory states, confer susceptibility to uncontrolled mucosal inflammation remain poorly understood.

Strong evidence supports UC and CD as complex genetic disorders with significant overlap and mandates systematic approaches to identify causal molecular events. **First**, Genome Wide Association Scans (GWAS) [9–19] and candidate gene approach [20–25] led to the identification of more than 30 susceptibility loci for CD and UC and identified "IBD-specific" gene variants within these loci (eg. *CARD15*, *TNFSF15*, *IL23R*, *ATG16L1*, *IRGM*, *PTPN2*). **Otherwise**, genome-wide arrays and subtractive hybridization studies identified hundreds of mRNAs with altered expression in non-inflamed [26,27] and in inflamed [28–32] colonic biopsies obtained from UC and CD patients. This provided valuable insights into dysregulated gene expression associated with IBD. In this connection, we hypothesized that dysregulated microRNA (miRNA) gene expression and/or pri-/pre- miRNA maturation may contribute to IBD pathogenesis.

miRNAs are small ($\sim$18–24 nt), non-coding RNAs which, by base-pairing to complementary sequences in the 3'-UTR of selected mRNA targets, prevent protein synthesis either by translational suppression [33,34] or by degradation of their target mRNAs [35,36]. miRNAs are regulators of early development, cell fate determination, differentiation, proliferation, apoptosis [37–39] and dysregulation of their expression has been involved in various human diseases such as cancer [40–44], developmental abnormalities [45], muscular disorders [46] and inflammatory diseases [47–51].

In the present paper, **our first objective** was to pinpoint alterations in the pattern of miRNA expression in the non-inflamed colonic mucosa of UC and CD patients relative to that of healthy subjects. Indeed, such altered miRNA expression in the quiescent colonic mucosa of IBD patients may account for epithelial dysfunction in the absence of epithelial damage (eg. ulcerations) and sensitize the mucosa to severe inflammation and infiltration of immune cells. **Our second objective** was to search whether dysregulated expression of several miRNAs may be coordinated and thus contribute to IBD susceptibility.

Results

In a first series of experiments, miRNA expression was quantified in right and left colon from healthy control subjects. Measuring the abundance of 321 mature human miRNA transcripts by real-time Q-PCR, preliminary analysis ($2^{-\Delta CT}$) showed that right and left colon displayed similar patterns of miRNA expression, as exemplified for a subset of miRNAs in Table S1.

In a second series of experiments, miRNA expression was measured by real-time Q-PCR in biopsies from UC and CD patients (Table 1; quiescent and inflamed mucosal tissues, Figure S1). Overall, miRNA expression varied continuously from -11.06 to $+20.31$ -fold (quiescent and inflamed CD biopsies) and from -7.50 to $+18.34$ -fold (quiescent and inflamed UC biopsies) when

Table 1. Characteristics of patients with CD or UC.

	Ulcerative Colitis	Cronh's Disease
N° of patients	8	8
Male/Female	5/3	4/4
Age (* y)		
Mean	45.9	37.6
Range	33–57	20–58
Disease duration (y)		
Mean	10.5	8.8
Range	1–21	0.5–23
# Medications (%)		
5 ASA	6 (75)	2 (25)
CS	-	2 (25)
AZA	1 (13)	2 (25)
MTX, IFX	-	1 (13)
CS, 5 ASA	1 (13)	-
None	-	1 (13)

*y, years;
#Medications : CS: steroids/5 ASA: 5 aminosalicylates/AZA: azathioprine/IFX: infliximab/MTX: methotrexate.

compared to healthy control subjects. However, a careful inspection of the data showed that even under our strictly controlled (i) biopsy selection (Figure S2), (ii) RT and (iii) Q-PCR conditions, miRNA expression levels were variable among patients (Figure S3). Thus, in order to avoid false/erroneous classification of miRNAs as up- and down- regulated in mucosal biopsies of IBD patients, only miRNAs with alterations of expression that fitted stringent thresholds ($2^{-\Delta\Delta CT}>5$-fold and $2^{-\Delta\Delta CT}<0.2$-fold, respectively) were considered.

miRNA expression is altered in both UC and CD

In order to check for specific modifications that may account for epithelial cell dysfunction in the quiescent colonic mucosa of IBD patients, we focused on biopsies scored grades 0 and 1 (both grades were observed in healthy controls and in quiescent UC and CD mucosa; Table S2). However, grades 2–4 (inflamed mucosa; *see* Figure S1) were also studied for comparison of both stages of the diseases.

According to our stringent criteria for the selection of miRNAs with altered expression, up- and down- regulations were balanced in UC (45.47% and 54.5%, respectively), whereas up-regulation was predominant (88.2%) in CD.

UC. 173 miRNAs were expressed above the level of detection ($C_T<35$). Of the 22 miRNAs that fit our stringent criteria, only 14 (7 up- and 7 down- regulated) exhibited significant differential expression when non-inflamed UC and healthy control tissues were compared ($0.001<p<0.05$; non parametric Mann-Whitney test), (Table S3, Figure 1A). With respect to cut-off values and statistical significance the expression of 9 miRNAs was dysregulated in both quiescent and inflamed UC mucosa and that of 1 miRNAs was specifically dysregulated in quiescent UC mucosa (mir-196a).

CD. 204 miRNAs were expressed above the level of detection. Of the 33 miRNAs that fit our stringent criteria, only 23 (all up-regulated) exhibited significant differential expression when non-inflamed CD and healthy control tissues were compared

(A) Ulcerative Colitis

Non-inflamed UC   Inflamed UC

1/5   9/17   4/6

mir-185
mir-196a
mir-214
mir-376a
mir-424

mir-15a
mir-26a
mir-29a
mir-29b
mir-30c
mir-126*
mir-127-3p
mir-324-3p

mir-1
mir-188-5p
mir-196b
mir-199a-3p
mir-199b-5p
mir-215
mir-320a
mir-346
mir-370

mir-7
mir-31
mir-135b
mir-200c
mir-223
mir-382

(B) Crohn's Disease

Non-inflamed CD   Inflamed CD

4/5   18/28   5/13

mir-9*
mir-30a*
mir-30c
mir-223
mir-451

mir-7
mir-26a
mir-29a
mir-29b
mir-30b
mir-34c-5p
mir-125b
mir-126*
mir-127-3p
mir-133b
mir-155
mir-185
mir-196a
mir-324-3p

mir-15a
mir-19a
mir-21
mir-22
mir-29c
mir-31
mir-106a
mir-146a
mir-146b-5p
mir-150
mir-152
mir-378
mir-379
mir-423-3p

let-7g
mir-9
mir-20b
mir-26b
mir-34a
mir-126
mir-130a
mir-130b
mir-181c
mir-375
mir-18a*
mir-200a*
mir-378*

(C) Ulcerative Colitis and Crohn's Disease

Non-inflamed UC   Non-inflamed CD

7/12   7/10   15/23

mir-1
mir-188-5p
mir-196b
mir-199a-3p
mir-199b-5p
mir-214
mir-215
mir-320a
mir-346
mir-370
mir-376a
mir-424

mir-15a
mir-26a
mir-29a
mir-29b
mir-30c
mir-126*
mir-127-3p
mir-185
mir-196a
mir-324-3p

mir-7
mir-19a
mir-22
mir-29c
mir-30b
mir-34c-5p
mir-106a
mir-125b
mir-133b
mir-152
mir-155
mir-378

mir-9*
mir-21
mir-30a*
mir-31
mir-146a
mir-146b-5p
mir-223
mir-379
mir-423-3p
mir-451

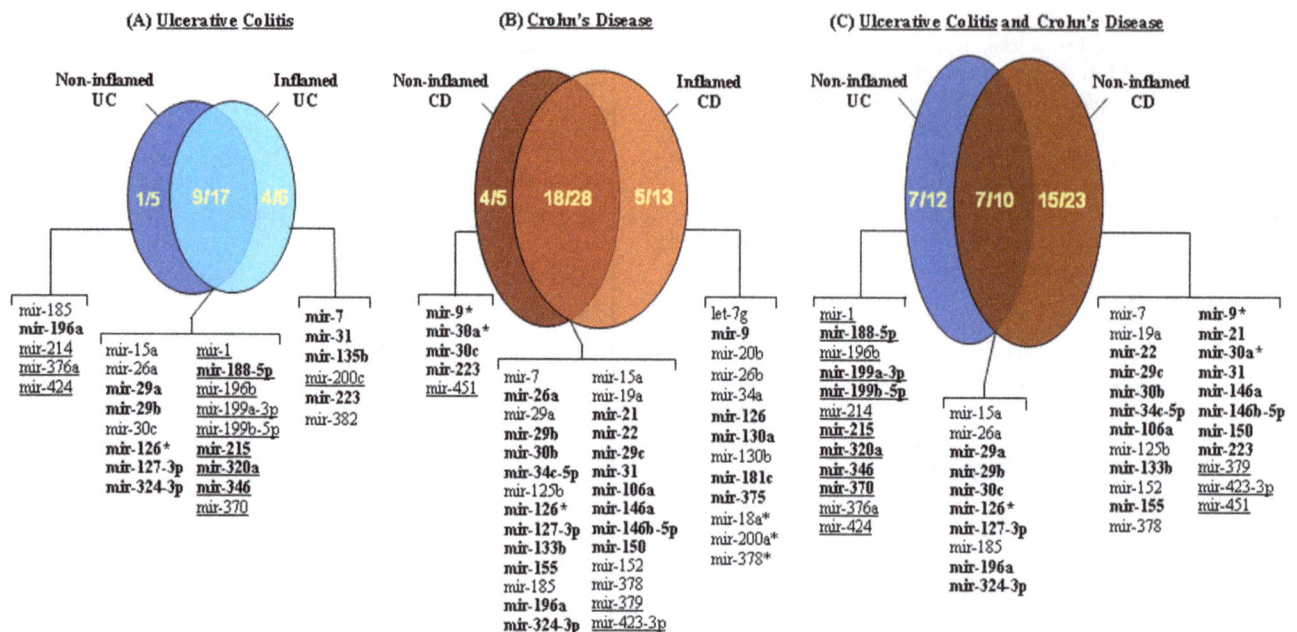

Figure 1. Disease- and stage- specific alterations of miRNA expression. miRNA expression was measured in non-inflamed and inflamed UC and CD tissues and computed vs. that measured in healthy controls. The total numbers of miRNAs that were underexpressed and overexpressed in non-inflamed (dark-colored ovals) or inflamed (light-colored ovals) IBD tissues, as well as those that were commonly altered in both states of the disease (intersect between light and dark-colored ovals) were determined. UC (A) or CD (B) tissues were considered independently. (C) miRNAs that were underexpressed and overexpressed in non-inflamed UC (dark-blue) or non-inflamed CD (dark-red), as well as those that were commonly altered in both diseases (intersect between ovals) were determined. Underexpressed miRNAs are underlined. Bolded characters, miRNA with statistically significant dysregulation of expression relative to healthy controls (p≤0.05).

$(0.002 < p < 0.05$; non parametric Mann-Whitney test), (Table S4, Figure 1B). With respect to cut-off values and statistical significance the expression of 18 miRNAs were dysregulated in both quiescent and inflamed CD mucosa and that of 4 miRNAs were specifically dysregulated in quiescent CD mucosa (mir-9*, mir-30a*, mir-30c, mir-223).

Finally, taking into account cut-off values and statistical significance, we also noticed alterations in miRNA expression specific to inflamed UC or CD tissues (4 and 5 miRNAs, respectively) (Figure 1A, B).

Common and specific alterations in miRNA expression in UC and CD

With respect to cut-off values and statistical significance 8 miRNAs shared common altered expression in non-inflamed CD and in non-inflamed UC (Figure 1C, Table S5), of which 6 (all but mir-30c, and mir-196a) were also overexpressed both in inflamed UC and in inflamed CD biopsies.

On the other hand, the expression of 6 miRNAs was statistically different in non-inflamed colonic biopsies of UC and CD patients (mir-150, $p = 0.0273$; mir-196b, $p = 0.0472$; mir-199a-3p, $p = 0.0472$; mir-199b-5p, $p = 0.0283$; mir-223, $p = 0.0357$ and mir-320a, $p = 0.0163$; non-parametric Mann-Whitney test) (Figure 2). These miRNAs, and an additional selection of 9 miRNAs (selected in an unsupervised manner using the Gene-Pattern "ComparativeMarkerSelection" module) (Owing to patent pending the identity of these miRNA is not disclosed in the manuscript) were tested for their ability to discriminate between UC and CD. Classification was performed with a supervised algorithm (GenePattern "KNNXValidation" module). Based on the clinical classification of our panel of patients as UC or CD, the

selection of 15 miRNAs was able to predict 15/16 patients in their true class (Table 2).

Altogether, these data unambiguously show that altered miRNA expression pre-exists in non-inflamed UC and CD mucosa.

Concerted regulation of miRNA expression in UC and CD

We then sought whether the altered levels of miRNA noticed in both quiescent UC and CD colonic mucosa could be accounted for by coordinated regulation(s) of miRNA expression. In silico clustering was achieved in an unsupervised manner using a K-Means algorithm, the expression data being partitioned into 20 distinct computational clusters. Interestingly, 7/8 miRNAs overexpressed both in non-inflamed UC and CD tissues (mir-26a, mir-29a, mir-29b, mir-30c, mir-126*, mir-127-3p, mir-324-3p), localized on different chromosomes, were assigned to a single computational cluster (cluster #7) when examining UC data, and to two such clusters (cluster #7: mir-26a, mir-30c, mir-127-3p, mir-324-3p and cluster #13: mir-29a, mir-29b, mir-126*) when CD data were inspected (Table 3). Moreover, five of these miRNAs (mir-26a, mir-29b, mir-126*, mir-127-3p, mir-324-3p) were also assigned to a single computational cluster when inflamed UC (cluster #7) and CD (cluster #13) data were classified. This suggested common regulation of expression for mir-26a, mir-29b, mir-126*, mir-127-3p and mir-324-3p.

Chromosomal localization of miRNA genes with altered expression

The chromosomal distribution of miRNA genes with altered expression in UC and CD mucosa was not even. Indeed, 9 chromosomes (1, 5, 9, 11, 14, 15, 17, 19 and X) housed ≥4 and up to 12 miRNA genes with dysregulated expression (overall: ~70%

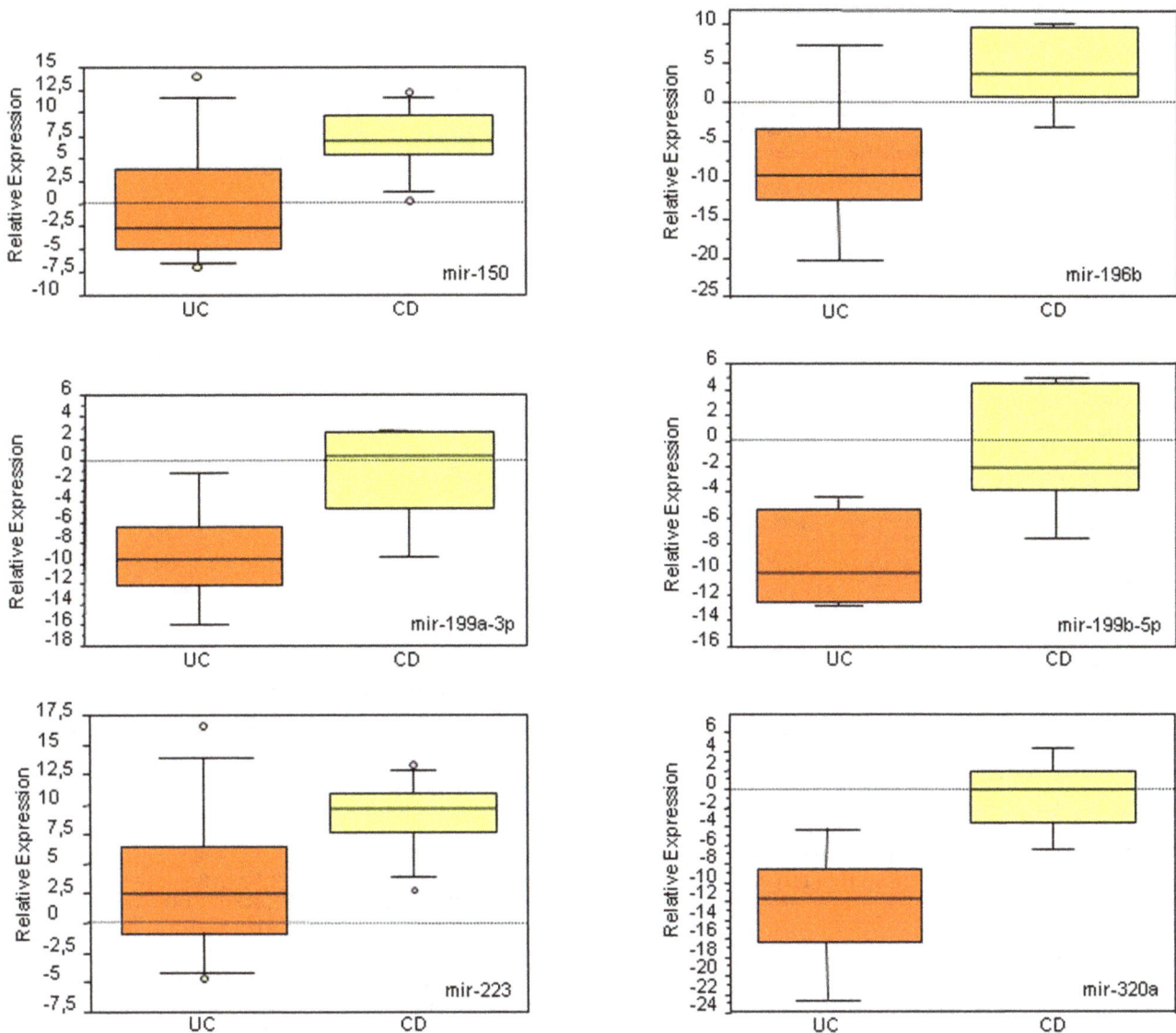

Figure 2. miRNAs with differentially altered expression in non-inflamed UC and CD tissues : Box-whisker plot analysis. miRNA expression was measured in non-inflamed colonic mucosa obtained from UC and CD patients (8 patients/IBD) and computed *vs.* that measured in healthy controls. Data corresponding to 6 miRNAs (mir-150, mir-196b, mir-199a-3p, mir-199b-5p, mir-223 and mir-320a) with statistically different alteration of expression in UC and CD mucosal tissues are presented as box-whisker plots [78] (box, 25–75%; whisker, 10–90%; line, median); $p < 0.05$.

of such miRNAs genes) (Table S6, Figure S4). The chromosomal loci where miRNA genes with dysregulated expression are localized encompass either one, two (miRNA duplexes) or more (miRNA clusters) distinct miRNA genes.

Interestingly, it could be observed that several miRNAs mapped within acknowledged IBD susceptibility loci (IBD-2, 3, 5 and 6), or colocalized with genetic variations identified in several GWAS studies that *(i)* account for part of the overall genetic susceptibility to CD and *(ii)* contribute to UC pathogenesis (Figure S5, Table S7). None mapped with IBD susceptibility loci 1, 4, 7, 8 and 9.

Otherwise, one chromosomal miRNA cluster (on chromosome 14q32.31) and several miRNA duplexes (6q13, 7q32.3, 9q34.11–q34.3, 15q26.1; 17p13.1–p13.3, 22q11.21, Xq26.2) were identified that map on chromosomal regions that have not been previously reported as IBD-susceptibility loci (Figure S5, Table 4). Interestingly, in the majority of loci, alterations of miRNA expression were observed in quiescent UC and CD tissues.

Alteration of miRNA expression: *in silico* characterization of target transcripts

Identification of a subset of 8 miRNAs that share common regulated overexpression in both UC and CD (*see* Table S5) could represent the first step towards the identification of regulatory networks, the dysregulation of which could be involved in the pathophysiology of IBD. *In silico*, 4094 genes (372 strictly down-regulated genes) stand as putative targets for these miRNAs.

Exploring the molecular functions associated to these gene products using The Gene Ontology, GeneCards and GeneNote data bases, we found associations to several biological processes (Figure 3). These include *(i)* cell proliferation (Cyclins D1, D2 and E1, PCNA, CDKs 6 and 8, GADD45A, RB1), *(ii)* apoptosis (BCL2, Caspase 2, C/EBP β,γ, DAPK, FOXO3, PTEN), *(iii)* autophagy (ATG 4a, 5 and 9a, Beclin-1, CDKN1B, IFNγ), *(iv)* extracellular matrix organization, cell adhesion and cell surface marker gene expression (COL(1,11,12,15,16)A1, Integrin-$\alpha_{1,2,3,5}$,

Table 2. Achievement of patient's class (UC or CD) prediction using the selection of 15 miRNAs.

Patient	True Class		Predicted Class	Confidence	Correct ?	
	Initial Diagnostic	Reassessment After Clinical Follow-up			Relative to Initial Diagnostic	After Clinical Follow-up/ Reassessment
CD_Quiescent_28	Cd	Not modified	Uc	1	false	
CD_Quiescent_102	Cd	Not modified	Cd	1	true	
CD_Quiescent_111	Cd	Not modified	Cd	1	true	
CD_Quiescent_120	Cd	Not modified	Cd	1	true	
CD_Quiescent_130	Cd	Not modified	Cd	0,7894	true	
CD_Quiescent_137	Cd	Not modified	Cd	1	true	
CD_Quiescent_158	Cd	Not modified	Cd	1	true	
CD_Quiescent_160	Cd	Not modified	Cd	1	true	
UC_Quiescent_107	Uc	Not modified	Uc	1	true	
UC_Quiescent_125	Uc	Not modified	Uc	0,8144	true	
UC_Quiescent_121	Uc	Not modified	Uc	1	true	
UC_Quiescent_114	Uc	Not modified	Uc	0,5339	true	
UC_Quiescent_109	Uc	Not modified	Uc	0,5508	true	
UC_Quiescent_13	**Uc**	**Cd**	**Cd**	0,6229	**false**	**true**
UC_Quiescent_15	Uc	Not modified	Uc	0,6415	true	
UC_Quiescent_132	Uc	Not modified	Uc	0,5176	true	

The 6 miRNAs that displayed significantly distinct alteration of expression in non-inflamed colonic biopsies of UC and CD patients and 9 additional miRNAs, which were selected in an unsupervised manner making use of the GenePattern "ComparativeMarkerSelection" module, were tested for their putative use as "biomarkers". The test was carried out using the "KNNXValidation" module computed on line from the GenePattern server. **Of note**, patient "UC_Quiescent_13", initially classified as UC on the basis of clinical criteria, was predicted as CD using our selection of 15 miRNAs. Interestingly its clinical follow-up for several years led to the reassessment of its clinical classification as CD.

Table 3. Concerted regulation of expression of miRNAs in non-inflamed and inflamed CD and UC tissues.

Overexpressed miRNA			
UC		**CD**	
Non-inflamed	**Inflamed**	**Non-inflamed**	**Inflamed**
Cluster #7 :	Cluster #7 :	Cluster #7 :	Cluster #13 :
mir-15a	mir-7	mir-7	**mir-26a**
mir-26a	**mir-26a**	**mir-26a**	**mir-29b**
mir-29a	mir-29a	mir-30b	**mir-126***
mir-29b	**mir-29b**	mir-30c	mir-155
mir-30c	mir-31	**mir-127-3p**	**mir-127-3p**
mir-126*	**mir-126***	mir-155	mir-185
mir-127-3p	**mir-127-3p**	mir-223	mir-196a
mir-324-3p	mir-135b	**mir-324-3p**	**mir-324-3p**
	mir-324-3p		mir-378
		Cluster #13 :	
		mir-29a	
		mir-29b	
		mir-126*	
		mir-196a	

Alterations in miRNA expression (8 UC, 8 CD patients) were clustered using a K-Means algorithm (computed on-line on the GenePattern server), independently in each IBD and for each state of the disease. Clusters that encompass several miRNAs with similarly up-regulated expression are highlighted (bold characters).

$\beta_{1,3}$, Laminin γ_1, MMPs 13 and 16, Keratin 5, NCAM1), *(v)* oxidative stress (GPX4, OXR1, OSXR1), *(vi)* the unfolded protein response (HSPA5, HSPA2, SERP1, XBP-1, EIF2AK3, ETF1) *(vii)* innate and adaptive immunity (IL1A, IL10, IL1R1, IL6R, IRAK2, p40^{phox}, TLR10, CXCL2, 12 and 14, CXCR4, NFATC3 and C4, PREX1). In addition, several of these genes are acknowledged IBD-susceptibility genes or are localized at replicated risk loci identified by GWAS (*eg.* ATG16L1, IL10, IL12B, JAK2, ARPC2, PTGER4, ZNF365, NKX2-3, PTPN2, PTPN22, C11orf30, ORMDL3, STAT3 (Table S8).

Discussion

In the present study, we have addressed the question of whether altered miRNA expression in quiescent UC and CD mucosa may be relevant to IBD pathogenesis. Our data allowed two major conclusions.

First. Alteration of miRNA expression was not confined to inflamed (grades 2–4), but preexisted in non-inflamed (grades 0 and 1) mucosa. Applying strictly controlled RT and real-time Q-PCR protocols and stringent cut-off values (>5-fold or <0.2-fold *vs.* healthy individuals), we identified 14 and 23 miRNAs with dysregulated expression in non-inflamed UC and CD biopsies, respectively, of which 8 were similarly dysregulated both in non-inflamed UC and CD biopsies. Our observation that mir-26a and 29a are up-regulated in quiescent UC mucosa has also been reported by Wu *et al.* [51]. In contrast, the other miRNAs (9/10, mir-629 was not tested in our screen) which were found to be up- (*eg.* mir-21, mir-126 and Let-7f) or down- (*eg.* mir-19b) regulated in [51] displayed only slight alterations in relative expression that did not match the stringent selection criteria we applied in our study. This suggests *(i)* that the discrepancies between both studies may

Table 4. Compilation of the sub-chromosomal regions where two or more miRNA genes with altered expression colocalize.

Chromsome	miRNA		Alteration of Expression			Duplex/Cluster
	Gene_Id	Locus	IBD_Type	Disease state	+/−	
6	30c-2	6q13	CD/UC	Quiescent/Quiescent	+	miRNA Duplex
	30a*	6q13	CD	Quiescent	+	
7	29a	7q.32.3	CD/UC	Both/Both	+	miRNA Duplex
	29b-2	7q.32.3	CD/UC		+	
9	199b-5p	9q34.11	UC	Both	−	miRNA Duplex
	126	9q34.3	CD	Inflamed	+	
	126*	9q34.3	CD/UC	Both/Both	+	
14	127-3p	14q32.31	CD/UC	Both/Both	+	miRNA Cluster
	370	14q32.31	UC	Both	−	
	382	14q32.31	UC	Inflamed	+	
15	7-2	15q26.1	UC	Inflamed	+	miRNA Duplex
	9-3	15q26.1	CD	Inflamed	+	
17	22	17p13.3	CD	Both	+	miRNA Duplex
	324-3p	17p13.1	CD/UC	Both/Both	+	
22	185	22q11.21	CD	Both	+	miRNA Duplex
	130b	22q11.21	CD	Inflamed	−	
X	106a	Xq26.2	CD	Both	+	miRNA Duplex
	20b	Xq26.2	CD	Inflamed	+	

Compilation of chromosomes and bands where colocalize 2 (miRNA Duplex) or more (miRNA Cluster) miRNA genes with altered expression relative to healthy controls in UC or CD tissues. Gene_Id, miRNA gene identification number; Locus, chromosomal band where the miRNA gene is localized; Quiescent, non-inflamed; Both, non-inflamed and inflamed; +/−, +: overexpression; −: underexpression.

be explained either by the differential sensitivity of the methods used for initial screening (microarray *vs.* real-time Q-PCR) and/or rather by the drastic cut-off value (>5-fold or <0.2-fold) we used to state altered miRNA expression in the present study and *(ii)* that the overlap in the alteration of miRNA expression observed in our study and in that reported by Wu *et al.* [51] may not have occurred only by chance. As far as we are aware, alteration of miRNA expression in non-inflamed CD colonic biopsies has not yet been reported.

Importantly, despite *(i)* the choice of a drastic cut-off that takes into account the variability in miRNA expression between IBD patients and *(ii)* the limited number of subjects kept for analysis in the present study, we could select miRNAs highly and significantly dysregulated in IBD relative to healthy controls. Interestingly, comparison of non-inflamed to inflamed tissues showed significant overlap in the alteration pattern of miRNA expression both in CD patients (this study) and UC (this study, [51]).

Altogether, these results support the notion that dysregulation of miRNA expression pre-exists in the quiescent colonic mucosa of UC and CD patients and may play a key role in the sensitization of the quiescent mucosa to environmental factors and/or to IBD inducers (ie. commensal flora), and *in fine* the onset and/or relapse of inflammation. Furthermore, they suggest that quiescent UC and CD mucosa already has distinct miRNA signatures which are not associated with significant variations in cellular contexts. Indeed, the quiescent colonic mucosa of IBD patients and that of healthy subjects were almost similar (grades 0 or 1 in both cases).

Since significant overlap was observed in the alteration of miRNA expression in quiescent UC and CD mucosa, our results also imply that several common molecular mechanisms may underlie the UC and CD pathogenic processes. Furthermore,

alteration of miRNA expression in quiescent IBD tissues is consistent with the notion that genetic variants that result in differential gene expression (*eg.* that of regulatory molecules such as miRNAs) as well as mutations in the open reading frame are expected to contribute to multifaceted diseases.

In this connection, one major drawback in investigating the dysregulation of miRNAs and of protein-coding genes expression in IBD tissues is related to cell type variations between samples (*eg.* inflamed *vs.* quiescent mucosa and normal healthy tissue). Indeed, inflamed mucosal tissue is characterized by a decreased number of epithelial cells, concomitant with an increased infiltration of inflammatory cells. This bias was taken into account in some genome wide cDNA microarray studies [26] but not in others [31]. For instance, decreased MICA (a gene expressed in intestinal epithelial cells) transcript expression was reported in inflamed CD [31] whereas flow cytometry and immuno-histochemistry identified strong MICA overexpression in intestinal epithelial cells of macroscopically involved areas of CD patients [52]. Similarly, it could be anticipated that the decreased level of mir-192 expression in inflamed mucosa of UC patients [51] may depend on cell-type heterogeneity between non-inflamed and inflamed mucosal tissues rather than on decreased gene expression (of note, in our study the slight decrease in mir-192 expression did not match our selection criteria in inflamed UC mucosa). Thus, the increase in MIP2α expression observed in [51] could be miRNA-independent and accounted for by increased TNFα secretion by immune infiltrating cells.

Finally, starting with a wide screen of 321 miRNAs, we could define *(i)* a selection of 8 miRNAs relevant in defining quiescent IBD *vs.* healthy mucosa and *(ii)* a distinct subset of 15 miRNAs (Patent pending) that allows discriminating between non-inflamed

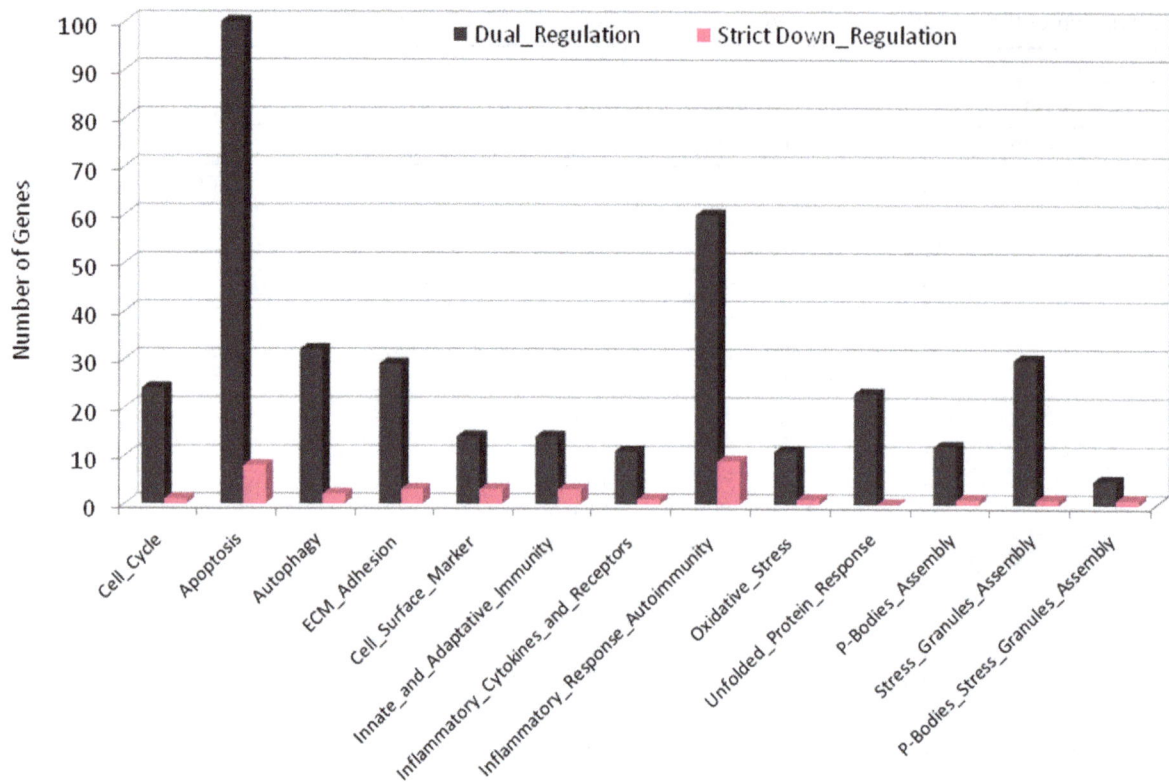

Figure 3. Alteration of miRNA expression in the colonic mucosa of UC and CD patients: *in silico* **characterization of target transcripts.** The exhaustive list of genes which are putatively targeted by the subset of 8 miRNAs that share common dysregulated expression both in quiescent UC and in quiescent CD was downloaded from the PITA catalog of predicted human microRNA targets (http://genie.weizmann.ac.il/pubs/mir07/mir07_data.html). The algorithm makes use of the parameter-free model for miRNA-target interaction described by Kertesz *et al.* [75]. The total number of genes involved in each single biological process is computed. Strict down regulation (light purple) stands for genes, the 3'-UTR of which interacts only with up-regulated miRNA(s).

UC and CD colonic mucosa and may define specific biomarkers relevant for UC and CD. Indeed on the basis of our panel of 16 patients, this selection of 15 miRNAs was able to predict 15/16 patients (94%) as UC or CD correctly. Such biomarkers may prove helpful as diagnostic tools of minimal invasivity (*eg.* for pediatric patients, incomplete colonoscopy) and as guidelines for surgical decisions. It can also be anticipated that miRNA signatures could be associated with different IBD profiles as prognostic biomarkers. This is out of the scope of the present study and deserves further studies on a larger cohort of patients.

Second. miRNAs play a major role in regulating coding-gene expression at the transcript and/or translational levels [34,36]. In this connection, we would like to emphasize that our study is the first one that reports the mapping of several miRNA genes with altered expression in quiescent UC and CD mucosa *(i)* at acknowledged IBD loci [53–55] or *(ii)* at loci conclusively associated with CD [11,16] } or UC [12,13,19] by GWAS studies. In this connection, we should like to emphasize that the co-localization of miRNA genes with dyregulated expression at chromosomal loci associated with IBD susceptibility does not occur only by chance. Indeed, our computations show that 1 miRNA gene (out of 321 tested) would be expected to be localized by chance in the vicinity of the 50 loci reported in [11,12,16–19] where 14 miRNA genes (14-fold more) with altered expression in quiescent UC and CD tissues map. In addition, even if 8 miRNA genes could map by chance within IBD susceptibility loci 1, 4, 7, 8 and 9, no miRNA genes with altered expression in quiescent UC and CD tissues were localized in these chromosomal regions

(although they encompass a total of 18 miRNA genes, the expression of which is not altered in IBD).

On this basis, we speculate that in addition to mutational events, IBD susceptibility might result from dysregulated miRNA expression in intestinal mucosa and to subsequent alteration of miRNA-dependent regulation of gene expression; consistent with the notion that not only allele variation, but also the alteration of regulatory processes that result in differential gene expression may contribute to multifaceted diseases.

Furthermore, our study characterizes band 14q32.31 as a cluster of 3 miRNA genes with altered expression in IBD. With the exception of mir-382, these miRNAs display altered expression in quiescent UC (mir-127-3p, mir-370) or in quiescent CD (mir-127-3p) mucosa. These miRNA genes are intergenic and constitute at least two distinct transcription units (mir-127 and mir-370). Alteration of miRNA expression within this sub-chromosomal region does not result from the overall chromosomal environment since *(i)* only the expression of 3 (UC) and 1 (CD) miRNAs was altered out of 38 localized within a DNA stretch of 44.74 kbp at 14q32.31, *(ii)* expression was either increased (mir-127-3p, CD/UC; mir-382, UC) or decreased (mir-370, UC) and *(iii)* expression was altered either in non-inflamed or in inflamed or in both states of the diseases. We speculate band 14q32.31 may represent a new, yet undefined IBD-susceptibility locus; this remains to be established and will be the subject of future studies.

Finally, the tight coordinated regulation of mir-26a, mir-29b, mir-126*, mir-127-3p and mir-324-3p (which genes are widespread on several chromosomes) in non-inflamed UC and CD mucosa also suggests that alteration of miRNA expression do contribute to the physiopathology of IBD. Interestingly, such concerted regulation of expression correlates with related biological functions. For instance, these miRNAs have been demonstrated to play roles either in cell cycle regulation, or in tumorigenesis in a broad spectrum of solid tumors (mir-26a, mir-29b, mir-127-3p and mir-324) [56–61], in the regulation of epithelial-mesenchymal transition and invasiveness (mir-126*) [62,63] or in the control of apoptosis (mir-29b and mir-126*) [64,65], in line with the higher than spontaneous occurrence of colorectal cancer (5-10%) in IBD patients. Of note, a recent study has reported that the mir-29 family of miRNAs regulates intestinal membrane permeability [66]. This observation should be connected with the increased gut permeability observed in IBD patients [67].

In silico studies emphasized that the transcripts targeted by the 8 miRNAs which share common overexpression in the quiescent colonic mucosa of both UC and CD patients correspond to genes that are involved/implicated in several cellular processes (*eg.* proliferation, apoptosis, autophagy, extracellular matrix organization, cell surface marker gene expression, oxidative stress, unfolded protein response, innate and adaptive immunity). Several of these genes stand as acknowledged IBD susceptibility genes or as genes of interest localized at convincingly replicated risk loci identified by GWAS (*eg.* ATG16L1, IL10, IL12B, JAK2, ARPC2, PTGER4, ZNF365, NKX2-3, PTPN2, PTPN22, C11orf30, ORMDL3, STAT3). However, an exhaustive identification of the genes targeted by UC- and/or CD- associated miRNAs (*eg.* common to or distinct between UC and CD), the demonstration of their actual regulation by miRNAs and the investigation of their influence on intestinal inflammation in experimental models of colitis is far beyond the scope of this paper and will be the subject of future studies.

Our study supports miRNAs as crucial players in the onset and/ or relapse of inflammation from quiescent mucosal tissues in UC and CD patients. It further highlights their putative role as contributors to IBD susceptibility and thus will help unravel the mechanisms (either distinct or shared between UC and CD) involved in relapsing (*eg.* identification of key targets and of gene networks). Finally, they may help develop new biomarkers to distinguish UC and CD at early stages.

Materials and Methods

IBD patients and controls

Colonic pinch biopsies were obtained in the course of endoscopical examination of patients with mild to severe CD and UC and of healthy control subjects undergoing screening colonoscopies (Table S2 for clinical details). Colonic biopsies were punctured from 24 CD, 18 UC and 19 healthy controls (*see* Figure S2). However, for the reasons outlined below (*see* paragraphs "Histopathological analyses" and "RNA isolation") and in Figure S2, the biopsies collected from some patients were not included in the study. Overall, expression of mature miRNAs was studied in inactive colonic mucosa of 8 patients with UC, 8 patients with CD and in 10 healthy control mucosa.

The diagnosis of UC and CD adhered to the criteria given by Lennard-Jones [68]. Clinical disease activity for CD and UC was assessed according to the Harvey-Bradshaw [69] and to the Colitis Activity (CAI) [70] indexes, respectively. In each IBD patient, endoscopically non-inflamed and inflamed areas of colonic tissue were punctured (5 biopsies/area). Non-inflamed and inflamed areas for biopsy collection were separated by more than 20 cm along the colon. Three biopsies from each area were allocated for

immediate RNAlater™ immersion then snap frozen and stored in liquid nitrogen, and two were set apart for histopathological examination. In healthy controls, 5 biopsies were punctured both in right and left colon and processed as above. The protocol was approved by the local Ethic Committee (Comité de Protection des Personnes -CPP- Ile de France IV n°2009/17 and AFFSSAPS D91534-80) and written informed consent was obtained from all patients.

Histopathological analyses

Biopsies were routinely stained with haematoxylin and eosin. Histological assessments of mucosal damage and inflammatory cells infiltration were graded by the same expert gastrointestinal pathologist (DCH) using a score previously validated to characterize the colonic involvement of both UC and CD [71]. Grades were as follows: 0, no evidence of inflammation (normal mucosa); 1, oedema and mild infiltration in the *lamina propria*; 2, crypt abscess and inflammation in the *lamina propria*; 3, severe inflammation with destructive crypt abscess and 4, severe inflammation with active ulceration. Grades 0–1 were considered as quiescent (or non-inflamed) mucosa. Grades 2–4 corresponded to various degrees of inflammation of the mucosa and were considered as active disease (Figure S1). Alterations in miRNA expression were studied following this histological dichotomy (0–1 *vs.* 2–4). IBD patients selected for miRNA analysis had both histologically assessed quiescent and inflammatory samples. 7 CD patients and 3 UC patients were excluded because their endoscopically quiescent colonic mucosa was classified as histologically active. 1 control patient with lymphocytic colitis was excluded (Figure S2).

RNA Isolation

Total RNA was extracted with TRIzol® Reagent (Invitrogen) then quantified using a ND-1000 NanoDrop spectrophotometer (NanoDrop Technologies) and purity/integrity was assessed using disposable RNA chips (Agilent RNA 6000 Nano LabChip kit) and an Agilent 2100 Bioanalyzer (Agilent Technologies, Waldbrunn, Germany). Only RNA preparations with RIN≥7 were further processed for analysis of miRNA expression. Nine CD, 7 UC and 8 controls with RNA preparations of insufficient purity (RIN<7) were excluded. Finally 8 CD, 8 UC and 10 controls with stringent homogeneity in histological assessment and RNA quality were selected for analysis (Figure S2).

Reverse-Transcription and Real-Time Q-PCR

The Human Early Access Release Kit (based on miRBase v 9.2; TaqMan® MicroRNA Assay; Applied Biosystems) designed to quantify 321 mature human miRNAs was used. cDNA was generated from 10 ng of total RNA using miRNA-specific stem-loop RT primers. Real-Time Q-PCR assays were performed according to the manufacturer's instructions using aliquots of cDNA equivalent to ~1.3 ng of total RNA and were run in a Light Cycler 480 (Roche Diagnostics).

Normalization of Real-Time Q-PCR results. Several RNAs (U6, U24, U48 and S18) were tested as putative standards and U6 (an ubiquitous small nuclear RNA) (Primer for U6 were included in the TaqMan® MicroRNA Assay) was found the most reliable. Expression of miRNAs was computed relative to that of U6 and a comparative threshold cycle method ($2^{-\Delta\Delta CT}$) [72] was used to compare non-inflamed and inflamed IBD tissues with healthy controls. Since the abundance of mature miRNA transcripts was expressed relative to that of the reference gene U6, we have checked that PCR efficiencies were identical for test (miRNAs) and reference (U6) transcripts, so that the comparison be accurate (*see* the MIQE guidelines; [73]).

CT, the fractional cycle number at which the amount of amplified target reaches a fixed threshold, was determined (default threshold settings were used in all instances). The cycle number above which the CT was considered as a false positive (cycle cut-off point) was set up at 35, as already argued in the literature dealing with limits of detection in Real-Time Quantitative- RT-PCR [74] (reviewed in [73]). $-\Delta\Delta CT$ was calculated as follows:

$$-\Delta\Delta CT = -(CT_{IBD} - \Delta CT_{healthycontrol})$$

where

$$\Delta CT_{healthcontrol} = (CT_{healthycontrol} - CT_{U6})$$

And

$$\Delta CT_{IBD} = (CT_{IBD} - CT_{U6})$$

Determination of cut-off values for miRNA over- and under- expression. Relative miRNA expressions ($2^{-\Delta\Delta CT}$) were computed as their log transformed ($10 \times \log_{10}$) values (after such computation up- and down- regulations were expressed as positive and negative values, respectively), and their means and standard deviations (SD_{miRNA}) were calculated independently for every miRNA, in each IBD at each stage of the disease. Box-whisker plots analysis of SD_{miRNA} pointed highly dispersed values among patients (Figure S3). Overall, when the data gathered from the two series of patients were considered (8 UC, 8 CD; non-inflamed and inflamed areas of colonic tissues), a mean value of 6.3 ± 1.4 ($mean_{Disp} \pm SD_{Disp}$) was calculated for the SD_{miRNA} values. Given such variation in relative miRNA expression, only those with mean $10 \times \log_{10} 2^{-\Delta\Delta CT} > 7$ and <-7 ($\pm |mean_{Disp} + 0.5\ SD_{Disp}|$) were considered as up- ($2^{-\Delta\Delta CT} > 5$-fold) and down- ($2^{-\Delta\Delta CT} < 0.2$-fold) regulated relative to healthy.

In silico prediction of miRNA targets

Exhaustive human miRNA targets were predicted using a parameter-free model for miRNA-target interaction. This model computes the difference between the free energy gained from the formation of the miRNA-target duplex (ΔG_{duplex}) and the energetic cost of unpairing the target (and proximal flanking sequences) to make it accessible to the miRNA (ΔG_{open}) [75].

We made use of the PITA catalog of predicted human microRNA targets (http://genie.weizmann.ac.il/pubs/mir07/mir07_data.html). The seed parameter settings described in Kertesz *et al.* [75] were followed: seeds of 8 bp in length, beginning at position 2 of the miRNA were chosen, seed conservation being set at 0.9. No mismatches or loops were allowed, but a single G:U wobble was permitted. In genes missing a 3' UTR annotation, 800 bp downstream of the annotated end of the coding sequence were used as the predicted 3' UTR. Flanks of 3 and 15 bp upstream and downstream the miRNA target, respectively, were considered in the computation of ΔG_{open}.

In some instances (mir-126*) predictions from the miRBase database (miRBase Targets Release Version v5; http://microrna.sanger.ac.uk/cgi-bin/targets/v5/mirna.pl?genome_id = 2964) were downloaded. These predictions combine the miRanda algorithm and the conservation of miRNA binding sites in orthologous transcripts from at least two species (http://microrna.sanger.ac.uk/targets/v5/info.html for details) [76].

Biological functions of the *in silico* predicted miRNA targets

We made use of the Gene Ontology (http://www.geneontology.org), GeneCards (http://www.genecards.org/) and GeneNote (http://bioinfo2.weizmann.ac.il/cgi-bin/genenote/home_page.pl) databases to document the biological functions of the genes that were predicted to be targeted by miRNAs with altered expression in quiescent UC and CD tissues (*see* Table S8).

Statistical analysis

Unpaired groups of values were compared according to the non-parametric Mann-Whitney test. Statistical significance was set at $p \leq 0.05$.

miRNA which shared closely related expression patterns were grouped according to K-means clustering [77] computed on line from the GenePattern Server. The specified number of clusters was set at 20.

When supervised class (UC or CD) prediction of individual patient's data was tested, we used a K Nearest Neighbors Classification algorithm with Leave-One-Out Cross-Validation (GenePattern "KNNXValidation" module). The class predictor was uniquely defined by the initial set of patients and marker miRNAs. The classifications were tested in leave-one-out cross-validation mode by iteratively leaving one sample out, training a classification on the remaining data and testing on the left out sample.

Supporting Information

Figure S1 Histological grading of disease activity in colonic biopsies. Hematoxylin and eosin staining of biopsies from non-inflamed and inflamed colonic mucosa (see Materials and Methods for details on histological grading). Note the progressive loss of intestinal epithelium with increasing grade of the disease (2–4) and the concomitant increase in the severity of inflammation/infiltration. Magnification, ×100.

Figure S2 Flow chart of sample selection. In order to exclude any bias in homogeneity among samples, biopsies of patients with endoscopically quiescent, but histologically active colonic mucosa were excluded. The histological dichotomy (grades 0–1 vs. 2–4) was strictly followed to study the alteration in miRNA gene expression. Similarly, 1 control patient with lymphocytic colitis was excluded. In all cases, RNA preparations of low integrity (RIN<7) were discarded.

Figure S3 Alteration of miRNA gene expression in non-inflamed and inflamed UC and CD tissues : Box-whisker plot analysis of standard deviations. miRNA expression was measured in non-inflamed and inflamed colonic mucosa obtained from patients with UC and CD (8 patients/IBD) and computed vs. that measured in healthy controls. The mean and standard deviation (SDmiRNA) of relative miRNA expression were then calculated for every miRNA, independently in each IBD for each state of the disease. SDmiRNA were then plotted as box-whisker plots (box, 25–75%; whisker, 10–90%; line, median) (1). 1 Tukey, J. W. (1977) in Exploratory Data Analysis (Addison-Wesley, Reading, MA), pp. 39–43.

Figure S4 Overview of the chromosomal distribution of miRNA genes with altered expression in IBD tissues: The total number of miRNA genes with altered expression was determined by chromosome. Negative and positive ordinates stand of over and under -expression, respectively.

Figure S5 Alteration of miRNA gene expression in IBD tissues: sub-chromosomal localization of the affected loci. Chromosomal bands where 2 (arrowheads) or more (squares) miRNA genes with altered expression colocalize are shown. Grey and light-red symbols represent loci where IBD susceptibility has yet been demonstrated by genetic means and previously unidentified loci, respectively.

Table S1 miRNA expression in left and right colon of healthy individuals. Relative miRNA expression ($10 \times \log 102^{-\Delta CT}$; see Materials and Methods) was calculated in the right and left colons independently. Note that miRNA expression was similar in both segments of the colon.

Table S2 Characteristics of patients with CD or UC and of healthy control individuals. * Sex: F : female/M : male; + disease location: C: colon/IC: ileocolonic/C+AP: colon and anoperineal lesions/R: right colon/S: sigmoid colon/LC: left colon; # Current treatment : CS: steroids/5 ASA: 5 aminosalicylates/AZA: azathioprine/IFX: infliximab/MTX: methotrexate.

Table S3 Alterations of miRNA expression in UC patients. Relative miRNA expression was computed vs. that measured in healthy controls and expressed as $10 \times \log 102^{-\Delta \Delta CT}$. Are only listed the miRNAs with relative expressions >7 or <−7 in non-inflamed UC tissues. When adequate, alteration of expression in inflamed UC is also mentioned. Access_N°, MIMAT identification number; Mean ± Sem (5–8 patients). Statistical significance (p values) was calculated relative to healthy control tissue using the non-parametric Mann-Whitney test. Bolded, miRNA with statistically significant dysregulation of expression in both quiescent and inflamed UC.

Table S4 Alterations of miRNA expression in CD patients. Relative miRNA expression was computed vs. that measured in healthy controls and expressed as $10 \times \log 102^{-\Delta \Delta CT}$. Are only listed the miRNAs with relative expressions >7 or <−7 in non-inflamed CD tissues. When adequate, alteration of expression in inflamed CD is also mentioned. Access_N°, MIMAT identification number; Mean ± Sem (5–8 patients). Statisticalsignificance (p values) was calculated relative to healthy control tissue using the non-parametric Mann-Whitney test. Bolded, miRNA with statistically significant dysregulation of expression both in quiescent and in inflamed CD.

Table S5 Shared alterations of miRNA expression in UC and CD patients. Relative miRNA expression was computed vs. that measured in healthy controls. miRNA with shared and significant overexpression ($10 \times \log 102^{-\Delta \Delta CT} > 7$) both in non-inflamed UC and in non-inflamed CD tissues are listed. Access_N°, MIMAT identification number; Mean ± Sem (5–8 patients). Italics (2 lower rows), miRNA that are not overexpressed in inflamed UC (mir-196a) or CD (mir-30c).

Table S6 Compilation of the characteristics of the miRNA with significantly altered expression in quiescent UC and CD colonic mucosa. Access_N°, MIMAT identification number; Gene-Id, miRNA gene identification number; Coordinates, coordinate of the miRNA gene on the chromosome [strand] (from http://www.mirbase.org/cgi-bin/mirna_summary.pl?org = hsa); Band, Chromosomal band where the miRNA gene is localized; Gene Context, presence or absence (intergenic) of overlap between the miRNA gene and another gene either on the same or on the opposite strand.

Table S7 Compilation of the sub-chromosomal regions where acknowledged IBD-susceptibility loci and miRNA genes with altered expression colocalize. Chromosomal locations where colocalize miRNA genes with altered expression relative to healthy controls in quiescent and/or inflamed UC or CD tissues and (i) acknowledged IBD susceptibility loci or (ii) replicated sub-chromosomal regions identified in GWAS are listed. The location of each IBD susceptibility loci is reminded. Gene_Id, miRNA gene identification number; Locus, chromosomal band where the miRNA gene is localized; Quiescent, non-inflamed; Both, non-inflamed and inflamed; +/−, +: overexpression; −: underexpression.

Table S8 Alteration of miRNA expression in the colonic mucosa of UC and CD patients: in silico characterization of target transcripts. The exhaustive list of genes which are putatively targeted by the subset of 8 miRNAs that share common dysregulated overexpression in both UC and CD was downloaded from the PITA catalog of predicted human microRNA targets (http://genie.weizmann.ac.il/pubs/mir07/mir07_data.html). The algorithm makes use of the parameter-free model for miRNA-target interaction described by Kertesz et al. (2007). Genes involved in a common biological process are listed together. Bold characters: strictly down regulated genes (the 3′-UTR of which interacts only with up-regulated miRNA(s))

Author Contributions

Conceived and designed the experiments: EOD. Performed the experiments: MF EP DCH FD. Analyzed the data: CR AG. Contributed reagents/materials/analysis tools: XT TA JCS YB. Wrote the paper: AG. Contributed to the experiments: CG. Expert gastrointestinal pathologist who assessed mucosal damage and inflammatory cells infiltration: DCH. Contributed to study design: RM ML.

References

1. Schreiber S, Rosenstiel P, Albrecht M, Hampe J, Krawczak M (2005) Genetics of Crohn disease, an archetypal inflammatory barrier disease. Nat Rev Genet 6: 376–88.

2. Kugathasan S, Amre D (2006) Inflammatory bowel disease–environmental modification and genetic determinants. Pediatr Clin North Am 53: 727–49.

3. Liu L, Li Y, Tollefsbol TO (2008) Gene-environment interactions and epigenetic basis of human diseases. Curr Issues Mol Biol 10: 25–36.

4. Bouma G, Strober W (2003) The immunological and genetic basis of inflammatory bowel disease. Nat Rev Immunol 3: 521–33.

5. Farmer RG, Easley KA, Rankin GB (1993) Clinical patterns, natural history, and progression of ulcerative colitis. A long-term follow-up of 1116 patients. Dig Dis Sci 38: 1137–46.

6. Rutgeerts P, Geboes K, Vantrappen G, Beyls J, Kerremans R, et al. (1990) Predictability of the postoperative course of Crohn's disease. Gastroenterology 99: 956–63.

7. Kaser A, Lee AH, Franke A, Glickman JN, Zeissig S, et al. (2008) XBP1 links ER stress to intestinal inflammation and confers genetic risk for human inflammatory bowel disease. Cell 134: 743–56.

8. Ahn SH, Shah YM, Inoue J, Morimura K, Kim I, et al. (2008) Hepatocyte nuclear factor 4alpha in the intestinal epithelial cells protects against inflammatory bowel disease. Inflamm Bowel Dis 14: 908–20.

9. Paavola-Sakki P, Ollikainen V, Helio T, Halme L, Turunen U, et al. (2003) Genome-wide search in Finnish families with inflammatory bowel disease provides evidence for novel susceptibility loci. Eur J Hum Genet 11: 112–20.

10. Vermeire S, Rutgeerts P (2005) Current status of genetics research in inflammatory bowel disease. Genes Immun 6: 637–45.

11. Barrett JC, Hansoul S, Nicolae DL, Cho JH, Duerr RH, et al. (2008) Genome-wide association defines more than 30 distinct susceptibility loci for Crohn's disease. Nat Genet 40: 955–62.

12. Franke A, Balschun T, Karlsen TH, Hedderich J, May S, et al. (2008) Replication of signals from recent studies of Crohn's disease identifies previously unknown disease loci for ulcerative colitis. Nat Genet 40: 713–5.

13. Franke A, Balschun T, Karlsen TH, Sventoraityte J, Nikolaus S, et al. (2008) Sequence variants in IL10, ARPC2 and multiple other loci contribute to ulcerative colitis susceptibility. Nat Genet 40: 1319–23.

14. Kugathasan S, Baldassano RN, Bradfield JP, Sleiman PM, Imielinski M, et al. (2008) Loci on 20q13 and 21q22 are associated with pediatric-onset inflammatory bowel disease. Nat Genet 40: 1211–5.

15. Mathew CG (2008) New links to the pathogenesis of Crohn disease provided by genome-wide association scans. Nat Rev Genet 9: 9–14.

16. Fisher SA, Tremelling M, Anderson CA, Gwilliam R, Bumpstead S, et al. (2008) Genetic determinants of ulcerative colitis include the ECM1 locus and five loci implicated in Crohn's disease. Nat Genet 40: 710–2.

17. Imielinski M, Baldassano RN, Griffiths A, Russell RK, Annese V, et al. (2009) Common variants at five new loci associated with early-onset inflammatory bowel disease. Nat Genet 41: 1335–40.

18. Asano K, Matsushita T, Umeno J, Hosono N, Takahashi A, et al. (2009) A genome-wide association study identifies three new susceptibility loci for ulcerative colitis in the Japanese population. Nat Genet 41: 1325–9.

19. Barrett JC, Lee JC, Lees CW, Prescott NJ, Anderson CA, et al. (2009) Genome-wide association study of ulcerative colitis identifies three new susceptibility loci, including the HNF4A region. Nat Genet 41: 1330–4.

20. Hugot JP, Chamaillard M, Zouali H, Lesage S, Cezard JP, et al. (2001) Association of NOD2 leucine-rich repeat variants with susceptibility to Crohn's disease. Nature 411: 599–603.

21. Parkes M, Barrett JC, Prescott NJ, Tremelling M, Anderson CA, et al. (2007) Sequence variants in the autophagy gene IRGM and multiple other replicating loci contribute to Crohn's disease susceptibility. Nat Genet 39: 830–2.

22. Hampe J, Franke A, Rosenstiel P, Till A, Teuber M, et al. (2007) A genome-wide association scan of nonsynonymous SNPs identifies a susceptibility variant for Crohn disease in ATG16L1. Nat Genet 39: 207–11.

23. Duerr RH, Taylor KD, Brant SR, Rioux JD, Silverberg MS, et al. (2006) A genome-wide association study identifies IL23R as an inflammatory bowel disease gene. Science 314: 1461–3.

24. Ogura Y, Bonen DK, Inohara N, Nicolae DL, Chen FF, et al. (2001) A frameshift mutation in NOD2 associated with susceptibility to Crohn's disease. Nature 411: 603–6.

25. Cho JH, Weaver CT (2007) The genetics of inflammatory bowel disease. Gastroenterology 133: 1327–39.

26. Noble CL, Abbas AR, Cornelius J, Lees CW, Ho GT, et al. (2008) Regional variation in gene expression in the healthy colon is dysregulated in ulcerative colitis. Gut 57: 1398–405.

27. Olsen J, Gerds TA, Seidelin JB, Csillag C, Bjerrum JT, et al. (2009) Diagnosis of ulcerative colitis before onset of inflammation by multivariate modeling of genome-wide gene expression data. Inflamm Bowel Dis 15: 1032–8.

28. Dooley TP, Curto EV, Reddy SP, Davis RL, Lambert GW, et al. (2004) Regulation of gene expression in inflammatory bowel disease and correlation with IBD drugs: screening by DNA microarrays. Inflamm Bowel Dis 10: 1–14.

29. Lawrance IC, Fiocchi C, Chakravarti S (2001) Ulcerative colitis and Crohn's disease: distinctive gene expression profiles and novel susceptibility candidate genes. Hum Mol Genet 10: 445–56.

30. Dieckgraefe BK, Stenson WF, Korzenik JR, Swanson PE, Harrington CA (2000) Analysis of mucosal gene expression in inflammatory bowel disease by parallel oligonucleotide arrays. Physiol Genomics 4: 1–11.

31. Costello CM, Mah N, Hasler R, Rosenstiel P, Waetzig GH, et al. (2005) Dissection of the inflammatory bowel disease transcriptome using genome-wide cDNA microarrays. PLoS Med 2: e199.

32. von Stein P, Lofberg R, Kuznetsov NV, Gielen AW, Persson JO, et al. (2008) Multigene analysis can discriminate between ulcerative colitis, Crohn's disease, and irritable bowel syndrome. Gastroenterology 134: 1869–81; quiz 2153–4.

33. Doench JG, Sharp PA (2004) Specificity of microRNA target selection in translational repression. Genes Dev 18: 504–11.

34. Flynt AS, Lai EC (2008) Biological principles of microRNA-mediated regulation: shared themes amid diversity. Nat Rev Genet 9: 831–42.

35. Wu L, Fan J, Belasco JG (2006) MicroRNAs direct rapid deadenylation of mRNA. Proc Natl Acad Sci U S A 103: 4034–9.

36. Filipowicz W, Bhattacharyya SN, Sonenberg N (2008) Mechanisms of post-transcriptional regulation by microRNAs: are the answers in sight? Nat Rev Genet 9: 102–14.

37. Reinhart BJ, Slack FJ, Basson M, Pasquinelli AE, Bettinger JC, et al. (2000) The 21-nucleotide let-7 RNA regulates developmental timing in Caenorhabditis elegans. Nature 403: 901–6.

38. Miska EA (2005) How microRNAs control cell division, differentiation and death. Curr Opin Genet Dev 15: 563–8.

39. Kapsimali M, Kloosterman WP, de Bruijn E, Rosa F, Plasterk RH, et al. (2007) MicroRNAs show a wide diversity of expression profiles in the developing and mature central nervous system. Genome Biol 8: R173.

40. Lu J, Getz G, Miska EA, Alvarez-Saavedra E, Lamb J, et al. (2005) MicroRNA expression profiles classify human cancers. Nature 435: 834–8.

41. Calin GA, Croce CM (2006) MicroRNA signatures in human cancers. Nat Rev Cancer 6: 857–66.

42. Volinia S, Calin GA, Liu CG, Ambs S, Cimmino A, et al. (2006) A microRNA expression signature of human solid tumors defines cancer gene targets. Proc Natl Acad Sci U S A 103: 2257–61.

43. Bandres E, Cubedo E, Agirre X, Malumbres R, Zarate R, et al. (2006) Identification by Real-time PCR of 13 mature microRNAs differentially expressed in colorectal cancer and non-tumoral tissues. Mol Cancer 5: 29.

44. Cummins JM, He Y, Leary RJ, Pagliarini R, Diaz LA, Jr., et al. (2006) The colorectal microRNAome. Proc Natl Acad Sci U S A 103: 3687–92.

45. Kloosterman WP, Lagendijk AK, Ketting RF, Moulton JD, Plasterk RH (2007) Targeted inhibition of miRNA maturation with morpholinos reveals a role for miR-375 in pancreatic islet development. PLoS Biol 5: e203.

46. Eisenberg I, Eran A, Nishino I, Moggio M, Lamperti C, et al. (2007) Distinctive patterns of microRNA expression in primary muscular disorders. Proc Natl Acad Sci U S A 104: 17016–21.

47. O'Connell RM, Taganov KD, Boldin MP, Cheng G, Baltimore D (2007) MicroRNA-155 is induced during the macrophage inflammatory response. Proc Natl Acad Sci U S A 104: 1604–9.

48. Moschos SA, Williams AE, Perry MM, Birrell MA, Belvisi MG, et al. (2007) Expression profiling in vivo demonstrates rapid changes in lung microRNA levels following lipopolysaccharide-induced inflammation but not in the anti-inflammatory action of glucocorticoids. BMC Genomics 8: 240.

49. Sonkoly E, Stahle M, Pivarcsi A (2008) MicroRNAs: novel regulators in skin inflammation. Clin Exp Dermatol 33: 312–5.

50. Sonkoly E, Pivarcsi A (2009) Advances in microRNAs: implications for immunity and inflammatory diseases. J Cell Mol Med 13: 24–38.

51. Wu F, Zikusoka M, Trindade A, Dassopoulos T, Harris ML, et al. (2008) MicroRNAs are differentially expressed in ulcerative colitis and alter expression of macrophage inflammatory peptide-2 alpha. Gastroenterology 135: 1624–35 e24.

52. Allez M, Tieng V, Nakazawa A, Treton X, Pacault V, et al. (2007) CD4+NKG2D+ T cells in Crohn's disease mediate inflammatory and cytotoxic responses through MICA interactions. Gastroenterology 132: 2346–58.

53. Bonen DK, Cho JH (2003) The genetics of inflammatory bowel disease. Gastroenterology 124: 521–36.

54. Van Limbergen J, Russell RK, Nimmo ER, Satsangi J (2007) The genetics of inflammatory bowel disease. Am J Gastroenterol 102: 2820–31.

55. Van Limbergen J, Wilson DC, Satsangi J (2009) The genetics of Crohn's disease. Annu Rev Genomics Hum Genet 10: 89–116.

56. Xu H, Cheung IY, Guo HF, Cheung NK (2009) MicroRNA miR-29 modulates expression of immunoinhibitory molecule B7-H3: potential implications for immune based therapy of human solid tumors. Cancer Res 69: 6275–81.

57. Kota J, Chivukula RR, O'Donnell KA, Wentzel EA, Montgomery CL, et al. (2009) Therapeutic microRNA delivery suppresses tumorigenesis in a murine liver cancer model. Cell 137: 1005–17.

58. Flavin R, Smyth P, Barrett C, Russell S, Wen H, et al. (2009) miR-29b expression is associated with disease-free survival in patients with ovarian serous carcinoma. Int J Gynecol Cancer 19: 641–7.

59. Sander S, Bullinger L, Wirth T (2009) Repressing the repressor: a new mode of MYC action in lymphomagenesis. Cell Cycle 8: 556–9.

60. Yan LX, Huang XF, Shao Q, Huang MY, Deng L, et al. (2008) MicroRNA miR-21 overexpression in human breast cancer is associated with advanced clinical stage, lymph node metastasis and patient poor prognosis. Rna 14: 2348–60.

61. Ferretti E, De Smaele E, Miele E, Laneve P, Po A, et al. (2008) Concerted microRNA control of Hedgehog signalling in cerebellar neuronal progenitor and tumour cells. Embo J 27: 2616–27.

62. Gebeshuber CA, Zatloukal K, Martinez J (2009) miR-29a suppresses tristetraprolin, which is a regulator of epithelial polarity and metastasis. EMBO Rep 10: 400–5.

63. Musiyenko A, Bitko V, Barik S (2008) Ectopic expression of miR-126*, an intronic product of the vascular endothelial EGF-like 7 gene, regulates prostein translation and invasiveness of prostate cancer LNCaP cells. J Mol Med 86: 313–22.

64. Park SY, Lee JH, Ha M, Nam JW, Kim VN (2009) miR-29 miRNAs activate p53 by targeting p85 alpha and CDC42. Nat Struct Mol Biol 16: 23–9.

65. Li Z, Lu J, Sun M, Mi S, Zhang H, et al. (2008) Distinct microRNA expression profiles in acute myeloid leukemia with common translocations. Proc Natl Acad Sci U S A 105: 15535–40.

66. Zhou Q, Souba WW, Croce CM, Verne GN (2010) MicroRNA-29a regulates intestinal membrane permeability in patients with irritable bowel syndrome. Gut 59: 775–84.

67. Hollander D (1999) Intestinal permeability, leaky gut, and intestinal disorders. Curr Gastroenterol Rep 1: 410–6.

68. Lennard-Jones JE (1989) Classification of inflammatory bowel disease. Scand J Gastroenterol Suppl 170: 2–6; discussion 16–9.

69. Harvey RF, Bradshaw JM (1980) A simple index of Crohn's-disease activity. Lancet 1: 514.

70. Xiao Li F, Sutherland LR (2002) Assessing disease activity and disease activity indices for inflammatory bowel disease. Curr Gastroenterol Rep 4: 490–6.

71. Gomes P, du Boulay C, Smith CL, Holdstock G (1986) Relationship between disease activity indices and colonoscopic findings in patients with colonic inflammatory bowel disease. Gut 27: 92–5.

72. Livak KJ, Schmittgen TD (2001) Analysis of relative gene expression data using real-time quantitative PCR and the 2(-Delta Delta C(T)) Method. Methods 25: 402–8.

73. Bustin SA, Benes V, Garson JA, Hellemans J, Huggett J, et al. (2009) The MIQE guidelines: minimum information for publication of quantitative real-time PCR experiments. Clin Chem 55: 611–22.

74. Burns M, Valdivia H (2008) Modelling the limit of detection in real-time quantitative PCR. Eur Food Res Technol 226: 1513–24.

75. Kertesz M, Iovino N, Unnerstall U, Gaul U, Segal E (2007) The role of site accessibility in microRNA target recognition. Nat Genet 39: 1278–84.

76. Megraw M, Sethupathy P, Corda B, Hatzigeorgiou AG (2007) miRGen: a database for the study of animal microRNA genomic organization and function. Nucleic Acids Res 35: D149–55.

77. MacQueen J. Some methods for classification and analysis of multivariate observations. In: Le Cam LMaN J, ed. Proceedings of the Fifth Berkeley Symposium on Mathematical Statistics and Probability. BerkeleyCalifonia: University of California Press 1967, 281–97.

78. Tukey JW. Box-and-Whisker Plots. Exploratory Data Analysis. ReadingMA: Addison-Wesley 1977, 39–43.

7

The Effects of Oral and Enteric *Campylobacter concisus* Strains on Expression of TLR4, MD-2, TLR2, TLR5 and COX-2 in HT-29 Cells

Yazan Ismail[1], Hoyul Lee[1], Stephen M. Riordan[2,3], Michael C. Grimm[4], Li Zhang[1]*

1 School of Biotechnology and Biomolecular Sciences, University of New South Wales, Sydney, New South Whales, Australia, 2 Gastrointestinal and Liver Unit, The Prince of Wales Hospital, Sydney, New South Whales, Australia, 3 Faculty of Medicine, University of New South Wales, Sydney, New South Whales, Australia, 4 St George Clinical School, University of New South Wales, Sydney, New South Whales, Australia

Abstract

Campylobacter concisus, a Gram-negative bacterium that colonizes the human oral cavity, has been shown to be associated with inflammatory bowel diseases (IBD). The effects of different *C. concisus* strains on intestinal epithelial expression of Toll like receptors (TLR) have not been investigated. This study examined the effects of *C. concisus* strains isolated from patients with IBD and controls on expression of TLR4, its co-receptor myeloid differentiation factor (MD)-2; TLR2, TLR5, cyclooxygenase-2 (COX-2) and interleukin (IL)-8 in HT-29 cells.   Fourteen oral and enteric *C. concisus* strains isolated from patients with IBD and healthy controls were co-incubated with HT-29 cells. Expression of TLR4, MD-2, TLR2, TLR5 and COX-2 in HT-29 cells in response to *C. concisus* infection was examined by Western blot, flow cytometry analysis and immunofluorescent staining visualized by confocal microscope. Production of IL-8 was evaluated by enzyme-linked immunosorbent assay.   Both oral and enteric *C. concisus* strains upregulated expression of TLR4 in HT-29 cells. The levels of glycosylated TLR4 (Gly-TLR4) and surface TLR4 induced by *C. concisus* strains isolated from patients with IBD were significantly higher than those induced by *C. concisus* strains isolated from the healthy controls. Four *C. concisus* strains isolated from patients with IBD induced more than two-fold increase of surface expression of MD-2. *C. concisus* did not affect expression of TLR2 and TLR5. All *C. concisus* strains induced production of IL-8 and COX-2 in HT-29 cells.   This study shows that some *C. concisus* strains, most from patients with IBD, upregulate surface expression of TLR4 and MD-2 in HT-29 cells. These data suggest that a potential role of specific *C. concisus* strains in modulating the intestinal epithelial responses to bacterial LPS needs to be investigated.

Editor: Markus M. Heimesaat, Charité, Campus Benjamin Franklin, Germany

Funding: This work was supported by the Broad Medical Research Program of the Broad Foundation (Grant no: IBD0273-R) and a faculty research grant from the University of New South Wales. Yazan Ismail is supported by a PhD scholarship from Al-Balaq' Applied University, Jordan. The funders had no role in study design, data collection and analysis, decision to publish, or preparation of the manuscript.

Competing Interests: The authors have declared that no competing interests exist.

* E-mail: L.Zhang@unsw.edu.au

Introduction

Campylobacter concisus is a Gram-negative bacterium commonly found in the human oral cavity [1,2]. *C. concisus* is motile by means of a single polar flagellum and requires H_2-enriched microaerobic conditions for growth [3].

C. concisus has been shown to be associated with inflammatory bowel disease (IBD) [4,5,6,7,8]. A significantly higher prevalence of *C. concisus* in intestinal biopsies and fecal samples of patients with IBD was detected as compared with controls [4,5,6,7]. IBD is a chronic inflammatory disorder of the gastrointestinal tract; its most common incidence is in adolescents and young adults [9,10]. The two major types of IBD are Crohn's disease (CD) and ulcerative colitis (UC). The aetiology of IBD is unknown. Multiple factors including intestinal microbiota, genetic factors, environmental factors and aberrant responses in the innate and adaptive immune system contribute to the development of IBD [9,10].

The intestinal microbiota play a key role in the development of IBD. Studies from both human and animal models of IBD have demonstrated that colitis does not occur in the absence of intestinal microbiota [11,12,13,14]. Furthermore, a breakdown in tolerance of the gut immune system to commensal intestinal bacteria in patients with IBD has been detected [15,16]. Despite the strong evidence supporting the important role of intestinal microbiota in the development of IBD, a causative agent(s) of human IBD remains elusive.

C. concisus colonizing the oral cavity has been shown to be a source of *C. concisus* colonizing the intestinal tissues in some patients with IBD [17]. Recently *C. concisus* was detected in fecal and saliva samples of domestic dogs and cats [18,19]. This bacterium has also been isolated from chicken and beef meat [20]. These data suggest that domestic pets, chicken and beef meat may also serve as a source of human intestinal colonization of *C. concisus*.

Despite its high prevalence in the intestinal tract of patients with IBD, whether *C. concisus* contributes to the pathogenesis of IBD is unknown. A number of studies have examined the effects of *C. concisus* on intestinal epithelial cells using *in vitro* cell culture models. Some oral and enteric *C. concisus* strains were shown to be invasive to Caco2 cells [5,17]. Increased intestinal epithelial permeability

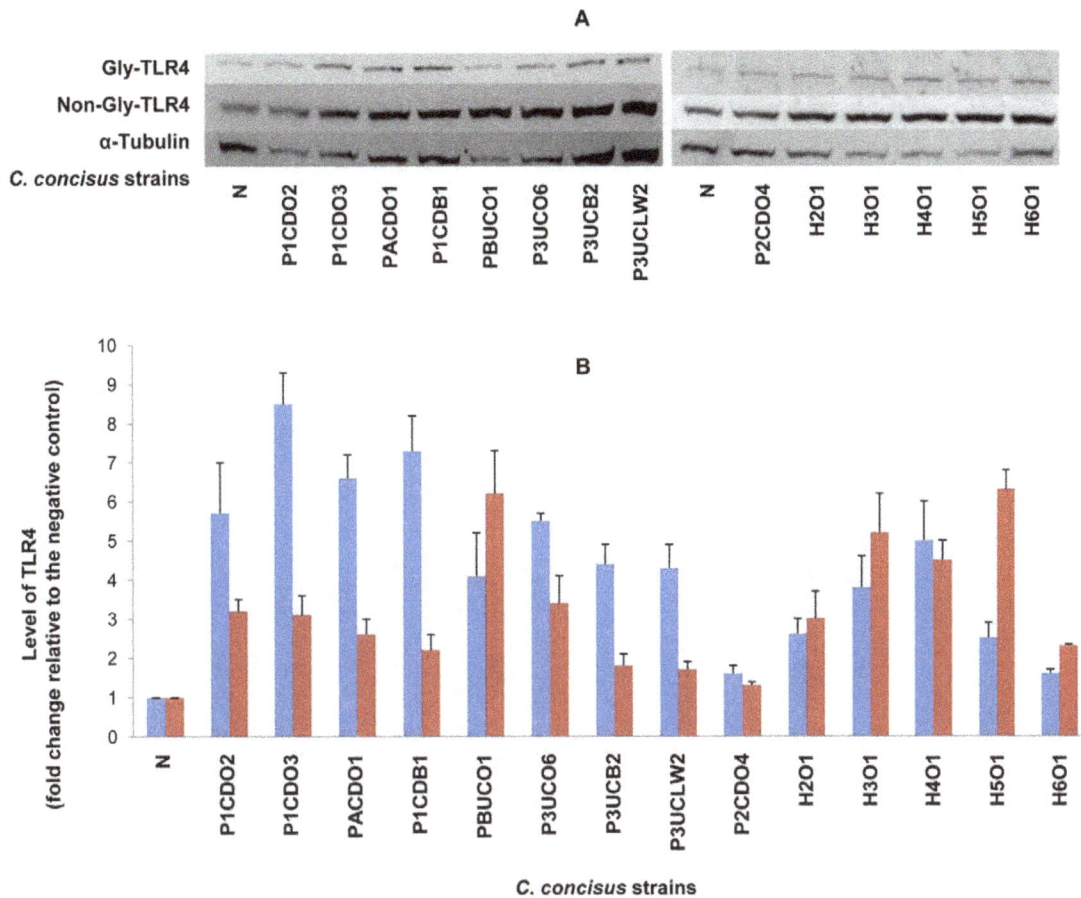

Figure 1. Detection of TLR4 by Western blot in HT-29 cells infected with *C. concisus* strains. HT-29 cells were lysed following incubation with *C. concisus* strains for 24 hours. Expression of TLR4 in HT-29 cells was detected by Western blot. Two bands, the Glycosylated TLR 4 (Gly-TLR4) and non-glycosylated TLR4 (Non-Gly-TLR4), were revealed on Western blot. The levels of Gly-TLR4 and Non-Gly-TLR4 of each sample were expressed as the fold change of the band intensity relative to the band intensity of the negative control (HT-29 cells without *C. concisus* infection), after normalization to the intensity of the internal control α-Tubulin of the same sample. A: Representative Western blot of Gly-TLR4 (120 kD), Non-Gly-TLR4 (95 kD) and α-Tubulin (55 kD). B: Level of Gly-TLR4 (blue column) and Non-Gly-TLR4 (red column) induced by different *C. concisus* strains; data were the average of triplicate experiments ± standard error. N: negative control. H2O1-H6O1: *C. concisus* strains isolated from healthy controls. The remaining nine *C. concisus* strains were from patients with IBD. The average level of Gly-TLR4 induced by *C. concisus* strains from patients with IBD was significantly higher than that induced by *C. concisus* strains from healthy controls ($P<0.05$).

and epithelial apoptosis were also observed following the incubation of Caco2 cells with both oral and enteric *C. concisus* strains [5,21]. Enteric *C. concisus* strains were shown to induce the production of IL-8 in HT-29 cells [5,22]. These data suggest that some *C. concisus* strains have a potential to cause enteric diseases.

The effects of *C. concisus* strains on intestinal epithelial expression of Toll like receptors (TLR) have not been investigated. A low level expression of TLR4 and its co-receptor myeloid differentiation factor (MD)-2 in intestinal epithelial cells under normal physiological conditions is a strategy of the intestinal immune system to avoid dysregulated inflammatory responses to bacterial lipopolysaccharide (LPS) [23]. In patients with IBD, increased levels of intestinal expression of TLR4 and other proinflammatory molecules such as cyclooxygenase-2 (COX-2) and interleukin (IL)-8 have been observed [24,25]. Examination of the effects of different *C. concisus* strains on intestinal epithelial expression of TLRs and other proinflamatory molecules will further shed light on whether some *C. concisus* strains have the potential to contribute to the pathogenesis of human enteric diseases including IBD. Given that *C. concisus* is a Gram-negative flagellated bacterium, in this study, we examined the effects of both oral and enteric *C.*

concisus strains isolated from patients with IBD and controls on intestinal epithelial expression of TLR4 and its co-receptor myeloid differentiation factor (MD)-2, which recognizes LPS found in Gram-negative bacteria, of TLR2, which recognizes bacterial lipoproteins, and of TLR5, which recognizes bacterial flagellin. Furthermore, the induction of COX-2 and IL-8 in HT-29 cells by both oral and enteric *C. concisus* strain was assessed.

Results

Expression of TLR4, MD-2, TLR2, TLR5 and COX-2 in HT-29 cells induced by different *C. concisus* strains detected by Western blot

On Western blot, TLR4, MD-2 and TLR2 revealed two protein bands (glycosylated and non-glycosylated proteins), TLR5 and COX-2 revealed one protein band. The intensity of each protein band detected by Western blot was normalized to the intensity of α-Tubulin (internal control) of the same sample. The levels of TLR4, MD-2, TLR2, TLR5 and COX-2 in each sample were expressed as the fold change of the normalized band intensity relative to the normalized band intensity of the negative control

A

B

C. concisus strains

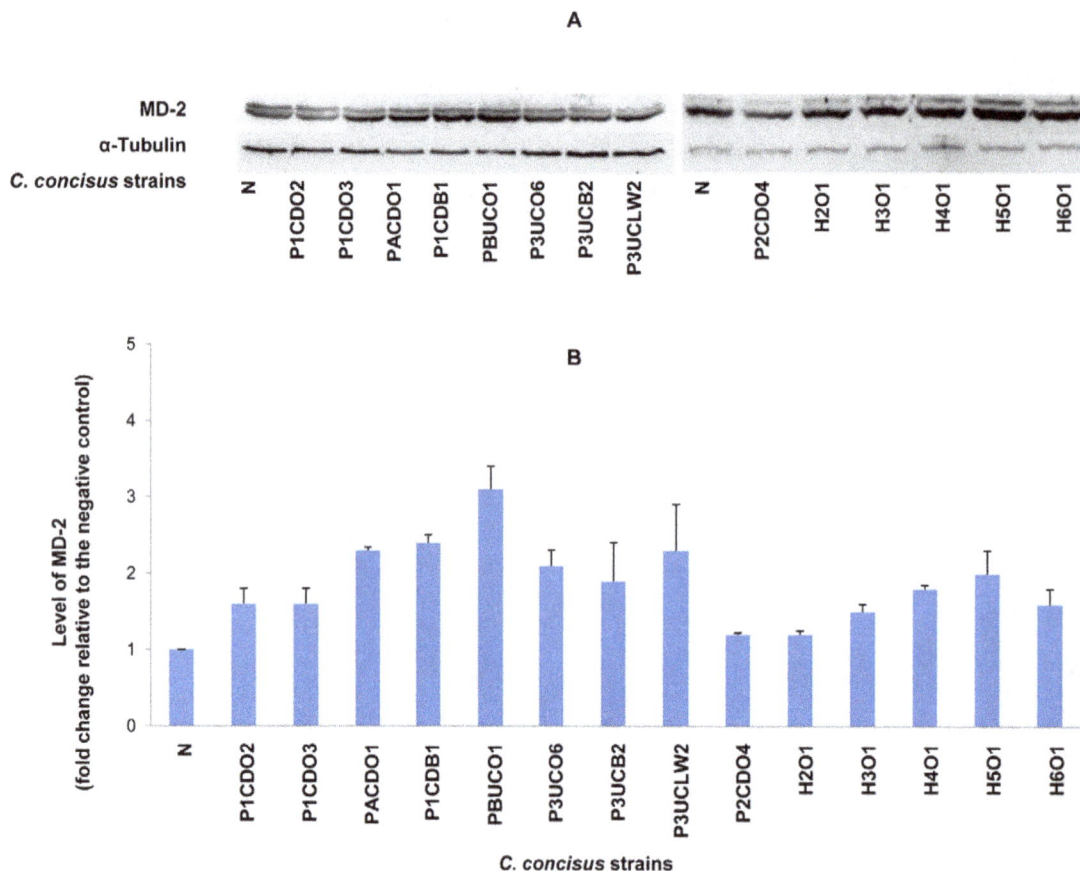

Figure 2. Detection of MD-2 by Western blot in HT-29 cells infected with *C. concisus* strains. HT-29 cells were lysed following incubation with *C. concisus* strains for 24 hours. Expression of MD-2 in HT-29 cells was detected by Western blot. Two bands, the Glycosylated MD-2 and non-glycosylated MD-2, were revealed on Western blot. Giving the close distance of Glycosylated MD-2 and non-glycosylated MD-2 protein bands which made it difficult to analyze the bands separately, these two protein bands were analyzed together. The level of MD-2 was expressed as the fold change of the normalized band intensity of a sample relative to the normalized band intensity of the negative control (HT-29 cells without *C. concisus* infection), after normalization to the intensity of the internal control α-Tubulin of the same sample. A: Representative Western blot of MD-2 (23–25 kD) and α-Tubulin (55 kD). B: Level of total MD-2 induced by different *C. concisus* strains; data were the average of triplicate experiments ± standard error. N: negative control. H2O1-H6O1: *C. concisus* strains isolated from healthy controls. The remaining nine *C. concisus* strains were from patients with IBD. The average level of MD-2 induced by *C. concisus* strains from patients with IBD was not significantly higher than that induced by *C. concisus* strains from healthy controls ($P>0.05$).

(HT-29 cells without *C. concisus* infection), which are shown in Table 1. For TLR4 and TLR2, the glycosylated receptors (Gly-TLR4 and Gly-TLR2) and the non-glycosylated receptors (Non-Gly-TLR4 and Non-Gly-TLR2) were analyzed separately. For MD-2, the glycosylated MD-2 and the non-glycosylated MD-2 were analyzed together, due to the narrow distance of glycosylated MD-2 and the non-glycosylated MD-2 bands on Western blot that made it difficult to analyze the two bands separately. The representative Western blot patterns and the schematic levels of TLR4, MD-2, TLR2, TLR5 and COX-2 are shown in Figure 1, Figure 2, Figure 3, Figure 4 and Figure 5 respectively.

C. concisus strains obtained from both patients with IBD and controls upregulated the expression of TLR4 in HT-29 cells. The levels of TLR4 induced by different *C. concisus* strains varied. Of the 14 *C. concisus* strains examined, 12 strains induced more than two-fold increase of expression of Gly-TLR4 and 11 strains induced more than two-fold increase of expression of Non-Gly-TLR4 (Figure 1 and Table 1). The average level of Gly-TLR4 induced by the nine *C. concisus* strains isolated from patients with IBD was significantly higher than that induced by the five *C. concisus* strains (H2O1-H6O1) isolated from healthy controls

(5.3 ± 0.7 vs 3.1 ± 0.6, $P<0.05$). The average level of Non-Gly-TLR4, induced by *C. concisus* strains from patients with IBD was not statistically different from that induced by the *C. concisus* strains from the healthy controls (2.8 ± 0.5 vs 4.3 ± 0.7, $P>0.05$). The average levels of Gly-TLR4 and Non-GlyTLR4 induced by the five oral *C. concisus* strains isolated from patients with IBD were 5.33 ± 2.33 and 3.31 ± 1.61 respectively, which were not significantly different from that induced by the three enteric *C. concisus* strains isolated from patients with IBD (5.33 ± 1.70 and 1.90 ± 0.27 respectively) ($P>0.05$).

Six *C. concisus* strains induced more than two-fold increase of expression of MD-2; five of these strains were from patients with IBD (Figure 2 and Table 1). The average level of MD-2 induced by *C. concisus* strains isolated from patients with IBD was not statistically different from that induced by *C. concisus* strains isolated from healthy controls (1.92 ± 0.15 vs 1.59 ± 0.21, $P>0.05$). The average level of MD-2 induced by the oral *C. concisus* strains isolated from patients with IBD was not statistically different from that induced by the enteric *C. concisus* strains isolated from patients with IBD (1.77 ± 0.20 vs 2.17 ± 0.14, $P>0.05$).

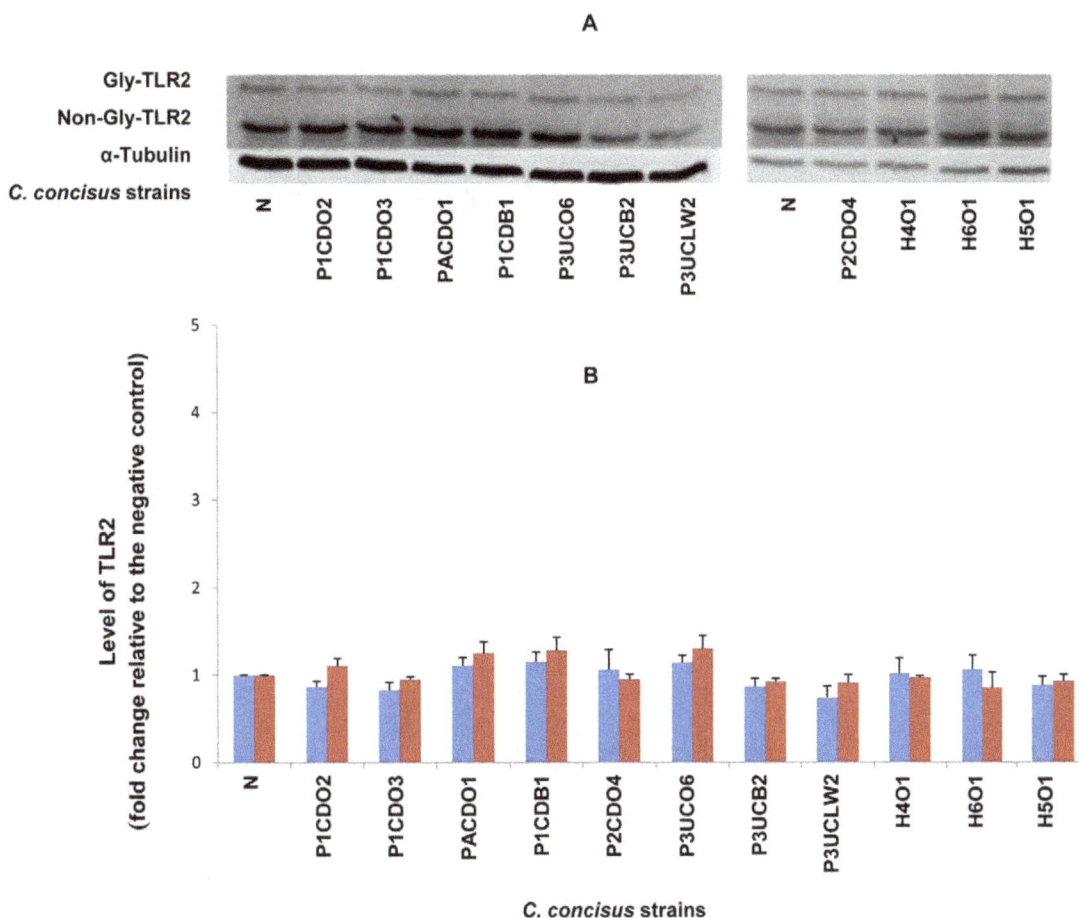

Figure 3. Detection of TLR2 by Western blot in HT-29 cells infected with *C. concisus* strains. HT-29 cells were lysed following incubation with *C. concisus* strains for 24 hours. Expression of TLR2 in HT-29 cells was detected by Western blot. Two bands, the Glycosylated TLR 2 (Gly-TLR4) and non-glycosylated TLR2 (Non-Gly-TLR4), were revealed on Western blot. The levels of Gly-TLR2 and Non-Gly-TLR2 of each sample were expressed as the fold change of the band intensity relative to the band intensity of the negative control (HT-29 cells without *C. concisus* infection), after normalization to the intensity of the internal control α-Tubulin of the same sample. A: Representative Western blot of Gly-TLR2 (100 kD), Non-Gly-TLR2 (90 kD) and α-Tubulin (55 kD). B: Level of Gly-TLR2 (blue column) and Non-Gly-TLR2 (red column) induced by different *C. concisus* strains; data were the average of triplicate experiments ± standard error. N: negative control. H2O1-H6O1: *C. concisus* strains isolated from healthy controls. The remaining *C. concisus* strains were from patients with IBD. The average levels of Gly-TLR2 and Non-Gly-TLR2 induced by *C. concisus* strains from patients with IBD were not significantly different that induced by *C. concisus* strains from healthy controls (*P*>0.05).

C. concisus strains did not affect the expression of TLR2 and TLR5 in HT-29 cells. The changes of TLR2 and TLR5 expression in HT-29 cells infected with *C. concisus* strains were all below two-fold in comparison to the levels of these two proteins in HT-29 cells without *C. concisus* infection (Figure 3, Figure 4 and Table 1).

Of the 14 *C. concisus* strains examined, eight strains isolated from patients with IBD induced more than two fold increase of expression of COX-2 (Figure 5, Table 1). The average level of COX-2 induced by *C. concisus* strains isolated from patients with IBD was significantly higher than that induced by *C. concisus* strains isolated from healthy controls (3.34±1.43 vs 1.66±0.30, *P*<0.05) (Figure 5, Table 1).

Expression of TLR4, MD-2, TLR2, TLR5 and COX-2 in HT-29 cells induced by different *C. concisus* strains detected by flow cytometry analysis

For flow cytometry analysis, the levels of surface TLR4, MD-2, TLR2 and TLR5 (non-permeabilized cells) and total TLR4, MD-2, TLR2, TLR5 and COX-2 (permeabilized cells) were expressed as the fold change of the mean channel fluorescence intensity (MFI) of HT-29 cells infected with a *C. concisus* strain relative to the MFI of the non-infected HT-29 cells (HT-29 cells without *C. concisus* infection).

All 11 *C. concisus* strains examined upregulated both surface expression and total expression of TLR4 in HT-29 cells (Figure 6 and Table 2). Nine strains induced more than two fold increase of surface expression of TLR4 (Table 2). The average level of surface TLR4 induced by *C. concisus* strains isolated from patients with IBD was significantly higher than that induced by *C. concisus* strains isolated from healthy controls (3.70±0.46 vs 1.93±0.05, *P*<0.05). The average level of total TLR4 induced by *C. concisus* strains isolated from patients with IBD was not statistically different from that induced by the *C. concisus* strains from the healthy controls (1.81±0.08 vs 1.63±0.05, *P*>0.05).

Four *C. concisus* strains isolated from patients with IBD, P1CDO2, P1CDO3, PACDO1 and P3UCB2, induced more than two-fold increase of surface expression of MD-2 (Figure 6 and Table 2). The average level of surface MD-2 induced by *C. concisus* strains isolated from patients with IBD was higher than that

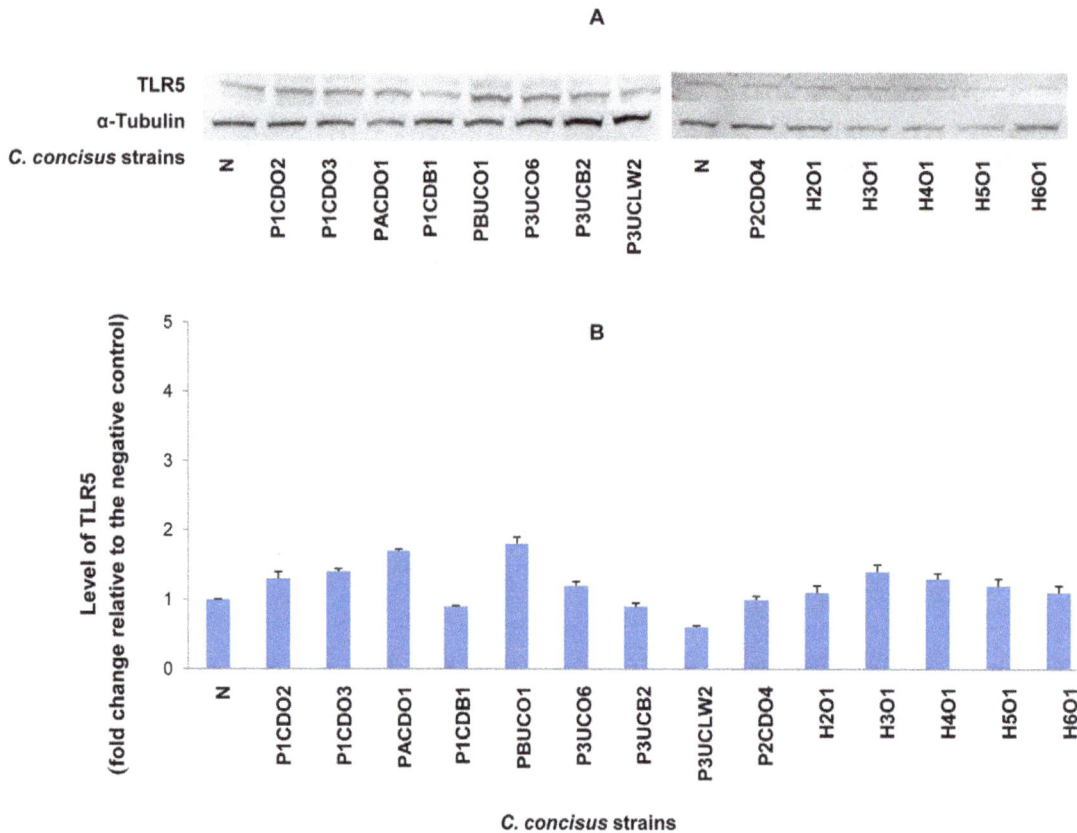

Figure 4. Detection of TLR5 by Western blot in HT-29 cells infected with *C. concisus* strains. HT-29 cells were lysed following incubation with *C. concisus* strains for 24 hours. Expression of TLR5 in HT-29 cells was detected by Western blot. One TLR 5 band was revealed on Western blot. The intensity of TLR5 of each sample was normalized to the intensity of the internal control α-Tubulin of the same sample. The level of TLR5 was expressed as the fold change of the normalized band intensity of a sample relative to the normalized band intensity of the negative control (HT-29 cells without *C. concisus*). A: Representative Western blot of TLR5 (110 kD) and α-Tubulin (55 kD). B: Levels of TLR5 induced by different *C. concisus* strains; data were the average of triplicate experiments ± standard error. N: negative control. H2O1-H6O2: *C. concisus* strains isolated from healthy controls. The remaining nine *C. concisus* strains were from patients with IBD. The average level of TLR5 induced by *C. concisus* strains from patients with IBD was not significantly higher than that induced by *C. concisus* strains from healthy controls ($P>0.05$).

induced by *C. concisus* strains isolated from healthy controls (2.10 ± 0.57 vs 1.36 ± 0.04). However, this was not statistically significant ($P = 0.059$). The average level of total MD-2 induced by *C. concisus* strains isolated from patients with IBD was not statistically different from that induced by *C. concisus* strains isolated from healthy controls (1.78 ± 0.17 vs 1.61 ± 0.19, $P>0.05$).

C. concisus strains did not affect the expression of TLR2 and TLR5 (Figure 6 and Table 2) in HT-29 cells.

All *C. concisus* strains induced an increased expression of COX-2 (Figure 6). However, the increment levels were all below two-fold (Table 2).

Confocal microscopy observation of TLR4, MD-2, TLR2, TLR5 and COX-2 in HT-29 cells

The effects of *C. concisus* strains on expression of TLR4, MD-2, TLR2, TLR5 and COX-2 in HT-29 cells were visualized by confocal microscopy analysis. Confocal microscopy images, which showed an increased expression of TLR4 and COX-2, a slightly increased expression of MD-2 and no change of TLR5 and TLR2 in HT-29 after coincubation with a representative *C. concisus* strain (P1CDB1) for 24 hours are shown in Figure 7.

IL-8 production in HT-29 cells induced by oral and enteric *C. concisus* strains

The concentrations of IL-8 in HT-29 cell culture supernatants were determined by enzyme linked immunosorbent assay (ELISA). The basal amount of IL-8 production by HT-29 cells (HT-29 cells without *C. concisus* infection) was subtracted from the concentration of IL-8 in each sample (HT-29 cells incubated with a *C. concisus* strain) and the results are shown in Figure 8A. The concentration of IL-8 induced by the positive control *Salmonella enterica* serovar Typhimurium LT2 (*Salmonella typhimurium*) was 903 ± 130 pg/ml. Both oral and enteric *C. concisus* strains isolated from patients with IBD and controls induced the production of IL-8. The concentrations (pg/ml) of IL-8 induced by different *C. concisus* strains at a multiplicity of infection (MOI) of 100 were 133 ± 31 for P1CDO2, 276 ± 20 for P1CDO3, 274 ± 9 for PACDO1, 171 ± 19 for P1CDB1, 148 ± 9 for PBUCO1, 234 ± 26 for P3UCO6, 244 ± 14 for P3UCB2, 344 ± 16 for P3UCLW2, 130 ± 11 for P2CDO4, 238 ± 23 for H2O1, 243 ± 36 for H3O1, 229 ± 43 for H4O1, 229 ± 13 for H5O1 and 288 ± 30 for H6O1 (Figure 8 A). The average concentration of IL-8 induced by *C. concisus* strains from patients with IBD was not significantly different from that induced by *C. concisus* strains from healthy controls (217 ± 24 vs 245 ± 11, $P>0.05$).

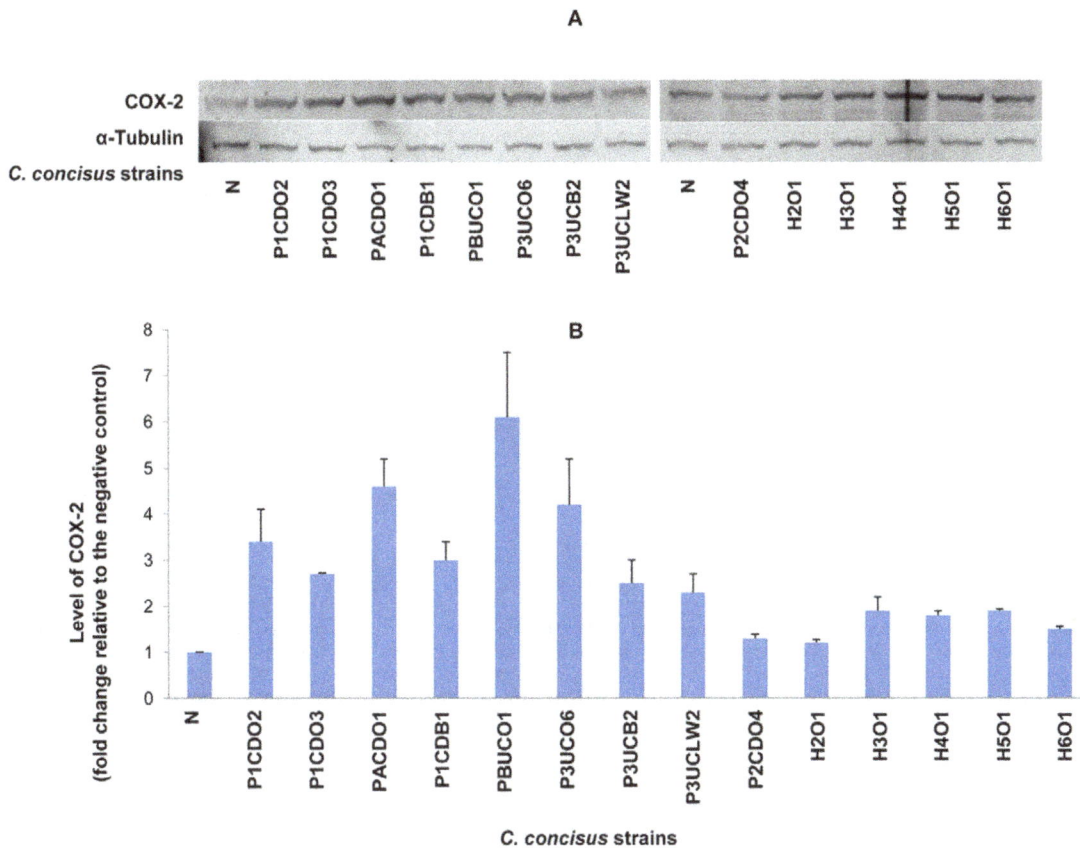

Figure 5. Detection of COX-2 by Western blot in HT-29 cells infected with *C. concisus* strains. HT-cells 29 were lysed following incubation with *C. concisus* strains for 24 hours. Expression of COX-2 in HT-29 cells was detected by Western blot. The intensity of COX-2 band of each sample was normalized to the intensity of the internal control α-Tubulin of the same sample. The level of COX-2 was expressed as the fold change of the normalized band intensity of a sample relative to the normalized band intensity of the negative control (HT-29 cells without *C. concisus* infection). A: Representative Western blot of COX-2 (70 kD) and α-Tubulin (55 kD). B: Levels of COX-2 induced by different *C. concisus* strains; data were the average of triplicate experiments ± standard error. N: negative control. H2O1-H6O1: *C. concisus* strains isolated from healthy controls. The remaining nine *C. concisus* strains were from patients with IBD. The average level of COX-2 induced by *C. concisus* strains from patients with IBD was significantly higher than that induced by *C. concisus* strains from healthy controls ($P<0.05$).

The relationship between the dose of *C. concisus* and the production of IL-8 in HT-29 cells was assessed by measurement of IL-8 concentrations in cell culture supernatants of HT-29 cells infected with three *C. concisus* strains, P1CDO2, P1CDO3 and P1CDB1, at four different MOIs (25, 50, 100 and 200). Concentrations of IL-8 induced by P1CDO2 *C. concisus* strain at the four MOIs were 217±11, 226±1, 276±12 and 482±45 respectively. Concentrations of IL-8 induced by P1CDO3 *C. concisus* strain at the four MOIs were 222±8, 220±8, 274±5 and 453±16 respectively. Concentrations of IL-8 induced by P1CDB1 *C. concisus* strain at the four MOIs were 157±6, 172±7, 171±11 and 292±25 respectively (Figure 8B).

Discussion

This study examined the effects of oral and enteric *C. concisus* strains isolated from patients with IBD and controls on intestinal epithelial expression of TLR4, MD-2, TLR2, TLR5, COX-2 and IL-8 using an *in vitro* cell culture model (HT-29 cells).

Functional membrane LPS receptor is a multiple protein complex including at least three proteins, TLR4, MD-2 and CD14 [26]. In physiological conditions, intestinal epithelial cells express a low level of LPS receptor proteins [23,24,27,28]. In patients with IBD, increased intestinal epithelial expression of

TLR4 has been detected [24]. In our study, we found that all *C. concisus* strains upregulated the expression of TLR4 in HT-29 cells. Furthermore, we found that most *C. concisus* strains isolated from patients with IBD, rather than those strains isolated from healthy controls, predominately upregulated surface expression of TLR4 and Gly-TLR4 (Figures 1 and 6, Tables 1 and 2). These data suggest that some *C. concisus* strains may have the potential to enhance the intestinal epithelial inflammatory responses to LPS derived from other bacterial species such as those from intestinal commensal bacteria. Further studies are needed to investigate this issue.

TLR4 glycosylation has been shown to be essential in forming the functional LPS receptor [26]. Upregulation of gastric epithelial expression of Gly-TLR4 by the gastric mucosal associated Gram-negative bacterium *Helicobacter pylori* was previously observed. In a study examining the effects of *H. pylori* LC11 and LC20 strains on expression of TLR4 in MKN45 gastric epithelial cells, Su *et al* found that *H. pylori* LC11 strain upregulated the expression of Gly-TLR4 at a much greater level than that induced by the LC20 strain [29]. The difference between these two strains is that LC11 contains the pathogenicity island [30]. The mechanisms by which some *C. concisus* strains more effectively upregulate Gly-TLR4 in HT-29 cells are currently unknown, which remains to be investigated.

Table 1. Expression of TLR4, MD-2, TLR2, TLR5 and COX-2 in HT-29 cells induced by *C. concisus* strains detected by Western blot.

	Gly-TLR4	Non-Gly-TLR4	MD-2	Gly-TLR2	Non-Gly-TLR2	TLR5	COX-2
P1CDO2	5.7±1.3	3.2±0.3	1.6±0.2	0.87±0.06	1.11±0.08	1.3±0.1	3.4±0.7
P1CDO3	8.5±0.8	3.1±0.5	1.6±0.2	0.83±0.09	0.95±0.03	1.4±0.04	2.7±0.02
PACDO1	6.6±0.6	2.6±0.4	2.3±0.04	1.11±0.09	1.25±0.13	1.7±0.02	4.6±0.6
P1CDB1	7.3±0.9	2.2±0.4	2.4±0.1	1.15±0.11	1.28±0.15	0.9±0.01	3.0±0.4
PBUCO1	4.1±1.1	6.2±1.1	3.1±0.3	ND	ND	1.8±0.1	6.1±1.4
P3UCO6	5.5±0.4	3.4±0.7	2.1±0.2	1.14±0.08	1.30±0.15	1.2±0.06	4.2±1.0
P3UCB2	4.4±0.5	1.8±0.3	1.9±0.5	0.87±0.09	0.92±0.04	0.9±0.05	2.5±0.5
P3UCLW2	4.3±0.6	1.7±0.2	2.3±0.6	0.74±0.13	0.91±0.09	0.6±0.02	2.3±0.4
P2CDO4	1.6±0.2	1.3±0.08	1.2±0.02	1.06±0.23	0.95±0.06	1.0±0.05	1.3±0.08
H2O1	2.6±0.4	3.0±0.7	1.2±0.05	ND	ND	1.1±0.1	1.2±0.07
H3O1	3.8±0.8	5.2±1.0	1.5±0.1	ND	ND	1.4±0.1	1.9±0.3
H4O1	5.0±1	4.5±0.5	1.8±0.05	1.02±0.17	0.97±0.02	1.3±0.08	1.8±0.1
H5O1	2.5±0.4	6.3±0.5	2.0±0.3	0.88±0.10	0.93±0.07	1.2±0.1	1.9±0.04
H6O1	1.6±0.1	2.3±0.03	1.6±0.2	1.06±0.16	0.85±0.18	1.1±0.1	1.5±0.05

The levels of molecules were expressed as the fold change of the band intensity of HT-29 cells infected with a *C. concisus* strain relative to the band intensity of the negative control (HT-29 cells without *C. concisus* infection), after normalization to the intensity of the internal control α-Tubulin of the same sample. Data were the average of triplicate experiments ± standard error. Gly: glycosylated. Non-Gly: non-glycosylated. Five *C. concisus* strains (H2O1-H6O1) were isolated from healthy controls; the remaining nine strains were from patients with IBD. P1CDB1, P3UCB2 and P3UCLW2 were enteric strains; the remaining 11 strains were oral strains.

Mucosal-associated bacterial species have different effects on TLR4 expression in HT-29 cells. In a study by Furrie *et al*, mRNA levels of TLR4 in HT-29 cells in response to six bacterial species isolated from intestinal biopsies, *Enterococcus faecalis*, *Escherichia coli*, *Peptostreptococcus anaerobium*, *Bifidobacterium longum*, *Bifidobacterium bifidum*, and *Bacteroides fragilis*, were assessed. This study showed that *E. coli* significantly reduced mRNA level of TLR4 and *E. faecalis* significantly increased the mRNA of TLR4 in HT-29 cells. The remaining four bacterial species did not significantly affect the expression of TLR4 in HT-29 cells [31].

MD-2 is a protein that is associated with the extracellular domain of TLR4, which enables TLR4 to function as the LPS receptor [32,33,34]. Increased intestinal epithelial expression and sera MD-2 activity in patients with IBD have been reported [35,36]. In our study, increased MD-2 expression in HT-29 cells following *C. concisus* infection was detected by both Western blot and flow cytometry analysis. However, the levels of increment of MD-2 induced by *C. concisus* were not as great as the increment of TLR4. Some *C. concisus* strains from patients with IBD induced more than two-fold increase of surface expression of MD-2 (Figure 6 and Table 2). Similar to TLR4 glycosylation, MD-2 glycosylation was also shown to be essential in maintaining the functional integrity of LPS receptor [26]. However, in our study we could not assess the levels of glycosylated MD-2 and non-glycosylated MD-2 separately due to the proximity of these two protein bands on Western blot.

TLR5 recognizes a conserved site on bacterial flagellin [37]. The flagellin of *S. typhimurium* is the major epithelial proinflammatory determinant; activating intestinal epithelial expression of TLR5 [38,39]. However, the flagellin of members of ε-Proteobacteria, which include genera of *Helicobacter*, *Campylobacter* and *Wollinella*, is able to evade recognition by TLR5, owing to altered amino acids at the TLR5 recognition site [40]. In our study *C. concisus* strains showed no or minimal effects on TLR5 expression in HT-29 cells (Figures 4 and 6). Previously we showed that *C. concisus* attached to Caco2 cells using their flagella [41]. The evasion of TLR5 would allow *C. concisus* to attach to the intestinal

epithelial cells using flagellum without the notice of the innate immune system, providing the opportunity for this bacterium to modulate the gut innate immune system as discussed above. TLR2 recognizes bacterial lipoproteins. In our study, we found that *C. concisus* did not affect the expression of TLR2 in HT-29 cells.

COX-2 is an inducible enzyme responsible for producing prostaglandins and other important inflammatory mediators [42,43]. Singer *et al* showed that COX-2 was not detected in normal colonic epithelial cells but was induced in patients with IBD [25]. COX-2 has also been shown to be associated with intestinal epithelial high fluid secretion induced by enteric pathogens [44,45]. In addition to its involvement in inflammation, COX-2 has been linked to several malignancies including colorectal cancer [46]. In this study, we found that *C. concisus* strains isolated from patients with IBD induced a significantly higher level of COX-2 in HT-29 cells in comparison to *C. concisus* strains isolated from healthy controls by Western blot. However through flow cytometry analysis, a low level of COX-2 increase induced by these *C. concisus* strains was detected. Furthermore, the increased levels of COX-2 induced by *C. concisus* strains isolated from patients with IBD and controls were not significantly different by flow cytometry analysis. As there may be discrepancies in the sensitivities of Western blot and flow cytometry techniques in the detection of low abundance proteins, it is unclear whether this may have an effect on the differing levels of COX-2 detected. Whether the increment of COX-2 induced by *C. concisus* has a biological impact remains to be examined.

The production of IL-8 induced by different *C. concisus* strains in HT-29 cells was investigated. In this study, we did not observe a correlation between the increased expression levels of TLR4 induced by different *C. concisus* strains and the production of IL-8 in HT-29 cells. The reason for this is not clear. One explanation is that in this study, whole bacteria were used in the induction of IL-8 in HT-29 cells. Given that IL-8 is induced by multiple bacterial components through multiple receptors and pathways, it is therefore difficult to correlate its expression levels to a single receptor. The second possibility is that different *C. concisus* strains

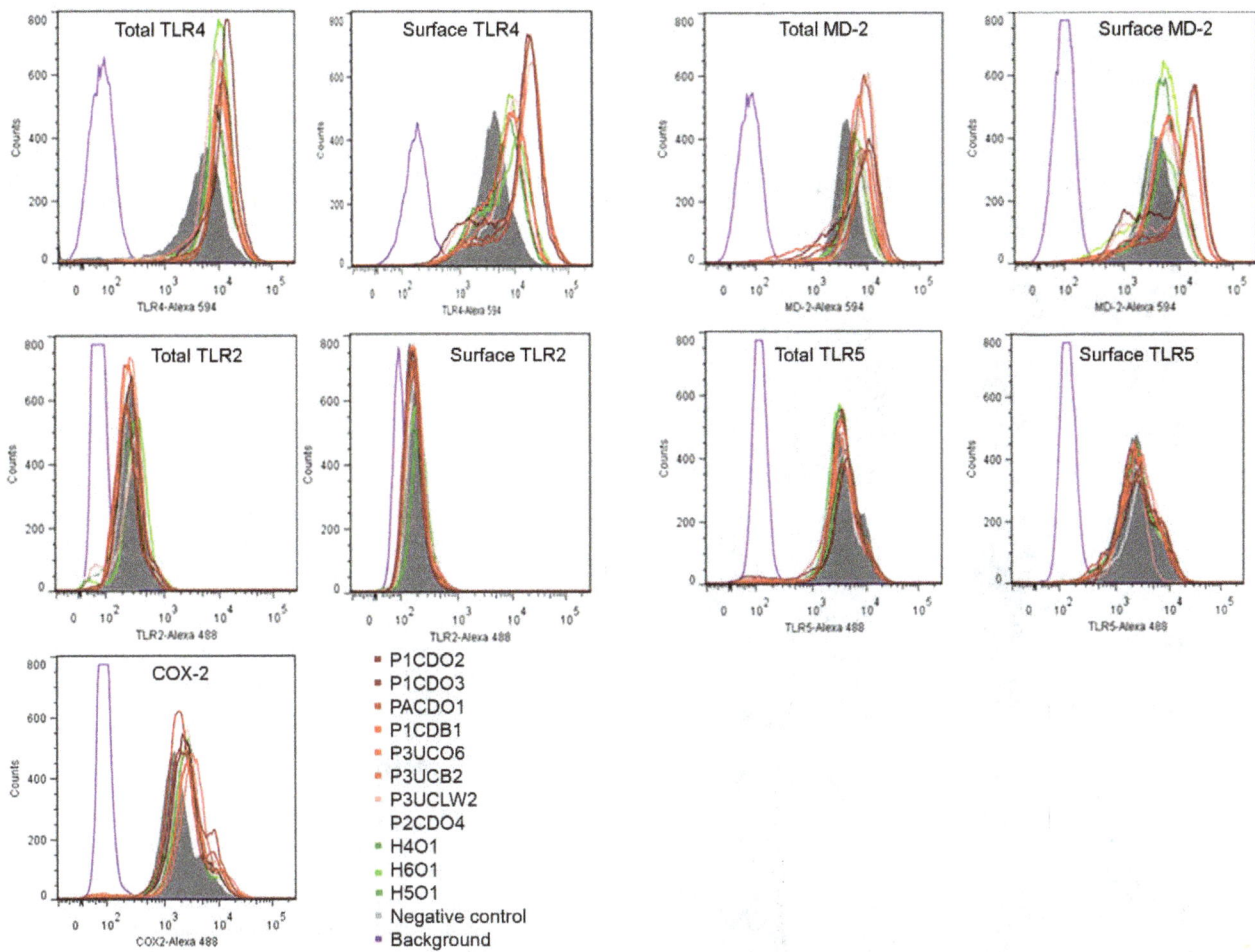

Figure 6. Detection of TLR4, MD-2, TLR2, TLR5 and COX-2 in HT-29 cells by flow cytometry analysis. Flow cytometry histogram showing the expression of surface and total TLR4, MD-2, TLR2, TLR5 and COX-2 in HT-29 cells with and without infection of *C. concisus* strains. A surface expression was measured from non-permeabilized cells and a total expression was measured from permeabilized cells. Background (purple) was from HT-29 cells that were not exposed to antibodies. Negative control (grey): HT-29 cells without *C. concisus* infection. H4O1, H5O1 and H6O1 were strains isolated from healthy controls (green); the remaining eight *C. concisus* strains were from patients with IBD (red).

Table 2. Expression of TLR4, MD-2, TLR2, TLR5 and COX-2 in HT-29 cells induced by *C. concisus* strains detected by flow cytometry.

Strain	Surface TLR4	Total TLR4	Surface MD-2	Total MD-2	Surface TLR2	Total TLR2	Surface TLR5	Total TLR5	COX-2
P1CDO2	4.18±0.56	2.10±0.19	2.46±0.32	1.87±0.07	1.11±0.16	0.99±0.02	1.11±0.06	1.16±0.11	1.43±0.08
P1CDO3	5.03±0.67	1.92±0.18	2.96±0.39	1.86±0.07	0.99±0.07	0.87±0.05	0.99±0.03	1.07±0.05	1.38±0.08
PACDO1	5.40±0.71	1.74±0.15	2.66±0.30	1.49±0.09	1.12±0.16	0.97±0.02	1.01±0.06	1.12±0.09	1.38±0.09
P1CDB1	3.50±0.26	2.12±0.09	1.90±0.18	1.69±0.08	1.13±0.14	0.94±0.04	0.91±0.12	1.08±0.05	1.53±0.04
P2CDO4	2.30±0.29	1.65±0.09	1.54±0.15	1.91±0.10	1.19±0.14	1.14±0.04	1.14±0.10	0.97±0.05	1.33±0.02
P3UCO6	2.23±0.22	1.62±0.11	1.51±0.04	2.00±0.17	1.32±0.33	1.28±0.24	1.13±0.03	1.06±0.05	1.58±0.13
P3UCB2	4.61±0.61	1.51±0.11	2.29±0.29	1.77±0.04	1.21±0.11	1.01±0.11	0.73±0.09	0.85±0.19	1.33±0.08
P3UCLW2	2.30±0.23	1.82±0.07	1.46±0.03	1.61±0.06	1.24±0.12	1.10±0.05	1.10±0.13	1.08±0.05	1.44±0.06
H4O1	1.84±0.20	1.64±0.08	1.36±0.06	1.68±0.10	1.20±0.19	0.95±0.04	1.02±0.06	0.97±0.04	1.45±0.03
H5O1	1.92±0.21	1.54±0.05	1.40±0.07	1.76±0.10	1.36±0.13	1.05±0.06	1.00±0.03	1.24±0.10	1.27±0.05
H6O1	2.02±0.23	1.71±0.09	1.32±0.05	1.40±0.07	1.14±0.11	1.17±0.04	1.02±0.05	0.96±0.04	1.35±0.07

The levels of molecules were expressed as the fold change of the mean channel fluorescence intensity (MFI) of HT-29 cells infected with a *C. concisus* strain relative to the MFI of the non-infected HT-29 cells (HT-29 cells without *C. concisus* infection). A surface expression was measured from non-permeabilized cells and a total expression was measured from permeabilized cells. Data were the average of triplicate experiments ± standard error. Three *C. concisus* strains (H4O1, H5O1 and H6O1) were isolated from healthy controls; the remaining eight strains were from patients with IBD. P1CDB1, P3UCB2 and P3UCLW2 were enteric strains; the remaining 11 strains were oral strains.

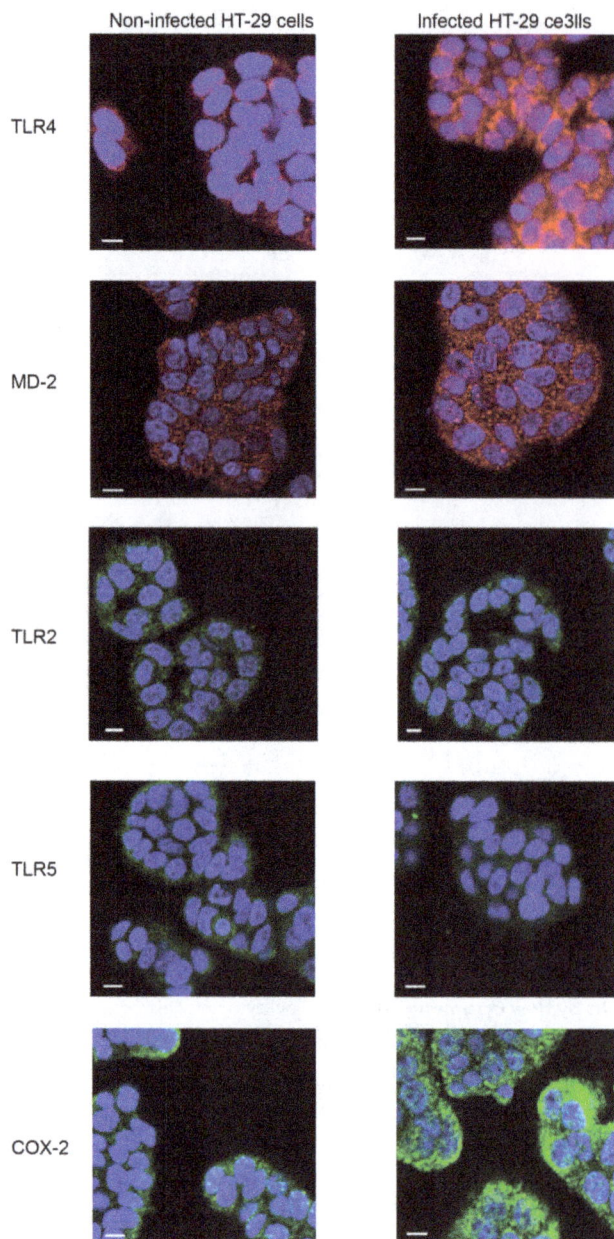

Figure 7. Confocal microscope image of TLR4, MD-2, TLR2, TLR5 and COX-2 expression in HT-29 cells with and without *C. concisu* infection. HT-29 cells were incubated with a representative *C. concisus* strain (P1CDB1) for 24 hours. Expression of TLR4, MD-2, TLR2, TLR5 and COX-2 in HT-29 cells with and without *C. concisus* infection were detected by immunostained using specific antibodies, followed by Alex Fluor conjugated secondary antibodies. The image was viewed using an Olympus FluoView FV1000 Confocal laser scanning microscope. The secondary antibodies used for detection of TLR4 and MD-2 were conjugated with Alexa Fluor 594 (emission colour red). The secondary antibodies used for detection of TLR2, TLR5 and COX-2 were conjugated with Alexa Fluor 488 (emission colour green). Scale Bar = 10 μm.

may have different types of LPS that vary in their abilities to induce proinflammatory mediators, which further complicates the matter of assessing the correlation between the levels of TLR4 and IL-8 between different *C. concisus* strains. This view is supported by many previous studies, as they showed that *C. concisus* is a bacterial

species with great diversity [17,47,48,49,50]. Future studies are required to investigate whether the upregulation of TLR4 by *C. concisus* enhances the intestinal epithelial inflammatory responses to LPS originating from intestinal commensal bacteria, enteric pathogens as well as varying *C. concisus* strains.

Examination of the relationship between *C. concisus* dose and the production of IL-8 in HT-29 cells showed that at lower MOIs (MOI 25–100), an increase in bacterial dose did not affect the production of IL-8. At higher MOIs (MOI 100–200), a bacterial dose dependent production of IL-8 in HT-29 cells was observed (Figure 8B). Interestingly, upregulation of TLR4 in HT-29 cells by *C. concisus* strains does not require a high dose of *C. concisus*. For example, we found that P1CDB1 strain upregulated TLR4 in HT-29 cells at a MOI of 5 and that the upregulation of TLR4 by P1CDB1 at a MOI of 100 was not as efficient as the upregulation of TLR4 by the same strain at a MOI of 25 (data not shown).

In summary, in this study we found that both oral and enteric *C. concisus* strains upregulated expression of TLR4 and MD-2 in HT-29 cells. Some *C. concisus* strains, most of them from patients with IBD, were more effective in regulating surface expression of TLR4 and MD-2, as well as Gly-TLR4. *C. concisus* infection in HT-29 cells did not affect the expression of TLR2 and TLR5. All *C. concisus* strains induced production of IL-8 and COX-2 in HT-29 cells. These data suggest that a potential role of specific *C. concisus* strains in modulating the intestinal epithelial responses to bacterial LPS needs to be investigated.

Materials and Methods

Ethics statement

C. concisus strains used in this study were isolated in our previous studies [2,4,7]. Ethics approvals were granted by the Ethics Committees of the University of New South Wales and the South East Sydney Area Health Service (Ethics Nos: HREC 09237/SESIAHS 09/078, HREC08335/SESIAHS(CHN)07/48 and HREC 06233/SESAHS (ES) 06/164). Written informed consent was obtained from the subjects or the parents/guardians of the minors.

C. concisus strains and cultivation conditions

Fourteen oral (isolated from saliva) and enteric (isolated from intestinal biopsies and feces) *C. concisus* strains we previously isolated were included in this study [2,4,7]. Details of the *C. concisus* strains used in this study were listed in Table 3.

All *C. concisus* isolates were grown in heart infusion broth (Oxoid, Hampshire, UK) containing 2.5% fetal blood serum (FBS) (Bovogen Biologicals, East Keilor, Australia) at 37°C with continuous agitation (120 rpm) under microaerobic condition. The microaerobic condition was generated using *Campylobacter* Gas Generating Kit (Oxoid).

Cultivation of HT-29 cells

Human intestinal epithelial cell line HT-29 cells (ATCC No. HTB-38), were maintained in McCoy's 5A medium (Invitrogen, California, USA) supplemented with 10% FBS (Bovogen Biologicals), 100 U/ml penicillin and 100 μg/ml streptomycin (Invitrogen). The cells were grown at 37°C in a humidified incubator containing 5% CO_2.

Antibodies used in this study

All antibodies used in this study were purchased from Santa Cruz Biotechnology Inc (Santa Cruz biotechnology Inc, California, USA). Primary antibodies used were polyclonal anti-TLR4 (sc-10741), anti-MD-2 (sc-20668), anti-TLR2 (sc-166900), anti-

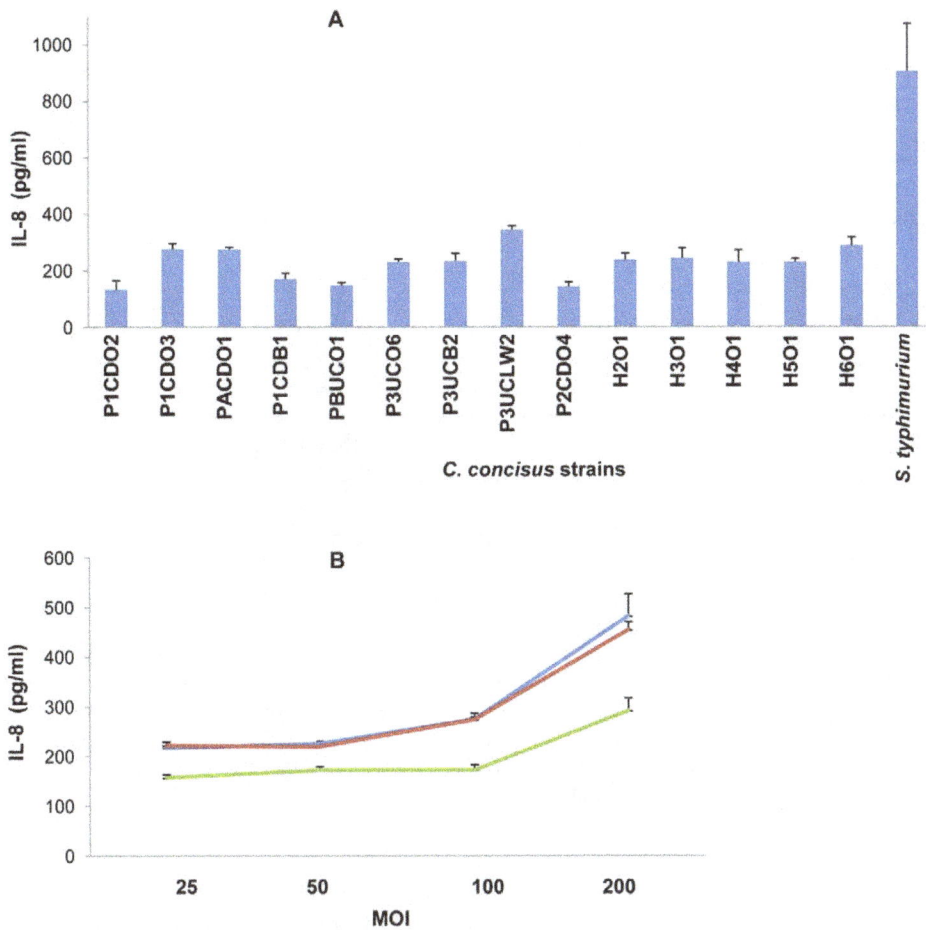

Figure 8. Production of IL-8 by HT-29 cells induced by *C. concisus* strains. A. HT-29 cells were incubated with *C. concisus* strains at a multiplicity of infection (MOI) of 100 for 24 hours. Concentrations of IL-8 in the cell culture supernatants were measured by ELISA. The basal production of IL-8 (HT-29 cells without *C. concisus* infection) has been subtracted from values shown in Figure 8A. Data were the average of triplicates ± standard error. The level of IL-8 induced by *C. concisus* strains from patients with IBD was not statistically different from that induced by *C. concisus* strains from the healthy controls (P>0.05). Five *C. concisus* strains (H2O1-H6O1) were isolated from healthy controls; the remaining nine strains were from patients with IBD. **B.** HT-29 cells were incubated with three *C. concisus* strains respectively at four different MOIs (25, 50, 100 and 200) for 24 hours. The three *C. concisus* strains used were P1CDO2 (blue), P1CDO3 (red) and P1CDB1 (green). Concentrations of IL-8 in the cell culture supernatants were measured by ELISA. The basal production of IL-8 (HT-29 cells without *C. concisus* infection) has been subtracted from values shown in Figure 8B. Data were the average of triplicates ± standard error.

TLR5 (sc-16243), anti-Cox-2 (sc-1746), and anti-α tubulin (sc-31779). Secondary antibodies conjugated with horseradish peroxidase (HRP) used for Western blot were bovine anti-goat IgG (sc-2352), goat anti-mouse IgG (sc-2031) and goat anti-rabbit IgG (sc-2054). Secondary antibodies used for flow cytometry analysis and immunostaining were Alexa Fluor® 488 donkey anti-goat IgG (A11055), Alexa Fluor® 488 goat anti-mouse IgG (A11029), and Alexa Fluor® 594 goat anti-rabbit IgG (A11037) (Invitrogen).

Western blot

Expression of TLR4, MD-2, TLR2, TLR5 and COX-2 in response to *C. concisus* infection in HT-29 cells was examined by Western blot. HT-29 cells at a concentration of 5×10^5 cell/ml were cultured in 6-well cell culture plates (3 ml cell suspension/well). The cells were grown for 48 hours. HT-29 cells were washed five times using Dulbecco's Phosphate-Buffered Saline (D-PBS) and then infected with *C. concisus* at a MOI of 25 in McCoy's 5A medium supplemented with 10% FBS without antibiotics. The

cells were further incubated for 24 hours. HT-29 cells without *C. concisus* infection were used as the negative control.

HT-29 cells were harvested from culture plates by scraping and washed with pre-cooled D-PBS. The cells were lysed using RIPA Buffer (50 mM Tris, 150 mM NaCl, 1% Triton X-100, 0.1% SDS) containing a mixture of protease inhibitors (Sigma-Aldrich, Castle Hill Australia). Whole cell lysates were centrifuged twice at 14000 relative centrifugal force (RCF) for 20 minutes at 4°C. Supernatant was collected and stored at −80°C till use. Protein concentrations were determined using Pierce® BCA Protein Assay Kit (Thermo Fisher Scientific, Scoresby, Australia).

C. concisus whole cell proteins (30 µg) were separated on 12% sodium dodecyl sulfate (SDS)-polyacrylamide gel under reducing conditions and transferred onto polyvinylidine difluoride (PVDF) membranes for two hour at 100 Volt in a cold room (4°C). PVDF Membrane were immersed in absolute methanol for five seconds then equilibrated in the transfer buffer for 10–20 minutes prior to be used for protein transfer. The transfer buffer consists of 0.3% (w/v) Tris base, 1.44% (w/v) glycine and 20% methanol (v/v).

Table 3. *C. concisus* strains used in this study.

Strain ID	Source	Clinical conditions
P1CDO2	Saliva	Crohn's disease
P1CDO3	Saliva	Crohn's disease
P1CDB1	Intestinal biopsy	Crohn's disease
PACDO1	Saliva	Crohn's disease
P3UCO6	Saliva	Ulcerative colitis
P3UCB2	Intestinal biopsy	Ulcerative colitis
P3UCLW2	Luminal washout	Ulcerative colitis
PBUCO1	Saliva	Ulcerative colitis
P2CDO4	Saliva	Crohn's disease
H2O1	Saliva	Healthy
H3O1	Saliva	Healthy
H4O1	Saliva	Healthy
H5O1	Saliva	Healthy
H6O1	Saliva	Healthy

These *C. concisus* strains were isolated from previous studies [2,4,7]. P1CDO2, P1CDO3 and P1CDB1 were isolated from a patient with CD. P3UCO6, P3UCB2 and P3UCLW2 were isolated from a patient with UC. The remaining strains were isolated from individual patients with IBD and healthy controls. P1CDB1 was named as UNSWCD and P1CDB1(UNSWCD) in previous studies [17,41].

The transfer buffer was pre-chilled on ice prior to use. Following protein transfer, PVDF membranes were blocked with 5% skim milk in washing buffer (0.05% Tween-20 in phosphate buffered saline (PBS)) for two hours then probed with primary antibodies (1:350) overnight at 4°C, followed by secondary antibodies conjugated with HRP (1:2500) for 90 minutes at room temperature (RT). Antibodies were diluted using blocking solution. The HRP-labeled antibodies were detected using Immun-Star^{TM} WesterC^{TM} Chemiluminescence Kits (Bio-Rad laboratory, Gladesville, Australia) and a LAS-3000 imaging system (Fujifilm). The intensities of protein bands were analyzed using Image J software (National institute of health, US). Western blot experiments were repeated three times. PVDF membranes were incubated with antibodies for the molecules examined (TLR4, MD-2, TLR2, TLR5 and COX-2) first, then stripped and re-incubacted with anti-alpha-tubulin antibody. One PVDF membrane was used for detection of one of the molecules examined.

Flow cytometry analysis

Expression of TLR4, MD-2, TLR2, TLR5 and COX-2 in HT-29 cells was detected by flow cytometry analysis. HT-29 cells (10 ml at 5×10^5 cell/ml) were seeded onto T-25 tissue culture flasks (Nunc, Roskilde, Denmark) for 24 hours, then infected with *C. concisus* at a MOI of 25 and further incubated for 24 hours. HT-29 cells without *C. concisus* infection were used as the negative control.

Following infection with *C. concisus*, HT-29 cells were washed twice with D-PBS and detached from culture flasks by incubating with 0.25% trypsin (Invitrogen) for five minutes (1 ml each flask), followed by deactivation of trypsin using McCoy's 5A medium supplemented with 10% FBS without antibiotics. The cells were washed twice with pre-cooled D-PBS by centrifugation at 300 RCF for 5 minutes at 4°C.

HT-29 cells were fixed for 12 minutes in 3.7% paraformaldehyde in PBS, then permeabilized for 10 minutes with 0.1% Triton X-100 in PBS when required to analyse the total expression of the

target protein in cells. HT-29 cells that were not permeabilized were used to analyse the surface expression of the target proteins. Cells were then washed twice using blocking solution (1% Bovine Serum albumin in PBS), and incubated with the blocking solution for 30 minutes at RT, HT-29 cells were then sequentially incubated at RT with a primary antibody (1:40) and an Alexa Fluor conjugated secondary antibody (5 µg/ml) for one hour and 45 minutes respectively. Primary and secondary antibodies were diluted by blocking solution. Cells were washed three times with the blocking solution between incubations for 10 minutes each time. Cells were collected after each wash by centrifugation at 300 RCF for 5 minutes at 4°C. HT-29 cells that were not exposed to antibodies were used to assess the background signal. Data were acquired by BD LSRFortessa^{TM} SORP cell analyser (BD Biosciences, San Jose, USA) and analysed in Flow Jo software (Tree star inc, OR, US). Flow cytometry experiments were in triplicate and repeated at least twice.

Immunofluorescence staining and confocal microscopy

Expression of TLR4, MD-2, TLR2, TLR5 and COX-2 in responses to *C. concisus* infection in HT-29 was visualized using immunofluorescence staining and confocal microscopy

HT-29 cells were seeded onto sterile cover-slips placed in 6-well cell culture plates (3 ml of cells at a concentration of 1×10^5 cell/ml) and allowed to grow for 48 hours. HT-29 cells were then infected with *C. concisus* at a MOI of 25 and incubated for further 24 hours. HT-29 cells without infection of *C. concisus* were used as negative control.

HT-29 cells grown on cover-slips were fixed in 3.7% paraformaldehyde (was diluted by PBS) for 17 minute at RT, permeabilized with 0.1% Triton X-100 in PBS for 10 minutes at RT. The cover-slips carrying HT-29 cells were blocked with 1% bovine serum albumin (Invitrogen) in PBS for one hour at RT. HT-29 cells were then sequentially incubated with a primary antibody (1:40) and an Alexa Fluor conjugated secondary antibody (5 µg/ml) for 75 minutes respectively, followed by staining with Hoechst 33342 (1.5 µg/ml) (Invitrogen) diluted in PBS for 12 minutes at RT. Both primary and secondary antibodies were diluted in blocking solution. The incubations with the secondary antibodies and the Hoechst 33342 were carried out in the dark at RT.

The cover slips were washed three times with PBS between incubations for 10 minutes at RT. The cover slips were mounted using AF1 antifadent (Citifluor Ltd, London, UK) and HT-29 cells were observed using an Olympus FluoView FV1000 Confocal laser scanning microscope.

Measurement of IL-8 in HT-29 cell culture supernatant by ELISA

To examine the production of IL-8 by HT-29 cells induced by *C. concisus*, HT-29 cells (5×10^5 cell/ml) were seeded in 24-well cell culture plates (1 ml/each well) and incubated for 48 hours. HT-29 cells were then infected with *C. concisus* and further incubated for 24 hours. Supernatants were collected and centrifuged twice for 2 minutes at 10,000 g. IL-8 secreted in the supernatants was measured by ELISA using Human IL-8 CytoSet^{TM} (Invitrogen) according to manufacturer's instructions.

Supernatant collected from HT-29 cells co-incubated with *S. typhimurium* (UNSW culture collection) and supernatant from HT-29 cells without bacterial infection were used as the positive and negative control respectively.

Statistic analysis

Data were analyzed by means of unpaired t test using GraphPad Prism version 5.1 (San Diego, CA). P-values below 0.05 (two tailed, 95% confidence interval) were considered significant.

References

1. Tanner ACR, Badger S, Lai CH, Listgarten MA, Visconti RA, et al. (1981) *Wolinella* gen-nov, *Wolinella-succinogenes* (Vibrio-succinogenes-wolin et-al) comb-nov, and description of bacteroides-gracilis sp-nov, *Wolinella-recta* sp-nov, *Campylobacter-concisus* sp-nov, and *Eikenella-corrodens* from humans with periodon-tal-disease. Int J Syst Bacteriol 31: 432–445.

2. Zhang L, Budiman V, Day AS, Mitchell H, Lemberg DA, et al. (2010) Isolation and detection of *Campylobacter concisus* from saliva of healthy individuals and patients with inflammatory bowel disease. J Clin Microbiol 48: 2965–2967.

3. Vandamme P, Dewhirst FE, Paster BJ, On SLW (2005) Genus I. *Campylobacter*. In: Garrity GM, Brenner DJ, Krieg NR, Staley JT, editors. Bergey's Manual of Syst Bacteriol. 2 ed. New York: Springer. pp. 1147–1160.

4. Zhang L, Man SM, Day AS, Leach ST, Lemberg DA, et al. (2009) Detection and isolation of Campylobacter species other than *C. jejuni* from children with Crohn's disease. J Clin Microbiol 47: 453–455.

5. Man SM, Zhang L, Day AS, Leach ST, Lemberg DA, et al. (2010) *Campylobacter concisus* and other *Campylobacter* species in children with newly diagnosed Crohn's disease. Inflamm Bowel Dis 16: 1008–1016.

6. Mukhopadhya I, Thomson JM, Hansen R, Berry SH, El-Omar EM, et al. (2011) Detection of *Campylobacter concisus* and other *Campylobacter* species in colonic biopsies from adults with ulcerative colitis. Plos One 6: e21490.

7. Mahendran V, Riordan S, Grimm M, Tran T, Major J, et al. (2011) Prevalence of *Campylobacter* species in adult Crohn's disease and the preferential colonization sites of *Campylobacter* species in the human intestine. Plos One 6: e25417.

8. Lastovica AJ (2009) Clinical relevance of *Campylobacter concisus* isolated from pediatric patients. J Clin Microbiol 47: 2360–2360.

9. Sartor RB (2008) Microbial influences in inflammatory bowel diseases. Gastroenterology 134: 577–594.

10. Kaser A, Zeissig S, Blumberg RS (2010) Inflammatory Bowel Disease. In: Paul WE, Littman DR, Yokoyama WM, editors. Ann Rev Immunol. pp. 573–621.

11. Taurog JD RJ, Croft JT, Simmons WA, Zhou M, Fernandez-Sueiro JL, Balish E, Hammer RE (1994) The germfree state prevents development of gut and joint inflammatory disease in HLA-B27 transgenic rats. J Exp Med 180: 2359–2364.

12. D'Haens GR, Geboes K, Peeters M, Baert F, Penninckx F, et al. (1998) Early lesions of recurrent Crohn's disease caused by infusion of intestinal contents in excluded ileum. Gastroenterology 114: 262–267.

13. Rutgeerts P, Goboes K, Peeters M, Hiele M, Penninckx F, et al. (1991) Effect of faecal stream diversion on recurrence of Crohn's disease in the neoterminal ileum. Lancet 338: 771–774.

14. Veltkamp C, Tonkonogy SL, De Jong YP, Albright C, Grenther WB, et al. (2001) Continuous stimulation by normal luminal bacteria is essential for the development and perpetuation of colitis in Tg is an element of 26 mice. Gastroenterology 120: 900–913.

15. Macpherson A, Khoo UY, Forgacs I, PhilpottHoward J, Bjarnason I (1996) Mucosal antibodies in inflammatory bowel disease are directed against intestinal bacteria. Gut 38: 365–375.

16. Duchmann R, Kaiser I, Hermann E, Mayet W, Ewe K, et al. (1995) Tolerance exists towards resident intestinal flora but is broken in active inflammatory bowel disease (IBD). Clin Exp Immunol 102: 448–455.

17. Ismail Y, Mahendran V, Octavia S, Day AS, Riordan SM, et al. (2012) Investigation of the enteric pathogenic potential of oral *Campylobacter concisus* strains Isolated from patients with inflammatory bowel disease. Plos One 7: e38217.

18. Chaban B, Ngeleka M, Hill JE (2010) Detection and quantification of 14 *Campylobacter* species in pet dogs reveals an increase in species richness in feces of diarrheic animals. BMC Microbiol 10: 73–79.

19. Petersen RF, Harrington CS, Kortegaard HE, On SLW (2007) A PCR-DGGE method for detection and identification of Campylobacter, Helicobacter, Arcobacter and related Epsilobacteria and its application to saliva samples from humans and domestic pets. J Appl Microbiol 103: 2601–2615.

20. Lynch OA, Cagney C, McDowell DA, Duffy G (2011) Occurrence of fastidious *Campylobacter* spp. in fresh meat and poultry using an adapted cultural protocol. Int J Food Microbiol 150: 171–177.

21. Nielsen HL, Nielsen H, Ejlertsen T, Engberg J, Gunzel D, et al. (2011) Oral and fecal *Campylobacter concisus* strains perturb barrier function by apoptosis induction in HT-29/b6 intestinal epithelial cells. Plos One 6: e23858.

22. Kalischuk LD, Inglis GD (2011) Comparative genotypic and pathogenic examination of *Campylobacter concisus* isolates from diarrheic and non-diarrheic humans. Bmc Microbiol 11: 53–66.

23. Abreu MT, Vora P, Faure E, Thomas LS, Arnold ET, et al. (2001) Decreased expression of toll-like receptor-4 and MD-2 correlates with intestinal epithelial cell protection against dysregulated proinflammatory gene expression in response to bacterial lipopolysaccharide. J Immunol 167: 1609–1616.

24. Cario E, Podolsky DK (2000) Differential alteration in intestinal epithelial cell expression of Toll-like receptor 3 (TLR3) and TLR4 in inflammatory bowel disease. Infect Immun 68: 7010–7017.

25. Singer, II, Kawka DW, Schloemann S, Tessner T, Riehl T, et al. (1998) Cyclooxygenase 2 is induced in colonic epithelial cells in inflammatory bowel disease. Gastroenterology 115: 297–306.

26. Correia JD, Ulevitch RJ (2002) MD-2 and TLR4 N-linked glycosylations are important for a functional lipopolysaccharide receptor. J Biol Chem 277: 1845–1854.

27. Grimm MC, Pavli P, Vandepol E, Doe WF (1995) Evidence for a CD14(+) population of monocytes in inflammatory bowel-disease mucosa-implications for pathogenesis. Clin Exp Immunol 100: 291–297.

28. Fusunyan RD, Nanthakumar NN, Baldeon ME, Walker WA (2001) Evidence for an immature immune response in the immature human intestine: Toll-like receptors on fetal enterocytes. Pediatr Res 49: 589–593.

29. Su B, Ceponis PJM, Lebel S, Huynh H, Sherman PM (2003) *Helicobacter pylori* activates toll-like receptor 4 expression in gastrointestinal epithelial cells. Infect Immun 71: 3496–3502.

30. Jones NL, Day AS, Jennings HA, Sherman PM (1999) *Helicobacter pylori* induces gastric epithelial cell apoptosis in association with increased Fas receptor expression. Infect Immun 67: 4237–4242.

31. Furrie E, Macfarlane S, Thomson G, Macfarlane GT (2005) Toll-like receptors-2,-3 and-4 expression patterns on human colon and their regulation by mucosal-associated bacteria. Immunol 115: 565–574.

32. Shimazu R, Akashi S, Ogata H, Nagai Y, Fukudome K, et al. (1999) MD-2, a molecule that confers lipopolysaccharide responsiveness on Toll-like receptor 4. J Exp Med 189: 1777–1782.

33. Nagai Y, Akashi S, Nagafuku M, Ogata M, Iwakura Y, et al. (2002) Essential role of MD-2 in LPS responsiveness and TLR4 distribution. Nat Immunol 3: 667–672.

34. Ohnishi T, Muroi M, Tanamoto K (2003) MD-2 is necessary for the Toll-like receptor 4 protein to undergo glycosylation essential for its translocation to the cell surface. Clin Diag Lab Immunol 10: 405–410.

35. Vamadevan AS, Fukata M, Arnold ET, Thomas LS, Hsu D, et al. (2010) Regulation of Toll-like receptor 4-associated MD-2 in intestinal epithelial cells: a comprehensive analysis. Innate Immun 16: 93–103.

36. Seksik P, Sokol H, Grondin V, Adrie C, Duboc H, et al. (2010) Sera from patients with Crohn's disease break bacterial lipopolysaccharide tolerance of human intestinal epithelial cells via MD-2 activity. Innate Immun 16: 381–390.

37. Smith KD, Andersen-Nissen E, Hayashi F, Strobe K, Bergman MA, et al. (2003) Toll-like receptor 5 recognizes a conserved site on flagellin required for protofilament formation and bacterial motility. Nat Immunol 4: 1247–1253.

38. Zeng H, Carlson AQ, Guo YW, Yu YM, Collier-Hyams LS, et al. (2003) Flagellin is the major proinflammatory determinant of enteropathogenic Salmonella. J Immunol 171: 3668–3674.

39. Gewirtz AT, Navas TA, Lyons S, Godowski PJ, Madara JL (2001) Cutting edge: Bacterial flagellin activates basolaterally expressed TLR5 to induce epithelial proinflammatory gene expression. J Immunol 167: 1882–1885.

40. Andersen-Nissen E, Smith KD, Strobe KL, Barrett SLR, Cookson BT, et al. (2005) Evasion of Toll-like receptor 5 by flagellated bacteria. Proc Natl Acad Sci USA 102: 9247–9252.

41. Man SM, Kaakoush NO, Leach ST, Nahidi L, Lu HK, et al. (2010) Host attachment, invasion, and stimulation of proinflammatory cytokines by *Campylobacter concisus* and other non-*Campylobacter jejuni Campylobacter* species. J Infect Dis 202: 1855–1865.

42. Williams CS, Mann M, DuBois RN (1999) The role of cyclooxygenases in inflammation, cancer, and development. Oncogene 18: 7908–7916.

43. Fukata M, Chen AL, Klepper A, Krishnareddy S, Vamadevan AS, et al. (2006) Cox-2 is regulated by Toll-like receptor-4 (TLR4) signaling: Role in proliferation and apoptosis in the intestine. Gastroenterology 131: 862–877.

44. Kim JM, Lee JY, Yoon YM, Oh YK, Kang JS, et al. (2006) *Bacteroides fragilis* enterotoxin induces cyclooxygenase-2 and fluid secretion in intestinal epithelial cells through NF-kappa B activation. Eur J Immunol 36: 2446–2456.

45. Bertelsen LS, Paesold G, Eckmann L, Barrett KE (2003) *Salmonella* infection induces a hypersecretory phenotype in human intestinal xenografts by inducing cyclooxygenase 2. Infect Immun 71: 2102–2109.

46. Thun MJ, Henley SJ, Patrono C (2002) Nonsteroidal anti-inflammatory drugs as anticancer agents: Mechanistic, pharmacologic, and clinical issues. J Natl Cancer Inst 94: 252–266.

47. Aabenhus R, On SLW, Siemer BL, Permin H, Andersen LP (2005) Delineation of *Campylobacter concisus* genomospecies by amplified fragment length polymorphism analysis and correlation of results with clinical data. J of Clin Microbiol 43: 5091–5096.

48. Vandamme P, Falsen E, Pot B, Hoste B, Kersters K, et al. (1989) Identification of EF group-22 Campylobacters from gastroenteritis cases as *Campylobacter concisus*. J Clin Microbiol 27: 1775–1781.

49. Matsheka MI, Lastovica AJ, Elisha BG (2001) Molecular identification of *Campylobacter concisus*. J Clin Microbiol 39: 3684–3689.

50. Bastyns K, Chapelle S, Vandamme P, Goossens H, Dewachter R (1995) Specific detection of *Campylobacter concisus* by PCR amplification of 23S rDNA areas. Mol Cell Probes 9: 247–250.

Author Contributions

Conceived and designed the experiments: YI HL LZ. Performed the experiments: YI HL. Analyzed the data: YI HL LZ. Wrote the paper: YI HL SMR MCG LZ.

8

Macrophages, Nitric Oxide and microRNAs are Associated with DNA Damage Response Pathway and Senescence in Inflammatory Bowel Disease

Jane J. Sohn[1], Aaron J. Schetter[1,9], Harris G. Yfantis[2,9], Lisa A. Ridnour[3], Izumi Horikawa[1], Mohammed A. Khan[1], Ana I. Robles[1], S. Perwez Hussain[1], Akiteru Goto[1], Elise D. Bowman[1], Lorne J. Hofseth[4], Jirina Bartkova[5], Jiri Bartek[5,6], Gerald N. Wogan[7], David A. Wink[3], Curtis C. Harris[1]*

1 Laboratory of Human Carcinogenesis, Center for Cancer Research, National Cancer Institute, Bethesda, Maryland, United States of America, 2 Pathology and Laboratory Medicine, Baltimore Veterans Affairs Medical Center, and Department of Pathology, University of Maryland School of Medicine, Baltimore, Maryland, United States of America, 3 Radiation Biology Branch, National Cancer Institute, Bethesda, Maryland, United States of America, 4 Department of Pharmaceutical and Biomedical Sciences, South Carolina College of Pharmacy, University of South Carolina, Columbia, South Carolina, United States of America, 5 Cancer Society Research Center, Copenhagen, Denmark, 6 Institute of Molecular and Translational Medicine, Faculty of Medicine and Dentistry, Palacky University, Olomouc, Czech Republic, 7 Department of Biological Engineering, Center for Environmental Health Sciences, Massachusetts Institute of Technology, Cambridge, Massachusetts, United States of America

Abstract

Background: Cellular senescence can be a functional barrier to carcinogenesis. We hypothesized that inflammation modulates carcinogenesis through senescence and DNA damage response (DDR). We examined the association between senescence and DDR with macrophage levels in inflammatory bowel disease (IBD). *In vitro* experiments tested the ability of macrophages to induce senescence in primary cells. Inflammation modulating microRNAs were identified in senescence colon tissue for further investigation.

Methodology/Principal Findings: Quantitative immunohistochemistry identified protein expression by colon cell type. Increased cellular senescence (HP1γ; P = 0.01) or DDR (γH2A.X; P = 0.031, phospho-Chk2, P = 0.014) was associated with high macrophage infiltration in UC. Co-culture with macrophages (ANA-1) induced senescence in >80% of primary cells (fibroblasts MRC5, WI38), illustrating that macrophages induce senescence. Interestingly, macrophage-induced senescence was partly dependent on nitric oxide synthase, and clinically relevant NO• levels alone induced senescence. NO• induced DDR *in vitro*, as detected by immunofluorescence. In contrast to UC, we noted in Crohn's disease (CD) that senescence (HP1γ; P<0.001) and DDR (γH2A.X; P<0.05, phospho-Chk2; P<0.001) were higher, and macrophages were not associated with senescence. We hypothesize that nitric oxide may modulate senescence in CD; epithelial cells of CD had higher levels of NOS2 expression than in UC (P = 0.001). Microarrays and quantitative-PCR identified miR-21 expression associated with macrophage infiltration and NOS2 expression.

Conclusions: Senescence was observed in IBD with senescence-associated β-galactosidase and HP1γ. Macrophages were associated with senescence and DDR in UC, and *in vitro* experiments with primary human cells showed that macrophages induce senescence, partly through NO•, and that NO• can induce DDR associated with senescence. Future experiments will investigate the role of NO• and miR-21 in senescence. This is the first study to implicate macrophages and nitrosative stress in a direct effect on senescence and DDR, which is relevant to many diseases of inflammation, cancer, and aging.

Editor: Benoit Foligne, Institut Pasteur de Lille, France

Funding: This research was supported by the Intramural Research Program of the National Cancer Institute. Dr. Sohn was supported by the Cancer Research Training Award Fellowship from the National Cancer Institute. Dr. Bartkova and Dr. Bartek were supported by the Danish Cancer Society, the Danish National Research Foundation, and the European Commission (projects: Infla-Care, Biomedreg and DDResponse). The funders had no role in study design, data collection and analysis, decision to publish, or preparation of the manuscript.

Competing Interests: The authors have declared that no competing interests exist.

* E-mail: Curtis_Harris@nih.gov

9 These authors contributed equally to this work.

Introduction

Inflammatory bowel disease (IBD) is associated with high morbidity, poor quality of life and an increased risk of colon cancer in over 3.5 million people in the United States and Europe, with a steadily growing prevalence in Asia [1]. The most important risk factors for colon cancer development in IBD patients are duration and extent of inflammation. Patients with ulcerative colitis (UC), a subtype of IBD, develop colon cancer with a five-fold overall relative risk compared to population controls [2]. Colon tissue from IBD patients has been used to study the relationship between inflammation and cancer, with an emphasis on DNA damage. IBD is associated with increased etheno-DNA adducts [3], microsatellite instability [4], p53 mutational load [5] and clonal expansion of cells with mutations in polyguanine tracts [6]. UC tissues show initial activation of p53 in response to nitric oxide (NO•) [7], and eventual inactivation of p53 with increasing mutation load [5], resulting in a pattern of mutation unique compared to spontaneous colon cancer [8].

Evidence suggests that senescence acts as a barrier to carcinogenesis in UC and that this barrier is reduced in dysplastic lesions [9]. Inflamed colons from UC patients have increased expression of the DNA damage response pathway (DDR) sensor protein γH2A.X [10], which leads to activation of the stress-associated p53 pathway. DDR is implicated in the induction of premature cellular senescence [11,12], independently of telomere length, which classically regulates senescence [13] in cellular aging. Prosenescent cytokines [14], WNT16 [15], and the Rb/p16 [16] pathway (through its induction of heterochromatin formation with HP1γ positive foci [17]), have all been implicated in premature cellular senescence. Premature cellular senescence halts carcinogenesis by limiting the proliferation of cells in the early stages of carcinogenesis [12,18–20]. Senescence during inflammation is not well studied, but experiments *in vitro* have shown increased p53 and p21, in response to oxidative stress induced senescence [21,22]. Elucidating the cause and outcome of inflammation-associated senescence is relevant for the 25% of human cancers associated with chronic inflammation and infection [23,24].

Macrophages are a key component of a chronic inflammatory response and constitute part of the heterogeneous population of cells in tumors. Macrophages and NO• has been implicated in the activation of p53 [7] in IBD and the activation of the Akt pathway in breast cancer [25]. In addition, tumor-associated macrophages are implicated in carcinogenesis [26,27]. We hypothesized that macrophages accelerate cellular senescence in epithelial cells at risk for carcinogenesis through the DNA damage pathway, in a NO• -dependent manner. NO• secreted by macrophages rapidly decreases in concentration with diffusion [28], thus cells may be exposed to different levels of NO• depending on distance from an NO• producing macrophage [29]. Stromal fibroblasts can be cellular targets of NO• and become senescent and secrete pro-inflammatory cytokines such as IL-6 and IL-8 [30]. We quantified macrophages in the lamina propria using quantitative immunohistochemistry (IHC) to identify macrophage numbers within the mucosa (i.e. macrophage infiltration). Levels of macrophage infiltration were correlated to DDR and senescence. Normal colonic epithelial cells can produce endogenous NO•, thus we also measured levels of NOS2 by IHC in the epithelium. Further, we determined if macrophages and NO• induce cellular senescence *in vitro*.

MicroRNAs (miRs) have been shown to be involved in nearly every biological process examined, including inflammation and senescence. To investigate the potential for miRs to be involved in macrophage or NOS2- induced senescence, we also evaluated the association of microRNAs with macrophage infiltration and NOS2 in IBD, and colonic adenomas.

Methods and Patients

Ethics Statement

This study was approved by the Institutional Review Board of the National Cancer Institute (OHSRP 3637, OHSRP 3961).

Tissues

Colon tissues from UC and CD patients and colon adenomas were obtained from the Cooperative Human Tissue Network (Philadelphia, PA; Table S1). Two samples with varying degrees of gross inflammation were taken from each patient. Normal colons were obtained from University of Maryland, with tissues collected within 2 hours of death from patients who died of traumatic causes, were donors for organ transplants, and had no diseases related to the colon or chronic inflammation (Department of Pathology, University of Maryland, Baltimore, MD). Consent for the use of the tissues for research purposes was provided by next of kin or legally responsible individual on behalf of the deceased prior to the autopsy being performed. Investigators were not provided with any personal identifiers for these tissues and all patients were anonymous. Detailed clinical history was not provided, and the information on the extent of disease involvement in the small and large bowels was limited.

Tissues for IHC were fixed in 10% neutral buffered formalin, and embedded in paraffin. Samples without epithelial cells were excluded. A total of 29 UC colons, and 32 CD colons, and 5 normal colons met these criteria.

Immunohistochemical Analysis

Immunohistochemistry (IHC) for DDR markers γH2A.X, phospho-Chk2, p53, and p21^{WAF1} was quantified by counting the number of positive epithelial cells versus total epithelial cells in three 250× magnification fields. An average of 3214 (UC) and 3178 epithelial cells (CD) were counted per sample in a blinded fashion by H. Y, a board certified pathologist. IHC for the monocyte and macrophage marker, CD68, was quantified by counting the number of stromal cells in the lamina propria. IHC for NOS2 was quantified by counting the number of epithelial and stromal cells in the lamina propria. Percent positivity was calculated by dividing the number of positive cells over total cells for each enumerated marker. For HP1γ, a combined score of intensity and distribution was used to score staining on a scale of 1–4 [31] to reflect the marked differences in both intensity and number of positive cells between UC and CD. All antibodies and further details are available in Materials and Methods S1. Antibodies for total Chk2 were tested by immunoblot for specificity (Figure S1) as described in the Materials and Methods S1.

Coculture and Cell Culture Treatment

Normal human fibroblast strains MRC-5 and WI-38 (Coriell Institute for Medical Research, Camden, NJ), and murine macrophage strain ANA-1 [32] were grown in phenol red-free DMEM supplemented with 10% FBS (Biofluids, Rockville, MD), 4 mM glutamine (Biofluids), penicillin (10 units/ml), and streptomycin (10 µg/ml, Biofluids).

Cocultures were established by seeding 2500 normal human fibroblasts and 833 macrophages per well (3:1 ratio) in a 6-well dish with 2 mL of media and cultured for 7 days. 200 µL of media was removed and replaced each day to replenish media contents. Fibroblasts were exposed to spermine NONOate (Sper/NO•; Sigma-Aldrich, St. Louis) as a NO• donor, or hydrogen peroxide (control) overnight (16 hrs) to evaluate induction of senescence in normal human fibroblasts. All experiments were repeated three times with three technical replicates for each repetition. At least 1500 cells were evaluated for senescence in each repetition using senescence-associated β-galactosidase (SA β-gal) buffer at pH 6.0 [33]. See Materials and Methods S1 for further details.

Results

UC and CD have Increased Macrophage Infiltration Compared to Normal Tissues

Both UC and CD had increased densities of macrophages, indicated by CD68+ cells, when compared to normal colons ($P<0.05$; Figure S2), reflective of the increased inflammation expected in UC and CD. UC and CD colons showed similar numbers of macrophages ($P>0.05$) compared to each other. The number of CD68+ cells was used to stratify tissues for this study; colons with macrophage numbers above the median were defined as having "high macrophage index".

Macrophage Infiltration is Positively Associated with Cellular Senescence in UC

We measured HP1γ as an indicator of cellular senescence in formalin-fixed paraffin-embedded (FFPE) tissue. HP1γ localizes to senescence-associated heterochromatin foci in vitro [17], and correlates to SAβ-gal [33] in fresh colonic adenomas [12]. High macrophage index was associated with elevated staining for HP1γ in colonic epithelial cells of UC patients ($P=0.01$). Macrophages in UC correlated with HP1γ in epithelial cells ($P=0.025$; Spearman $=0.43$), indicating that macrophage infiltration is associated with senescence in nearby epithelial cells. In contrast, CD colonic epithelial cells had higher levels of HP1γ than UC ($P<0.001$; Figure 1A). HP1γ was not associated with high macrophage index in CD patients (Figure 1A), suggesting there may be other factors contributing to senescence in CD versus UC. Examples of strong HP1γ in CD, moderate staining in UC, and negative staining in normal tissues is shown (Figure 1B–D). Strong staining in colon adenoma (positive control) is shown in Figure S3E.

We next examined senescence-associated β-galactosidase (SAβ-gal) activity in frozen sections of UC and CD patients to confirm the presence of cellular senescence because enzyme activity is considered the gold standard. Fresh tissue is optimal for testing enzyme activity, but only archival frozen tissue was available for this study. Long-term storage of archival tissue may degrade enzyme activity, leading to false negatives, yet we were able to detect SAβ-gal activity in 13/21 (62%) UC and in 14/38 (37%) CD colons, illustrating for the first time that SAβ-gal-associated senescence is present in IBD tissue (Figure S3A-D). Immortalized normal human fibroblasts treated with Nutlin-3A [34] were used as positive controls.

Activation of DDR (γ-H2A.X and Phospho-Chk2) is Higher in CD and UC than in Normal Tissue

We determined levels of DDR markers associated with premature senescence [11,12] by IHC in the epithelial cells of IBD and normal colons. UC and CD colons showed increased levels of γH2A.X ($P<0.05$; $P<0.001$), phospho-Chk2 ($P<0.01$, $P<0.001$), p53 ($P<0.01$), and p21 ($P<0.05$) when compared to normal colons (Figure 2A). No increase was observed in total Chk2 in IBD versus normal colons, consistent with previous data that Chk2 is unchanged during colon carcinogenesis [11].

We found that UC colons had lower levels of DDR compared to CD, based on γH2A.X ($P<0.05$) and phospho-Chk2 ($P<0.001$) staining. No differences were observed in total Chk2, p53 or p21 between CD and UC (Figure 2A). Examples of staining patterns are shown in Figure S4.

Macrophages are Positively Associated with Activation of DDR in UC

We examined if high macrophage index was associated with activation of DDR. In UC patients, high macrophage index was associated with increased γH2A.X ($P=0.031$) and phospho-Chk2 ($P=0.014$; Figure 2B) in colonic epithelium. No significant differences were observed for p53, or p21, although p21 was marginally increased in tissues with higher macrophage index (Figure 2B). In colons from CD patients, macrophage index was not associated with either activation of the DDR pathway or immunopositivity of p21 (Figure S5).

We hypothesized that macrophages directly induce senescence, based on the data from UC tissues. To test this, we performed the following in vitro experiments with macrophages and primary human cells.

Macrophages cause NO• Induced Cellular Senescence in vitro

To investigate the role of macrophages in the induction of senescence in vitro, normal, primary human fibroblast strains MRC5 and WI38 were cocultured with macrophages for 7 days and evaluated by the SA-βgal assay. Fibroblasts are relevant because senescent stromal cells can produce proinflammatory cytokines that may influence the senescent state of epithelial cells. Approximately eighty percent of fibroblasts cocultured with macrophages were positive for SA-βgal, and showed more senescent blue-stained cells compared to fibroblasts grown alone (Figure 3A; WI38, $P=0.002$; MRC5, $P=0.003$).

To determine if NO• produced by macrophages may be capable of inducing senescence in stromal fibroblasts, macrophages and fibroblasts were cocultured in media with and without the NO• synthase inhibitor N-nitro-l-arginine methyl ester (L-NAME, 500 μM, Sigma-Aldrich, St. Louis). DAF-FM diacetate (4-amino-5-methylamino-2′, 7′-difluorofluorescein diacetate; DAF, Invitrogen, Carlsbad) was used to assess the amount of NO• diffused into the media of cocultured cells. As expected, L-NAME led to decreased NO• present in the media of cocultures (Figure 3B; WI38, $P=0.008$, MRC5; $P=0.03$). After exposure to coculture, fibroblasts were fixed and stained for SA-βgal activity at pH 6.0, resulting in blue substrate in senescent cells (Figure S6.) Cocultures grown in the presence of L-NAME showed decreased blue SA-βgal positive cells (Figure 3A; WI38, $P=0.002$; MRC5, $P=0.003$). This suggested that NO• is at least partially responsible for macrophage-induced senescence.

To determine if NO• alone could induce cellular senescence, normal human fibroblasts were exposed to clinically relevant levels of NO• and examined for SA-βgal activity. To achieve target steady state levels of 4.5 nM, 15 nM and 50 nM NO•, fibroblasts were incubated with 0.9 μM, 3 μM and 10 μM of the NO• donor Spermine NONOate (Sper/NO•). These doses were chosen because they are consistent with known levels of steady state NO• secreted by macrophages in vitro [35,36] and levels of NO• detected in ulcerative colitis [37]. NO• concentrations at or below 50 nM are below the limit of detection for our NO• gas analyzer. To confirm that Sper/NO• was producing NO• levels near our target concentration, we measured NO• produced by 100 μM Sper/NO• (expected concentration of 500 nM NO•) and found steady state levels of 380 nM NO• at 4 hours (Figure S7; SD ± 35 nM; n = 3), similar to the expected concentrations calculated from our previously published data [29]. Treatment with 3 μM and 10 μM, but not 0.9 μM, Sper/NO• induced enlarged SA-βgal positive cells ($P<0.0001$; Figure 3C; Figure S6). Thus, levels of

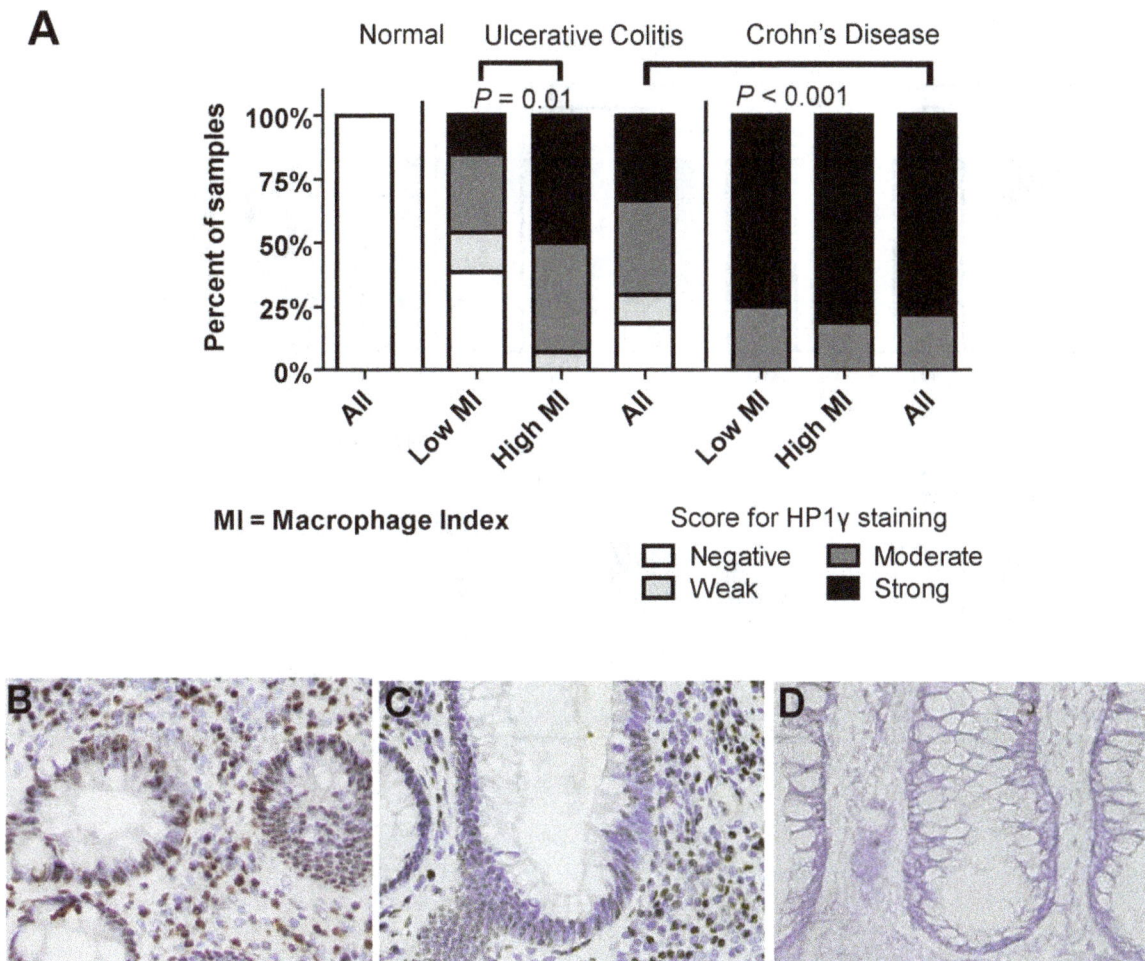

Figure 1. Senescence is induced in inflammatory bowel disease colons in association with infiltrating macrophages. Senescent epithelial cells were identified by HP1γ immunohistochemistry. Categorical scores reflecting intensity and distribution are shown as negative, weak, moderate, and strong. A) Colons from normal patients were negative for senescence-associated HP1γ. Ulcerative colitis and Crohn's disease colonic epithelial cells were positive for HP1γ. Crohn's disease colons had a greater percentage of HP1γ positive cells than ulcerative colitis colons (P<0.001). HP1γ was associated with high macrophage index (P = 0.01) in ulcerative colitis colons, but no such difference was observed within Crohn's disease. B) A representative picture of a Crohn's colitis crypt with strong HP1γ, C) a representative picture of ulcerative colitis crypt with weak staining, and D) a representative picture of normal autopsy tissue with negative staining. All are shown at 400× magnification. Epithelial and stromal HP1γ positive staining cells are shown in brown, with blue-purple hematoxylin counter stain in surrounding cells.

NO• that are physiologically relevant to IBD induce senescence in a dose-dependent manner.

To determine if DDR is upregulated in cells induced into senescence by NO•, we performed immunofluorescence for γH2A.X in MRC5 cells treated with 10 μM Sper/NO•. Indeed, Sper/NO• treated cells showed increased levels of γH2A.X foci, compared to untreated control cells (Figure S8.).

Higher Levels of NOS2 Expression in CD Correlates with Higher Levels of Senescence-associated HP1γ

Macrophages were associated with senescence in epithelial cells in UC, but thus far we could not identify a driver of senescence in CD. Based on our *in vitro* studies that identified NO• as an inducer or senescence, we hypothesized that NO•, secreted by macrophages and produced by epithelial cells themselves may modulate senescence. To study this model of extracellular and intracellular-induced senescence, IHC for NOS2 was performed on tissue. Significantly more epithelial cells were positive for NOS2 in CD than in UC (Figure 4; P = 0.0017) while no significant difference

was observed comparing stromal cells of CD and UC. Increased levels of epithelial NOS2 in CD were consistent with an increase in senescence-associated HP1γ in CD compared to UC (Figure 1A). We were not able to stratify CD tissues to investigate if epithelial cell NOS2 expression correlated with senescence because all CD tissues had high senescence, possibly due to the combined effects of NO• from macrophages and intracellular NO• from epithelial cells. There are no primary epithelial cells of a colonic origin to test our proposal that NO• from epithelial cells is directly related to senescence *in vitro*. We introduce the hypothesis that intracellular (epithelial) NO• may be involved in senescence in CD, and this may be tested should appropriate model systems become available.

MicroRNAs are Associated with NOS2 and Senescence

After establishing that macrophages are associated with senescence in UC, and directly induce senescence in an NO•-dependent fashion *in vitro*, we performed microRNA microarray expression analysis on RNA extracted from both UC and CD tissues to identify candidate microRNAs which may have a role in

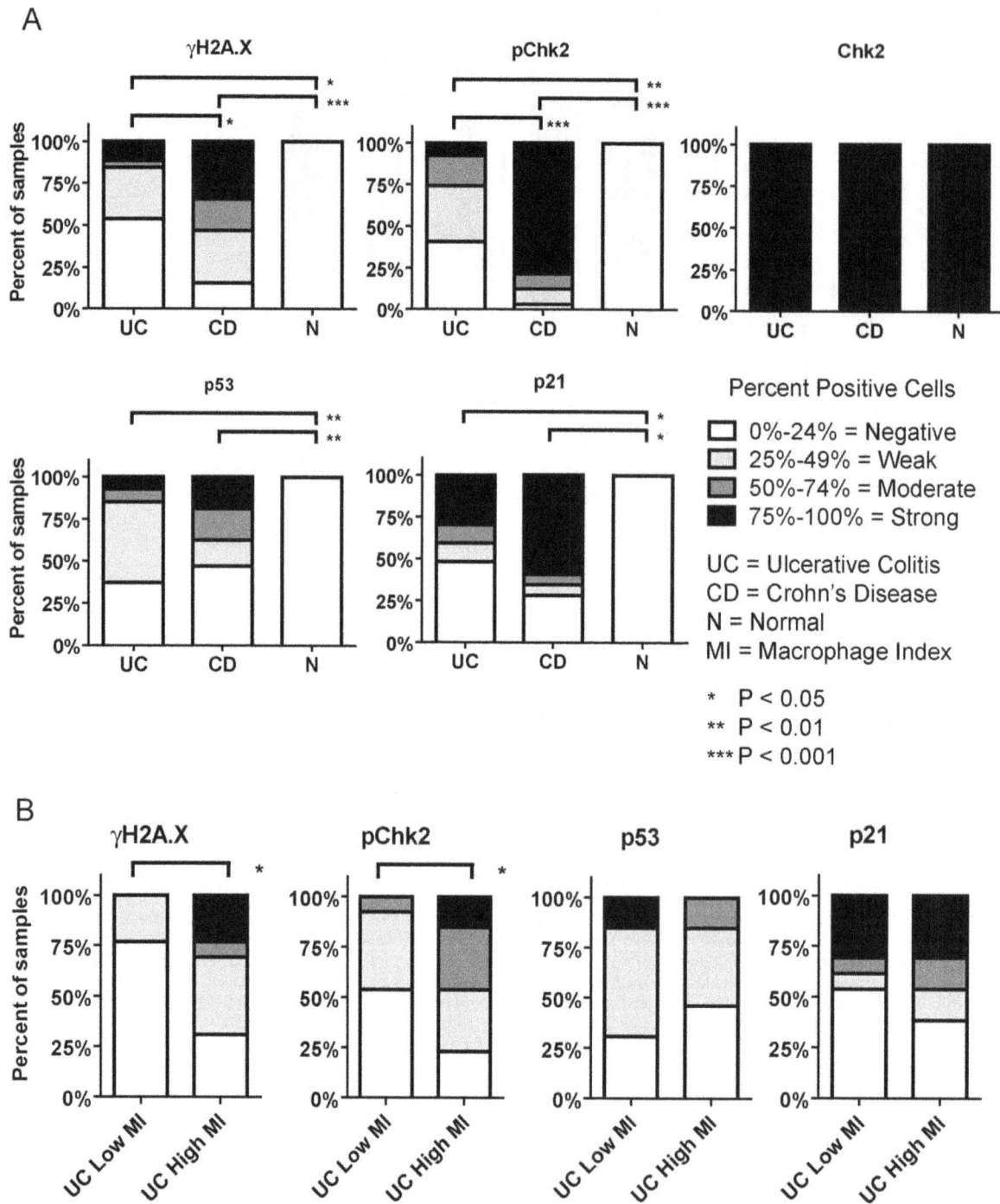

Figure 2. DNA damage response pathway and p21 are upregulated in inflammatory bowel disease and the DNA Damage response pathway is associated with high macrophage infiltration in ulcerative colitis. (A) Normal, ulcerative colitis, and Crohn's disease colons were analyzed by immunostaining to determine the percent of positive epithelial cells for γ-H2A.X, phospho-Chk2, Chk2, p53 and p21. Data is shown by the percent of total samples with 0–24%, 25–49%, 50–74%, and 75–100% cell positivity. Normal colonic epithelial cells had low, or 0–24% cell positivity, for all markers. Both Crohn's disease and ulcerative colitis colons had increased levels of γ-H2A.X ($P<0.001$; $P<0.05$), phospho-Chk2 ($P<0.01$; $P<0.001$), p53 ($P<0.01$) and p21 ($P<0.05$) compared to normal colon. Tissues from Crohn's disease patients showed higher levels of γH2A.X ($P<0.05$), phospho-Chk2 ($P<0.001$) than in ulcerative colitis. No differences were detected in levels of total Chk2 between ulcerative colitis, Crohn's disease, and normal colons, as expected. (B) Analysis of γH2A.X, phospho-Chk2, p53, and p21 in ulcerative colitis colonic epithelial cells was stratified by macrophage infiltration index to determine if macrophage infiltration in the lamina propria was associated with induction of the DNA damage response pathway and p21 activation. Colons with macrophage numbers above the median were defined as having high macrophage index, while those with macrophage numbers below the median were defined as having low macrophage index (i.e., low cellular densities). High macrophage index was associated with increased γH2A.X ($P=0.031$) and phospho-Chk2 ($P=0.014$). No significant differences were observed for p53 and p21 with respect to macrophage index.

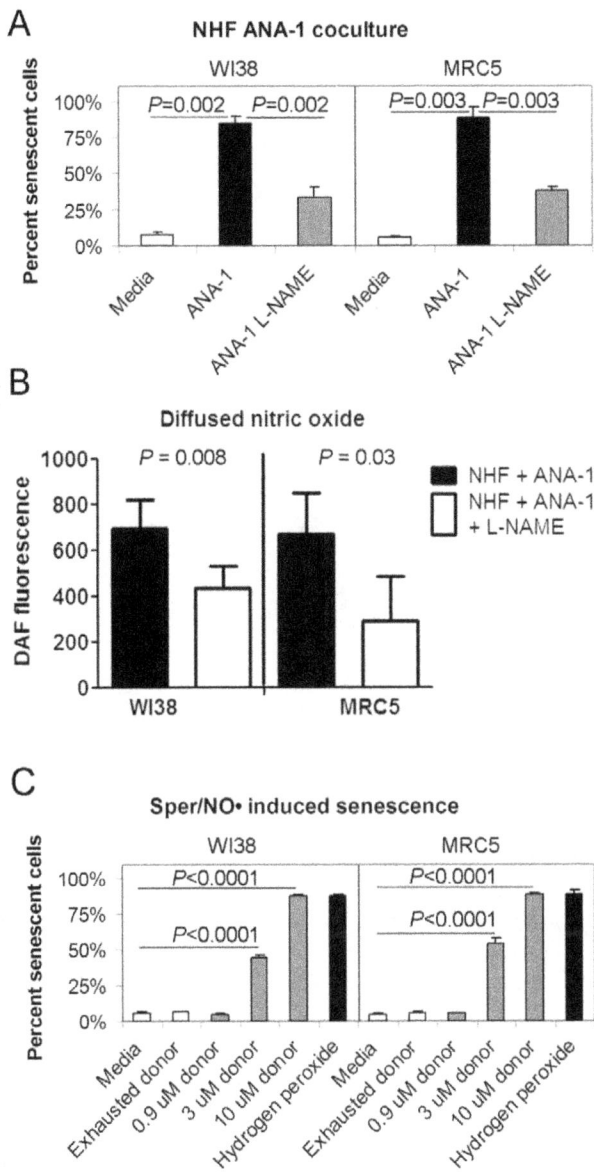

Figure 3. Senescence is induced by either macrophages or NO• in primary normal human fibroblasts in culture. Normal human fibroblasts (WI38 and MRC5) were grown in coculture with murine macrophages (ANA-1), or with the NO• donor spermine NONOate (Sper/NO•). Senescence-associated β-galactosidase activity was used to determine to the percent of senescent fibroblasts divided by the number of total fibroblasts. Results are shown from three experiments, with each experiment done in triplicate. (A) Normal human fibroblasts were cocultured with macrophages, with and without the NO• synthase inhibitor L-NAME (500 µM). Macrophages induced senescence in WI38 and MRC5 cells. Senescence was partially abrogated by L-NAME in WI38 and MRC5 cells. (B) The NO• synthase inhibitor L-NAME reduces diffused NO• in media of cocultures comprised of normal human fibroblasts (WI38 or MRC5) and macrophages (ANA-1). 100 µl of media from three separate cocultures was aliquoted with 100 µL of 5 µM of DAF in 96-well plates. Plates were read for DAF-fluorescence as an indicator of NO•. Addition of the NO• inhibitor L-NAME resulted in decreased levels of NO• in both WI38 (P=0.008) and MRC5 (P=0.03) cells. Fluorescence measurements from cocultures were normalized by subtracting the DAF fluorescence measured in media from wells with fibroblasts only. (C) Fibroblasts were dosed with 0.09 µM, 3 µM and 10 µM Sper/NO•, Sper/NO• that was previously incubated in media with sodium hydroxide (vehicle) for 48 hours (exhausted donor), and media alone (negative control) overnight (16 hrs). These concentrations

were selected to achieve steady state concentrations of 4.5 nM, 15 nM and 50 nM NO• respectively. 10 µM and 3 µM Sper/NO• induced significant levels of senescence (P<0.0001). Exhausted Sper/NO• (negative control) and 0.09 µM Sper/NO• did not induce significant levels of senescence when compared to media alone. Hydrogen peroxide (200 µM; 2 hrs) was used as a positive control.

senescence. We measured the expression of NOS2 and the macrophage marker, CD68 by qRT-PCR and analyzed associations between these and microRNA expression levels. We identified 6 microRNAs (miR-21, miR-17, miR-146a, miR-126, miR-223 and miR-221) that were associated with NOS2 expression (P<0.001, FDR <5%) indicating that these microRNAs are potentially involved in NO• associated senescence (Figure 5, Table S2). While no microRNAs were associated with CD68 expression at the stringent statistical cutoff of P<0.001, a more lenient cutoff identified 5 microRNAs that were associated with CD68 (P<0.05), including miR-21, providing evidence that miR-21 may be involved in both macrophage and NOS2 induced senescence.

Colon adenomas are premalignant lesions in which high levels of cellular senescence serves as a barrier to a malignant transformation [12,38]. In order to identify microRNAs whose expression is associated with cellular senescence in multiple disease states, we examined microRNAs expression patterns in senescent adenomas to compare to senescent-associated microRNAs from UC and CD. As expected, adenomas expressed high levels of senescence-associated HP1γ (Figure S3E) and we previously have shown that these adenomas are positive for SA-βgal [39]. This confirms high levels of cellular senescence in these tissues. We next performed microRNA microarray profiling of colonic adenomas and paired normal tissue, and compared these results with our findings in IBD. Among the 31 microRNAs altered in adenomas (Figure 5, Table S3), miR-21 had the highest fold change increase in adenomas, consistent with our previous qRT-PCR data on miR-21 in adenomas [40]. MiR-21 was the only microRNA that was associated with both NOS2 and CD68 in IBD; thus miR-21 is commonly associated with macrophages linked to senescence in IBD and *in vitro*, and NO• which induces senescence *in vitro*. We have previously reported that miR-21 expression is associated with NOS2 expression in colon cancer [41] providing more confidence that this association is relevant. This suggests a potential role for this microRNA in NO• and inflammation-associated senescence, and future investigations will focus on the possible role of miR-21 *in vivo*, and mechanistic experiments *in vitro* to show direct effects that cannot be tested in human tissue. Interestingly, miR-17 was commonly altered in adenomas and associated with NOS2 in IBD while miR-181b was altered in adenomas and associated with CD68.

Conclusions

Cellular senescence is one of the many links between aging and cancer, and may occur through several mechanisms including telomere dysfunction and oncogenic stress [42]. UC has been theorized to be a disease of cellular aging, based on evidence of telomere attrition and chromosomal instability [10,43]. We found that senescence-associated HP1γ expression in colonic epithelia was increased in UC colons in association with a high number of macrophages. This association is consistent with the hypothesis that macrophages may directly or indirectly induce cellular senescence in adjacent epithelial cells, which we observed *in vitro*. Our findings suggest that in addition to cell intrinsic mechanisms such as replicative telomere shortening, microenvironmental cues such as infiltrating immune cells and their derived factors may

A   **NOS2 Expression**

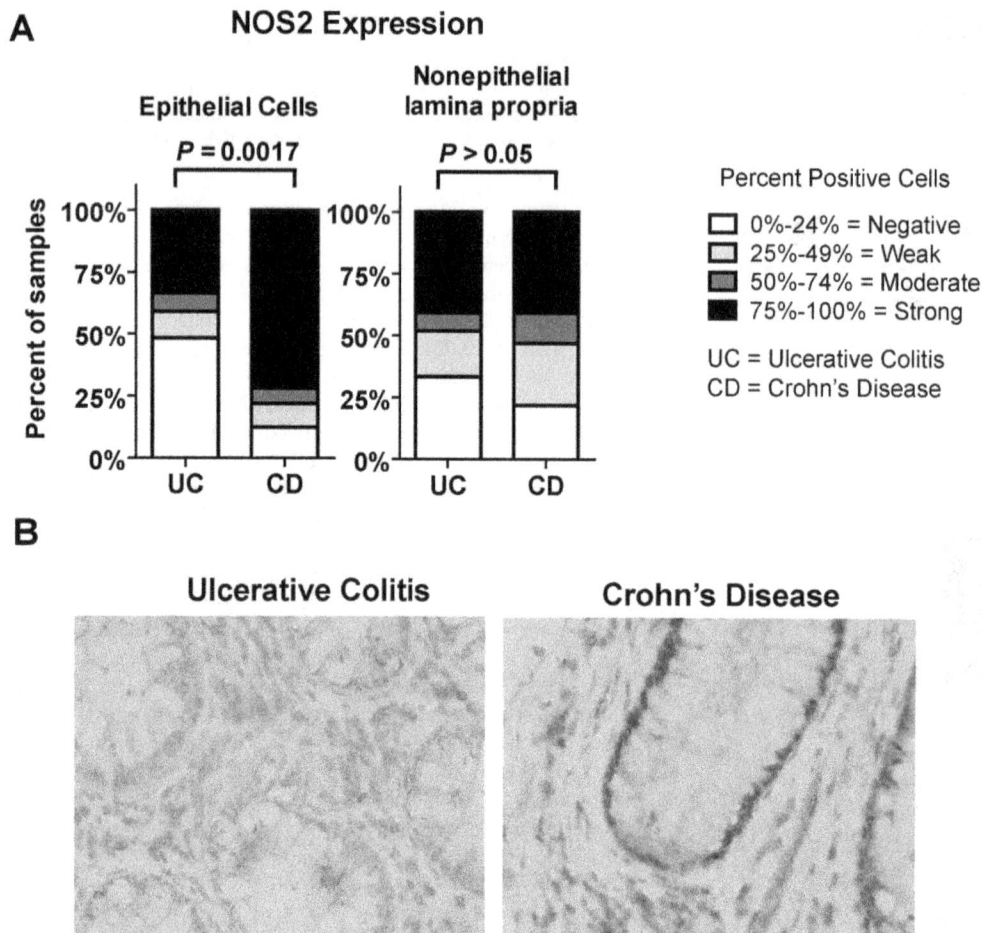

Figure 4. Epithelial cells in Crohn's disease colon show higher levels of anti-NOS2 immunoreactivity than epithelial cells in ulcerative colitis colon. Immunohistochemistry for NOS2 was performed as a possible indicator of NO• produced in the colon of ulcerative colitis and Crohn's disease patients. (A) Colonic epithelial cells had higher NOS2 expression in ulcerative colitis than Crohn's disease ($P = 0.0013$) colons as shown by the percent of samples with positive cells while there was no significant difference in NOS2 expressing cells in the lamina propria. (B) Representative pictures show an ulcerative colitis section with low (0–24% positive) epithelial NOS2, and a Crohn's disease section with high (75–100% positive) epithelial NOS2.

regulate epithelial cell senescence in cancer-prone lesions. This is consistent with a recent report associating high levels of infiltrating lymphocytes with telomere shortening and senescence in UC [44]. Stromal senescent fibroblasts can also secrete proinflammatory cytokines, e.g., IL-6, IL-8 and Gro-α [45] that can contribute to IBD, consistent with our observations.

High macrophage infiltration was associated with increases in the DDR sensor molecule γH2A.X, an indicator of active DNA damage response signaling by upstream DDR kinases including ATM and ATR [46,47], and phosphorylation of downstream stress response protein Chk2 in colonic epithelial cells of inflamed, cancer-prone tissue of UC patients. The increased level of γ-H2A.X in UC colon, when compared to normal colon, is consistent with a previous report [10] and suggests that DDR may lead to cellular senescence in a proinflammatory environment. It is not clear if the DDR response associated with macrophages *in vivo*, and induced by NO• *in vitro*, is pro- or anti-carcinogenic, but DDR has previously been hypothesized to be an anti-cancer barrier [11]. It is possible that macrophages and/or NO• induce the DDR pathway leading to cellular senescence, and limiting proliferation of cells as a barrier to cancer. Alternatively, senescent cells in the microenvironment may themselves be

procarcinogenic by secreting cytokines including IL-6, IL-8, IL-1α and IL-1β [38,48].

Our *in vitro* data suggest that macrophages induce cellular senescence in a NO• dependent manner. Macrophages or clinically relevant concentrations of NO• induce cellular senescence in normal human fibroblasts and the NO• synthase inhibitor L-NAME proportionally reduced both NO• and senescence. L-NAME is often considered a nonselective NO• synthase inhibitor, but it has been previously shown to more efficiently block NO• production from NOS3. NOS3 is known to be important in the regulation of NOS2 expression [49], thus we hypothesize that L-NAME may decrease the amount of NO• by inhibiting NOS3 activity and down regulating NOS2 expression. This may be especially relevant at the low levels of steady state NO• (50–100 nmol) expected with 10 μM of Sper/NO• [50]. NO• has been implicated in the activation of the DDR pathway in cell lines and primary cells of patients with Barrett's esophagus. Specifically, NO• donor MAHMA-NONOate induces γH2A.X in Barrett's esophagus non-dysplastic, high-grade dysplastic, and adenocarcinoma cell lines [51]. Interestingly, Dickey *et al.* have shown that NO• induces γH2A.X *in vitro*, and that γH2A.X is induced in unexposed cells adjacent to cells exposed to irradiation [52]. We

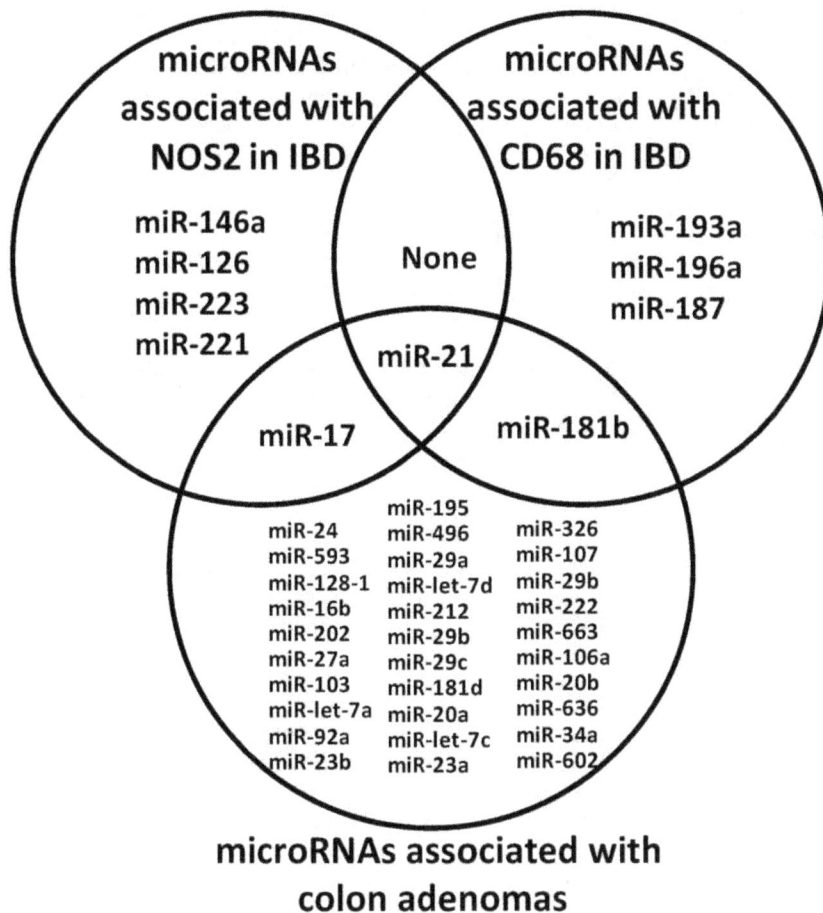

Figure 5. Association of microRNAs with NOS2 and CD68 expression in IBD and microRNAs altered in colon adenomas. The Venn diagram displays microRNAs that were significantly associated with the mRNA expression of NOS2 ($P<0.001$) and CD68 ($P<0.05$) and those microRNAs that are altered in colon adenomas ($P<0.001$) based on microRNA microarray profiling. MiR-21 was found to be associated in all three comparisons suggesting a potential role for this microRNA in senescence.

have also shown that NO• induces γH2A.X in normal human fibroblasts.

NOS2 is increased in colon adenomas [8]; when NOS2 is overexpressed in p53 wild type cells, p53 accumulates and induces a negative feedback loop that down regulates NOS2 expression to decrease nitrosative stress [53]. In contrast, NOS2 overexpression of NOS2 in p53 mutant cells leads to increased angiogenesis and tumorigenicity of human cancer cells as xenografts in immuno-suppressed mice [54]. We hypothesize that NOS2 expression in IBD patients with intact and activated p53 serves as a barrier to carcinogenesis, based on the literature and our *in vitro* data that NO• induces senescence and DDR. However, once p53 is inactivated in IBD by mutation [5], nitrosative stress induced by NOS2 may not induce senescence due to loss of p53, and may become procarcinogenic. We plan to investigate these hypotheses should *in vitro* models with primary epithelial cells lines become available.

The miR-146a/b family of microRNAs that are elevated in senescent fibroblasts and thought to modulate senescence through effects on IL-6 and IL-8 [55]. We find that miR-146 expression correlates to NOS2 expression levels in IBD tissues, consistent with a role for miR-146 and NO• in senescence. MiR-21 is an oncogenic microRNA with known roles in inflammation, cell proliferation and tumorigenesis. We found that miR-21 expression is associated with high NOS2 and CD68 expression in UC and

CD, as well as colon adenomas. Mir-21 has previously been shown to be increased in active ulcerative colitis [56] and upregulated during DNA damage by hydrogen peroxide and ionizing radiation associated with reactive oxygen species [57]. Inflammatory stimuli, such as *Corynebacterium parvum*-induced inflammation in mice, results in elevated levels of miR-21 [58]. MiR-21 can activate the NO• pathway *in vitro* [59] and miR-21 levels can be regulated by NF-kappaB [60]. Our data suggests that miR-21 may have a role in senescence, although future studies are needed to confirm these results in a second population using a more sensitive assay like RT-PCR, and in *in vitro* studies to show a direct effect. While at first a role in senescence may seem counterintuitive given the oncogenic role of miR-21, other oncogenes, including RAS [61], have roles in oncogene-induced senescence. Interestingly, the RAS pathway has been shown to increase miR-21 expression [62], and NO• can activate the RAS pathway [63]. Therefore, it is possible that in IBD, NO• leads to RAS activation and miR-21 transcription that is in part responsible for senescence in IBD. Future studies should explore if miR-21 is induced by NO• in a RAS-dependent manner and contributes to senescence.

Our study revealed a significance difference in senescence between CD and UC; higher HP1γ-associated senescence was observed in CD than in UC, and may reflect a critical difference between these two chronic inflammatory diseases. Genome wide association studies have shown thus far that some susceptibility loci are shared by both UC and CD, while others are solely associated with one but not the other disease [64–67]. For example, inflammatory pathways involving IL-23/IL-17 are both implicated in UC and CD, but *NOD2* is associated solely with CD. *NOD2* is required for tolerization of macrophages to bacterial peptides, including ligands for TLR2 and TLR4 [68]. Macrophages from CD Leu1007insC Nod2 homozygote individuals fail to develop tolerance to repeated stimulation with ligands, leading to the production of TNFα, IL-1β, and IL-8 [68]. Mice carrying a similar variant of NOD2 have elevated levels of NF-kappaB and IL-1βin response to MDP [69]. TNFα and IL-1β both contribute to NOS2 expression and NO• production *in vivo* [35], and IL-8 has been shown to be a prosenescent cytokine important to senescence induced by DNA damage [48]. The presence of senescence cells can cause age-related, chronic conditions in addition to inhibiting carcinogenesis [70]. We summarize these data in a model (Figure S9), and propose that regulation of NO• by proinflammatory cytokines contributes to up regulation of the DNA damage response pathway and senescence based on our *in vitro* assays.

Our findings related to inflammatory bowel disease may be applicable to other precancerous states associated with inflammation, and also those associated with oncogenic stress. Macrophages have long been implicated in association with tumors [27], and many questions remain on how immunity is involved in carcinogenesis. Before now, there had been no direct connection established between macrophages or NO• and senescence. Future studies may focus on the modulation of senescence through immune response to improve cancer outcome.

Supporting Information

Figure S1 Antibodies against phospho-Chk2 (Thr68) and Chk2 are specific. HCT116 Chk2−/− and parental Chk2+/+ isogenic cell lines (generously given by the Vogelstein Laboratory) growing in log phase were exposed to 12 Gy of ionizing radiation to induce phospho-Chk2, and harvested 1 hour later. Lysates from Chk2+/+ cells (0 Gy; lane 1, 12 Gy; lane 2), and lysates from Chk2−/− cells (0 Gy; lane 3, 12 Gy; lane 4) are indicated by numbers below each immunoblot. Antibody for (A) phospho-Chk2 (Thr68) used for immunohistochemistry, was determined to be specific by immunoblot, as illustrated by the appropriate sized band detected in irradiated Chk+/+ cells only. (B) Specificity of the Chk2 (clone 273) antibody was confirmed, as shown by the darkest band detected in only Chk2+/+ cells, regardless of irradiation. (C) Additional total Chk2 antibodies (clone 270; Stressgen) and (D) ascites from clone 273 (generously given by Jiri Bartek) were tested to confirm the results. Immunocytochemistry was also performed with (E) phospho-Chk2 (Thr68) and (F) Chk2 (clone 273) antibodies, with similar results. (IR− = 0 Gy gamma-irradiation, IR+ = 12 Gy gamma-irradiation).

Figure S2 Inflammatory bowel disease colons have increased macrophage infiltration in the lamina propria compared to normal colons. Macrophages were identified with anti-CD68 immunohistochemistry and quantified by enumerating the number of positive brown cells in the lamina propria. Ulcerative colitis and Crohn's disease colons had an increased number of macrophages compared to normal colons (ANOVA, $P = 0.02$; Dunn's $P < 0.05$ for both comparisons). There was no significant difference in the number of macrophages between colons from ulcerative colitis and Crohn's disease patients.

Figure S3 Senescent cells are detectable by both immunohistochemistry for HP1γ and enzyme activity for senescence associated β-galactosidase in inflammatory bowel disease. A) A representative picture of senescence associated β-galactosidase positivity is shown in frozen sections from ulcerative colitis colon. Colonic epithelial cells showed distinct cytoplasmic blue staining at 100× and B) 400× magnification. (C) Cells of the lamina propria, adjacent to epithelial cells, also stained blue for SAβ-gal activity at 100× and (D) 400× magnification. E) A representative picture of colon adenoma tissue stained for HP1γ.

Figure S4 Examples of immunohistochemistry for DNA damage response and p53-stress response markers. Examples from inflammatory bowel disease colon sections were chosen to emphasize differences reflected in cell counts (represented in Figure 2). Positive cells are indicated by brown nuclear stain (DAB) and negative cells are shown with blue counterstaining (Hematoxylin). Positive staining for γH2A.X, phospho-Chk2, Chk2, p53, and p21 was nuclear. For normal tissues, areas with well-oriented crypts were available, and these are illustrated with the lumen oriented toward the top of the panel. A summary of this data is shown in Figure 2.

Figure S5 Crohn's disease colons show no difference in DNA damage or p53 activation in association with macrophage index. Tissues from Crohn's disease patients were evaluated by immunohistochemistry for γ-H2A.X, phospho-Chk2, total p53 and p21. Staining is not associated with low and high macrophage index ($P > 0.05$).

Figure S6 Macrophages and nitric oxide induce senescence in primary human fibroblasts. Representative pictures are shown of positive (blue) and negative (white) cells, indicative of senescence-associated β-galactosidase (SA-βgal) enzyme activity. A) A low density of normal human fibroblasts (MRC5) were cocultured with macrophages (ANA-1) in 6-well plates at a ratio of 3:1, respectively. Cocultures were allowed to grow for 7 days with and without the nitric oxide inhibitor L-NAME (500 μM). Macrophages induced cellular senescence in fibroblasts, as shown by the enlarged, blue, SA-βgal positive cells. L-NAME partially abrogated the induction of senescence in fibroblasts. Cells grown in media only were negative for SA-βgal. (B) Normal human fibroblasts were incubated with 10 μM, 3 μM, and 0.9 μM Spermine NONOate (Sper/NO•) over night (16 hrs). After treatment, the cells were fixed and stained for SA-βgal. Treatment with 10 μM and 3 μM Sper/NO• induced a significant number of enlarged, SA-βgal positive cells, when compared cells grown in media alone (negative control). Treatment with 0.9 μM Sper/NO• did not induce significant levels of SA-βgal positive cells. Hydrogen peroxide (positive control; 200 μM) induced SA-βgal activity.

Figure S7 Steady state nitric oxide was highest at 381 nM at 4 hours, and nitric oxide was decayed by 6 hours. The decay of Spermine NONOate (Sper/NO•) was determined by measuring steady state nitric oxide on a nitric oxide gas analyzer. A 100 μl aliquot of 100 μM of Sper/NO• in serum-free media was aspirated by gas-free syringe into the sampling chamber at 0, 0.75, 1.5, 2, 4, and 6 hour time points.

Figure S8 Nitric oxide induces DNA damage response in primary human fibroblasts in culture. Normal human fibroblasts (MRC5) were incubated with media alone (negative control) or 10 μM Spermine NONOate (donor) and assayed for γH2A.X foci by immunofluorescence as indicated by FITC (green) fluorescence. DAPI (purple blue) was used to identify nuclei, and this image was overlaid with FITC top create a composite. (A, C, E,) Cells grown in media alone were negative for γH2A.X.foci at 400× magnification. (G) Enlargement of a single cell treated with media alone (indicated by the red box in panel C) shows that there is very little FITC fluorescence for γH2A.X. (B, D, F) Cells treated with donor Sper/NO• became enlarged and failed to divide, leading to a low density of cells. Due to the low cell density, it was difficult to capture multiple cells in one 400× magnification field, thus each panel is a composite of four pictures of one single cell each. Each cell shows positive FITC fluorescence for γH2A.X foci. (H) Enlargement of a single cell treated with Sper/NO• (indicated by the red box in panel D) shows distinct focal fluorescence. Panels are shown at 400× magnification except for γH2A.X high magnification panels (G, H), which show an enlarged section (red rectangle) from the γH2A.X panels (C, D).

Figure S9 Proposed model of DNA damage response and senescence resulting from a polymorphism in NOD2/CARD 15 carried by Crohn's disease patients. Previous studies have illustrated that a polymorphism in NOD2 carried by Crohn's disease patients results in the loss of tolerization to bacterial peptide, including TLR2 and TLR4 ligands upon restimulation. [68] This may result in the production of NF-κB and proinflammatory cytokines that are part of a chronic inflammatory response. [69] Cytokines IL-1β and TNF-α can lead to the induction of NOS2 to secrete nitric oxide. [35] Our data suggest that nitric oxide may induce DNA damage and result in cellular senescence.

Table S1 Characteristics of the study populations. [1]CHTN, Cooperative Human Tissue Network.

Table S2 MicroRNAs are associated with NOS2 and CD68 expression in Ulcerative Colitis (UC) and Crohn's Disease (CD) tissues. NOS2 and CD68 expression levels were dichotomized based on median expression levels. Class comparison analyses identified microRNAs that were differentially expressed when comparing high vs low expressing groups for NOS2 and CD68. FDR, False discovery rate.

Table S3 MicroRNAs that are altered in colon adenomas compared to adjacent nonadenoma tissue. Class comparison analyses identified microRNAs that were differentially expressed in colon adenomas. FDR, False discovery rate.

Materials and Methods S1 These are methods that describe the protocols for immunohistochemical anaylsis, coculture and cell culture studies, statistical analysis, senescence-associated β-galactosidase studies, nitric oxide quantification, immunofluorescence, RNA isolation, microRNA profiling and qRTPCR.

Acknowledgments

We acknowledge Dr. Krista Zanetti for her advice on statistics, Dr. Tia Bobo for her technical help, and Dr. Sharon Pine and Dr. Stefan Ambs for thoughtful discussions.

Author Contributions

Conceived and designed the experiments: JJS AJS LAR IH AIR SPH GNW DAW CCH. Performed the experiments: JJS AJS LAR MAK AIR EDB. Analyzed the data: JJS AJS HGY LAR IH AIR SPH AG LJH J. Bartkova J. Bartek GNW DAW CCH. Contributed reagents/materials/analysis tools: LAR DAW J. Bartkova J. Bartek. Wrote the paper: JJS AJS AIR GNW DAW CCH.

References

1. Loftus EV Jr (2004) Clinical epidemiology of inflammatory bowel disease: Incidence, prevalence, and environmental influences. Gastroenterology 126: 1504–1517.

2. Ekbom A, Helmick C, Zack M, Adami HO (1990) Ulcerative colitis and colorectal cancer. A population-based study. N Engl J Med 323: 1228–1233.

3. Nair J, Gansauge F, Beger H, Dolara P, Winde G, et al. (2006) Increased etheno-DNA adducts in affected tissues of patients suffering from Crohn's disease, ulcerative colitis, and chronic pancreatitis. Antioxid Redox Signal 8: 1003–1010.

4. Hofseth LJ, Khan MA, Ambrose M, Nikolayeva O, Xu-Welliver M, et al. (2003) The adaptive imbalance in base excision-repair enzymes generates microsatellite instability in chronic inflammation. J Clin Invest 112: 1887–1894.

5. Hussain SP, Amstad P, Raja K, Ambs S, Nagashima M, et al. (2000) Increased p53 mutation load in noncancerous colon tissue from ulcerative colitis: a cancer-prone chronic inflammatory disease. Cancer Res 60: 3333–3337.

6. Salk JJ, Salipante SJ, Risques RA, Crispin DA, Li L, et al. (2009) Clonal expansions in ulcerative colitis identify patients with neoplasia. Proc Natl Acad Sci U S A.

7. Hofseth LJ, Saito S, Hussain SP, Espey MG, Miranda KM, et al. (2003) Nitric oxide-induced cellular stress and p53 activation in chronic inflammation. Proc Natl Acad Sci U S A 100: 143–148.

8. Ambs S, Bennett WP, Merriam WG, Ogunfusika MO, Oser SM, et al. (1999) Relationship between p53 mutations and inducible nitric oxide synthase expression in human colorectal cancer. J Natl Cancer Inst 91: 86–88.

9. Risques RA, Lai LA, Himmetoglu C, Ebaee A, Li L, et al. (2011) Ulcerative colitis-associated colorectal cancer arises in a field of short telomeres, senescence, and inflammation. Cancer Res 71: 1669–1679. 0008-5472.CAN-10-1966 [pii];10.1158/0008-5472.CAN-10-1966 [doi].

10. Risques RA, Lai LA, Brentnall TA, Li L, Feng Z, et al. (2008) Ulcerative colitis is a disease of accelerated colon aging: evidence from telomere attrition and DNA damage. Gastroenterology 135: 410–418.

11. Bartkova J, Horejsi Z, Koed K, Kramer A, Tort F, et al. (2005) DNA damage response as a candidate anti-cancer barrier in early human tumorigenesis. Nature 434: 864–870.

12. Bartkova J, Rezaei N, Liontos M, Karakaidos P, Kletsas D, et al. (2006) Oncogene-induced senescence is part of the tumorigenesis barrier imposed by DNA damage checkpoints. Nature 444: 633–637.

13. Jones CJ, Kipling D, Morris M, Hepburn P, Skinner J, et al. (2000) Evidence for a telomere-independent "clock" limiting RAS oncogene-driven proliferation of human thyroid epithelial cells. Mol Cell Biol 20: 5690–5699.

14. Campisi J, Yaswen P (2009) Aging and cancer cell biology, 2009. Aging Cell 8: 221–225.

15. Binet R, Ythier D, Robles AI, Collado M, Larrieu D, et al. (2009) WNT16B is a new marker of cellular senescence that regulates p53 activity and the phosphoinositide 3-kinase/AKT pathway. Cancer Res 69: 9183–9191.

16. Serrano M, Lin AW, McCurrach ME, Beach D, Lowe SW (1997) Oncogenic ras provokes premature cell senescence associated with accumulation of p53 and p16INK4a. Cell 88: 593–602.

17. Narita M, Nunez S, Heard E, Narita M, Lin AW, et al. (2003) Rb-mediated heterochromatin formation and silencing of E2F target genes during cellular senescence. Cell 113: 703–716. S009286740300401X [pii].

18. Xue W, Zender L, Miething C, Dickins RA, Hernando E, et al. (2007) Senescence and tumour clearance is triggered by p53 restoration in murine liver carcinomas. Nature 445: 656–660.

19. Schmitt CA, Fridman JS, Yang M, Lee S, Baranov E, et al. (2002) A senescence program controlled by p53 and p16INK4a contributes to the outcome of cancer therapy. Cell 109: 335–346.

20. Di Micco R, Fumagalli M, Cicalese A, Piccinin S, Gasparini P, et al. (2006) Oncogene-induced senescence is a DNA damage response triggered by DNA hyper-replication. Nature 444: 638–642.

21. Rai P, Onder TT, Young JJ, McFaline JL, Pang B, et al. (2009) Continuous elimination of oxidized nucleotides is necessary to prevent rapid onset of cellular senescence. Proc Natl Acad Sci U S A 106: 169–174.

22. Favetta LA, Robert C, King WA, Betts DH (2004) Expression profiles of p53 and p66shc during oxidative stress-induced senescence in fetal bovine fibroblasts. Exp Cell Res 299: 36–48.

23. Hussain SP, Harris CC (2007) Inflammation and cancer: an ancient link with novel potentials. Int J Cancer 121: 2373–2380.

24. Stewart B, Kleihues P (2003) The Causes of Cancer. In: World Cancer Report. Lyon: IARC Press. 56–61.

25. Prueitt RL, Boersma BJ, Howe TM, Goodman JE, Thomas DD, et al. (2007) Inflammation and IGF-I activate the Akt pathway in breast cancer. Int J Cancer 120: 796–805.

26. Mantovani A, Schioppa T, Porta C, Allavena P, Sica A (2006) Role of tumor-associated macrophages in tumor progression and invasion. Cancer Metastasis Rev 25: 315–322.

27. Pollard JW (2009) Trophic macrophages in development and disease. Nat Rev Immunol 9: 259–270.

28. Thomas DD, Ridnour LA, Isenberg JS, Flores-Santana W, Switzer CH, et al. (2008) The chemical biology of nitric oxide: implications in cellular signaling. Free Radic Biol Med 45: 18–31. S0891-5849(08)00175-5 [pii];10.1016/j.freeradbiomed.2008.03.020 [doi].

29. Thomas DD, Espey MG, Ridnour LA, Hofseth LJ, Mancardi D, et al. (2004) Hypoxic inducible factor 1alpha, extracellular signal-regulated kinase, and p53 are regulated by distinct threshold concentrations of nitric oxide. Proc Natl Acad Sci U S A 101: 8894–8899.

30. Campisi J, Andersen JK, Kapahi P, Melov S (2011) Cellular senescence: A link between cancer and age-related degenerative disease? Semin Cancer Biol. S1044-579X(11)00050-2 [pii];10.1016/j.semcancer.2011.09.001 [doi].

31. Boersma BJ, Howe TM, Goodman JE, Yfantis HG, Lee DH, et al. (2006) Association of breast cancer outcome with status of p53 and MDM2 SNP309. J Natl Cancer Inst 98: 911–919.

32. Cox GW, Mathieson BJ, Gandino L, Blasi E, Radzioch D, et al. (1989) Heterogeneity of hematopoietic cells immortalized by v-myc/v-raf recombinant retrovirus infection of bone marrow or fetal liver. J Natl Cancer Inst 81: 1492–1496.

33. Dimri GP, Lee X, Basile G, Acosta M, Scott G, et al. (1995) A biomarker that identifies senescent human cells in culture and in aging skin in vivo. Proc Natl Acad Sci U S A 92: 9363–9367.

34. Kumamoto K, Spillare EA, Fujita K, Horikawa I, Yamashita T, et al. (2008) Nutlin-3a activates p53 to both down-regulate inhibitor of growth 2 and up-regulate mir-34a, mir-34b, and mir-34c expression, and induce senescence. Cancer Res 68: 3193–3203.

35. Espey MG, Miranda KM, Pluta RM, Wink DA (2000) Nitrosative capacity of macrophages is dependent on nitric-oxide synthase induction signals. J Biol Chem 275: 11341–11347.

36. Ridnour LA, Windhausen AN, Isenberg JS, Yeung N, Thomas DD, et al. (2007) Nitric oxide regulates matrix metalloproteinase-9 activity by guanylyl-cyclase-dependent and -independent pathways. Proc Natl Acad Sci U S A 104: 16898–16903. 0702761104 [pii];10.1073/pnas.0702761104 [doi].

37. Lundberg JO, Hellstrom PM, Lundberg JM, Alving K (1994) Greatly increased luminal nitric oxide in ulcerative colitis. Lancet 344: 1673–1674.

38. Kuilman T, Michaloglou C, Vredeveld LC, Douma S, van Doorn R, et al. (2008) Oncogene-induced senescence relayed by an interleukin-dependent inflammatory network. Cell 133: 1019–1031.

39. Fujita K, Mondal AM, Horikawa I, Nguyen GH, Kumamoto K, et al. (2009) p53 isoforms Delta133p53 and p53beta are endogenous regulators of replicative cellular senescence. Nat Cell Biol 11: 1135–1142.

40. Schetter AJ, Leung SY, Sohn JJ, Zanetti KA, Bowman ED, et al. (2008) MicroRNA expression profiles associated with prognosis and therapeutic outcome in colon adenocarcinoma. JAMA 299: 425–436.

41. Schetter AJ, Nguyen GH, Bowman ED, Mathe EA, Yuen ST, et al. (2009) Association of inflammation-related and microRNA gene expression with cancer-specific mortality of colon adenocarcinoma. Clin Cancer Res 15: 5878–5887.

42. DePinho RA (2000) The age of cancer. Nature 408: 248–254.

43. O'Sullivan JN, Bronner MP, Brentnall TA, Finley JC, Shen WT, et al. (2002) Chromosomal instability in ulcerative colitis is related to telomere shortening. Nat Genet 32: 280–284.

44. Risques RA, Lai LA, Himmetoglu C, Ebaee A, Li L, et al. (2011) Ulcerative colitis-associated colorectal cancer arises in a field of short telomeres, senescence, and inflammation. Cancer Res 71: 1669–1679. 0008-5472.CAN-10-1966 [pii];10.1158/0008-5472.CAN-10-1966 [doi].

45. Campisi J, Andersen JK, Kapahi P, Melov S (2011) Cellular senescence: A link between cancer and age-related degenerative disease? Semin Cancer Biol. S1044-579X(11)00050-2 [pii];10.1016/j.semcancer.2011.09.001 [doi].

46. Rogakou EP, Pilch DR, Orr AH, Ivanova VS, Bonner WM (1998) DNA double-stranded breaks induce histone H2AX phosphorylation on serine 139. J Biol Chem 273: 5858–5868.

47. Jackson SP, Bartek J (2009) The DNA-damage response in human biology and disease. Nature 461: 1071–1078.

48. Coppe JP, Patil CK, Rodier F, Sun Y, Munoz DP, et al. (2008) Senescence-associated secretory phenotypes reveal cell-nonautonomous functions of oncogenic RAS and the p53 tumor suppressor. PLoS Biol 6: 2853–2868.

49. Connelly L, Jacobs AT, Palacios-Callender M, Moncada S, Hobbs AJ (2003) Macrophage endothelial nitric-oxide synthase autoregulates cellular activation and pro-inflammatory protein expression. J Biol Chem 278: 26480–26487.

50. Thomas DD, Ridnour LA, Espey MG, Donzelli S, Ambs S, et al. (2006) Superoxide fluxes limit nitric oxide-induced signaling. J Biol Chem 281: 25984–25993.

51. Clemons NJ, McColl KE, Fitzgerald RC (2007) Nitric oxide and acid induce double-strand DNA breaks in Barrett's esophagus carcinogenesis via distinct mechanisms. Gastroenterology 133: 1198–1209.

52. Dickey JS, Baird BJ, Redon CE, Sokolov MV, Sedelnikova OA, et al. (2009) Intercellular communication of cellular stress monitored by gamma-H2AX induction. Carcinogenesis 30: 1686–1695. bgp192 [pii];10.1093/carcin/bgp192 [doi].

53. Forrester K, Ambs S, Lupold SE, Kapust RB, Spillare EA, et al. (1996) Nitric oxide-induced p53 accumulation and regulation of inducible nitric oxide synthase expression by wild-type p53. Proc Natl Acad Sci U S A 93: 2442–2447.

54. Ambs S, Merriam WG, Ogunfusika MO, Bennett WP, Ishibe N, et al. (1998) p53 and vascular endothelial growth factor regulate tumor growth of NOS2-expressing human carcinoma cells. Nat Med 4: 1371–1376.

55. Bhaumik D, Scott GK, Schokrpur S, Patil CK, Orjalo AV, et al. (2009) MicroRNAs miR-146a/b negatively modulate the senescence-associated inflammatory mediators IL-6 and IL-8. Aging (Albany NY) 1: 402–411.

56. Wu F, Zikusoka M, Trindade A, Dassopoulos T, Harris ML, et al. (2008) MicroRNAs are differentially expressed in ulcerative colitis and alter expression of macrophage inflammatory peptide-2 alpha. Gastroenterology 135: 1624–1635.

57. Simone NL, Soule BP, Ly D, Saleh AD, Savage JE, et al. (2009) Ionizing radiation-induced oxidative stress alters miRNA expression. PLoS One 4: e6377.

58. Mathe E, Nguyen GH, Funamizu N, He P, Moake M, et al. (2011) Inflammation regulates microRNA expression in cooperation with p53 and nitric oxide. Int J Cancer. 10.1002/ijc.26403 [doi].

59. Weber M, Baker MB, Moore JP, Searles CD (2010) MiR-21 is induced in endothelial cells by shear stress and modulates apoptosis and eNOS activity. Biochem Biophys Res Commun 393: 643–648. S0006-291X(10)00256-1 [pii];10.1016/j.bbrc.2010.02.045 [doi].

60. Shin VY, Jin H, Ng EK, Cheng AS, Chong WW, et al. (2011) NF-kappaB targets miR-16 and miR-21 in gastric cancer: involvement of prostaglandin E receptors. Carcinogenesis 32: 240–245. bgq240 [pii];10.1093/carcin/bgq240 [doi].

61. DeNicola GM, Tuveson DA (2009) RAS in cellular transformation and senescence. Eur J Cancer 45 Suppl 1: 211–216. S0959-8049(09)70036-X [pii];10.1016/S0959-8049(09)70036-X [doi].

62. Frezzetti D, Menna MD, Zoppoli P, Guerra C, Ferraro A, et al. (2011) Upregulation of miR-21 by Ras in vivo and its role in tumor growth. Oncogene 30: 275–286. onc2010416 [pii];10.1038/onc.2010.416 [doi].

63. Oliveira CJ, Schindler F, Ventura AM, Morais MS, Arai RJ, et al. (2003) Nitric oxide and cGMP activate the Ras-MAP kinase pathway-stimulating protein tyrosine phosphorylation in rabbit aortic endothelial cells. Free Radic Biol Med 35: 381–396. S0891584903003113 [pii].

64. Abraham C, Cho JH (2009) Inflammatory bowel disease. N Engl J Med 361: 2066–2078.

65. McGovern DP, Gardet A, Torkvist L, Goyette P, Essers J, et al. (2010) Genome-wide association identifies multiple ulcerative colitis susceptibility loci. Nat Genet 42: 332–337.

66. Franke A, McGovern DP, Barrett JC, Wang K, Radford-Smith GL, et al. (2010) Genome-wide meta-analysis increases to 71 the number of confirmed Crohn's disease susceptibility loci. Nat Genet 42: 1118–1125. ng.717 [pii];10.1038/ng.717 [doi].

67. Rivas MA, Beaudoin M, Gardet A, Stevens C, Sharma Y, et al. (2011) Deep resequencing of GWAS loci identifies independent rare variants associated with inflammatory bowel disease. Nat Genet 43: 1066–1073. ng.952 [pii];10.1038/ng.952 [doi].

68. Hedl M, Li J, Cho JH, Abraham C (2007) Chronic stimulation of Nod2 mediates tolerance to bacterial products. Proc Natl Acad Sci U S A 104: 19440–19445.

69. Maeda S, Hsu LC, Liu H, Bankston LA, Iimura M, et al. (2005) Nod2 mutation in Crohn's disease potentiates NF-kappaB activity and IL-1beta processing. Science 307: 734–738.

70. Baker DJ, Wijshake T, Tchkonia T, LeBrasseur NK, Childs BG, et al. (2011) Clearance of p16Ink4a-positive senescent cells delays ageing-associated disorders. Nature 479: 232–236. nature10600 [pii];10.1038/nature10600 [doi].

9

Disease Activity in Inflammatory Bowel Disease is Associated with Increased Risk of Myocardial Infarction, Stroke and Cardiovascular Death

Søren Lund Kristensen[1,2]*, **Ole Ahlehoff**[1,2], **Jesper Lindhardsen**[1], **Rune Erichsen**[3], **Gunnar Vagn Jensen**[2], **Christian Torp-Pedersen**[1], **Ole Haagen Nielsen**[4], **Gunnar Hilmar Gislason**[1], **Peter Riis Hansen**[1]

1 Department of Cardiology, Copenhagen University Hospital Gentofte, Hellerup, Denmark, 2 Department of Cardiology, Copenhagen University Hospital Roskilde, Roskilde, Denmark, 3 Department of Clinical Epidemiology, Aarhus University Hospital, Denmark, 4 Department of Gastroenterology, Copenhagen University Hospital Herlev, Herlev, Denmark

Abstract

Purpose: Chronic inflammatory diseases have been linked to increased risk of atherothrombotic events, but the risk associated with inflammatory bowel disease (IBD) is unclear. We therefore examined the risk of myocardial infarction (MI), stroke, and cardiovascular death in patients with IBD.

Methods: In a nationwide Danish population-based setting, a cohort of patients with incident IBD between 1996 and 2009 were identified in national registers. Hospitalizations with IBD as primary diagnosis, initiation of biological treatment and dispensed prescriptions of corticosteroids were all used as surrogate markers for disease activity, with flares classified as the first 120 days after diagnosis of IBD, and 120 days after a new corticosteroid prescription, biological treatment or IBD hospitalization, respectively. Continued corticosteroid prescriptions or IBD hospitalizations were defined as persistent activity, and periods free of such events were defined as remissions. Poisson regression was used to examine risk of MI, stroke, and cardiovascular death using a matched population-based comparison cohort as reference

Results: We identified 20,795 IBD patients with a mean age of 40.3 years that were matched according to age and sex with 199,978 controls. During the study period, there were 365 patients with MI, 454 with stroke, and 778 with cardiovascular death. Patients with IBD had an overall increased risk of MI (rate ratio [RR] 1.17 [95% confidence interval 1.05–1.31]), stroke (RR 1.15 [1.04–1.27], and cardiovascular death (RR 1.35 [1.25–1.45]). During flares and persistent IBD activity the RRs of MI increased to 1.49 (1.16–1.93) and 2.05 (1.58–2.65), the RRs of stroke to 1.53 (1.22–1.92) and 1.55 (1.18–2.04) and for cardiovascular death 2.32 (2.01–2.68) and 2.50 (2.14–2.92). In remission periods, the risk of MI, stroke and cardiovascular death was similar to controls.

Conclusion: Inflammatory bowel disease is associated with increased risk of MI, stroke, and cardiovascular death during periods with active disease.

Editor: Adrian V. Hernandez, Universidad Peruana de Ciencias Aplicadas (UPC), Peru

Funding: The study was supported by Department of Cardiology, Copenhagen University Hospital Gentofte, DK-2900, and Department of Cardiology, Copenhagen University Roskilde, DK-4000, Denmark. SL Kristensen has received donations from the foundations of Eva and Henry Fränkel and Snedkermester Sophus Jacobsen. The funders had no role in study design, data collection and analysis, decision to publish, or preparation of the manuscript.

Competing Interests: The authors have declared that no competing interests exist.

* E-mail: slk@heart.dk

Introduction

The pivotal role of inflammatory mechanisms in the progression of atherosclerosis has fuelled research aimed at whether diseases characterized by chronic inflammation, including inflammatory bowel disease (IBD), carry an increased risk of cardiovascular disease [1,2]. Indeed, an increased incidence of MI and stroke has been demonstrated in patients with rheumatoid arthritis, psoriasis, and systemic lupus erythematosus [3–5]._ENREF_3 In patients with IBD, however, studies on the risk of atherothrombotic disease are less conclusive [6–9]. Despite these inconclusive findings, it is

well-established that patients with IBD have increased risk of developing venous thromboembolic events, and recent evidence has shown that this risk is particularly elevated during periods of increased disease activity [10,11]. These findings are consistent with studies linking active inflammation to a general prothrombotic state [12–14]. IBD including the two main entities ulcerative colitis (UC) and Crohn's disease (CD) has an estimated prevalence of 2.2 million persons in Europe alone, and linkage between IBD and atherothrombotic disease could potentially have a major impact on the management of these patients [15]. We therefore investigated the risk of MI, stroke, and cardiovascular death in patients with IBD with correlation to disease activity in a nationwide Danish cohort.

Methods

Data sources

The study was conducted and reported in accordance with the Strengthening the Reporting of Observational studies in Epidemiology (STROBE) recommendations [16]._ENREF_15 Each resident in Denmark is given a unique and permanent personal civil registration number at birth or immigration, which enables linkage on individual level across nationwide registers. We used information on date of birth, migration, and socioeconomic status from the civil registration system. Data on morbidity were included from the National Patient Register, holding diagnoses listed according to the international classification of diseases, 8th revision (ICD-8) until 1994, and the 10th revision (ICD-10) thereafter. The National Patient Register contains information on all hospital admissions (since 1978) and outpatient activities (from 1995) and at discharge each admission is registered by one primary diagnose and, if appropriate one or more secondary diagnoses [17]. The Danish Register of Medicinal Product Statistics (the national prescription register) holds complete information on all prescriptions claimed from Danish pharmacies since 1995, and each prescription is registered according to the international Anatomical Therapeutical Chemical (ATC) classification. As drug expenses in Denmark are partially reimbursed by the government-financed health care system, Danish pharmacies are required to register each dispensed prescription in the national prescription registry, which ensures complete and accurate registration [18]. Deaths are registered in the National Cause of Death Register with one primary, and if appropriate, one or more underlying or contributing causes of death. Socioeconomic status was divided into quintiles, based on mean annual taxed income in the 5 years prior to inclusion.

Study population - Cohort entry and follow-up

In the present matched cohort study we defined IBD cases as all individuals aged ≥15 years who received a first diagnosis of IBD, i.e. CD (K50 and 563.01) or UC (K51 and 569.04+563.01), during the period 1996–2009 in combination with a dispensed prescription for pharmacological IBD treatment, including one or more of the following agents (ATC codes): 5-aminosalicylic acid (A07EC02), sulfasalazine (A07EC01), oral corticosteroids (H02AB06), budesonide (A07EA), azathioprine (L04AX01), 6-mercaptopurine (L01BB02) and methotrexate (L01BA01) within one year before the time of diagnosis and hereafter. The index dates of IBD cases were the date of IBD ICD-10 code and drug prescription, whichever came last. Initiation of biological treatment with anti-tumor necrosis factor-α (TNF) agents was defined by the Danish procedural code (BHJ18A). Surgery for IBD was defined by procedure codes (KJF [colon and small intestine], KJG and KJH [perianal area] in combination with IBD-diagnosis). The IBD diagnoses in the National Patient Registry have been found to be accurate [19]. Patients with a diagnosis of IBD, MI or stroke prior to index date were excluded. Also, individuals with a history of prescribed IBD medication (apart from corticosteroids) more than a year prior to IBD diagnosis were excluded. Each IBD patient was matched with 10 controls from the general population at time of inclusion according to age and gender. Controls with a history of MI, stroke or IBD diagnoses were excluded as well. Study subjects were followed from inclusion (index date) until MI, stroke, emigration, death or end of follow-up. Patients with a

diagnosis of both UC and CD were identified as having unclassified IBD.

IBD activity

Hospitalizations with IBD as primary diagnosis, initiation of anti-TNF treatment and dispensed prescription of corticosteroids were used as surrogate markers for disease activity. An IBD flare was defined as a 120 days period starting at the day of initiation of corticosteroid treatment, biological treatment and/or hospitalization for IBD, following 120 days free of corticosteroid prescription or hospitalizations due to IBD (Fig.1) [10]. The first 120 days after study inclusion were likewise defined as a flare period. We further defined periods of persistent activity, as those which succeeded flare periods if additional hospitalizations, anti-TNF treatment or corticosteroid prescriptions had taken place within the 120 days from flare start. Remission periods started 120 days after last hospitalization, anti-TNF treatment or corticosteroid prescription and ended at the time of reinitiating of corticosteroid treatment or hospitalization. We also did sensitivity analyses where corticosteroid prescriptions were excluded as an activity marker.

Co-morbidity and medical treatment

We assessed the presence of co-morbidity at study entry by hospitalization for the following prespecified diagnoses in the 5 years preceding study inclusion (ICD-10 and ICD-8 codes): Cardiac dysrhythmia (I44–I49 and 427.3, 427.4, 427.5, 427.6, 427.9), diabetes (E10–E14 and 250), chronic obstructive pulmonary disease (J42, J44 and 490–492), renal disease (N03, N04, N17, N18, N19, R34, I12, I13 and 582–588), hypertension (I10–I15 and 400–404), venous thromboembolic disease (I26, I80, I82 and 415, 453 excluding I80.8, I80.0 and I82.0), and heart failure (I42, I43, I50 and 110, 517)._ENREF_19Use of the following drugs (ATC codes) was defined at study inclusion : Glucose-lowering agents (A10), statins (C10A), loop diuretics (C03C), platelet inhibitors (B01AC), vitamin K antagonists (B01AA) and we identified patients with hypertension by treatment with at least two of the following classes of antihypertensive drugs: α-adrenergic blockers (C02A, C02B, C02C), non-loop diuretics (C02DA, C02L, C03A, C03B, C03D, C03E, C03X, C07C, C07D, C08G, C09BA, C09DA, C09XA52), vasodilators (C02DB, C02DD, C02DG), β blockers (C07), calcium channel blockers (C07F, C08, C09BB, C09DB), and renin-angiotensin system inhibitors (C09). Similarly we defined diabetes by either the hospital diagnosis (E10–E14) or use of glucose-lowering agents (A10). All information on cardiovascular medication and co-morbidity were continually updated throughout the follow-up period.

Study endpoints

The following endpoints (ICD-10 codes) were used: MI (I21–I22), stroke (I60–I61, I63–I64), cardiovascular death (I00–I99) and a secondary composite endpoint of MI, stroke and cardiovascular death. The stroke and MI codes have previously been validated in the National Patient Register [20,21].

Statistical analysis

Baseline characteristic were summarized as means with standard deviations for continuous variables and frequencies and percentages for categorical variables. Incidence rates (IRs) are presented per 1000 person-years. To estimate rate ratios (RRs) and 95% confidence intervals (CIs) for MI, stroke, cardiovascular death, and the composite endpoint, we fitted multivariable Poisson regression models in patients with IBD using the matched controls as reference. The models were adjusted for confounding factors,

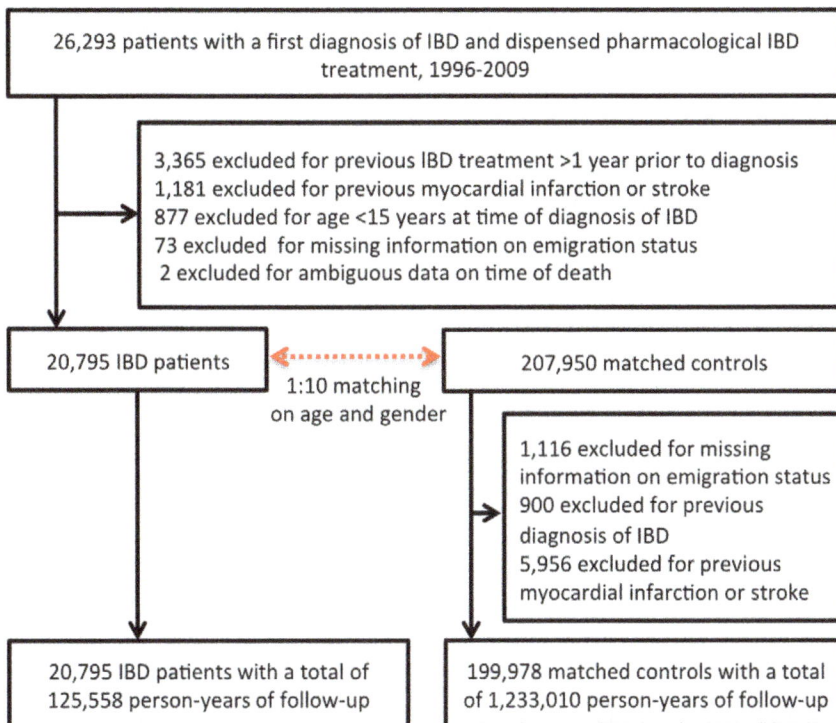

Figure 1. Example of disease activity periods and hospitalizations in apatient with inflammatory bowel disease (IBD) throughout the study period.

including socioeconomic status, and gender. Age, co-morbidity, use of cardiovascular medication (antihypertensive treatment, statins, loop diuretics, vitamin K antagonists), lipid-lowering agents, glucose-lowering medication, and IBD disease activity status were included as time-dependent variables. Subjects lost to follow-up due to emigration from Denmark were censored at time of emigration. To address potential differences in risk of cardiovascular disease in patients with CD, UC or unspecified IBD we evaluated overall risk and disease activity related risk for each endpoint in an IBD subtype-stratified analysis. In addition, we changed the flare duration to assess the potential impact of flare-definition on the risk estimates. We did subgroup analyses of patients that received anti-TNF agents (BHJ18A) and other immunomodulators including 6-mercaptopurine (L01BA01), aza-thioprine (L01BB02), and/or methotrexate (L04AX). We also did a subgroup analysis where we evaluated the influence of nine predefined risk factors (prior venous thromboembolism, heart failure, cardiac arrhythmias, chronic obstructive pulmonary disease [COPD], renal disease, hypertension, diabetes, and use of loop diuretics, lipid-lowering agents, and vitamin K antagonists) and stratified all IBD patients in groups of 0 (reference group), 1–2 or ≥3 risk factors. SAS version 9.2 and Stata version 11.1 were used for statistical analyses. Risk set matching was performed with Greedy matching macro (last accessed 5 September 2012 at http://mayoresearch.mayo.edu/mayo/research/biostat/upload/gmatch.sas). We tested model assumptions, including the linearity of continuous variables and absence of interactions, and found them to be valid unless otherwise specified. Evaluation of the significance of an unmeasured confounder was made using the "rule out" approach for all reported results [22].

Ethics

Register-based studies do not require ethical approval in Denmark as individual patients cannot be identified from the encrypted data that are available. The Danish Data protection agency approved the study (reference no. 2007-58-0015, international reference: GEH-2010-001).

Results

A total of 26,293 IBD patients were identified with in the study period. After exclusion of patients with prior IBD, MI or stroke, the final study population included 20,795 patients (Fig. 2). A total of 199,978 matched controls were enrolled in the study.

Patient characteristics at index are displayed in Table 1. The mean age of the study population was 43.8 (SD 18.7) years, and 54.5 % were women. Loss to follow-up due to emigration was 2.0 % among the included IBD cases and 3.5 % among controls. The frequencies of co-morbidities were significantly higher among IBD patients compared to the matched controls, and use of cardiovascular drugs and glucose-lowering agents at baseline was significantly higher in the IBD group. Distribution of IBD disease activity is shown in table 2.

We observed a total of 365 MIs, 454 strokes and 778 cardiovascular deaths in the IBD cohort as compared to 2,389 MIs, 3,327 strokes and 4,738 cardiovascular deaths in the matched control group during follow-up.

IRs for MI were 2.93 (95% CI 2.64–3.24) and 1.95 (1.87–2.03) per 1000 person-years for IBD patients and matched controls. The risk of MI was increased both in unadjusted and adjusted analyses, with an adjusted overall risk of RR 1.17 (1.05–1.31). During flares RR was 1.49 (1.16–1.93) and during persistent activity the RR was 2.05 (1.58–2.65) (Fig. 3 and Table 3). During remission the RR for MI was not increased (1.01 [0.89–1.15]) and it was significantly

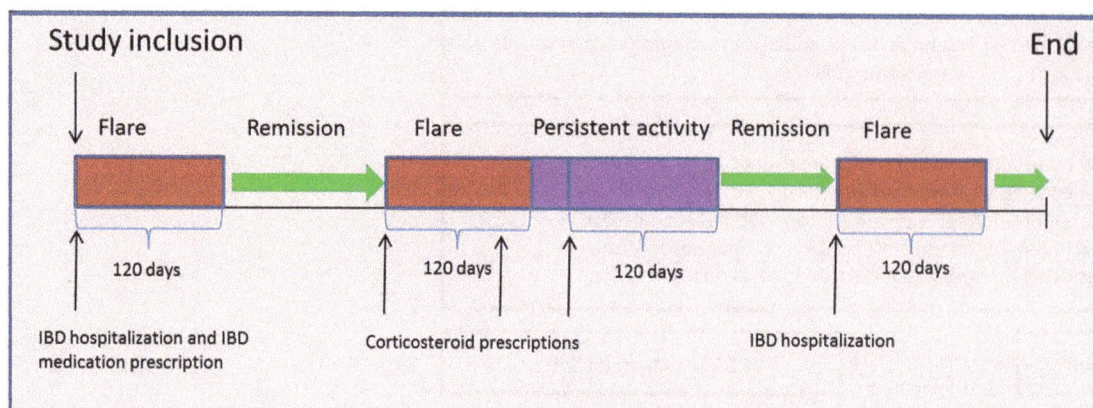

Figure 2. Flowchart for the study population, IBD: Inflammatory bowel disease.

lower than RRs during flares (p = 0.005) and in periods with persistent activity of IBD (p<0.0001).

The incidence of stroke was also highest during periods of flares (IR 5.60 [4.48–7.00]) and persistent activity (IR 8.60 [6.57–11.25]) and as compared to controls (IR 2.72 [2.62–2.81]). The overall adjusted RR for stroke was 1.15 (1.04–1.27), and the risk was evenly increased in periods of flare and persistent activity with RR 1.53 (1.22–1.92) and RR 1.55 (1.18–2.04). Again, the risk during remission was negligible with RR 1.04(0.92–1.16) and significantly

lower than periods with persistent activity (p = 0.008) and flares (p = 0.003)

Concerning cardiovascular death the IRs were markedly increased during flares (IR 13.89 [12.06–16.01]) and persistent activity (IR 26.91 [23.13.31.30]) compared to remission (IR 3.96 [3.60–4.36]) and matched controls (IR 3.84 [3.73–3.95]). The augmented risk in the IBD cohort was prominent for cardiovascular death with an overall increased RR of 1.35 (1.25–1.45) in the adjusted analysis. The risk of cardiovascular death was more than two-fold increased both in periods of flares (RR 2.32 [2.01–2.68])

Table 1. Baseline characteristics of the study population. IBD: inflammatory bowel disease.

	IBD patients n = 20,795	Controls n = 199,978	p -value
Male (%)	9,455 (45.5)	90,439 (45.2)	
Female (%)	11,340 (54.5)	109,539 (54.8)	
Age, years mean (SD)	43.8 (18.7)	43.1 (18.7)	
Mean follow-up time, years	6.04	6.17	
No. of patient-years	125,558	1,233,010	
Ulcerative colitis (%)	13,622 (65.5)	–	
Crohns disease (%)	4,732 (22.8)	–	
Unspecific IBD (%)	2,441 (11.7)	–	
Treatment (%)			
Antihypertensive treatment	1,806 (8.7)	10,362 (5.2)	<0.001
Statin	871 (4.2)	5,337 (2.7)	<0.001
Platelet inhibitor	1,222 (5.9)	6,845 (3.4)	<0.001
Loop diuretic	829 (4.0)	3,968 (2.0)	<0.001
Vitamin K antagonist	233 (1.1)	1,255 (0.6)	<0.001
Glucose-lowering medication	479 (2.3)	3,527 (1.8)	<0.001
Co morbidity (%)			
Cardiac dysrhythmia	409 (2.0)	1,938 (1.0)	<0.001
Heart failure	221 (1.1)	761 (0.4)	<0.001
Renal disease	102 (0.5)	275 (0.1)	<0.001
Diabetes	375 (1.8)	155 (0.1)	<0.001
Hypertension	635 (3.1)	2,335 (1.2)	<0.001
Venous thromboembolism	195 (0.9)	868 (0.4)	<0.001
Chronic obstructive pulmonary disease	403 (1.9)	1,125 (0.6)	<0.001

Table 2. Disease activity periods and follow-up time in study cohort with inflammatory bowel disease (IBD).

	Disease activity periods (n [%])	Mean duration (days)	Total duration of follow-up in IBD population (person-years)
Flare	42,685 (42.8)	117.0	13,674 (10.9)
Persistent activity	17,542 (17.6)	128.4	6,166 (4.9)
Remission	39,547 (29.1)	976.4	105,718 (84.2)
Total	99,774 (100)	459.6	125,558(100)

and periods of persistent activity (RR 2.50 [2.14–2.92]). Again, the RRs were higher for flares and periods with persistent activity in comparison with remission periods (both p<0.0001). For IBD in remission, the risk was similar to matched controls (RR 0.98 [0.89–1.09]; p = 0.96). Finally for the composite endpoint of MI, stroke, and cardiovascular death, the RR was 1.97 (1.74–2.22) during flares and 2.07 (1.80–2.39) in periods with persistent activity. Once more there was no increased risk during remission RR 1.00 (0.93–1.08).

We saw no differences in cardiovascular risk between men and women with IBD, and we observed no interaction between IBD subtypes and the cardiovascular risk stratified by disease activity. The overall risk was similar for MI and augmented for stroke and cardiovascular death in CD patients as compared to UC patients (MI: RR 1.35 [1.03–1.77] vs. 1.17 [1.03–1.33] p = 0.81, stroke: RR 1.37 [1.10–1.72] vs. 1.10 [1.02–1.19] p = 0.02 and cardiovascular death: RR 1.63 [1.36–1.95] vs. 1.25 [1.14–1.37] p = 0.04). In IBD activity analyses without corticosteroid prescriptions as activity marker, we found that the higher cardiovascular risk in periods of IBD disease activity persisted (not shown). When we removed hospitalization from our IBD disease activity definition, we found similar risks of MI (RR 1.43 [1.09–1.87] vs. 1.49 [1.16–1.93]) and stroke (RR 1.46 [1.15–1.86] vs. 1.53 [1.22–1.92]) during flares. Additionally we compared the risk 120 days after surgery due to pancolitis (K51.0) and proctitis (K51.2) in UC patients, and surgery for isolated colon disease (K50.1) versus more

widespread CD disease (K50.8) in CD patients, respectively. In general, we found elevated risks during this period (all RRs >2) but due to low number of events no significant differences were found between the aforementioned groups (not shown).

When we reduced flare length to 60 days, the risk for the composite endpoint in periods with persistent activity was RR 2.67 (2.25–3.18) and during flares RR 2.08 (1.82–2.37). Also, when flare duration was increased to 180 days the corresponding RR was 1.92 (1.68–2.20) in periods with persistent activity and RR 1.75 (1.57–1.98) during flares. We identified 679 (3.3 %) patients who received anti-TNF agents in the period from inclusion to end of study. These patients were younger (median [IQR] age 27.6 [20.7–37.6] years) and had shorter (median 1.2 years) follow up time than the general IBD cohort. We found no cardiovascular events among the patients treated with anti-TNF agents within the study period.

In total 6,017 patients (28.9 %) who received treatment with 6-mercaptopurine, azathioprine and/or methotrexate. In these subjects, we found no significant differences on the risks of MI, stroke and cardiovascular death as compared to the total IBD population (MI: RR 1.15 vs. 1.17 p = 0.88, stroke RR 1.16 vs. 1.14 p = 0.79 and cardiovascular death RR: 1.23 vs. 1.35 p = 0.33). In a sensitivity analysis where we excluded patients with COPD, we found the overall risks of the cardiovascular endpoints for IBD patients essentially unchanged (MI: RR 1.16 [1.03–1.32] vs. 1.18 [1.05–1.31]], stroke: RR 1.15 [1.04–1.27] vs.

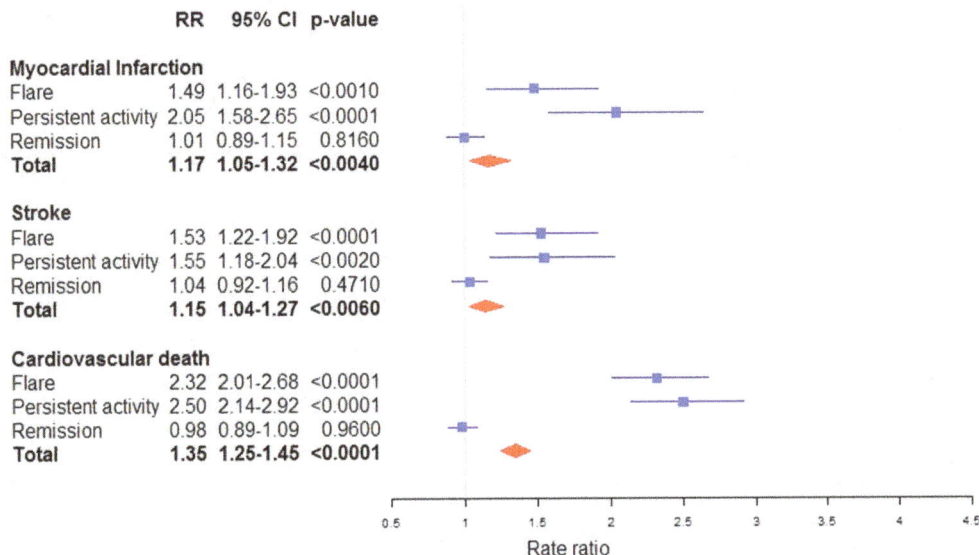

Figure 3. Risk of myocardial infarction, stroke and cardiovascular death stratified by inflammatory bowel disease activity. CI: confidence interval. RR: Rate ratio.

Table 3. Number of events, incidence rates per 1000 person-years, adjusted rate ratios (RRs) and 95% confidence intervals (CIs).

	Number of events	Incidence rate (unadjusted)	95% CI	RR	95% CI
Myocardial infarction					
Ulcerative colitis	272	3.42	3.03–3.85	1.17	1.03–1.33
Crohns disease	61	2.16	1.68–2.78	1.35	1.03–1.77
Unspecific IBD	32	1.89	1.33–2.67	1.05	0.76–1.48
IBD total	365	2.93	2.64–3.24	1.17	1.05–1.31
Age>45 years	334	7.08	6.36–7.89	1.18	1.05–1.32
Flare	60	4.36	3.38–5.61	1.49	1.16–1.93
Persistent activity	60	9.73	7.56–12.53	2.05	1.58–2.65
Remission	245	2.34	2.06–2.65	1.01	0.89–1.15
Controls	2,389	1.95	1.87–2.03	ref.	–
Stroke					
Ulcerative colitis	309	3.88	3.47–4.34	1.10	1.02–1.19
Crohns disease	89	3.17	2.57–3.90	1.37	1.10–1.72
Unspecific IBD	56	3.30	2.54–4.29	1.41	1.06–1.88
IBD total	454	3.64	3.32–3.99	1.15	1.04–1.27
Age>45 years	410	8.71	7.90–9.59	1.15	1.03–1.27
Flare	77	5.60	4.48–7.00	1.53	1.22–1.92
Persistent activity	53	8.60	6.57–11.25	1.55	1.18–2.04
Remission	324	3.09	2.77–3.45	1.04	0.92–1.16
Controls	3,327	2.72	2.62–2.81	ref.	–
Cardiovascular death					
Ulcerative colitis	540	6.73	6.19–7.32	1.25	1.14–1.37
Crohns disease	148	5.23	4.45–6.14	1.63	1.36–1.95
Unspecific IBD	90	5.28	4.30–6.49	1.69	1.34–2.13
IBD total	778	6.20	5.78–6.65	1.35	1.25–1.45
Age>45 years	758	15.85	14.76–17.02	1.29	1.22–1.37
Flare	192	13.89	12.06–16.01	2.32	2.01–2.68
Persistent activity	168	26.91	23.13–31.30	2.50	2.14–2.92
Remission	418	3.96	3.60–4.36	0.98	0.89–1.09
Controls	4,738	3.84	3.73–3.95	ref.	–
Composite endpoint					
Ulcerative colitis	869	10.99	10.28–11.74	1.17	1.09–1.26
Crohns disease	229	8.18	7.19–9.31	1.48	1.28–1.70
Unspecific IBD	138	8.18	6.92–9.67	1.38	1.15–1.65
IBD total	1,236	9.97	9.43–10.54	1.24	1.16–1.31
Age>45 years	1,155	24.87	23.47–26.34	1.26	1.18–1.34
Flare	266	19.41	17.22–21.89	1.97	1.74–2.22
Persistent activity	205	33.67	29.36–38.60	2.07	1.80–2.39
Remission	765	7.35	6.84–7.88	1.00	0.93–1.08
Controls	8,056	6.60	6.46–6.75	ref.	–

The composite endpoint was myocardial infarction, stroke and cardiovascular death combined. IBD: inflammatory bowel disease. The model was adjusted for age, gender, co-morbidity, cardiovascular medication and socioeconomic status.

1.15 [1.04–1.27]], and cardiovascular death: RR 1.33 [1.22–1.45] vs. 1.28 [1.18–1.38]).

When we compared IBD patients with and without present cardiovascular risk factors, particularly the risk of MI was correlated to presence of risk factors, with RRs 9.09 (7.89–10.49) and 23.14 (20.00–26.77) when comparing 0 vs. 1–2, and

0 vs. ≥3 risk factors, respectively. The corresponding RRs were somewhat lower for stroke (RR 5.29 [4.80–5.87] and RR 8.21 [7.39–9.12]) and cardiovascular death (RR 2.41 [2.24–2.60] and RR 4.36 [4.04–4.70]). IBD patients without any notable cardiovascular risk factors at the time of events comprised 9.0 % of MIs, 13.2 % of strokes, and 11.8 % of cardiovascular deaths.

Discussion

This present study examined the incidence of MI, stroke, and cardiovascular death in a nationwide cohort of more than 20,000 patients with a new onset of IBD who were followed for a mean period of 6 years. Compared to controls, we found that the risks of MI, stroke, and cardiovascular death were significantly increased during periods of IBD activity including flares and persistent activity, whereas there was no increased risk of these adverse outcomes during periods of IBD remission. The observed IBD activity-dependent increased risk suggests that systemic inflammation contributes to the pathophysiological mechanisms leading to atherothrombosis and the results parallel recent findings of IBD activity-dependent augmented risk of venous thromboembolic disease [10,11]. Patients with CD had a higher risk of stroke and cardiovascular death as compared to UC, but we found a parallel relative risk increase regardless of IBD entity during periods with IBD activity (flares and persistent activity).

While increased risk of venous thromboembolic events in subjects with IBD is now well-established, the risk of athero-thrombotic disease including MI and stroke has been the topic of debate [6–12]. For example, a 2007 meta-analysis of 11 studies including roughly 14,000 IBD patients _ENREF_22_ENREF_22-found no increased risk of cardiovascular mortality [23]. In line with this result, two recent registry-based studies of around 17,000 and 25,000 IBD patients, respectively, reported that the risk of MI in IBD patients was comparable to matched IBD-free controls [7,8]. However, a Canadian study of 8,000 IBD patients showed an increased risk of ischaemic heart disease (RR 1.26 [1.11–1.44]), whereas increased risk of stroke was only significant among CD patients (RR 1.26 [1.04–1.53]) [24]. In addition, in a cohort of 8,000 patients with CD from the UK General Practice Research Database, an increased risk of stroke in patients <50 years (odds ratio 2.93 [1.44–5.98]) was observed, but no increased overall risk of stroke among older patients [6]. Moreover, a retrospective single-center cohort study of around 350 IBD patients found an increased risk of coronary artery disease [25].

The current results add considerably to the existing literature by demonstrating a significantly increased risk of MI, stroke, and cardiovascular death in a large and unselected population of patients with IBD. A novel finding was that the risk was related to IBD activity with highest risk during flares and periods of persistent activity, while in remission periods the risk of MI and stroke was only marginally increased and in the latter periods the risk of cardiovascular death was comparable to the reference population. In agreement with our results, a study from the same nationwide population published during the preparation of our manuscript also reported an increased risk of ischaemic heart disease including MI in patients with IBD, with particularly high risk in the first 3 months after IBD diagnosis and in patients with a history of treatment with oral corticosteroids [26]. Importantly, that study did not examine the risk of stroke and cardiovascular death, and did not specifically explore the risk associated with different activity of IBD as done in the present study. Moreover, the primary outcome of that study, i.e. ischaemic heart disease, has not been validated in the Danish National Patient Register. These differences notwithstanding, the results clearly suggest that the systemic inflammatory burden in subjects with IBD may be an important determinant of atherothrombotic risk. In agreement with this contention, a disease severity-dependent increased risk of MI and stroke has also been found in patients with other chronic inflammatory diseases, including rheumatoid arthritis and psoriasis [27,28].

Atherosclerosis is a chronic inflammatory disease characterized by inflammation both in the arterial wall and systemically in the body, and atherothrombotic disease is associated with increased inflammation as exemplified by elevated levels of C-reactive protein [2,29,30]. Indeed, the inflammatory state involves many unspecific mechanisms including release of cytokines and other mediators (including tumor necrosis factor alpha, interleukin-1, and platelet activating factor) which may contribute to shifting the hemostatic balance towards a prothrombotic state [2]. IBD is also characterized by an inappropriate immuno-inflammatory activation, and the pathophysiological processes in the colonic wall in patients with IBD share many features with the processes in the arterial wall during progression of atherosclerosis and, ultimately, atherosclerotic plaque rupture and thrombosis [12,31–35]._EN-REF_21_ENREF_21 Reports that IBD is associated with subclinical atherosclerosis, including endothelial dysfunction and increased carotid intima-media thickness, together with athero-genic alterations of the lipid profile, lend additional support to the current finding of an increased risk of atherothrombotic disease in these patients [14,34,36,37]. Although the increased risk of atherothrombotic disease associated with IBD activity may be explained in part by an increased inflammatory activity, other contributory mechanisms should be considered as well, e.g., increased use of corticosteroids, and susceptibility to surgical interventions and infections during periods of augmented IBD activity. Specifically, corticosteroids may have pro-thrombotic effects, but it remains controversial if use of these drugs adds to the risk of atherothrombotic disease in patients with IBD or other chronic inflammatory diseases.[38]_ENREF_30 We also made a sensitivity analysis with exclusion of COPD patients and found no alterations in the overall results. Among the patients who received TNF inhibitors within the study period, we found no cardiovascular events. Whether this was due to the anti-inflammatory effects of anti-TNF agents or caused by the low median age and short follow-up time of these patients warrants further investigations. We found similar cardiovascular risk in the 6,017 IBD patients who received treatment with azathioprine, 6-mercaptopurine, and/or methotrexate as compared to the total IBD population. Whether this result reflects that these drugs truly had no effects on cardiovascular outcomes or that such effects were confounded by the selection of patients with more severe IBD is unclear at present.

Our subgroup analysis which stratified IBD patients according to presence of cardiovascular risk factors showed a strong correlation between the number of risk factors and the risk of adverse cardiovascular endpoints. Only approximately 10 % of cardiovascular events occurred in IBD patients with no notable risk factors at the time of the event.

Strengths and limitations

The major strength of this study was the large number of IBD patients included and the completeness of data that covered the entire population of Denmark independent of race, socioeconomic status, age, or participation in health insurance programs. Also, the IBD, MI, and stroke diagnoses have been validated in the National Patient Register, with a sensitivity of 94% for both the CD and UC diagnoses and positive predictive values of 97% and 90%, respectively, and for MI a positive predictive value for MI of 93.6 % and sensitivity of 77.6 % [19,23]. For stroke the positive predictive value ranged from 73 % for cerebral hemorrhage to 95 % for ischaemic stroke [22]. Moreover, the number of patients identified by IBD treatment agents in combination with diagnosis of IBD used for establishing the IBD diagnosis and the observed number of incident IBD patients corresponded closely to those observed in previous Danish studies [39]. Also, we were able to adjust for concomitant cardiovascular medication and co-morbidities.

The main study limitation was inherent to the observational design which precludes conclusions on causality and allows for confounding. The higher prevalence of co-morbidities found among IBD-patients could be related, in part, to their more frequent contact to the health care system and hence increased likelihood of a receiving other diagnoses and treatment (detection bias). We lacked information on important cardiovascular risk factors, e.g. lipid levels, obesity, blood pressure, and smoking, although some of these unmeasured risk factors were adjusted for, in part, by use of time-dependent surrogates including medical treatment (e.g. statins for hyperlipidaemia and antihypertensive agents for hypertension) and diagnoses (e.g. COPD for smoking). Adjustment for socioeconomic status at baseline is also likely to have integrated factors such as obesity and smoking. In addition, detection bias may have contributed to increased prevalence of co-morbidities in IBD patients owing to more frequent medical control in these subjects. These limitations notwithstanding, our study design that focused on the importance of IBD disease activity for the cardiovascular risk is likely to have reduced the importance of confounders.

Misclassifications of risk factors such as untreated hypertension, diabetes, or dyslipidaemia may be present and result in unmeasured confounding. The definition of hypertension used has been validated in a randomly selected cohort of people from the Danish population aged ≥ 16 years, with a positive predictive value of 80% and specificity of 94.7 % [40].

An unmeasured confounder, must be prevalent, unevenly distributed and carry a very high risk to nullify the findings, for example the increased cardiovascular risk during flare periods. We estimated that such a confounder should have a prevalence of 20% and increase RR by a factor of >2 for MI and stroke, and >6 for cardiovascular death. Comparable estimates for hypothetical 'rule out' confounders were apparent for persistent activity, rendering its existence unlikely [22] . Finally, our definition of active IBD in terms of flares and persistent activity from corticosteroid prescriptions and primary IBD hospitalizations was arbitrary, as was the assumption that a flare leaves the patient at risk for 120 days. Nevertheless, although the length and duration of risk is likely to vary for each individual and more precise evaluation on a patient level would be advantageous, the 120 day period has been used earlier for assessment of the IBD activity-dependent risk of venous thromboembolic events [10]. Halving the flare duration to 60 days increased the relative risk both during flares and persistent activity, whereas a 50 % increase of flare duration to 180 days led to slightly reduced relative risks (not shown). In sensitivity analyses excluding the use of corticosteroids as an activity marker, the elevated cardiovascular risk in periods of flares persisted, which indicated some robustness in our definition of IBD activity.

Conclusions

This nationwide study of IBD patients found a significantly increased risk of MI, stroke, and cardiovascular mortality as compared to matched controls. This risk was predominantly present in periods of IBD activity, including flares and persistent activity, whereas the risk was insignificantly raised for MI and stroke and not increased for cardiovascular death during remission disease stages. The results suggest that effective treatment of IBD aimed at disease remission may reduce cardiovascular risk in these patients, and that treatment strategies for atherothrombotic risk reduction during periods of IBD activity should be explored.

Author Contributions

Conceived and designed the experiments: SLK PRH GHG OHN CTP OA RE JL GVJ. Performed the experiments: SLK PRH GHG OHN OA RE JL GVJ. Analyzed the data: SLK PRH GHG OHN CTP OA RE JL GVJ. Wrote the paper: SLK PRH GHG OHN CTP OA RE JL GVJ .

References

1. Ross R (1999) Atherosclerosis--an inflammatory disease. N Engl J Med 340: 115–126.
2. Hansson GK (2005) Inflammation, atherosclerosis, and coronary artery disease. N Engl J Med 352: 1685–1695.
3. Ahlehoff O, Gislason GH, Charlot M, Jorgensen CH, Lindhardsen J, et al. (2011) Psoriasis is associated with clinically significant cardiovascular risk: a Danish nationwide cohort study. J Intern Med 270: 147–157.
4. Meune C, Touze E, Trinquart L, Allanore Y (2009) Trends in cardiovascular mortality in patients with rheumatoid arthritis over 50 years: a systematic review and meta-analysis of cohort studies. Rheumatology (Oxford) 48: 1309–1313.
5. Svenungsson E, Jensen-Urstad K, Heimburger M, Silveira A, Hamsten A, et al. (2001) Risk factors for cardiovascular disease in systemic lupus erythematosus. Circulation 104: 1887–1893.
6. Andersohn F, Waring M, Garbe E (2010) Risk of ischemic stroke in patients with Crohn's disease: a population-based nested case-control study. Inflamm Bowel Dis 16: 1387–1392.
7. Ha C, Magowan S, Accortt NA, Chen J, Stone CD (2009) Risk of arterial thrombotic events in inflammatory bowel disease. Am J Gastroenterol 104: 1445–1451.
8. Osterman MT, Yang YX, Brensinger C, Forde KA, Lichtenstein GR, et al. (2011) No increased risk of myocardial infarction among patients with ulcerative colitis or Crohn's disease. Clin Gastroenterol Hepatol 9: 875–880.
9. Gandhi S, Narula N, Marshall JK, Farkouh M (2012) Are Patients with Inflammatory Bowel Disease at Increased Risk of Coronary Artery Disease? Am J Med.
10. Grainge MJ, West J, Card TR (2010) Venous thromboembolism during active disease and remission in inflammatory bowel disease: a cohort study. Lancet 375: 657–663.
11. Kappelman MD, Horvath-Puho E, Sandler RS, Rubin DT, Ullman TA, et al. (2011) Thromboembolic risk among Danish children and adults with inflammatory bowel diseases: a population-based nationwide study. Gut 60: 937–943.
12. Zitomersky NL, Verhave M, Trenor CC, 3rd (2011) Thrombosis and inflammatory bowel disease: a call for improved awareness and prevention. Inflamm Bowel Dis 17: 458–470.
13. Ageno W, Dentali F (2008) Venous thromboembolism and arterial thromboembolism. Many similarities, far beyond thrombosis per se. Thromb Haemost 100: 181–183.
14. Gresele P, Momi S, Migliacci R (2010) Endothelium, venous thromboembolism and ischaemic cardiovascular events. Thromb Haemost 103: 56–61.
15. Loftus EV, Jr. (2004) Clinical epidemiology of inflammatory bowel disease: Incidence, prevalence, and environmental influences. Gastroenterology 126: 1504–1517.
16. von Elm E, Altman DG, Egger M, Pocock SJ, Gotzsche PC, et al. (2007) The Strengthening the Reporting of Observational Studies in Epidemiology (STROBE) statement: guidelines for reporting observational studies. Lancet 370: 1453–1457.
17. Kildemoes HW, Sorensen HT, Hallas J (2011) The Danish National Prescription Registry. Scand J Public Health 39: 38–41.
18. Gaist D, Sorensen HT, Hallas J (1997) The Danish prescription registries. Dan Med Bull 44: 445–448.
19. Fonager K, Sorensen HT, Rasmussen SN, Moller-Petersen J, Vyberg M (1996) Assessment of the diagnoses of Crohn's disease and ulcerative colitis in a Danish hospital information system. Scand J Gastroenterol 31: 154–159.
20. Krarup LH, Boysen G, Janjua H, Prescott E, Truelsen T (2007) Validity of stroke diagnoses in a National Register of Patients. Neuroepidemiology 28: 150–154.
21. Madsen M, Davidsen M, Rasmussen S, Abildstrom SZ, Osler M (2003) The validity of the diagnosis of acute myocardial infarction in routine statistics: a comparison of mortality and hospital discharge data with the Danish MONICA registry. J Clin Epidemiol 56: 124–130.
22. Schneeweiss S (2006) Sensitivity analysis and external adjustment for unmeasured confounders in epidemiologic database studies of therapeutics. Pharmacoepidemiol Drug Saf 15: 291–303.
23. Dorn SD, Sandler RS (2007) Inflammatory bowel disease is not a risk factor for cardiovascular disease mortality: results from a systematic review and meta-analysis. Am J Gastroenterol 102: 662–667.
24. Bernstein CN, Wajda A, Blanchard JF (2008) The incidence of arterial thromboembolic diseases in inflammatory bowel disease: a population-based study. Clin Gastroenterol Hepatol 6: 41–45.

25. Yarur AJ, Deshpande AR, Pechman DM, Tamariz L, Abreu MT, et al. (2011) Inflammatory bowel disease is associated with an increased incidence of cardiovascular events. Am J Gastroenterol 106: 741–747.

26. Rungoe C, Basit S, Ranthe MF, Wohlfahrt J, Langholz E, et al. (2012) Risk of ischaemic heart disease in patients with inflammatory bowel disease: a nationwide Danish cohort study. Gut.

27. Solomon DH, Kremer J, Curtis JR, Hochberg MC, Reed G, et al. (2010) Explaining the cardiovascular risk associated with rheumatoid arthritis: traditional risk factors versus markers of rheumatoid arthritis severity. Ann Rheum Dis 69: 1920–1925.

28. Ahlehoff O, Gislason GH, Jorgensen CH, Lindhardsen J, Charlot M, et al. (2012) Psoriasis and risk of atrial fibrillation and ischaemic stroke: a Danish Nationwide Cohort Study. Eur Heart J 33: 2054–2064.

29. Libby P, Ridker PM, Hansson GK (2009) Inflammation in atherosclerosis: from pathophysiology to practice. J Am Coll Cardiol 54: 2129–2138.

30. Kaptoge S, Di Angelantonio E, Lowe G, Pepys MB, Thompson SG, et al. (2010) C-reactive protein concentration and risk of coronary heart disease, stroke, and mortality: an individual participant meta-analysis. Lancet 375: 132–140.

31. Baumgart DC, Carding SR (2007) Inflammatory bowel disease: cause and immunobiology. Lancet 369: 1627–1640.

32. Irving PM, Pasi KJ, Rampton DS (2005) Thrombosis and inflammatory bowel disease. Clin Gastroenterol Hepatol 3: 617–628.

33. Abraham C, Cho JH (2009) Inflammatory bowel disease. N Engl J Med 361: 2066–2078.

34. van Leuven SI, Hezemans R, Levels JH, Snoek S, Stokkers PC, et al. (2007) Enhanced atherogenesis and altered high density lipoprotein in patients with Crohn's disease. J Lipid Res 48: 2640–2646.

35. Strober W, Fuss IJ (2011) Proinflammatory cytokines in the pathogenesis of inflammatory bowel diseases. Gastroenterology 140: 1756–1767.

36. Roifman I, Sun YC, Fedwick JP, Panaccione R, Buret AG, et al. (2009) Evidence of endothelial dysfunction in patients with inflammatory bowel disease. Clin Gastroenterol Hepatol 7: 175–182.

37. Dagli N, Poyrazoglu OK, Dagli AF, Sahbaz F, Karaca I, et al. (2010) Is inflammatory bowel disease a risk factor for early atherosclerosis? Angiology 61: 198–204.

38. Walker BR (2007) Glucocorticoids and cardiovascular disease. Eur J Endocrinol 157: 545–559.

39. Vind I, Riis L, Jess T, Knudsen E, Pedersen N, et al. (2006) Increasing incidences of inflammatory bowel disease and decreasing surgery rates in Copenhagen City and County, 2003–2005: a population-based study from the Danish Crohn colitis database. Am J Gastroenterol 101: 1274–1282.

40. Olesen JB, Lip GY, Hansen ML, Hansen PR, Tolstrup JS, et al. (2011) Validation of risk stratification schemes for predicting stroke and thromboembolism in patients with atrial fibrillation: nationwide cohort study. BMJ 342: d124.

10

A Comprehensive Evaluation of Colonic Mucosal Isolates of *Sutterella wadsworthensis* from Inflammatory Bowel Disease

Indrani Mukhopadhya[1,9], Richard Hansen[1,2,9], Charlotte E. Nicholl[1], Yazeid A. Alhaidan[1], John M. Thomson[1], Susan H. Berry[1], Craig Pattinson[3], David A. Stead[3], Richard K. Russell[4], Emad M. El-Omar[1], Georgina L. Hold[1]*

1 Gastrointestinal Research Group, Division of Applied Medicine, University of Aberdeen, Foresterhill, Aberdeen, United Kingdom, 2 Child Health, University of Aberdeen, Royal Aberdeen Children's Hospital, Foresterhill, Aberdeen, United Kingdom, 3 Aberdeen Proteomics Group, Institute of Medical Sciences, University of Aberdeen, Foresterhill, Aberdeen, United Kingdom, 4 Department of Paediatric Gastroenterology, Royal Hospital for Sick Children, Glasgow, United Kingdom

Abstract

Inflammatory bowel disease (IBD) arises in genetically susceptible individuals as a result of an unidentified environmental trigger, possibly a hitherto unknown bacterial pathogen. Twenty-six clinical isolates of *Sutterella wadsworthensis* were obtained from 134 adults and 61 pediatric patients undergoing colonoscopy, of whom 69 and 29 respectively had IBD. *S. wadsworthensis* was initially more frequently isolated from IBD subjects, hence this comprehensive study was undertaken to elucidate its role in IBD. Utilizing these samples, a newly designed PCR was developed, to study the prevalence of this bacterium in adult patients with ulcerative colitis (UC). *Sutterella wadsworthensis* was detected in 83.8% of adult patients with UC as opposed to 86.1% of control subjects (p = 0.64). Selected strains from IBD cases and controls were studied to elicit morphological, proteomic, genotypic and pathogenic differences. This study reports Scanning Electron Microscopy (SEM) appearances and characteristic MALDI-TOF MS protein profiles of *S. wadsworthensis* for the very first time. SEM showed that the bacterium is pleomorphic, existing in predominantly two morphological forms, long rods and coccobacilli. No differences were noted in the MALDI-TOF mass spectrometry proteomic analysis. There was no distinct clustering of strains identified from cases and controls on sequence analysis. Cytokine response after monocyte challenge with strains from patients with IBD and controls did not yield any significant differences. Our studies indicate that *S. wadsworthensis* is unlikely to play a role in the pathogenesis of IBD. Strains from cases of IBD could not be distinguished from those identified from controls.

Editor: Stefan Bereswill, Charité-University Medicine Berlin, Germany

Funding: This work was funded by a Clinical Academic Training Fellowship from the Chief Scientist Office in Scotland (CAF/08/01), which also funded the salary of RH and the Broad Medical Research Program (Grant number IBD-0178). JMT was supported by grants from the GI Research Unit, Aberdeen Royal Infirmary. The Royal Hospital for Sick Children, Glasgow IBD team is generously supported by the Catherine McEwan Foundation. RKR has received support from a Medical Research Council patient research cohorts initiative grant (G0800675) for Paediatric Inflammatory Bowel Disease Cohort and Treatment Study (PICTS). The funders had no role in study design, data collection and analysis, decision to publish, or preparation of the manuscript.

Competing Interests: The authors have declared that no competing interests exist.

* E-mail: g.l.hold@abdn.ac.uk.

9 These authors contributed equally to this work.

Introduction

Inflammatory bowel disease (IBD) is an idiopathic inflammatory disorder that is comprised of two major phenotypes, Crohn's disease (CD) and ulcerative colitis (UC). The understanding of its aetiopathogenesis has taken rapid strides in the last decade, with current investigations focusing heavily on aberrations in host-microbe interactions at the luminal intestinal surface. Genetic defects in pathogen recognition and primary handling of microbes by the innate immune system compounded with distinct changes in the luminal microbiome or dysbiosis form the current backbone of this pathogenic hypothesis [1,2]. Despite this, researchers in the field have been striving to identify and delineate a solitary microorganism that can explain the initiation and perpetuation of this chronic inflammatory process.

In this regard, anaerobic and microaerophilic bacteria residing in the intestinal lumen have often been the neglected species,

primarily on account of the intrinsic difficulty in culturing and isolating these organisms by using traditional microbiological techniques. Molecular studies have demonstrated that a substantial proportion of bacterial species (up to 30–40% of dominant species) in patients with active IBD belong to phylogenetic groups that are unusual when compared to healthy subjects [3,4]. With this premise in mind, our laboratory has focused on enhanced and improved bacteriological conditions for the optimum growth of microaerophilic bacteria from colonic biopsy samples [5,6]. In our pilot studies we noted the unusual preponderance of the rare microaerophilic Gram negative bacterium *Sutterella wadsworthensis* from cultures of biopsy samples from patients with IBD. This unusual organism has been encountered before by Mangin *et al.* who used 16S rRNA gene sequencing to create molecular inventories of the dominant fecal bacteria in four CD patients and four controls. They found that bacterial species which were not commonly dominant in healthy individuals were over-represented in CD. One of these species included *S. wadsworthensis*, which belonged to the dominant microbiota of one of the four CD patients [7].

These bacteria were first reported when performing biochemical characterization and susceptibility testing of *Campylobacter gracilis* clinical isolates from patients with diverse infections of the GI tract [8]. These organisms could be differentiated from *C. gracilis* mainly by their bile resistance and cell wall fatty acid patterns. 16S rRNA gene sequencing confirmed that these unusual organisms were not related phylogenetically to any of the *Campylobacters*, including *C. gracilis*, with the closest taxa belonging to unrelated aerobes. This was ratified by a subsequent report which demonstrated that the majority of *S. wadsworthensis* strains were isolated from GI infections, only occasionally being isolated from non-abdominal specimens, and were more likely to be involved in serious infections than *C. gracilis* [9]. The supposition was that *S. wadsworthensis* was a putative human pathogen. Three other species, *Sutterella stercoricanis*, *Sutterella morbirenis* and *Sutterella parvirubra* belonging to the same genera have subsequently been identified from canine and human feces [10,11].

The role of this group of bacteria has not been clearly elucidated in the aetiopathogenesis of IBD. This study has for the first time outlined the role of *S. wadsworthensis* in patients with IBD and performed a comprehensive phenotypic, genotypic, proteomic and pathogenetic characterization of this bacterial species, which will serve as a useful benchmark for future studies.

Methods

Study subjects, specimen collection and processing

Adult patients were recruited from the Department of Gastroenterology at the Aberdeen Royal Infirmary. These subjects were recruited for a previous study looking at the role of enterohepatic *Helicobacter* in UC [5]. A total of sixty-nine patients with a diagnosis of UC made on the basis of histology of colonoscopic biopsies were recruited and assessed. Sixty-five healthy controls were contacted prior to their index colonoscopy as part of the bowel cancer screening programme and recruited for the study if they had documented absence of both macroscopic and microscopic inflammation. Children were recruited from the Departments of Paediatric Gastroenterology, Hepatology and Nutrition at the Royal Aberdeen Children's Hospital and the Royal Hospital for Sick Children (Yorkhill), Glasgow as part of an ongoing study to investigate the role of microaerophilic colonic microbiota in *de-novo* paediatric IBD (Bacteria in Inflammatory bowel disease in Scottish Children Undergoing Investigation before Treatment: BISCUIT study). Twenty-nine paediatric patients with newly-presenting, treatment naïve IBD and thirty-two paediatric controls undergoing routine colonoscopy were included in this present study [12]. The extent and severity of disease was assigned using the Montreal criteria [13]. Subjects were excluded if they received antibiotics within three months prior to recruitment. Mucosal colonic biopsies were obtained during the colonoscopy procedures. One to two biopsies were used for culture work and the rest were then transferred to a −80°C freezer for storage pending DNA extraction and analysis.

Ethics

Ethical approval for the study was granted by the North of Scotland Research Ethics Service, UK (reference numbers 04/S0802/8 and 09/S0802/24). Written informed consent was obtained from all adult subjects and from the parents of all paediatric subjects in the study. Informed assent was also obtained from older children who were deemed capable of understanding the nature of the study.

Bacterial strains

Sutterella wadsworthensis strains. A total of twenty-seven *S. wadsworthensis* strains were used in this study. The type strain, DSM 14016 (=ATCC 51579) was obtained from the German Collection of Microorganisms and Cell Cultures (DSMZ). Another twenty-six *S. wadsworthensis* strains obtained during the course of this study were also examined.

Other bacterial strains. Twenty-eight other bacterial strains were used in this study, obtained from international culture collections as well as from clinical and environmental sources: *Campylobacter jejuni* (NCTC 11351), *Campylobacter upsaliensis* (NCTC 11540), *Campylobacter fetus* (NCTC 10842), *Campylobacter lari* (NCTC 11352), *Campylobacter coli* (clinical isolate), *Campylobacter concisus* (clinical isolate), *Helicobacter pylori* (ATCC 700392), *Helicobacter hepaticus* (ATCC 51449), *Helicobacter cholecystitis* (ATCC 700242), *Helicobacter canis* (ATCC 51402), *Helicobacter canadensis* (ATCC 700968), *Escherichia coli* (NCIMB 12201), Pseudomonas *fluorescences* (clinical isolate), *Pseudomonas aeruginosa* (ATCC 27853), *Shigella sonnei* (25931 clinical isolate), *Proteus mirabilis* (NCTC 3177), *Proteus vulgaris* (NCTC 4157), *Salmonella enteritidis* (NCTC 12694), *Salmonella typhimurium* (NCIMB 13284), *Staphylococus aureus* (NCIMB 12702), *Bacillus cereus* (ATCC 10876), *Enterococcus faecalis* (NCIMB 13280), *Enterobacter aerogenes* (NCIMB 10102), *Listeria monocytogenes* (clinical isolate), *Fusobacterium nucleotum* (clinical isolate), *Klebsiella pneumonia* (NCIMB 13281), *Acinetobacter calcoaceticus* (clinical isolate), *Yersinia fredericksenii* (NCIMB 2124), and *Aeromonas caviae* (clinical isolate).

Sutterella wadsworthensis growth conditions

S. wadsworthensis isolates were obtained by culturing 1–2 mucosal biopsy samples on five selective plates, the details of which are listed in Table 1. Biopsies were first ground in brucella broth before the resultant suspension was added to the plates. 50 μl was added to each plate with the exception of the filtered blood plate where 200 μl was first passed through a 0.45 μm filter. Cultures were incubated in a micro-aerophilic atmosphere, comprising of 5.9% oxygen, 7.2% carbon dioxide, 3.6% hydrogen and 83.3% nitrogen at 37°C. This atmosphere was generated using Anoxomat® Atmosphere Generating System, from Mart® Microbiology b.v. (9200 JB Drachten, Netherlands). Plates were reviewed twice weekly for up to one month. Any bacterial isolate deemed Gram-negative and oxygen sensitive (by virtue of failed subculture in room air) was identified by sequencing of the 16S rRNA gene and sequence search on NCBI BLAST (http://blast.ncbi.nlm.nih.gov/Blast.cgi).

Genotypic Characterization

DNA Extraction. Genomic DNA was extracted from the colonic mucosal biopsies using the QIAamp DNA Mini Kit (Qiagen, Crawley, UK) according to an established modification of the manufacturer's instructions, optimised in-house for colonic biopsy tissue as described previously [5].

S. wadsworthensis specific primer design. For the design of a new *S. wadsworthensis* -specific primer, 16S rRNA gene sequences of all the *S. wadsworthensis* strains and other related bacterial strains were obtained from the NCBI database (http://www.ncbi.nlm.nih.gov) for multiple alignment. Nearly full length 16S rRNA sequences of *S. wadsworthensis* strains isolated from clinical specimens in this study were also used for the alignment analysis. Several primer sequences were initially designed by using

Table 1. Culture media used in the study.

Media Name	Base	Additives	Volume of biopsy suspension added	Reference
Blood agar	Blood Agar	Nil	50μmol	-
Blood Agar	Blood Agar	Nil	200μmol through 0.45μm filter	-
Skirrow	Blood Agar	Polymyxin B, Trimethoprim, Vancomycin	50μmol	[27]
CVA	Blood Agar	Amphotericin, Cefoperazone, Vancomycin	50μmol	[28]
Helicobacter	Blood Agar	Amphotericin, Bacitracin, Nalidixic acid, Polymyxin B, Vancomycin	50μmol	[29]
Campylobacte	Blood Agar	Trimethoprim, Vancomycin	50μmol	[30]

the Primer 3 software [14] and then the most suitable one was identified manually using the BioEdit software package (version 7.0.5.3) (http://www.mbio.ncsu.edu/BioEdit/bioedit.html). The downloaded *S. wadsworthensis* specific sequences were aligned with the newly designed primer sequences and the ones that matched to the highly conserved 16S rRNA gene sequences of the target species but were variable among the other bacterial species, were selected. The 20 base pair *S. wadsworthensis* specific primer sequences designed (SWF and SWR) are outlined in Table 2. The primer sequences were then subjected to BLAST analysis against all the other sequences within the BLAST database to ensure that at least one of the primers did not share any identical sequence with any microorganisms other than S. *wadsworthensis*.

Optimization of *S. wadsworthensis* PCR assay. The specificity of the newly developed *S. wadsworthensis* primer pair was tested against a wide panel of bacterial species as listed earlier in the methods section. The PCR assay was tested using 40 ng of bacterial DNA in a 50 μl reaction mixture consisting of 10 pmol of each primer (SWF and SWR [Sigma-Aldrich, UK]), 1X PCR buffer (Roche, UK), 250 nM of each deoxy-nucleotide-triphosphate (Bioline, UK), 2 mM $MgCl_2$ (Roche, UK) and 1 U of Taq polymerase (Roche,UK). The sensitivity of the PCR assay was determined by serially diluting a known quantity of target DNA (50 ng/μl to 0.005 pg/ μl) to detect the minimum concentration that would yield a visible amplicon after gel electrophoresis.

Restriction fragment length polymorphism (RFLP) analysis was also done using the 555 bp *S. wadsworthensis*-specific PCR products using *EcoR* I and *Hha* I enymes to confirm that the PCR products were from a single bacterial species.

Sequence Analysis. Sequencing was done on an Applied Biosystems model 3730 automated capillary DNA sequencer using the *S. wadsworthensis* - specific primers SWF and SWR or 16S rRNA specific universal bacterial primers for the whole gene amplification of the *S. wadsworthensis* strains. The sequences obtained were compared to those of the National Center for Biotechnology Information GenBank database using the basic local alignment search tool (BLAST) search program. Multiple alignments and

phylogenetic analysis were performed using Bioedit (http://www.mbio.ncsu.edu/BioEdit/bioedit.html) (version 7.0.5.3) and a dendogram was constructed using MEGA version 4 software [15]. The evolutionary distances were calculated according to Kimura's two-parameter model. A phylogenetic tree was inferred using the neighbor-joining algorithm, and the tree topology was statistically evaluated by 1,000 bootstrap resamplings.

GenBank Sequence Submission. All 16S rRNA gene sequences derived from the sequencing of *S. wadsworthensis*-specific PCR products were submitted to GenBank with the accession numbers from JN664092-JN664117.

Phenotypic Characterization

Basic biochemical tests including Gram staining, catalase, urease and oxidase tests were conducted using conventional manual methods to characterize the isolates. The strains were further characterized using the API Campy commercial biochemical kit according to the manufacturer's instructions (BioMerieux, La Balme Les Grottes, France). The purpose of using the API kits in this study was not to identify or name the bacteria, but to use the biochemical tests to further characterize the *S. wadsworthensis* strains. By comparing the resultant biochemical profiles, any potential differences between the strains might be elicited. Of all the API kits available it was assumed that API Campy would yield the best results, as *S. wadsworthensis* is phenotypically similar to *Campylobacter* species.

Scanning Electron Microscopy (SEM)

S. wadsworthensis strains were harvested for SEM. Bacterial cells were suspended in 2% Glutaraldehyde in 0.1 M sodium Cacodylate buffer (pH 7.2) for 3 hours to be fixed. The fixed cell suspensions were then applied to glass coverslips coated with poly-L-lysine and allowed to adhere for five minutes. Coverslips were then rinsed with water and post-fixed with 1% Osmium tetroxide (OsO4) for 30 minutes. They were next rinsed with water and dehydrated through a graded ethanol series (60%, 80%, and 90%) for 10 minutes each. The sample was then left for 30 minutes in absolute ethanol with ethanol changes every 10 minutes. The coverslips were kept in Hexamethyldisilazane (HMDS) Sigma® for 10 minutes, and left to dry overnight. Next day, the specimen was coated with gold using automated sputter coater EMITECH K550 (Emitech limited, Ashford, Kent) and samples were transferred to view *S. wadsworthensis* using SEM.

Proteomic Characterization

To complement the phenotypic and genotypic methods, matrix-associated laser desorption/ionisation - time of flight mass

Table 2. Sequences of PCR primers designed in this study.

Primer name	Sequence	Reference
SWF	5'- GAC GAA AAG GGA TGC GAT AA - 3'	This study
SWR	5'- CTG GCA TGT CAA GGC TAG GT- 3'	This study

spectrometry (MALDI-TOF MS) was performed to further characterize selected *S. wadsworthensis* strains.

Sample preparation. A total of 11 bacterial strains were analyzed by MALDI-TOF MS: eight *S. wadsworthensis* isolates (4 strains obtained from healthy controls and 4 strains from IBD patients), the *S. wadsworthensis* type strain DSM 14016, *C. jejuni* and *C. concisus* strains. Approximately 5-10 mg (half a plastic loop) of bacterial cells were harvested from fresh blood agar plates and proteins were extracted as described by Alispahic *et al.* (2010) [16]. The protein extract (supernatant) was diluted, with 30% acetonitrile in 0.1% trifluoracetic acid (Applied Biosystems, UK) in water. Subsequently, 1 μl of diluted supernatant was mixed with 1 μl of matrix solution (10 mg HCCA (α-cyano-4-hydroxycinnamic acid) matrix (Bruker Daltonics, Germany) to 1 ml of a solution comprising: 500 μl acetonitrile, 475 μl UHQ water and 25 μl trifluoroacetic acid). 1 μl of the sample-matrix mixture was pipetted onto a MALDI ground steel target plate (Bruker Daltonics) and left to dry on air.

MALDI-TOF MS. Mass spectra were acquired using an ultrafleXtreme™ series MALDI-TOF MS (Bruker Daltonics), equipped with a 1 kHz smartbeam-II™ nitrogen laser (λ = 337 nm). Spectra were recorded using the linear positive mode for masses in the range of 2 kDa to 20 kDa. The parameter settings were as follows: ion source 1, 25 kV; ion source 2, 23.85 kV; lens, 6.5 kV; pulse ion extraction time, 160 ns. A low-mass gate of 800 Da was used. Insulin, ubiquitin, cytochrome C and myoglobin were used as external calibrants, enabling a mass accuracy of ±0.5 parts per 1000. Laser power and the number of laser shots per sample were varied by the operator for optimal performance.

Data analysis. Mass spectra were processed prior to visual inspection using FlexAnalysis 3.3 software (Bruker Daltonics). This included smoothing, baseline subtraction and intensity normalisation. MALDI BioTyper software 2.0 (Bruker Daltonics) was used to generate pseudo gel view representations of each spectrum. The mass spectra and corresponding pseudo gel images for each bacterial strain were then visually inspected and compared.

Preparation of monocytes and *S. wadsworthensis* (whole cell) stimulation studies

Whole venous blood was collected from six adult healthy individuals who were not on any medications. The blood was diluted 1:1 in RPMI 1640 (Sigma-Aldrich), layered onto Histopaque-1077 (Sigma-Aldrich), and centrifuged at 800×g for 30 min. Peripheral blood mononuclear cells were removed from the interface and monocytes were prepared as published earlier [17]. The effect of *S. wadsworthensis* whole cell preparations was assessed by stimulating the monocytes for up to 24 hours. Seven *S. wadsworthensis* strains (4 strains obtained from healthy controls and 3 strains from IBD patients) were used in this study along with an *E. coli* (S1041) as a positive control. Unstimulated monocytes were used as a negative control.

Cytometric bead array

In order to assess whether the whole cell preparations induced an inflammatory response, levels of TNF-α in culture supernatant were measured at the different time points using a human inflammatory cytokine cytometric bead array (CBA;BD Biosciences). Samples were analyzed on a multifluorescence BD FACSCalibur™ flow cytometer using BD CellQuest™ software and BD™ cytometric bead array software. Standard curves were generated using FCAP Array Software™. Sample results were then calculated by comparing sample CBA results to the respective

standard curve. All CBA work was performed in duplicate and cytokine levels induced by stimulation were calculated by subtracting unstimulated cytokine levels from each stimulated value and expressing TNF-α levels as a fold-change relative to TNF-α levels derived from *E. coli* stimulations.

Statistical Analysis

Statistical analysis was performed using the Pearson Chi Squared, 2-tailed test or the Fisher's exact test wherever appropriate, utilizing Graph Pad software (San Diego, CA).

Results

Assessment of *S. wadsworthensis* prevalence in mucosal colonic biopsies

Clinical information of the study population. The mean age of the sixty-nine patients with UC was 45.6±27.8 years and 46.4% were male as opposed to the sixty-five control patients whose mean age was 64.2±5.6 years and 59.3% of these subjects were male. There was a statistically significant difference in age between the UC cohort and the control group (p<0.0001). At the time of colonoscopy the adult patients were classified as extensive (24.6%), left sided (63.8%) and proctitis (11.6%) according to the Montreal criteria. During recruitment 10.1% of patients were in clinical remission (S0), 23.2% had mild UC (S1), 46.4% had moderate UC (S2) and the remaining 20.3% had severe UC (S3). A total of 115 biopsy sites were analyzed from UC patients. Twenty-four (34.8%) subjects had a single site analyzed and forty-five (65.2%) had more than one biopsy site assessed. A single biopsy site was analyzed from each control subject. The adult patients served as clinical sources for the isolation of *S. wadsworthensis*. The newly developed PCR was utilized to detect the presence of *S. wadsworthensis* from mucosal biopsies from these patients.

The paediatric IBD patients (n = 29, male 62.1%) had a median age of 12.2 years (interquartile range, IQR, 9.8, 14.1 years) at the time of recruitment out of which fifteen had CD, nine UC and five IBD-unclassified. The paediatric control patients (n = 32, male 78.1%) had a mean age of 10.8 years (IQR, 8.3, 12.7 years) at the time of index colonoscopy. The paediatric cohort was primarily utilized as a source for isolation of *S. wadsworthensis*, which was then utilized to develop and standardize the detection PCR.

A total of twenty-six *S. wadsworthensis* strains were isolated from the mucosal colonic biopsy samples of the above mentioned study populations. The majority of the clinical strains were obtained from paediatric patients, ten from control and seven from IBD patients. Six strains were obtained from adult IBD patients and three from adult control patients.

Evaluation of the sensitivity and specificity of the newly developed *S. wadsworthensis* -specific PCR assay. Twenty-seven strains of *S. wadsworthensis* and twenty-eight other bacterial strains representing a broad spectrum of bacterial species were screened to test for the specificity of the newly designed species-specific primers. The primer pair produced an intense band of ≈555 bp from all the *S. wadsworthensis* strains (Figure 1). No amplicon was observed from any of the other bacterial strains tested. For detection of *S. wadsworthensis* DNA from mucosal biopsy samples a nested PCR approach was taken where the first round PCR was done using universal bacterial primers (27F and 1492R) [18] followed by a second round of PCR using the *S. wadsworthensis*–specific SWF and SWR primers. The optimal thermal cycling conditions required to obtain specificity for the *S. wadsworthensis*-specific PCR were: 94°C for 5 minutes, 30 cycles of 94°C for 30 seconds, 58°C for 30 seconds, and 72°C for 2

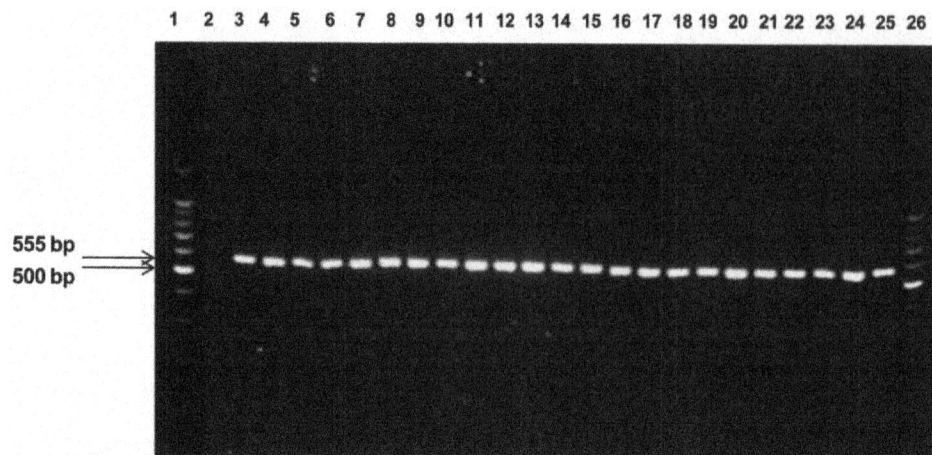

Figure 1. Amplification of *S. wadsworthensis* DNA from reference and clinical strains using the SW-F and SW-R primers. The assay amplified a product of ≈555 bp in size. Lane 1:100 bp marker, Lane 2: negative control (no DNA), Lane 3: *S. wadsworthensis* DSM 14016, Lane 4 – Lane 25: *S. wadsworthensis* isolate SW1, SW2, SW4, SW5, SW6, SW7, SW8, SW9, SW10, SW11, SW12, SW13, SW14, SW15, SW16, SW17, SW18, SW19, SW20, SW21, SW22, SW23, Lane 26:100 bp marker.

minutes, followed by 72°C for 15 minutes. The optimized PCR was able to detect 0.5 pg/μl of *S. wadsworthensis* DNA (Figure 2).

The RFLP analysis of all the *S. wadsworthensis*–specific PCR products also showed the expected banding pattern of 327 bp and 228 bp for *EcoR* 1 digestion and 420 bp and 135 bp for *Hha* I digestion respectively.

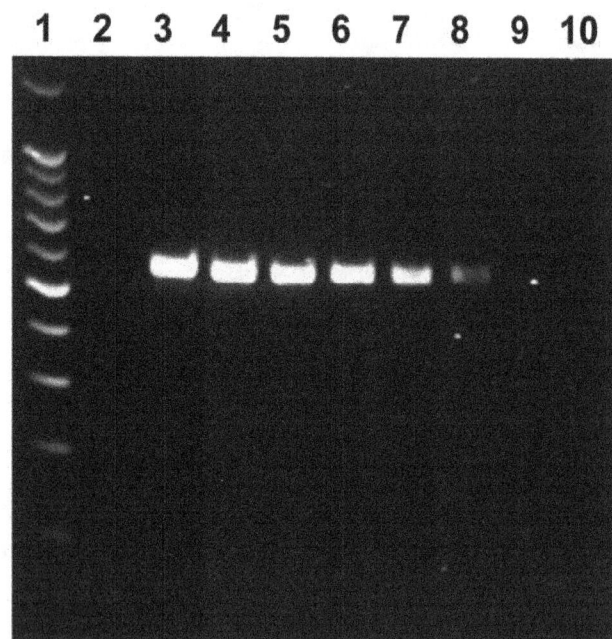

Figure 2. Limit of detection for the newly developed *S. wadsworthensis*-specific nested PCR assay. The PCR assay was able to detect 0.5 pg of *S. wadsworthensis* DNA. Lane 1: 100 bp marker, Lane 2: negative control (no DNA), Lane 3: *S. wadsworthensis* DNA 50 ng/μl, Lane 4: *S. wadsworthensis* DNA 5 ng/μl, Lane 5: *S. wadsworthensis* DNA 0.5 ng/μl, Lane 6: *S. wadsworthensis* DNA 50 pg/μl, Lane 7:*S. wadsworthensis* DNA 5 pg/μl, Lane 8: *S. wadsworthensis* DNA 0.5 pg/μl, Lane 9: *S. wadsworthensis* DNA 0.05 pg/μl, Lane 10: *S. wadsworthensis* DNA 0.005 pg/μl.

Prevalence of *S. wadsworthensis* in adults with UC using species-specific PCR. All the adult mucosal biopsy samples were screened using the newly developed and optimized *S. wadsworthensis*-specific PCR. *S. wadsworthensis* was detected in fifty-seven of the sixty-nine subjects with ulcerative colitis and fifty-six of the sixty-five controls. The prevalence of *S. wadsworthensis* in the UC population was 83.8% which was similar to that in the controls, 86.1% (p = 0.64). There was no statistically-significant difference in the prevalence of *S. wadsworthensis* in male subjects as opposed to female patients. Furthermore, no age related differences could be demonstrated. Looking specifically at patients with UC, no statistically-significant differences were noted in the prevalence of *S. wadsworthensis* with respect to extent or severity of UC according to the Montreal classification.

Phylogenetic Analysis. A phylogenetic tree was constructed based on nearly full-length (~1400 bp) 16S rRNA gene sequences of the *S. wadsworthensis* strains isolated from this study and sequences of *S. wadsworthensis* strains and other *Sutterella* species available in GenBank (Figure 3). All the *S. wadsworthensis* sequences derived from this study clustered closely with the other *S. wadsworthensis* sequences from GenBank and presented the highest (99–100%) sequence identity to the *S. wadsworthensis* type strain ATCC 51579. The *S. wadsworthensis* strains from different geographical locations (strain ATCC 51579, strain WAL 7877 and strain WAL 9054 originating from USA and the strains from this study being from the UK) did not cluster into different lineages. Also, *S. wadsworthensis* sequences analyzed from the UC and the healthy controls did not cluster into separate groups in the dendrogram. The GenBank derived sequences from the *S. parvirubra*, *S. stercoricanis* and *S. morbirenis* strains each grouped into different clusters in the dendrogram confirming different species.

Characterization of *S. wadsworthensis* isolates to detect strain difference

As the PCR results revealed almost universal prevalence of *S. wadsworthensis* in both IBD cases and controls, we hypothesised that there may be differences between the strains isolated from the two groups and so went on to study their phenotypic, morphological, proteomic and pathogenic profiles.

Phenotypic Characterization. *S. wadsworthensis* was found to be a Gram-negative pleomorphic rod shaped organism with

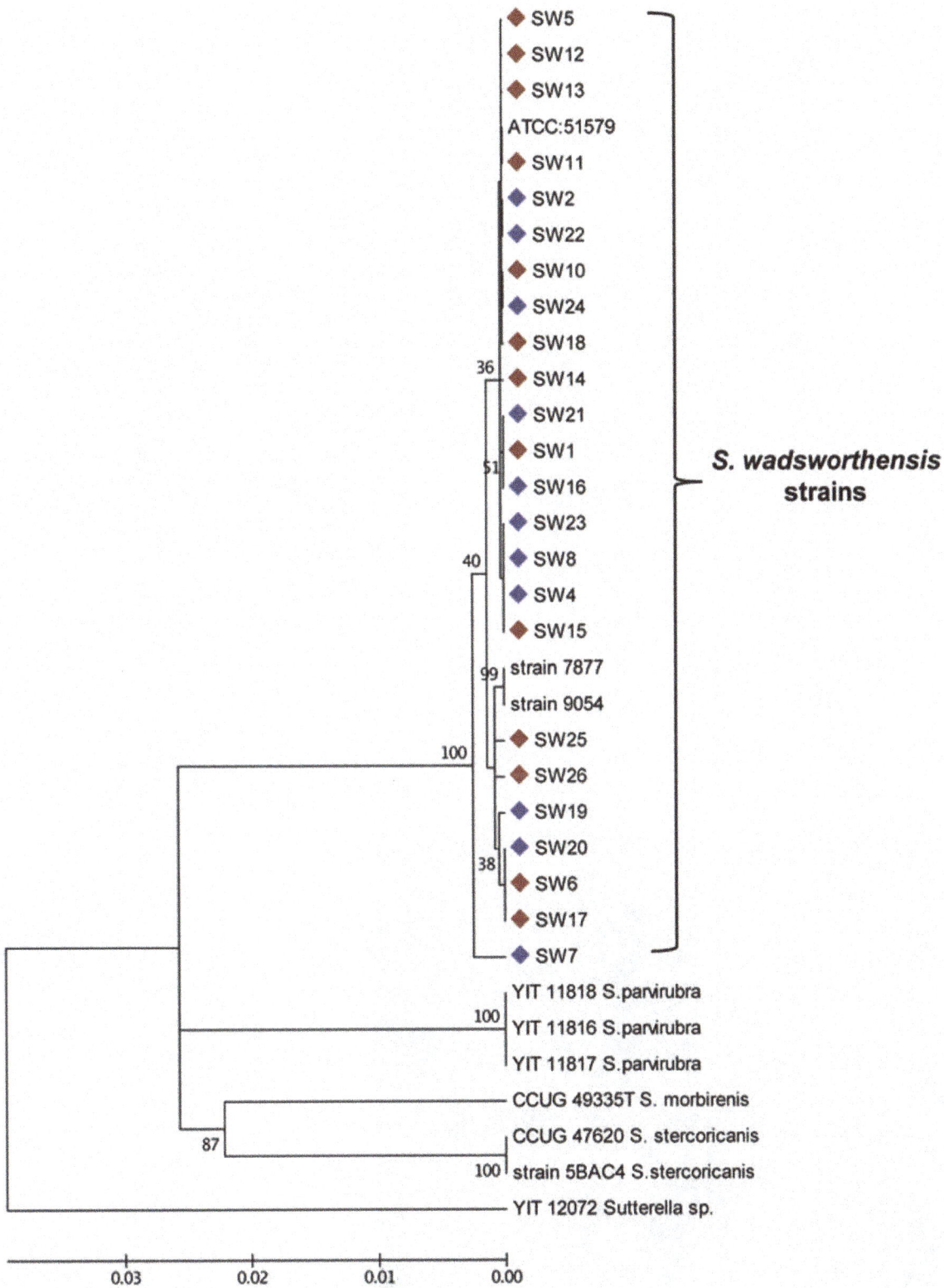

Figure 3. Phylogenetic tree constructed using nearly full-length (~1400 bp) sequences of the 16S rRNA gene of *S. wadsworthensis* strains from UC and controls alongside other *Sutterella* sequences available in GenBank. The evolutionary history was inferred using the Neighbor-Joining method. The percentage of replicate trees in which the associated taxa clustered together in the bootstrap test (1000 replicates) are shown next to the branches. The tree is drawn to scale, with branch lengths in the same units as those of the evolutionary distances used to infer the phylogenetic tree. The *S. wadsworthenis* isolates from IBD cases are marked in red and those from controls are marked in blue.

different morphological structures seen on Gram stain, even though the *S. wadsworthensis* cultures were pure. All *S. wadsworthensis* strains tested negative for catalase, urease and oxidase tests. The API Campy kit results showed that all the *S. wadsworthensis* strains tested (9 clinical isolates and the type strain) were positive for the EST, ArgA and AspA tests, indicating they possess the enzymes esterase, L-arginine arylamidase and L-aspartate arylamidase respectively. The only discrepant result between the *S. wadsworthensis* strains was for the HIP test; four strains, including the type strain, tested positive and six strains were found to be negative. This tested the ability of the bacteria to hydrolyse sodium hippurate. A positive result indicated the presence of the enzyme hippurate hydrolase. All the assimilation tests on the second half of the strips were negative for all *S. wadsworthensis* strains.

SEM. Under conventional light microscopy, there were clearly two different morphologies for *S. wadsworthensis*. For this reason, an intensive literature search for *S. wadsworthensis* electron micrographs was done. However, there were no published electron micrograph images available to answer the morphology question. Due to this, two *S. wadsworthensis* strains (SW9 from control and SW13 from IBD) were selected for SEM. The SEM images clearly indicated lattice formation (Figure 4A) and two distinct morphologies of this bacterium: a long rod (nearly 4µm) and a short cocco-bacillus (nearly 1µm) (Figure 4B). Interestingly, there were also cells with filamentous shape (Figure 4C) and a helical form was also observed (Figure 4D).

MALDI-TOF MS. Matrix-associated laser desorption/ ionization – time of flight mass spectrometry (MALDI-TOF MS) is a well-established technique in proteomics for the analysis of proteins and peptides. Profiling of proteins by MALDI-TOF MS has been developed as a rapid and sensitive technique for microorganism identification [16]. In the MALDI Biotyper system developed by Bruker Daltonics, MALDI-TOF mass

spectra of small proteins (range 2–20 kDa) acquired directly from smears of cells or their extracts are compared with reference spectra in the MALDI Biotyper database. The most recent MALDI Biotyper 2.0 database available (version 3.1.2, dated 28 January 2011, containing reference spectra for 3740 microorganisms) did not contain any information on *S. wadsworthensis*. The purpose of MALDI-TOF MS in this study, as with the API testing kit, was not to identify the bacterial strains but to further characterize them and elicit any differences between them.

Out of the eleven strains tested, triplicate samples of the first six bacterial strains analyzed by MALDI-TOF MS were analyzed to assess how reproducible the method was. All three replicates for these six strains produced almost identical results, so it was decided that obtaining a single mass spectrum for each of the remaining five strains would be sufficient. The remaining five strains were analyzed and the mass spectra for all 11 strains were obtained. It was immediately apparent that there was a characteristic *S. wadsworthensis* pattern that all of the strains conformed to (Figure 5A). Notably there was a dominant peak at approximately 9400Da which was common to all *S. wadsworthensis* strains (Figure 5B). The *Campylobacter* strains on the other hand, produced different patterns of peaks, with *C. jejuni* producing a dominant double peak at approximately 9500Da and 10300Da (data not shown).

Monocyte challenge. A human monocyte challenge system was used to assess the immunogenicity of different *S. wadsworthensis* strains. A survival test was performed to examine the ability of *S. wadsworthensis* strains to survive when exposed to the oxygen present in the monocyte stimulation experimental setup. This showed that >50% of *S. wadsworthensis* cells survived for four hours. Seven *S. wadsworthensis* strains and an *E. coli* strain were inoculated onto monocytes that were obtained from six healthy

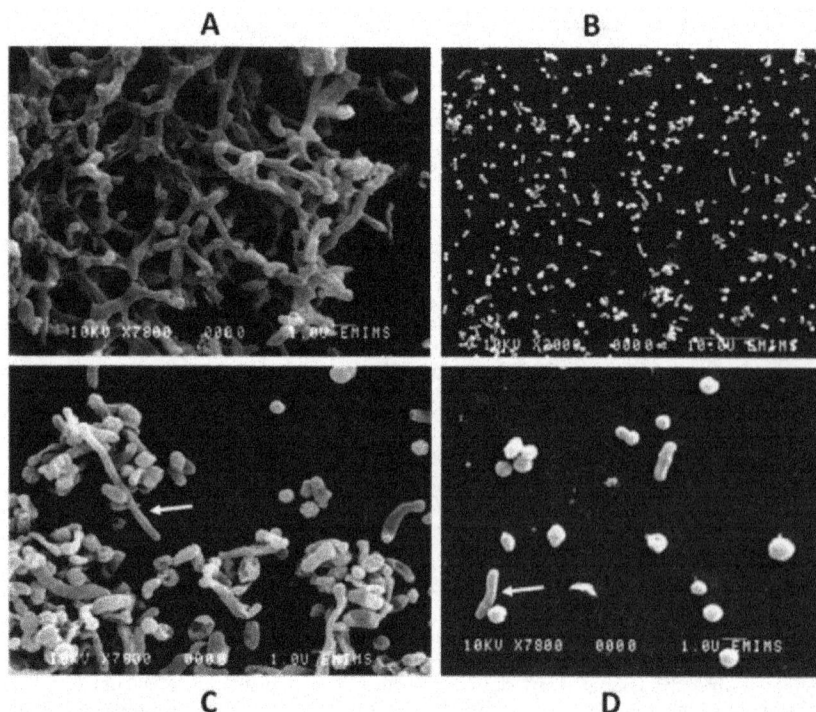

Figure 4. Scanning electron microscopy (SEM) images of *S. wadsworthensis* showing different morphologies for this organism. Small and large, filamentous and helical bacteria forms were observed. A) *S. wadsworthensis* cells formed as a lattice B) Different *Sutterella* cell morphologies C) Filamentous bacterial form D) Helical bacterial form.

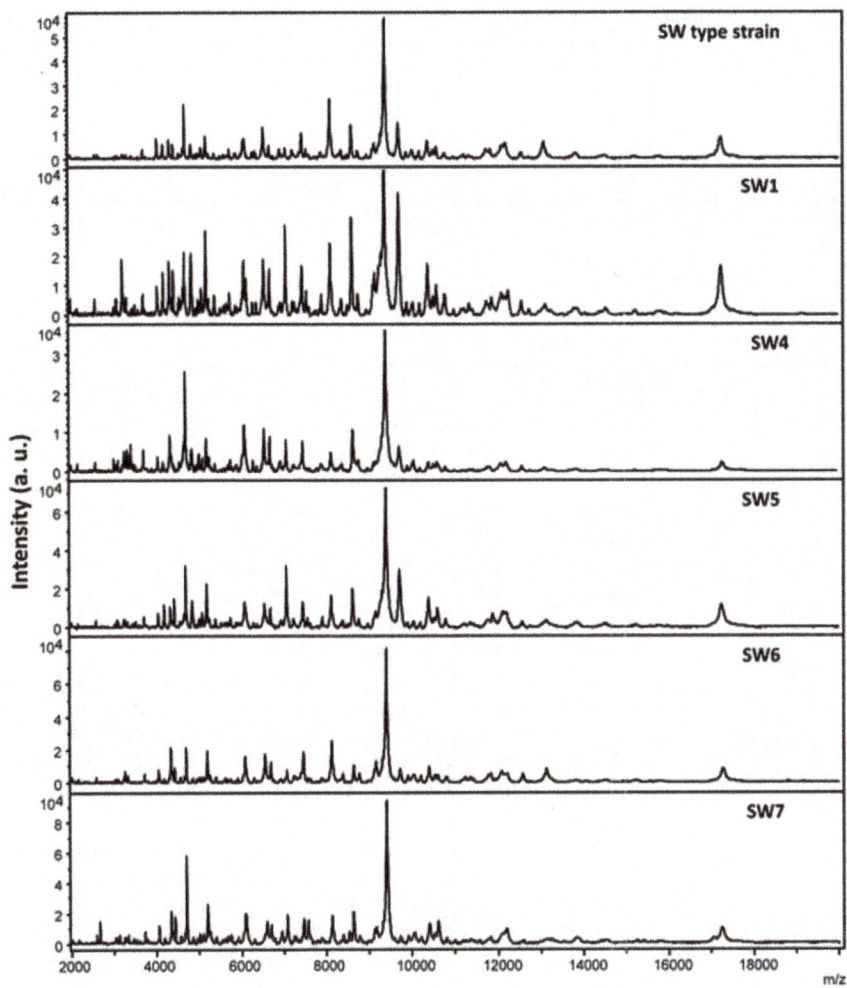

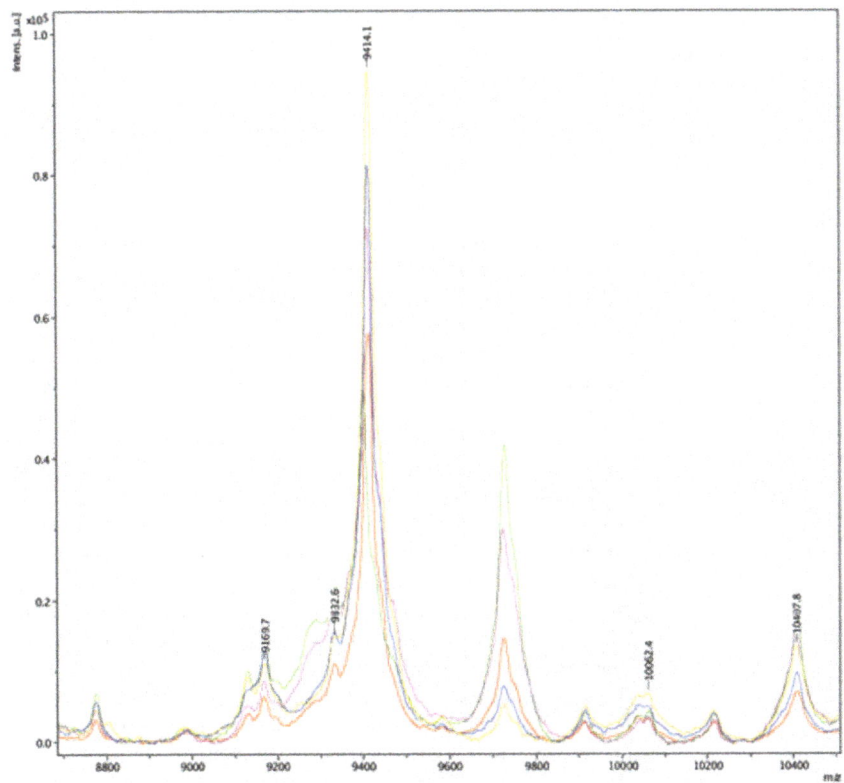

Figure 5. Mass spectra obtained for *S. wadsworthensis* strains. (A) Spectra obtained for 6 *S. wadsworthensis* strains: *S. wadsworthensis* type strain, SW1, SW4, SW5, SW6 and SW7. All of the *S. wadsworthensis* strains conform to a common pattern. a.u. arbitrary unit; m/z, mass-to-charge ratio; Da, Daltons; (B) Overlaid spectra of five *S. wadsworthensis* strains overlaid. This is a close-up of the mass spectra from 8,700 Da to 10,500 Da. It shows how closely each *S. wadsworthensis* mass spectrum, aside from intensity, matches the others. a.u., arbitrary unit; m/z, mass-to-charge ratio; Da, daltons.

volunteers. Levels of TNF-α were measured at 4 hours of stimulation. All *S. wadsworthensis* strains induced TNF-α cytokine production from the human monocytes. Compared to the *E. coli* strain used *S. wadsworthensis* strains induced higher levels of TNF-α production over the first 4 hours although subsequent measurements at 24 hours indicated that TNF-α levels remained detectable in *E. coli* stimulated monocytes but that TNF-α was not detectable in *S. wadsworthensis* stimulated wells, most likely because of the death of *S. wadsworthensis* organisms (Table 3).

Discussion

The role of *S. wadsworthensis* in human gastrointestinal diseases has been documented in the past but its specific involvement in inflammatory bowel disease has never been firmly established [8,9]. The fortuitous isolation of this unusual bacterial strain from mucosal biopsies of patients with IBD prompted a series of experiments that have been outlined in this paper and has culminated in detailed characterization of this putative pathogen. Despite this detailed microbial analysis no specific differences have been identified between cases and controls. However, this negative result does not preclude the importance of successful isolation of this fastidious organism from colonic biopsy samples by adhering to a strict microaerophilic culture environment and stringent growth conditions. Our study provides an important proof of concept that will enable future studies to satisfy Koch's postulates to tie in other luminal microaerophilic bacteria as causative factors in IBD.

This is the first report of the appearances of this bacterial species under scanning electron microscopy (SEM). As opposed to previous descriptions, the bacteria are pleomorphic, with strains existing in predominantly two morphological forms, long rods and coccobacilli. Filamentous and helical forms were also documented. The bacteria appeared in clusters on Gram stain and this was further corroborated with the appearance of a lattice type network on SEM. The functional role of this lattice formation is unclear, but given the high prevalence of this organism that we have demonstrated in the human colonic mucosa, further investigation of the interaction of *S. wadsworthensis* in the complex luminal

microbiota may be of interest. This lattice structural network may paradoxically harbour either commensal bacteria or pathogenic bacterial strains in close juxtaposition to the epithelial surface with diametrically opposite consequences.

All *S. wadsworthensis* strains were negative for urease, catalase and oxidase, consistent with the initial description by Wexler et al [8]. The authors had described *S. wadsworthensis* as asaccharolytic, and certainly none of the sugar assimilation tests from the API kit were found to be positive [8]. As *S. wadsworthensis* is phenotypically closely related to the *Campylobacter* genus, the API Campy kit, specifically for the identification of *Campylobacter* species was trialed. This yielded more promising results. All of the *S. wadsworthensis* strains tested were positive for the EST, ArgA and AspA tests, meaning they possessed the enzymes esterase, L-arginine arylamidase and L-aspartate arylamidase respectively. Esterases are often required to breakdown dietary residue and are mostly derived from the intestinal microbiota, with *E. coli*, *Bifidobacterium* and *Lactobacillus* species all known to be sources [19]. Colonic esterases have been shown to release powerful antioxidants, present in cereal bran, from complex ester-linked structures which could otherwise not be absorbed [20]. It is possible that the esterases produced by *S. wadsworthensis* have a similar role.

This study utilized a newly developed PCR to detect the presence of *S. wadsworthensis* in a subset of adult patients with UC and adult control patients. The rates of detection was similar in both these groups (83.8% vs. 86.1%, $p = 0.64$), suggesting that this bacterial strain is probably a commensal. The only other study that has looked at the prevalence of this pathogen in patients with gastrointestinal disease was by Engberg et al. who used PCR and DNA sequencing of the 16S rRNA gene to characterize bacterial populations in fecal samples [21]. They detected *S. wadsworthensis* in only 7 out of 1483 (0.47%) patients with GI disorders, and only 1 out of 107 (0.93%) healthy individuals. This wide disparity in prevalence between this study and our cohort of patients and controls suggests that *S. wadsworthensis* is closely adherent to the mucosal lining and is more likely to be identified from biopsy samples as opposed to feces. Additionally, this newly designed PCR for this bacterial strain was validated using the type strain of *S. wadsworthensis* as well as several related bacterial strains and will form a useful tool in future studies.

Despite similar rates of detection of *S. wadsworthensis* from patients with IBD and controls, our clinical isolates gave us an excellent opportunity to further characterize this organism. Several bacterial species have been noted to have distinctly different phenotypic and genotypic profiles when isolated from patients with clinical disease as opposed to controls. This has been recently documented in *Campylobacter concisus* and mucosa associated *E. coli* wherein distinct genomospecies have been documented with varying pathogenic potential [22,23]. Sequence analysis of strains identified during the study from cases and controls did not cluster in distinct groups confirming that this phenomenon does not extend to *S. wadsworthensis*.

Proteomic analysis of *S. wadsworthensis* strains utilizing MALDI-TOF MS is being reported for the first time in this paper. MALDI-TOF MS has recently emerged as an alternative to phenotypic and genotypic methods for the fast and reliable identification of

Table 3. TNF-α levels (depicted as percentage) derived from human monocytes (N = 6) exposed to whole cell preparations of various *S. wadsworthensis* strains.

	SW1	SW2	SW3	SW7	SW8	SW9	SW13
Volunteer A	3	407	62	43	64	92	128
Volunteer B	0	651	184	108	200	178	NT
Volunteer C	17	120	908	125	120	120	NT
Volunteer D	747	924	197	360	350	541	NT
Volunteer E	163	625	117	237	237	429	NT
Volunteer F	NT	NT	NT	NT	NT	NT	139

TNF-α production in the supernatant was determined after 4 hours of stimulation. The cytokine amounts shown are expressed as a percentage of the cytokine induction by whole cell *E. coli* preparations. NT = not tested.

microorganisms down to the species level [16,24,25,26]. It can be used to classify closely related bacteria, which may be indistinguishable by conventional methods [24]. It was therefore employed to investigate the diversity of the *S. wadsworthensis* protein profiles. A characteristic pattern was clearly demonstrated on the analysis of *S. wadsworthensis* strains, with a dominant peak at approximately 9400Da. Although no major differences were detected between the strains, MALDI-TOF MS proved to be a highly sensitive and reproducible method for the characterization of the bacterial mass spectra. Very small mass of sample were required, which was ideal for analyzing the slow and modest growing *S. wadsworthensis*. This finding will provide a useful reference for future studies and an alternative to genotypic methods like 16S rRNA gene sequencing.

The *in-vitro* cytokine analysis after monocyte challenge failed to show any distinct differences between strains isolated from patients with IBD and controls. This last finding essentially closes the loop in the series of studies looking at the possible role of *S. wadsworthensis* in IBD. Our experiments have conclusively shown that the prevalence of this bacterium is similar in IBD patients and controls and that there is no phenotypic, genotypic, proteomic or pathogenic characteristic to distinguish bacteria isolated from

these two groups of patients. It is quite likely that *S. wadsworthensis* is a commensal and a harmless bystander amidst the inflammatory cascade that is typical of inflammatory bowel disease.

Acknowledgments

We would like to thank all adult gastroenterologists (Aberdeen Royal Infirmary) and paediatric gastroenterologists (Royal Aberdeen Children's Hospital and Royal Hospital for Sick Children, Glasgow) for their assistance in recruiting patients to this study. We would also like to thank the patients, children and families who gave their time and consent to participate in this research.

We gratefully acknowledge the technical assistance of Mr Ian Davidson for help with MALDI-TOF MS and Mr Kevin MacKenzie for expertise in SEM. We also thank Bruker Daltonics for providing the MALDI BioTyper software.

Author Contributions

Conceived and designed the experiments: IM RH EME-O GLH. Performed the experiments: IM RH CEN YAA SHB CP DAS. Analyzed the data: IM RH JMT RKR GLH. Contributed reagents/materials/analysis tools: JMT RKR EME-O. Wrote the paper: IM RH GLH.

References

1. Hansen R, Thomson JM, El-Omar EM, Hold GL (2010) The role of infection in the aetiology of inflammatory bowel disease. J Gastroenterol 45: 266–276.

2. Khor B, Gardet A, Xavier RJ (2011) Genetics and pathogenesis of inflammatory bowel disease. Nature 474: 307–317.

3. Marteau P (2009) Bacterial flora in inflammatory bowel disease. Dig Dis 27(Suppl 1): 99–103.

4. Sokol H, Seksik P, Rigottier-Gois L, Lay C, Lepage P, et al. (2006) Specificities of the fecal microbiota in inflammatory bowel disease. Inflamm Bowel Dis 12: 106–111.

5. Thomson JM, Hansen R, Berry SH, Hope ME, Murray GI, et al. (2011) Enterohepatic helicobacter in ulcerative colitis: potential pathogenic entities? PLoS One 6: e17184.

6. Mukhopadhya I, Thomson JM, Hansen R, Berry SH, El-Omar EM, et al. (2011) Detection of Campylobacter concisus and Other Campylobacter Species in Colonic Biopsies from Adults with Ulcerative Colitis. PLoS One 6: e21490.

7. Mangin I, Bonnet R, Seksik P, Rigottier-Gois L, Sutren M, et al. (2004) Molecular inventory of faecal microflora in patients with Crohn's disease. FEMS Microbiol Ecol 50: 25–36.

8. Wexler HM, Reeves D, Summanen PH, Molitoris E, McTeague M, et al. (1996) Sutterella wadsworthensis gen. nov., sp. nov., bile-resistant microaerophilic Campylobacter gracilis-like clinical isolates. Int J Syst Bacteriol 46: 252–258.

9. Molitoris E, Wexler HM, Finegold SM (1997) Sources and antimicrobial susceptibilities of Campylobacter gracilis and Sutterella wadsworthensis. Clin Infect Dis 25(Suppl 2): S264–265.

10. Sakon H, Nagai F, Morotomi M, Tanaka R (2008) Sutterella parvirubra sp. nov. and Megamonas funiformis sp. nov., isolated from human faeces. Int J Syst Evol Microbiol 58: 970–975.

11. Greetham HL, Collins MD, Gibson GR, Giffard C, Falsen E, et al. (2004) Sutterella stercoricanis sp. nov., isolated from canine faeces. Int J Syst Evol Microbiol 54: 1581–1584.

12. Hansen R, Mukhopadhya I, Russell RK, Bisset WM, Berry SH, Thomson JM, El-Omar EM, Hold LG (2011) The role of microaerophilic colonic mucosal bacteria in de novo paediatric inflammatory bowel disease. Gut 60(Suppl 1): A147.

13. Silverberg MS, Satsangi J, Ahmad T, Arnott ID, Bernstein CN, et al. (2005) Toward an integrated clinical, molecular and serological classification of inflammatory bowel disease: Report of a Working Party of the 2005 Montreal World Congress of Gastroenterology. Can J Gastroenterol 19(Suppl A): 5–36.

14. Rozen S, Skaletsky H (2000) Primer3 on the WWW for general users and for biologist programmers. Methods Mol Biol 132: 365–386.

15. Kumar S, Tamura K, Nei M (2004) MEGA3: Integrated software for Molecular Evolutionary Genetics Analysis and sequence alignment. Brief Bioinform 5: 150–163.

16. Alispahic M, Hummel K, Jandreski-Cvetkovic D, Nobauer K, Razzazi-Fazeli E, et al. (2010) Species-specific identification and differentiation of Arcobacter, Helicobacter and Campylobacter by full-spectral matrix-associated laser

desorption/ionization time of flight mass spectrometry analysis. J Med Microbiol 59: 295–301.

17. Haag AF, Wehmeier S, Muszynski A, Kerscher B, Fletcher V, et al. (2011) Biochemical characterization of Sinorhizobium meliloti mutants reveals gene products involved in the biosynthesis of the unusual lipid A very long-chain fatty acid. J Biol Chem 286: 17455–17466.

18. Hold GL, Pryde SE, Russell VJ, Furrie E, Flint HJ (2002) Assessment of microbial diversity in human colonic samples by 16S rDNA sequence analysis. FEMS Microbiol Ecol 39: 33–39.

19. Selma MV, Espin JC, Tomas-Barberan FA (2009) Interaction between phenolics and gut microbiota: role in human health. J Agric Food Chem 57: 6485–6501.

20. Andreasen MF, Kroon PA, Williamson G, Garcia-Conesa MT (2001) Esterase activity able to hydrolyze dietary antioxidant hydroxycinnamates is distributed along the intestine of mammals. J Agric Food Chem 49: 5679–5684.

21. Engberg J, On SL, Harrington CS, Gerner-Smidt P (2000) Prevalence of Campylobacter, Arcobacter, Helicobacter, and Sutterella spp. in human fecal samples as estimated by a reevaluation of isolation methods for Campylobacters. J Clin Microbiol 38: 286–291.

22. Kalischuk LD, Inglis GD (2011) Comparative genotypic and pathogenic examination of Campylobacter concisus isolates from diarrheic and non-diarrheic humans. BMC Microbiol 11: 53.

23. Schippa S, Conte MP, Borrelli O, Iebba V, Aleandri M, et al. (2009) Dominant genotypes in mucosa-associated Escherichia coli strains from pediatric patients with inflammatory bowel disease. Inflamm Bowel Dis 15: 661–672.

24. Ilina EN, Borovskaya AD, Malakhova MM, Vereshchagin VA, Kubanova AA, et al. (2009) Direct bacterial profiling by matrix-assisted laser desorption-ionization time-of-flight mass spectrometry for identification of pathogenic Neisseria. J Mol Diagn 11: 75–86.

25. Lasch P, Beyer W, Nattermann H, Stammler M, Siegbrecht E, et al. (2009) Identification of Bacillus anthracis by using matrix-assisted laser desorption ionization-time of flight mass spectrometry and artificial neural networks. Appl Environ Microbiol 75: 7229–7242.

26. Kolinska R, Drevinek M, Jakubu V, Zemlickova H (2008) Species identification of Campylobacter jejuni ssp. jejuni and C. coli by matrix-assisted laser desorption/ionization time-of-flight mass spectrometry and PCR. Folia Microbiol (Praha) 53: 403–409.

27. Skirrow MB (1977) Campylobacter enteritis: a "new" disease. Br Med J 2: 9–11.

28. Reller LB, Merritt S, Reimer LG (1983) Controlled evaluation of an improved selective medium for isolation of Campylobacter jejuni from human feces [abstract] 83rd Annu Meet Am Soc Microbiol: C274: 357.

29. Fox JG, Dewhirst FE, Shen Z, Feng Y, Taylor NS, et al. (1998) Hepatic Helicobacter species identified in bile and gallbladder tissue from Chileans with chronic cholecystitis. Gastroenterology 114: 755–763.

30. Zhang L, Man SM, Day AS, Leach ST, Lemberg DA, et al. (2009) Detection and isolation of Campylobacter species other than C. jejuni from children with Crohn's disease. J Clin Microbiol 47: 453–455.

11

Role of Mast Cells in Inflammatory Bowel Disease and Inflammation-Associated Colorectal Neoplasia in IL-10-Deficient Mice

Maciej Chichlowski[1], Greg S. Westwood[1], Soman N. Abraham[1,2,3], Laura P. Hale[1,4]*

1 Department of Pathology, Duke University Medical Center, Durham, North Carolina, United States of America, **2** Department of Molecular Genetics and Microbiology, Duke University Medical Center, Durham, North Carolina, United States of America, **3** Department of Immunology, Duke University Medical Center, Durham, North Carolina, United States of America, **4** The Human Vaccine Institute, Duke University Medical Center, Durham, North Carolina, United States of America

Abstract

Background: Inflammatory bowel disease (IBD) is hypothesized to result from stimulation of immune responses against resident intestinal bacteria within a genetically susceptible host. Mast cells may play a critical role in IBD pathogenesis, since they are typically located just beneath the intestinal mucosal barrier and can be activated by bacterial antigens.

Methodology/Principal Findings: This study investigated effects of mast cells on inflammation and associated neoplasia in IBD-susceptible interleukin (IL)-10-deficient mice with and without mast cells. IL-10-deficient mast cells produced more pro-inflammatory cytokines *in vitro* both constitutively and when triggered, compared with wild type mast cells. However despite this enhanced *in vitro* response, mast cell-sufficient $Il10^{-/-}$ mice actually had decreased cecal expression of tumor necrosis factor (TNF) and interferon (IFN)-γ mRNA, suggesting that mast cells regulate inflammation *in vivo*. Mast cell deficiency predisposed $Il10^{-/-}$ mice to the development of spontaneous colitis and resulted in increased intestinal permeability *in vivo* that preceded the development of colon inflammation. However, mast cell deficiency did not affect the severity of IBD triggered by non-steroidal anti-inflammatory agents (NSAID) exposure or helicobacter infection that also affect intestinal permeability.

Conclusions/Significance: Mast cells thus appear to have a primarily protective role within the colonic microenvironment by enhancing the efficacy of the mucosal barrier. In addition, although mast cells were previously implicated in progression of sporadic colon cancers, mast cells did not affect the incidence or severity of colonic neoplasia in this inflammation-associated model.

Editor: Derya Unutmaz, New York University, United States of America

Funding: This work was funded by the National Institutes of Health R21-DK075522 and 1R01-CA115480. The funders had no role in study design, data collection and analysis, decision to publish, or preparation of the manuscript.

Competing Interests: The authors have declared that no competing interests exist.

* E-mail: laura.hale@duke.edu

Introduction

Inflammatory bowel disease (IBD) is characterized by aberrant immune responses against microorganisms that are present in the intestine. Debilitating clinical symptoms of pain and diarrhea result from intestinal mucosal damage that is driven by the continuous activation of the mucosal immune system by enteric bacteria. A variety of genetic, microbial, and environmental factors have been identified that increase susceptibility to IBD in both animal models and humans. Based on this data, we have proposed that the development of IBD requires three factors [1]. First, bacterial antigens and adjuvants must be present within the intestine. This factor is not easily modifiable, since potentially colitogenic bacterial antigens and adjuvants are present within the intestine of all humans and all mice that are not kept in germ-free facilities. Second, the mucosal barrier must be defective so that the bacterial antigens and adjuvants present within the intestine can come in contact with the innate and adaptive immune cells to generate responses. And third, the host must have a defect in immune regulation that allows induction of sustained immune responses against these antigens. This three-factor model can potentially explain how the known susceptibility alleles and IBD-related triggers in existing murine models result in the development of chronic colitis. The model also predicts that colitis can potentially be prevented or treated by interventions that favor maintenance of appropriate immune regulation and/or enhancement of mucosal barrier function.

Most of the currently used IBD treatments target the immune regulatory pathways, but resulting immunosuppression can increase patient risk for developing opportunistic infections and/or treatment-related lymphomas. Mechanisms that govern the barrier function of the intestinal mucosa are thus of great interest to identify potential targets for novel IBD therapies that can add or synergize with existing therapies. A number of murine models of intestinal inflammation have been established [1,2]. One very commonly used model uses mice deficient in interleukin (IL)-10.

These mice have defects in immune regulation and develop chronic enterocolitis with loss of tolerance to bacterial stimuli when triggered by environmental exposures that decrease mucosal barrier function [3,4,5,6].

Mast cells are innate immune cells that can potentially contribute to IBD through their pro- inflammatory activity and/ or effects on immunoregulation. Their pattern recognition molecules allow them to readily recognize and rapidly respond to bacteria that breach the epithelium [7]. Upon activation, mast cells can immediately release large amounts of pro-inflammatory cytokines that are contained in pre-formed granules [8] and can continue to synthesize and release a wide array of pro-inflammatory mediators *de novo*. Mast cells thus rapidly and selectively produce appropriate mediators that enhance effector-cell recruitment and complement other effector components of the immune system [9]. For example, mast cell-derived mediators can contribute to colitis severity by enhancing neutrophil influx and thus perpetuating ongoing inflammation. However mast cells have also been documented to have anti-inflammatory or immunosuppressive functions, such that they can serve to either enhance or to limit innate or adaptive immune responses, depending on the context [10].

Mast cells are physically located adjacent to the intestinal epithelium, so their activation may also affect the function of the mucosal barrier. The presence of mast cells or the mast cell-produced proteinase *Mcpt4* (chymase) was recently shown to enhance the permeability of jejunal segments studied *ex vivo* [8]. The same study showed that mast cell-deficient $Kit^{W-sh/W-sh}$ (sash) mice have changes in small intestinal architecture, including increased crypt depth, decreased migration of epithelial cells up the villus, and decreased expression of the tight junction protein claudin-3 compared to wild type mice [8]. Claudin-3 is an important sealing protein and its loss from colon tissue has been correlated with lack of tight junction integrity [11]. Mast cells have also been shown to mediate increased intestinal permeability caused by exposure to stress neuropeptides (e.g. corticotropin-releasing factor or sauvagine) *in vitro* [12]. Several studies have shown increased numbers of mast cells or increased release of mast cell mediators from actively inflamed colon of IBD patients compared with non-inflamed colon or normal controls [13,14,15,16], suggesting a potential role for mast cells in the pathogenesis of IBD. However, specific *in vivo* data relating to mechanisms by which mast cells may influence IBD pathogenesis remains limited.

In view of the the well known role of mast cells in exacerbating inflammatory diseases such as arthritis, allergy, and asthma [17,18,19] and the potential of mast cells to contribute to one or more of the three factors that affect development of IBD, we hypothesized that mast cells might play a prominent role in the pathogenesis of IBD. We used a well-established model of IBD, based on IL-10-deficient mice with and without added mast cell deficiency to test this hypothesis.

Results

Mediator response is elevated in Il10$^{-/-}$ mast cells, but absence of mast cells does not affect the severity of IBD triggered by piroxicam in Il10$^{-/-}$ mice

The purpose of these studies was to determine the role of mast cells in the pathogenesis of IBD. *Il10*$^{-/-}$ mice were used, since they are highly susceptible to developing IBD when subjected to conditions that enhance mucosal permeability. Since IL-10 can also directly affect the function of immune cells including mast cells [20], bone marrow-derived mast cells (BMMC) from wild-type

(WT) and *Il10*$^{-/-}$ mice were first compared to determine how IL-10 deficiency affected the ability of BMMC to produce other inflammatory mediators. Similar mast cell survival and % degranulation *in vitro* were observed for WT vs. *Il10*$^{-/-}$ BMMC after the treatment with IgE + cross-linking with anti-IgE. Exposure to enteric bacteria (cecal contents) did not cause significant degranulation of either wild type or *Il10*$^{-/-}$ mast cells and also did not affect mast cell survival (data not shown). However, *Il10*$^{-/-}$ BMMC produced higher baseline levels of IL-6, MCP-1, and MIP-1α in the absence of stimulation (buffer-treated cells) than did WT BMMC (Figure 1). Levels of IL-6 and MCP-1 secretion following IgE-induced degranulation were further increased in *Il10*$^{-/-}$ BMMC compared with WT BMMC (Figure 1). Exposure of BMMC to enteric bacteria (cecal contents) triggered a pattern of cytokine production distinct from that triggered by IgE stimulation, with increased production of tumor necrosis factor (TNF) by *Il10*$^{-/-}$ compared with WT BMMC ($p<0.05$), but decreased or unchanged production of MCP-1, IL-6, and MIP-1α (Figure 1). The increased baseline and stimulated production of pro-inflammatory cytokines by *Il10*$^{-/-}$ BMMC to both classic (e.g. IgE) and IBD-relevant (e.g. enteric bacteria) activation stimuli *in vitro* suggested that *Il10*$^{-/-}$ mast cells might be particularly potent in stimulating inflammatory reactions in the gut following breakdown of the mucosal barrier *in vivo*.

Exposure to the non-steroidal anti-inflammatory agent (NSAID) piroxicam uniformly triggers the development of IBD in *Il10*$^{-/-}$ mice by enhancing apoptosis of mucosal epithelial cells, resulting in barrier breakdown that massively exposes immune cells in the lamina propria to bacterial antigens [5]. Mice variously deficient in IL-10 and mast cells received 200 ppm piroxicam for 7 days and then were observed for 16 additional days prior to assessment of colon inflammation. Wild type mice did not develop chronic colitis when exposed to piroxicam (mean histologic scores ± SEM = 7±2; Figure 2). Mast cell-deficient sash mice also did not develop colitis following piroxicam exposure, either with or without reconstitution with WT BMMC (Figure 2). As reported previously [5], IL-10-deficient mice developed moderate to severe colitis when exposed to piroxicam (mean histologic scores ± SEM = 30±5; Figure 2). *Il10*$^{-/-}$ mice with mast cell deficiency due to the Kit^{W-sh}/Kit^{W-sh} mutation (DKO mice), DKO mice reconstituted with WT BMMC, and DKO mice reconstituted with *Il10*$^{-/-}$ BMMC also developed moderate to severe colitis when exposed to piroxicam, with severity that statistically did not differ from that seen in mast cell-sufficient *Il10*$^{-/-}$ mice (p = 0.14, 0.34, and 0.93, respectively; Figure 2). Thus, even though *Il10*$^{-/-}$ mast cells produce elevated levels of inflammatory mediators when stimulated *in vitro*, the absence of mast cells does not affect the severity of IBD triggered by exposure of *Il10*$^{-/-}$ mice to the mucosal barrier-damaging NSAID piroxicam.

Mast cells modulate production of pro-inflammatory mediators in vivo, but absence of mast cells does not affect the severity of helicobacter-triggered IBD in Il10$^{-/-}$ mice

In vivo activation responses of mast cells may differ from their responses *in vitro* due to the complexities of the *in vivo* colonic microenvironment. To address this issue, we determined the effect of mast cells on the inflammatory milieu in IBD-susceptible and control mice with mucosal barrier compromise due to helicobacter infection. Colon tissues from *Il10*$^{-/-}$, DKO, sash, and TNF-deficient mice with and without co-infection by *H. typhlonius* and *H. rodentium* were analyzed for inflammation severity and for the production of selected cytokines by real time reverse transcriptase

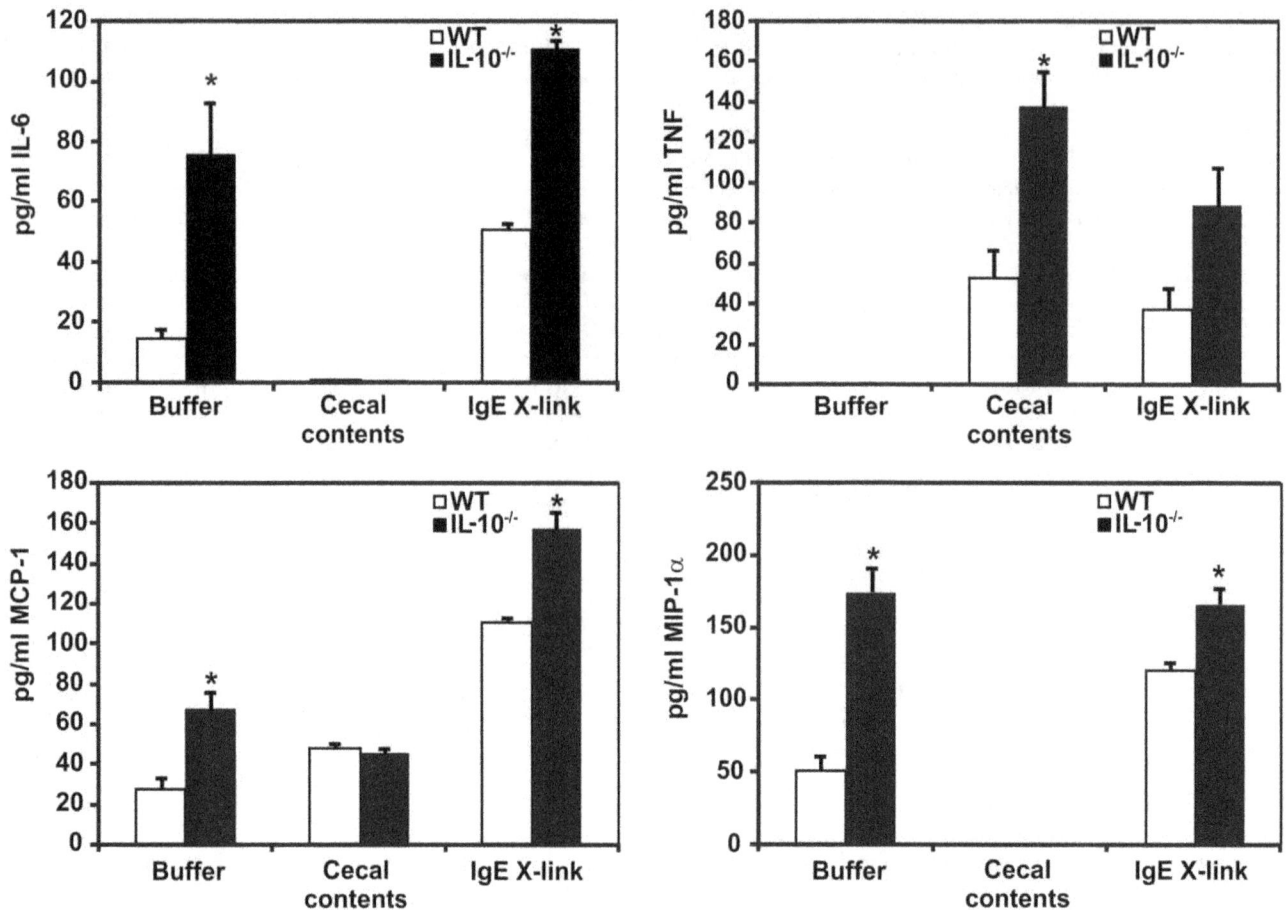

Figure 1. BMMC cytokine production after stimulation with IgE or enteric bacteria. BMMC were stimulated for 4 hrs, then media was harvested for cytokine analysis via Luminex bead-based fluorescent immunoassays. $Il10^{-/-}$ BMMC make more IL-6, MCP-1, and MIP-1α constitutively (buffer treatment) and following IgE stimulation than WT BMMC ($p<0.05$). Exposure to enteric bacteria in cecal contents triggers a different pattern of cytokine expression, with higher TNF production by $Il10^{-/-}$ vs. WT BMMC. Data shown is the mean ± SEM for 3–5 independent experiments. * indicates $p \leq 0.05$ vs. WT.

polymerase chain reaction (PCR) at 4–5 wks after infection. At this time point, $Il10^{-/-}$ and DKO mice have severe chronic colitis, while $Tnf^{-/-}$ and mast cell-deficient sash mice do not (Figure 3). DKO mice had significantly increased production of mRNA encoding TNF and interferon (IFN)-γ, with strong trends toward increased IL-4 and IL-12/23p40 compared with mast cell-sufficient $Il10^{-/-}$ mice (Figure 4). Elevated levels of IL-4 were also seen in sash mice singly deficient in mast cells and in TNF-deficient mice that do not develop colitis under these conditions, compared with $Il10^{-/-}$ mice that develop severe colitis (Figure 4). Thus, tissue from DKO mice with colitis showed increased production of pro-inflammatory cytokines compared with mice singly deficient in IL-10, mast cells, or TNF. This demonstrates that mast cells play a role in down-regulating production of pro-inflammatory cytokines within the inflamed colon, at this relatively early time point in the course of chronic colitis.

To determine how mast cells affected the long-term severity of IBD in helicobacter-infected mice that had sustained mucosal barrier dysfunction, $Il10^{-/-}$ and DKO mice were infected with *H. rodentium* and *H. typhlonius* and monitored for up to 27 wks post-infection. Infected $Il10^{-/-}$ and DKO mice both demonstrated severe colitis that was slightly increased in the absence of mast cells (mean histologic score $=43\pm1$ in $Il10^{-/-}$ mice vs. 48 ± 2 in DKO mice; $p=0.03$) (Figure 5A). However, this slight

difference in colitis severity did not translate into a difference in survival based on presence or absence of mast cells (p = 0.29; Figure 5B).

Mast cells do not affect inflammation-associated colonic neoplasia in helicobacter-infected $Il10^{-/-}$ mice

Colonic inflammation has previously been shown to predispose to the development of malignancy, both in humans and in murine models of IBD [6,21]. Mast cells have also been shown to affect the incidence and severity of neoplasia in models of sporadic colon cancers [22,23]. Therefore, the effect of mast cells on inflammation-associated neoplasia was also investigated in $Il10^{-/-}$ mice with colitis triggered by helicobacter infection. Sixty three percent of $Il10^{-/-}$ mice (n = 24) developed colorectal neoplasia by 18 ± 1 weeks after IBD triggering, with an average of 3 ± 2 neoplastic lesions per mouse (range = 1–6) (Figure 6A and B). Similarly, 62% (n = 21) of DKO mice had colorectal neoplasia 17 ± 1 weeks after IBD triggering, with an average of 2 ± 1 neoplastic lesions per mouse (range = 1–6) (Figure 6C and D). Half of these neoplastic lesions were invasive at the time of detection in both groups. Thus mast cells do not affect the incidence of inflammation-associated neoplasia in $Il10^{-/-}$ mice with severe long-standing compromise of the mucosal barrier due to helicobacter infection.

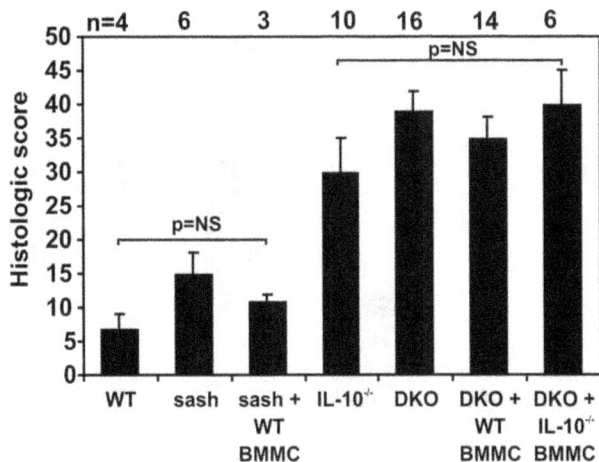

Figure 2. Mast cells do not affect the severity of colitis triggered by piroxicam. Mice of the indicated genotypes ± reconstitution with WT or $Il10^{-/-}$ BMMC received 200 ppm piroxicam ×7 days to trigger the onset of colitis. Tissue was harvested for histologic analysis 16 d later. WT or sash mice ± reconstitution with WT BMMC did not develop colitis in this study. Mice deficient in IL-10 uniformly developed colitis, however the presence or absence of mast cells and whether or not the mast cells could produce IL-10 did not affect the severity of inflammation.

Absence of mast cells predisposes to spontaneous development of IBD in Il10$^{-/-}$ mice

Since we did not see any contributory role for mast cells in actively induced inflammatory responses in gut of $Il10^{-/-}$ mice, we investigated whether mast cells had a role in the spontaneous development of IBD in $Il10^{-/-}$ vs. DKO mice. All mice were documented to remain free of helicobacter infection throughout the study. Whereas most mast cell-sufficient $Il10^{-/-}$ mice did not develop colitis by 9 months of age (mean histologic score ± SEM = 13±2), most DKO mice developed at least moderate colitis

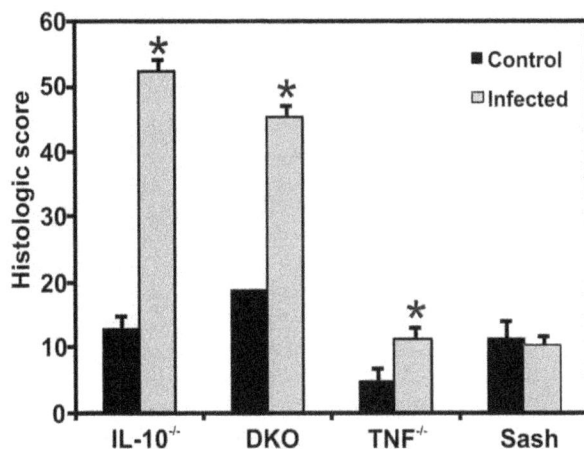

Figure 3. Mast cells do not affect early colitis severity in Helicobacter-infected Il10$^{-/-}$ mice. Both IL-10-deficient and DKO mice exhibited severe colonic inflammation when infected with *H. rodentium* and *H. typhlonius* for 30 d (n = 3 for $Il10^{-/-}$ and n = 4 for DKO mice) compared to $Tnf^{-/-}$ and sash mice (n = 4 each) (p<0.001 for both $Il10^{-/-}$ and DKO vs. $Tnf^{-/-}$ and sash). * indicates p<0.01, comparing control (non-infected) and infected mice of a given genotype.

(mean ± SEM histologic score = 27±4) (Figure 7). These DKO mice were significantly younger (31±2 wks; range = 25–38 wks; n = 10) than the $Il10^{-/-}$ mice studied (36±1 wks; range 34–36 wks; n = 15; p = 0.02) due to more frequent occurrence of rectal prolapse (an indicator of severe IBD) in DKO mice that led to euthanasia for humane reasons prior to the planned study endpoint. Overall, these results demonstrate that mast cells protect $Il10^{-/-}$ mice against the development of spontaneous colitis.

Mast cells enhance epithelial barrier function

$Il10^{-/-}$ mice have defects in immune regulation due to their genetic deficiency of IL-10 and their intestines contain potentially colitogenic antigens and adjuvants derived from their commensal intestinal microbiota. The three factor model presented earlier thus predicts that colitis will develop when the mucosal barrier is compromised, a prediction supported by the ability of NSAIDs and helicobacter infection to trigger colitis in these mice. Our finding that absence of mast cells predisposed to spontaneous development of IBD in $Il10^{-/-}$ mice suggested that absence of mast cells might also decrease the effectiveness of the mucosal barrier.

A quantitative assessment of barrier function was performed to determine the effect of mast cells on intestinal permeability. Phenol red dye was administered orally to $Il10^{-/-}$ vs. DKO mice *in vivo* and the amount of dye recovered in urine was measured as an indicator of intestinal paracellular permeability. DKO mice exhibited higher permeability as indicated by increased dye recovery (Figure 8B) compared to $Il10^{-/-}$ mice (Figure 8A; p = 0.02). Histologic scores indicated minimal to no inflammation in the animals tested (mean histologic score ± SEM = 7±1 (n = 33) for DKO and 15±3 (n = 18) for $Il10^{-/-}$ mice). The increased intestinal permeability of DKO mice was due to the Kit^{W-sh} mutation that results in absence of mast cells, since it was also seen in sash mice that lacked mast cells, but were wild type with respect to IL-10 expression (Figure 8C). Taken together, these studies indicate that mice that lack mast cells have increased intestinal permeability. Furthermore, the data clearly show that the decreased barrier integrity observed in DKO relative to $Il10^{-/-}$ mice occurs prior to, rather than in response to, the development of colon inflammation.

Discussion

Although mast cells are best known for their pathogenic over-responses in immune-mediated diseases such as allergy and asthma, their protective role in innate immune responses is underscored by high susceptibility of mice deficient in mast cells to fatal infections with enteric bacteria [24,25]. Mast cells aid the development of antigen-specific cellular and humoral adaptive immune responses by stimulating lymph node swelling and sequestration [26]. The data presented here suggest that mast cells also enhance intestinal mucosal barrier function *in vivo* and can protect against spontaneous development of IBD in susceptible mouse strains.

Intestinal epithelial barrier function is regulated by epithelial cells, innate and adaptive immunity, and the enteric nervous system and dysregulation of any of these alters the barrier [27]. Several mast cell-derived mediators, including histamine, serotonin, arachidonic acid, and mast cell proteinases have been shown to affect intestinal epithelial function, including ion channel conductance and activation/inhibition of secretion of electrolytes and mucus [8,27,28]. Our results show that mast cell-deficient sash and DKO mice had increased the baseline paracellular permeability of the intestine *in vivo*, independent of IL-10 status (Figure 8).

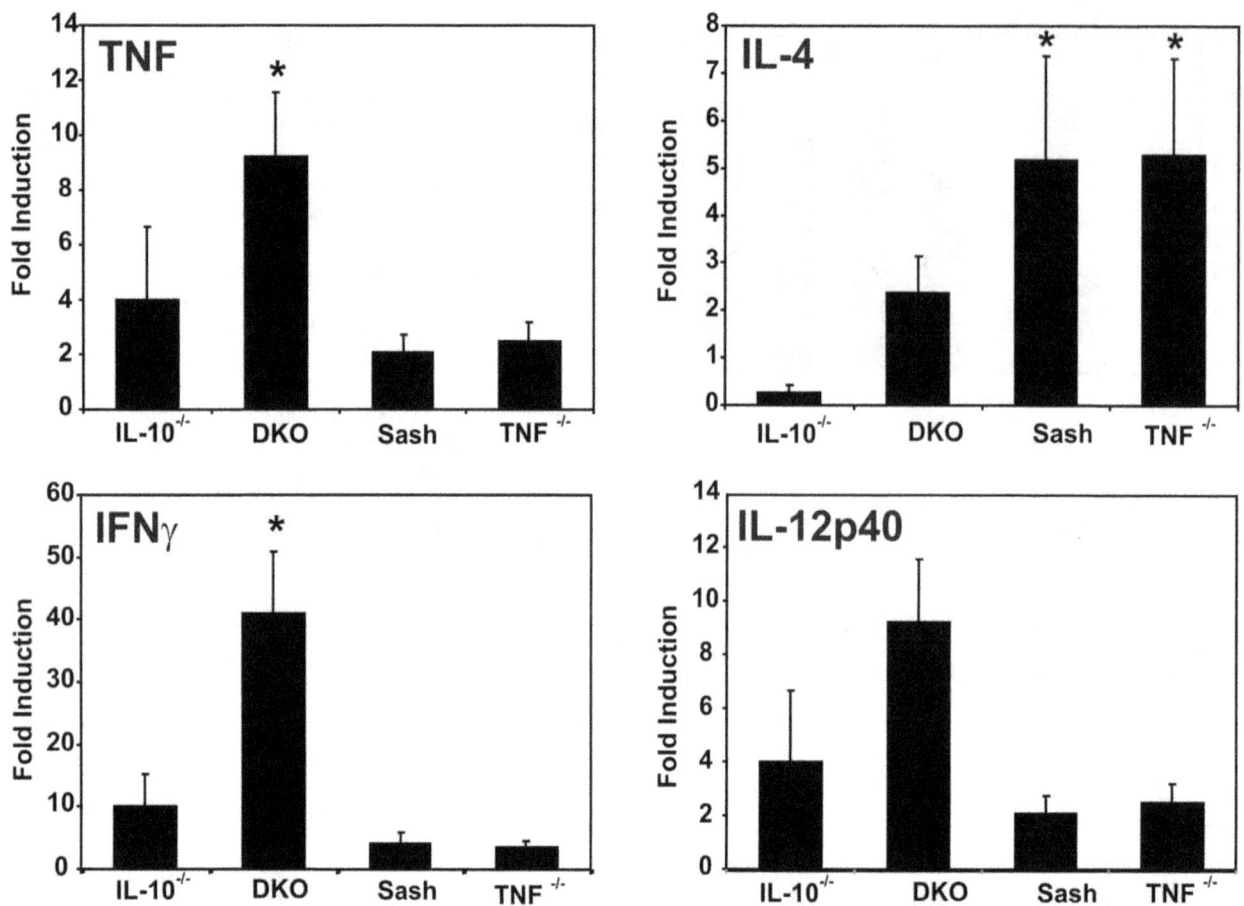

Figure 4. Mast cells modulate pro-inflammatory cytokine mRNA expression in inflamed cecal tissues. Cytokine mRNA expression in cecal tissue of mice of the indicated genotypes harvested after 5 weeks of infection with *H. rodentium* and *H. typhlonius* was measured by real-time PCR, normalized to β-actin and expressed as fold-induction relative to non-infected cecal tissue of the same genotype. Bars represent 5–6 mice per genotype. * indicates $p<0.05$ compared to $Il10^{-/-}$ mice. Infected DKO mice have increased expression of Th1 cytokines (TNF, IFN-γ) and a trend towards increased Th2 (IL-4) and Th17-inducing cytokines (IL-12/23p40) compared with mast cell-sufficient $Il10^{-/-}$ mice.

In addition to increased intestinal permeability, the data presented also show that mast cell-deficient DKO mice are at increased risk for spontaneous development of IBD compared to mast cell-sufficient $Il10^{-/-}$ mice. These results parallel previous studies in humans demonstrating that patients with IBD and 10–25% of their first degree relatives have increased paracellular permeability relative to controls and that relapse of quiescent IBD was often preceded by increased intestinal permeability [29,30,31]. Interestingly, the $Il10^{-/-}$ mice in our study had low gut permeability even at the relatively advanced ages of 30–35 wks. Others have shown that $Il10^{-/-}$ mice develop increased gut permeability prior to development of colitis [32]. However, the lack of barrier dysfunction in the 30–35 wk old $Il10^{-/-}$ mice reported here (Figure 8) correlates very well with the low incidence of spontaneous colitis (2 of $15 = 13\%$) that we observed in 36 wk old $Il10^{-/-}$ mice (Figure 7).

A recent report by Groschwitz *et al* [8] showed that jejunal tissue from mast cell-deficient mice had *decreased* baseline permeability *ex vivo* compared to jejunal tissue from wild type mice. Our data differs since it represents an integration of the permeability of non-manipulated tissues throughout the gastrointestinal tract of live mice. The permeability characteristics of small intestine and colon are known to be different with respect to water as well as a variety of nutrients. Our *in vivo* studies also include potential contributions

from different mast cell subsets that may be present in different parts of the intestinal tract, bacterial-mucosal interactions, leukocyte trafficking, and transient inflammation that can also affect net intestinal permeability *in vivo*. It is also possible that mast cells contribute differentially to homeostatic versus inflammation-induced barrier function. For example, during the normal non-inflamed state, mast cells may increase permeability (as reported by Groschwitz *et al.* [8]) to optimize small intestinal absorption of nutrients and antigens and to facilitate cellular interaction important for both digestive and immune system functions. However, mast cells may limit inflammation-induced barrier dysfunction by rapidly responding to pathogens that cross the mucosal barrier. The specific types of mast cells present and the quantity and type of mediators they release upon activation are likely to be critical in regulating their net effect [33].

We found that mast cell-sufficient $Il10^{-/-}$ mice demonstrated decreased mucosal production of several pro-inflammatory cytokines (TNF, IFNγ, and IL12/23p40) compared with mice singly deficient in IL-10, mast cells, or TNF (Figure 4). Several previous studies using murine models have shown these pro-inflammatory cytokines can directly increase intestinal epithelial permeability by inducing disassembly of epithelial cell tight junctions (reviewed in [1]). Based on current understanding of tight junction function, the decrease in claudin-3 documented in

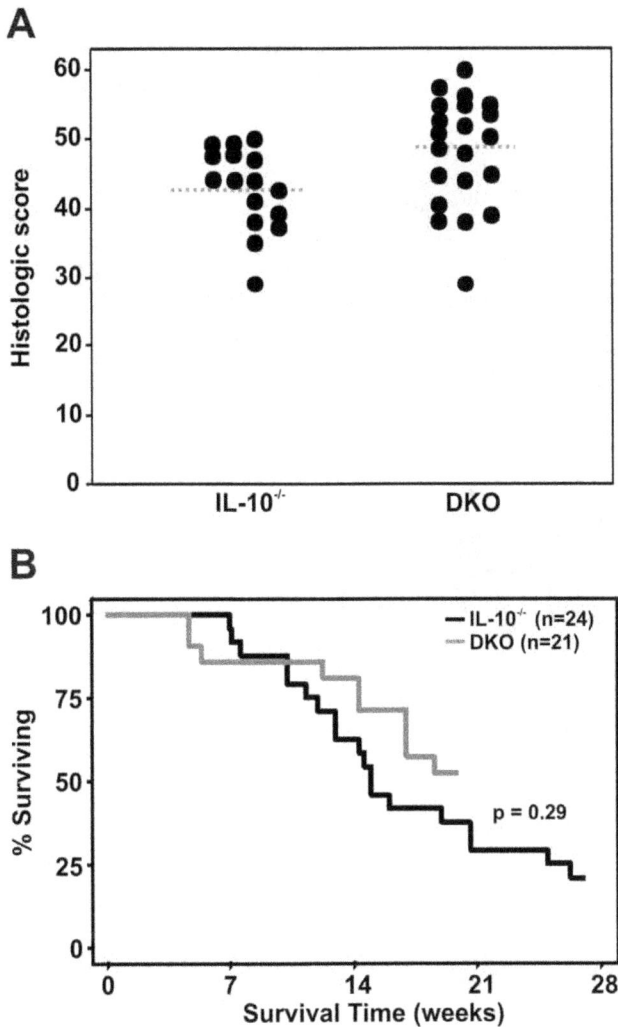

Figure 5. Mast cells do not affect long-term colitis severity in Helicobacter-infected $Il10^{-/-}$ mice. $Il10^{-/-}$ mice with (n = 21) and without (n = 24) genetic deficiency of mast cells were infected with *H. rodentium* and *H. typhlonius* and monitored for up to 27 wks. DKO mice had a small increase in histologic score compared with mice deficient in IL-10 alone (A; p = 0.03), but there was no difference in survival between DKO and mast cell-sufficient $Il10^{-/-}$ mice (B).

intestinal tissues from mast cell-deficient sash mice [8] would be expected to increase the *in vivo* permeability of their intestinal tissues *in vivo* [11]. Perturbation of tight junctions and increased mucosal permeability and activation of the mucosal immune system have been shown to affect the severity of mucosal inflammation in humans [34,35,36]. However, since effect of mast cells on the mucosal barrier likely results from a balance of multiple effector and immunoregulatory functions [10], more studies will be required to precisely determine the mechanisms involved.

The Kit^{W-sh} allele that renders sash mice mast cell-deficient contains an inversion that abolishes Kit expression in mast cells and melanocytes but does not affect Kit expression in most other cell types [37]. Recent work has further identified that this inversion also inhibits the production of corin, a proteinase responsible for the activation of atrial natriuretic peptide [38]. It is also possible that the increased permeability may be due to this or to other factors in sash mice that render them susceptible to inflammation independent of

their mast cell deficiency. However, we note that, despite their increased intestinal permeability, mice bearing the Kit^{W-sh} mutation alone do not have added susceptibility to IBD in the absence of concomitant IL-10 deficiency. Furthermore, reconstitution of $Il10^{-/-}$ mice also homozygous for the Kit^{W-sh} mutation (DKO) mice with mast cells does not affect IBD severity (Figures 2 and 3).

Since mast cells protect $Il10^{-/-}$ mice from spontaneous IBD, their failure to influence the severity of inflammation triggered by exposure of $Il10^{-/-}$ mice to piroxicam or co-infection with *H. rodentium* and *H. typhlonius* may seem paradoxical at first glance. However, this result is predicted by the three factor model of IBD pathogenesis presented earlier [1]. $Il10^{-/-}$ mice have bacteria within their intestine and their IL-10 deficiency results in defective immunoregulation. The model thus predicts that colitis will develop when the mucosal barrier is compromised. Exposure to piroxicam or infection with helicobacter already compromises mucosal barrier sufficiently to result in colitis. Thus further compromise of the barrier by mast cell deficiency would be predicted to have little to no additional effect, as was observed experimentally. Additional studies using mice with mast cell deficiency and/or alterations in intestinal permeability derived via other mechanisms will be useful for further confirming (or disproving) this hypothesized mechanism.

We also found that the presence or absence of mast cells had no effect on the incidence or progression of inflammation-associated colon cancers in $Il10^{-/-}$ mice with colitis. There is currently controversy in the literature regarding the role of mast cells in tumor progression in the colon. Mice with a genetic susceptibility to intestinal neoplasia (Apc^{Min}) had a greater frequency and size of adenomas in the absence of mast cells, suggesting a protective function for mast cells in colorectal carcinogenesis [23]. However, another report [22] showed recently that mast cells were required for the growth of adenomatous polyps in mice. Of note, both of these studies used different strains of mice genetically susceptible to polyp formation in models with minimal inflammation. Mast cells may thus have varying effects on the inflammatory milieu in these models based on any additional environmental triggers of intestinal inflammation that may be present.

In summary, our studies suggest that mast cells have primarily a protective role within the colonic microenvironment, serving to enhance barrier function and limit spontaneous inflammation. However, the presence of mast cells is insufficient to affect the severity of IBD triggered by massive disruption of the mucosal barrier and does not affect the development and progression of colorectal neoplasia associated with severe IBD.

Materials and Methods

Ethics Statement

All animal studies were approved by the Institutional Animal Care and Use Committee of Duke University, an institution accredited by the Association for Assessment and Accreditation of Laboratory Animal Care (AAALAC) International. The protocol numbers covering this work were A225-06-07 and A151-09-05.

Animal Studies

Breeding pairs of IL-10-deficient mice (strain name = B6.129P2-$Il10^{tm1Cgn}/J$, stock # 002251), sash mice (strain name = B6.Cg-Kit^{W-sh}/HNihrJaeBsmJ; stock #005051), mice transgenic for global expression of green fluorescent protein (GFP) (strain name = C57BL/6-Tg(UBC-GFP)30Scha/J; stock # 004353), and mice deficient in TNF (strain name = B6.129S6-Tnf$^{tm1Gkl}/J$; stock # 005540) were obtained from Jackson Laboratories (Bar Harbor, ME). IL-10-deficient mice have been documented to be highly

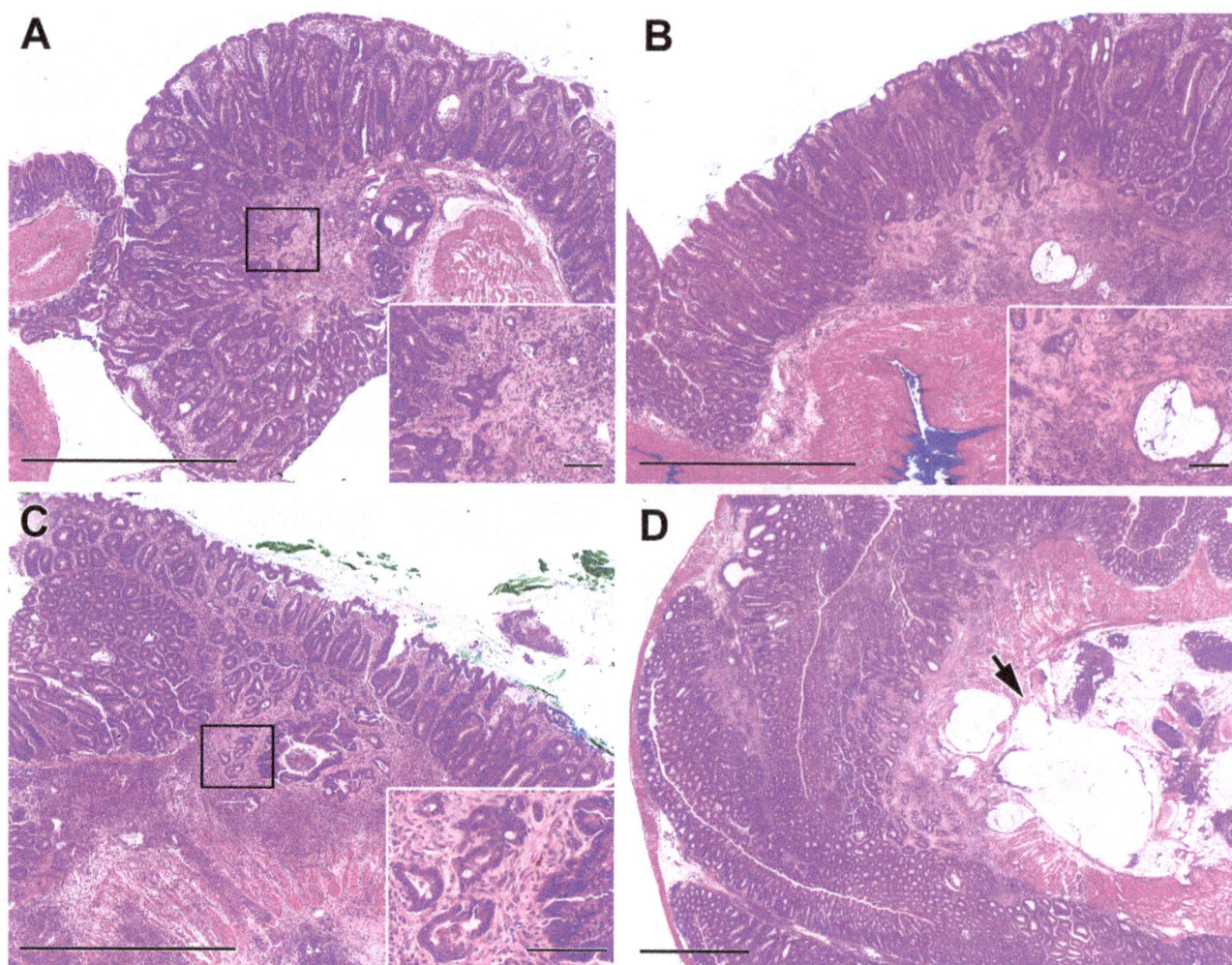

Figure 6. Colon histology and neoplasia in *Helicobacter*-infected and non-infected *Il10*$^{-/-}$ and DKO adult mice. Helicobacter-infected *Il10*$^{-/-}$ (A, B) and DKO mice (C, D) uniformly exhibited mucosal hyperplasia with prominent inflammatory infiltrates. Examples of neoplastic lesions seen in the long-term study are shown. The arrow in D indicates malignant glands that have invaded into the serosa. Bar represents 1 mm in the large panels and 100 µm in the insets.

susceptible to developing IBD, either spontaneously or in response to triggers such as infection with intestinal helicobacter species or exposure to NSAIDs that damage their mucosal barrier [4,5,6,39]. The Kit^{W-sh} allele contains an inversion located proximal to the Kit locus that abolishes Kit expression in mast cells and melanocytes but does not affect Kit expression in germ cells or erythrocytes [37]. Thus, although sash mice are white and lack mast cells, they can be propagated as homozygotes with normal litter sizes [40]. *Il10*$^{-/-}$ and sash strains were crossed to generate DKO mice that were IBD-susceptible and lacked mast cells. All of these strains were on the C57BL/6 background.

Mice were housed in polycarbonate micro-isolator cages in individually ventilated racks under BSL-2 conditions, with access to food and water *ad libitum*. Mice were observed daily for clinical signs of distress and weight was monitored three times per week. Humane endpoints included >15% loss of body weight and development of rectal prolapse, a well-recognized complication of chronic inflammation in the colon.

Sentinel mice exposed repetitively to dirty bedding from the mice used in this study were negative for parasites by microscopic exam, negative for *Citrobacter rodentium* by fecal culture, and

negative by serology for a panel of 22 murine protozoal, bacterial, and viral pathogens, including murine parvovirus, murine hepatitis virus, and murine norovirus. All mice not intentionally infected with Helicobacter *spp.* were confirmed to be Helicobacter-free by PCR of feces using a species-specific primer.

Models of Inflammatory Bowel Disease

For studies of spontaneous colitis, cohorts of mice were housed under specific pathogen-free conditions and euthanized for histologic scoring of colon inflammation if they experienced >15% loss of body weight, rectal prolapse, or reached pre-determined time points. Some cohorts of mice were exposed to 200 ppm piroxicam in powdered LabDiet 5001 chow (Purina, Framingham, MA) for 7 days to trigger the onset of colitis as previously described [6]. Based on measured food consumption, the dose of piroxicam averaged 40 mg/kg/day (range 21–62 mg/kg/day over 35 cage-days). The mice were then placed back on pelleted 5001 chow without piroxicam and observed for an additional 16 days before euthanasia for histologic scoring of colon inflammation. For studies of colitis triggered by helicobacter infection, 6–8 wk old mice were infected with *H. typhlonius* (clinical isolate DU-01) [41]

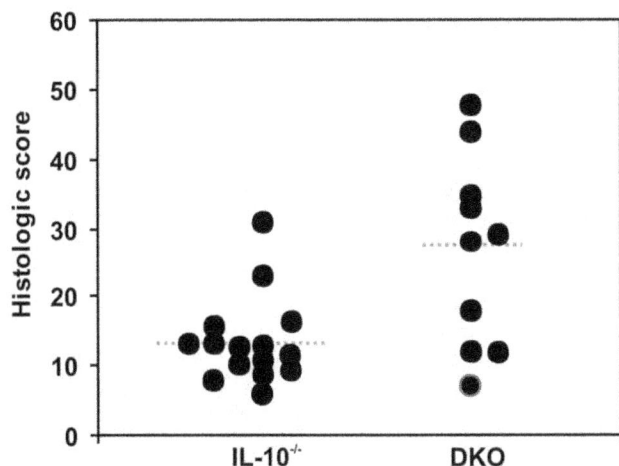

Figure 7. Severity of spontaneous IBD in specific pathogen-free $Il10^{-/-}$ and DKO mice. $Il10^{-/-}$ mice on the C57BL/6 background rarely developed spontaneous colitis by 36 weeks of age when housed under clean conditions, free from specific pathogens including Helicobacter *spp.* (mean histologic scores ± SEM = 13±2; n = 15). In contrast, DKO mice that lacked mast cells frequently developed spontaneous colitis (mean histologic scores = 27±4; n = 10; p = 0.02), which was evident at an earlier age (31±2 wks vs. 36±1 wks; p = 0.02) compared with $Il10^{-/-}$ mice.

and *H. rodentium* (MIT 95–1707 = ATCC type strain 700285) [42] by gavage of a single dose of 500 μl culture (generally 10^8 organisms) as previously described [6]. Infection was confirmed 7 days post-infection (PI) by quantitative real time PCR of feces (see below). Similar numbers of helicobacter organisms were present in feces on day 7 post-infection for $Il10^{-/-}$ mice infected with 10^4, 10^6, or 10^8 organisms and all infected mice developed severe colitis (data not shown). Thus the severity of colonic inflammation was insensitive to inoculum size over the range of 10^4–10^8 helicobacter organisms due to their rapid *in vivo* multiplication. Mice were euthanized by CO_2 asphyxiation in accordance with the American Veterinary Medical Association Recommendations on Euthanasia if they developed 15% body weight loss, rectal prolapse, or at 25–36 wks after infection. All mice in this study were evaluated pathologically for both colitis and neoplasia.

Tissue collection

After euthanasia, the digestive tract from stomach to anus was removed and divided into segments representing the stomach, cecum, and proximal, mid-, distal, and terminal colon/rectum. Portions of each gastrointestinal segment were rinsed briefly with PBS to remove non-adherent organisms. Tissues for molecular analysis were immediately frozen and stored at -20°C for subsequent quantitation of mRNAs or associated *Helicobacter* organisms by quantitative real-time PCR. The remaining tissues were fixed in Carnoy's solution for 2–4 hrs, then processed and embedded into paraffin.

Histological Scoring

The severity of colonic inflammation and incidence of colon neoplasia seen in hematoxylin and eosin-stained sections was scored by a board-certified pathologist blinded to experimental group. Histologic scores were calculated as described ([43]; modified from [44]), using a scale that takes into account mucosal changes in 5 different bowel segments, including hyperplasia and ulceration, degree of inflammation, and % of each bowel segment

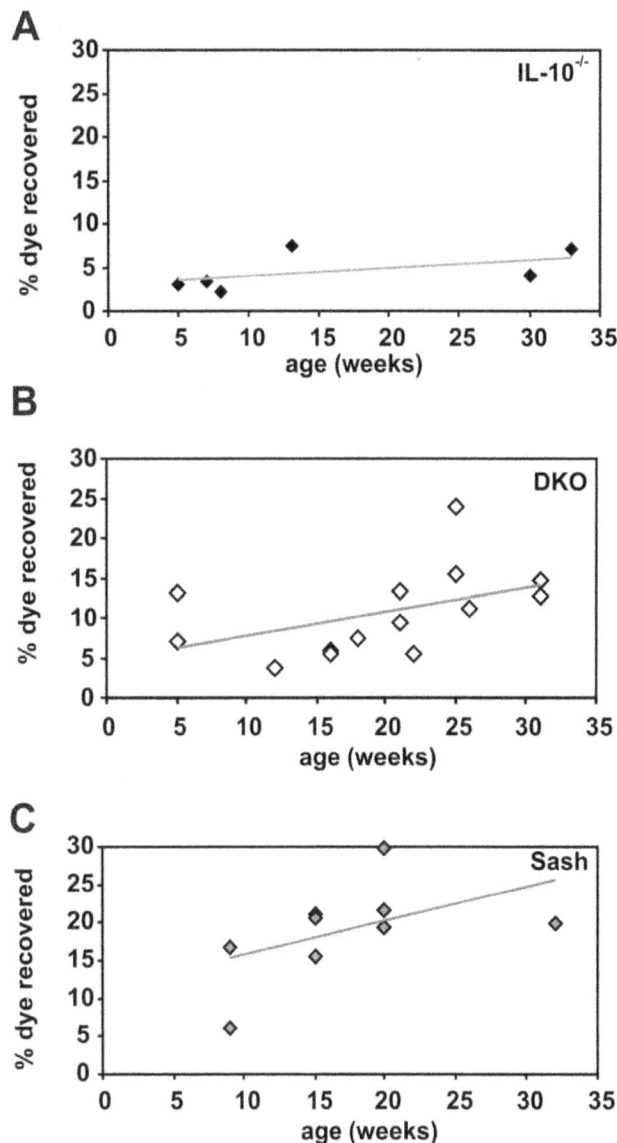

Figure 8. Permeability of the intestinal barrier in $IL-10^{-/-}$ and DKO mice. Mice of the indicated ages and genotypes were gavaged with phenol red and the amount of dye absorbed was determined by spectrophotometric measurement of urine. Each point shown represents the average of 2–4 mice tested in a single experiment. Mast cell-deficient DKO and sash mice had significantly increased dye recovery compared with $Il10^{-/-}$ mice (p = 0.02 for differences in data point elevation via linear regression analysis). The total numbers of mice tested were: $Il10^{-/-}$ (n = 14), DKO (n = 18), and sash (n = 22).

affected by these changes. Using this scale, the maximum score is 75 and a score >12 indicates the presence of colitis.

Neoplastic lesions were classified according to a consensus report for intestinal neoplasia in mouse models as gastrointestinal intraepithelial neoplasia or invasive carcinoma [45]. The category of gastrointestinal intraepithelial neoplasia is synonymous with atypical hyperplasia, atypia, microadenoma, carcinoma *in situ*, and dysplasia, which are non-invasive neoplastic lesions. A diagnosis of invasive carcinoma required the presence of a desmoplastic response to differentiate invasion from mucosal herniation or pseudoinvasion. Regions of neoplasia that were separated by regions of normal mucosa were scored as separate lesions.

Real-time PCR Assays

For detection of helicobacter organisms, DNA was extracted from 40 mg frozen tissue or 20 mg feces using the DNeasy Tissue kit (Qiagen, Valencia, CA). Real-time PCR was performed to quantify the relative concentrations of fecal and mucosa-associated *H. rodentium* and *H. typhlonius* organisms per milligram of feces or tissue based on comparison with a standard, as described previously [6].

For analysis of cytokine expression, total RNA was extracted from ~30 mg cecal tissue using the RNA extraction kit (Ambion, Austin, TX). Complementary DNA (cDNA) was synthesized using 1 μg of RNA through a reverse transcription reaction (Applied Biosystems, Foster City, CA). Real-time PCR quantitative mRNA analyses were performed using SYBR green fluorescence (Stratagene, Cedar Creek, TX). The standard PCR conditions were 95°C for 10 min, 40 cycles for 1 min at 94°C, 56°C for 1 min and 72°C for 2 min, followed by the standard denaturation curve. The primer sequences used in this analysis were modified from Cardoso *et al.* [46] and were as follows: β-actin (fwd, 5'-AGT TGC GTT TTA CAC CCT TT-3'; rev, 5'-AAG CCA TGC CAA TGT TGT CT-3'), IL-4 (fwd, 5'-CTG ACG GCA CAG AGC TAT TGA-3'; rev, 5'-TAT GCG AAG CAC CTT GGA AGC-3'), TNF (fwd, 5'-TGT GCT CAG AGC TTT CAA CAA-3'; rev, 5'-CTT GAT GGT GGT GCA TGA GA-3'), IL-12p40 (fwd, 5'-AGC ACC AGC TTC TTC ATC AGG-3'; rev, 5'-GCG CTG GAT TCG AAC AAA G- 3'), IFN-γ (fwd, 5'-GCA TCT TGG CTT TGC AGC T-3' ; rev, 5'-CTT TTT TCG CCT TGC TGT TG-3'). SYBR Green PCR Master Mix (Stratagene, Cedar Creek, TX), specific primers, and cDNA template were used in each reaction. The relative mRNA amount of each sample was calculated based on its threshold cycle, Ct, in comparison to the Ct of housekeeping gene β-actin. The results for cytokine mRNAs were demonstrated as mRNA expression relative to non-infected mice of the same genotype. The purity of amplified product was determined as a single peak of dissociation curve. Negative controls without RNA were also performed.

Culture and In vitro Stimulation of Mast Cells

To obtain BMMC, mouse femurs were flushed with RPMI 1640 media using a 22G needle and 10 ml syringe. The bone marrow cells were cultured for 4 weeks in RPMI 1640 (Invitrogen, Carlsbad, CA) containing 10% fetal bovine serum, essential and non-essential amino acids, 100 U/ml penicillin, 100 μg/ml streptomycin, 10 mM HEPES, 5.5×10^{-5} M 2-mercaptoethanol, 10 ng/ml stem cell factor, and 5 ng/ml IL-3 (R&D Systems, Minneapolis, MN) to stimulate mast cell differentiation. Non-adherent cells were harvested to flasks containing fresh media once weekly. The percentage of mast cells was determined by performing a differential on a cytocentrifuge preparation stained with a modified Wright-Giemsa stain; % of mast cells averaged 95%. 10^7 BMMC in 100 μl

PBS were injected intraperitoneally to reconstitute mast cell-deficient mice, which were used 12 wks after reconstitution.

The *in vitro* reactivity of BMMC derived from C57BL/6 wild type or $Il10^{-/-}$ mice was compared by measuring degranulation, viability, and cytokine production post-degranulation. BMMC (1×10^6 cells/well) in Tyrode's buffer were sensitized by overnight incubation with 1 μg/ml IgE then stimulated by cross-linking with 1 μg/ml goat anti-mouse IgE (BD, San Jose, CA) or by incubation with a mixture of enteric bacterial antigens prepared as 100 mg cecal contents per ml of saline or Tyrode's buffer then filtered at 0.2 μm. Degranulation was assessed by β-hexoseaminidase activity using a colorimetric substrate assay as previously described [47]. Viability after degranulation was measured using a tetrazolium-based colorimetric assay (CellTiter96 Aqueous, Promega, Madison, WI). Media was harvested from some wells 4 hrs after stimulation for measurement of cytokine content using a Luminex bead-based multiplex fluorescent immunoassay (BioRad, Hercules, CA).

Intestinal permeability

The permeability of the mucosal layer was assessed using phenolsulfonphthalein (phenol red) [48]. Under normal conditions, phenol red is not absorbed in the intestine. However under conditions of increased intestinal permeability, the dye is absorbed then excreted in the urine. The urinary dye recovery was measured after administration of 2 μmol (~700 μg) phenol red in 0.5 ml of saline by oral gavage. Groups of 2–4 animals were placed in metabolic caging that is optimized to separate urine from feces. Urine was collected for 18 hrs, alkalinized extracts were prepared, and the phenol red content of each sample was determined spectrophotometrically at 560 nm by comparison to standards of known concentration. The urinary recovery of phenol red was expressed as percent of the dose administered.

Statistical Analysis

Statistical comparison of groups was performed using Student's t-test. Survival rates were calculated using Kaplan-Meier test with *p*-values calculated using the log rank test. Linear regression was performed using GraphPad prism software. A value of $p \leq 0.05$ was considered to be significant.

Acknowledgments

The authors would like to thank Paula K. Greer and Chau T. Trinh for expert technical assistance.

Author Contributions

Conceived and designed the experiments: SNA LPH. Performed the experiments: MC GSW LPH. Analyzed the data: MC LPH. Contributed reagents/materials/analysis tools: SNA. Wrote the paper: MC SNA LPH.

References

1. Chichlowski M, Hale LP (2008) Bacterial-mucosal interactions in inflammatory bowel disease—an alliance gone bad. Am J Physiol Gastrointest Liver Physiol 295: G1139–1149.

2. Sollid LM, Johansen F-E (2008) Animal Models of Inflammatory Bowel Disease at the Dawn of the New Genetics Era. PLoS Med 5: e198.

3. Inaba Y, Ashida T, Ito T, Ishikawa C, Tanabe H, et al. (2010) Expression of the antimicrobial peptide alpha-defensin/cryptdins in intestinal crypts decreases at the initial phase of intestinal inflammation in a model of inflammatory bowel disease, IL-10-deficient mice. Inflammatory Bowel Diseases 9999: NA.

4. Kühn R, Löhler J, Rennick D, Rajewsky K, Müller W (1993) Interleukin-10-deficient mice develop chronic enterocolitis. Cell 75(2): 263–274.

5. Hale LP, Gottfried MR, Swidsinski A (2005) Piroxicam treatment of IL-10-deficient mice enhances colonic epithelial apoptosis and mucosal exposure to intestinal bacteria. Inflamm Bowel Dis 11: 1060–1069.

6. Chichlowski M, Sharp JM, Vanderford DA, Myles MH, Hale LP (2008) Helicobacter typhlonius and Helicobacter rodentium differentially affect the severity of colon inflammation and inflammation-associated neoplasia in IL10-deficient mice. Comp Med 58(6): 534–541.

7. Hofmann AM, Abraham SN (2009) New roles for mast cells in modulating allergic reactions and immunity against pathogens. Current Opinion in Immunology 21: 679–686.

8. Groschwitz KR, Ahrens R, Osterfeld H, Gurish MF, Han X, et al. (2009) Mast cells regulate homeostatic intestinal epithelial migration and barrier function by a chymase/Mcpt4-dependent mechanism. Proceedings of the National Academy of Sciences 106: 22381–22386.

9. Mekori YA, Metcalfe DD (1999) Mast cell-T cell interactions. J Allergy Clin Immunol 104: 517–523.

10. Galli SJ, Grimbaldeston M, Tsai M (2008) Immunomodulatory mast cells: negative, as well as positive, regulators of immunity. Nat Rev Immunol 8: 478–486.

11. Thuijls G, Derikx JPM, Haan J-Jd, Grootjans J, Bruïne Ad, et al. (2010) Urine-based Detection of Intestinal Tight Junction Loss. Journal of Clinical Gastroenterology 44: e14–e19. 10.1097/MCG.1090b1013e31819f35652.

12. Santos J, Yates D, Guilarte M, Vicario M, Alonso C, et al. (2008) Stress neuropeptides evoke epithelial responses via mast cell activation in the rat colon. Psychoneuroendocrinology 33: 1248–1256.

13. Fox CC, Lazenby AJ, Moore WC, Yardley JH, Bayless TM, et al. (1990) Enhancement of human intestinal mast cell mediator release in active ulcerative colitis. Gastroenterology 99: 119–124.

14. Raithel M, Matek M, Baenkler HW, Jorde W, Hahn EG (1995) Mucosal histamine content and histamine secretion in Crohn's disease, ulcerative colitis and allergic enteropathy. Int Arch Allergy Immunol 108(2): 127–133.

15. Heatley RV, Calcraft BJ, Rhodes J, Owen E, Evans BK (1975) Disodium cromoglycate in the treatment of chronic proctitis. Gut 16: 559–563.

16. Nolte H, Spjeldnaes N, Kruse A, Windelborg B (1990) Histamine release from gut mast cells from patients with inflammatory bowel diseases. Gut 31: 791–794.

17. Lee DM, Friend DS, Gurish MF, Benoist C, Mathis D, et al. (2002) Mast Cells: A Cellular Link Between Autoantibodies and Inflammatory Arthritis. Science 297: 1689–1692.

18. Galli SJ, Tsai M, Piliponsky AM (2008) The development of allergic inflammation. Nature 454: 445–454.

19. Hamid Q, Tulic M (2009) Immunobiology of Asthma. Annual Review of Physiology 71: 489–507.

20. Kalesnikoff J, Galli SJ (2008) New developments in mast cell biology. Nat Immunol 9: 1215–1223.

21. Eaden JA, Abrams KR, Mayberry JF (2001) The risk of colorectal cancer in ulcerative colitis: a meta-analysis. Gut 48(4): 526–535.

22. Gounaris E, Erdman SE, Restaino C, Gurish MF, Friend DS, et al. (2007) Mast cells are an essential hematopoietic component for polyp development. Proceedings of the National Academy of Sciences 104: 19977–19982.

23. Sinnamon MJ, Carter KJ, Sims LP, LaFleur B, Fingleton B, et al. (2008) A protective role of mast cells in intestinal tumorigenesis. Carcinogenesis 29: 880–886.

24. Echtenacher B, Männel DN, Hültner L (1996) Critical protective role of mast cells in a model of acute septic peritonitis. Nature 381: 75–77.

25. Malaviya R, Ikeda T, Ross E, Abraham SN (1996) Mast cell modulation of neutrophil influx and bacterial clearance at sites of infection through TNF-alpha. Nature 381: 77–80.

26. McLachlan JB, Hart JP, Pizzo SV, Shelburne CP, Staats HF, et al. (2003) Mast cell-derived tumor necrosis factor induces hypertrophy of draining lymph nodes during infection. Nat Immunol 4: 1199–1205.

27. Wood JD (2004) Enteric neuroimmunophysiology and pathophysiology. Gastroenterology 127: 635–657.

28. Bischoff S (2009) Physiological and pathophysiological functions of intestinal mast cells. Seminars in Immunopathology 31: 185–205.

29. Suenaert P, Bulteel V, Lemmens L, Noman M, Geypens B, et al. (2002) Anti-tumor necrosis factor treatment restores the gut barrier in Crohn's disease. Am J Gastroenterol 97: 2000–2004.

30. Peeters M, Geypens B, Claus D, Nevens H, Ghoos Y, et al. (1997) Clustering of increased small intestinal permeability in families with Crohn's disease. Gastroenterology 113: 802–807.

31. Söderholm JD, Olaison G, Lindberg E, Hannestad U, Vindels A, et al. (1999) Different intestinal permeability patterns in relatives and spouses of patients with Crohn's disease: an inherited defect in mucosal defence? Gut 44: 96–100.

32. Madsen KL, Malfair D, Gray D, Doyle JS, Jewell LD, et al. (1999) Interleukin-10 gene-deficient mice develop a primary intestinal permeability defect in response to enteric microflora. Inflamm Bowel Dis 5(4): 262–270.

33. Weidner N, Austen KF (1991) Ultrastructural and Immunohistochemical Characterization of Normal Mast Cells at Multiple Body Sites. J Investig Dermatol 96: 26S–31S.

34. Gibson P, Rosella O, Nov R, Young G (1995) Colonic epithelium is diffusely abnormal in ulcerative colitis and colorectal cancer. Gut 36: 857–863.

35. Hollander D, Vadheim CM, Brettholz E, Petersen GM, Delahunty T, et al. (1986) Increased intestinal permeability in patients with Crohn's disease and their relatives. A possible etiologic factor. Ann Intern Med 105(6): 883–885.

36. Gassler N, Rohr C, Schneider A, Kartenbeck J, Bach A, et al. (2001) Inflammatory bowel disease is associated with changes of enterocytic junctions. Am J Physiol Gastrointest Liver Physiol 281: G216–228.

37. Berrozpe G, Timokhina I, Yukl S, Tajima Y, Ono M, et al. (1999) The Wsh, W57, and Ph Kit Expression Mutations Define Tissue-Specific Control Elements Located Between -23 and -154 kb Upstream of Kit. Blood 94: 2658–2666.

38. Nigrovic PA, Gray DHD, Jones T, Hallgren J, Kuo FC, et al. (2008) Genetic Inversion in Mast Cell-Deficient Wsh Mice Interrupts Corin and Manifests as Hematopoietic and Cardiac Aberrancy. Am J Pathol 173: 1693–1701.

39. Berg DJ, Zhang J, Weinstock JV, Ismail HF, Earle KA, et al. (2002) Rapid development of colitis in NSAID-treated IL-10-deficient mice. Gastroenterology 123: 1527–1542.

40. Wolters PJ, Clair JM-S, Lewis CC, Villalta SA, Baluk P, et al. (2005) Tissue-selective mast cell reconstitution and differential lung gene expression in mast cell-deficient Kit^{W-sh}/Kit^{W-sh} sash mice. Clinical & Experimental Allergy 35: 82–88.

41. Hale LP, Perera D, Gottfried MR, Maggio-Price L, Srinivasan S, et al. (2007) Neonatal Co-Infection with Helicobacter Species Markedly Accelerates the Development of Inflammation-Associated Colonic Neoplasia in IL-10$^{-/-}$ Mice. Helicobacter 12: 598–604.

42. Shen Z, Fox JG, Dewhirst FE, Paster BJ, Foltz CJ, et al. (1997) Helicobacter rodentium sp. nov., a urease-negative Helicobacter species isolated from laboratory mice. Int J Syst Bacteriol 47: 627–634.

43. Hale LP, Greer PK, Trinh CT, Gottfried MR (2005) Treatment with oral bromelain decreases colonic inflammation in the IL-10-deficient murine model of inflammatory bowel disease. Clinical Immunology 116: 135–142.

44. Burich A, Hershberg R, Waggie K, Zeng W, Brabb T, et al. (2001) Helicobacter-induced inflammatory bowel disease in IL-10- and T cell-deficient mice. Am J Physiol Gastrointest Liver Physiol 281: G764–778.

45. Boivin GP, Washington K, Yang K, Ward JM, Pretlow TP, et al. (2003) Pathology of mouse models of intestinal cancer: Consensus report and recommendations. Gastroenterology 124: 762–777.

46. Cardoso CR, Teixeira G, Provinciatto PR, Godoi DF, Ferreira BR, et al. (2008) Modulation of mucosal immunity in a murine model of food-induced intestinal inflammation. Clinical & Experimental Allergy 38: 338–349.

47. Shin J-S, Shelburne CP, Jin C, LeFurgey EA, Abraham SN (2006) Harboring of Particulate Allergens within Secretory Compartments by Mast Cells following IgE/Fc{epsilon}RI-Lipid Raft-Mediated Phagocytosis. J Immunol 177: 5791–5800.

48. Nakamura J, Takada S, Ueda S, Hamaura T, Yamamoto A, et al. (1985) Assessment of pharmaceutical excipient-induced gastrointestinal mucosal damage in rats in vivo by measuring the permeation of phenolsulfonphthalein. Chem Pharm Bull 33(8): 3527–3529.

12

Associations between Genetic Polymorphisms in *IL-33, IL1R1* and Risk for Inflammatory Bowel Disease

Anna Latiano[1]*, **Orazio Palmieri**[1], **Luca Pastorelli**[2,8], **Maurizio Vecchi**[2,8], **Theresa T. Pizarro**[3], **Fabrizio Bossa**[1], **Giuseppe Merla**[4], **Bartolomeo Augello**[4], **Tiziana Latiano**[1], **Giuseppe Corritore**[1], **Alessia Settesoldi**[5], **Maria Rosa Valvano**[1], **Renata D'Incà**[6], **Laura Stronati**[7], **Vito Annese**[5], **Angelo Andriulli**[1]

1 Division of Gastroenterology, IRCCS 'Casa Sollievo della Sofferenza', San Giovanni Rotondo, Italy, 2 Gastroenterology and Gastrointestinal Endoscopy Unit, IRCCS Policlinico San Donato, San Donato Milanese, Italy, 3 Department of Pathology, Case Western Reserve University School of Medicine, Cleveland, Ohio, United States of America, 4 Medical Genetic Unit, IRCCS 'Casa Sollievo della Sofferenza', San Giovanni Rotondo, Italy, 5 Gastroenterology Unit, AOU Careggi Hospital, Florence, Italy, 6 Department of Surgical and Gastroenterological Sciences, University of Padua, Padua, Italy, 7 Department of Radiobiology and Human Health, Italian National Agency for New Technologies, Energy and Sustainable Economic Development (ENEA), Rome, Italy, 8 Department of Medical and Surgical Sciences, University of Milan, Milan, Italy

Abstract

Background: Recent evidence suggests that the IL-33/IL1RL1 axis plays a critical role in several autoimmune and inflammatory disorders; however, its mechanistic role in inflammatory bowel disease (IBD) has not been clearly defined. We investigated the contribution of *IL-33* and *IL1RL1* polymorphisms to IBD risk, and possible correlations with phenotype in an Italian cohort of adult and pediatric patients.

Methods: We evaluated the association of six SNPs in *IL-33* and *IL1RL1* genes, in 805 Crohn's disease (CD), 816 ulcerative colitis (UC), and 752 controls, using Taqman. IL-33 and IL1RL1 mRNA expression was also analyzed.

Results: Significant allele and genotype associations with *IL-33* rs3939286 were found in CD ($P = 0.004$; $P = 0.035$) and UC patients ($P = 0.002$; $P = 0.038$). After stratifying the cohort for age at diagnosis, the differences remained significant only in the IBD adult-onset. Significant associations were also obtained in CD patients with two *IL1RL1* polymorphisms (rs13015714 and rs2058660, $P < 0.015$). By combining homo- and heterozygous carriers of the rs13015714 risk allele, differences were still significant for both CD adult- and pediatric-onset. Upon genotype-phenotype evaluation, an increased frequency of extensive colitis in adult UC ($P = 0.019$) and in steroid-responsive pediatric patients ($P = 0.024$) carrying the *IL-33* rs3939286 risk genotype, was observed. mRNA expression of *IL-33* and *IL1RL1* in inflamed IBD biopsy samples was significantly increased.

Conclusions: Common *IL-33* and *IL1RL1* polymorphisms contribute to the risk of IBD in an Italian cohort of adult and pediatric patients, with some influence on sub-phenotypes.

Editor: Mathias Chamaillard, INSERM, France

Funding: This work was supported by the Italian Ministry of the Health grants: RC1102GA33, RC1102GA34, RC1202GA38 and GR-2008-1144485. The funders had no role in study design, data collection and analysis, decision to publish, or preparation of the manuscript.

Competing Interests: The authors have declared that no competing interests exist.

* E-mail: a.latiano@operapadrepio.it

Introduction

Intestinal mucosal inflammation is a highly regulated process, with a wide repertoire of pro- and anti-inflammatory molecules mediating distinct phases of gut immune responses. Pathologic, chronic intestinal inflammation may arise from an imbalance between different players within this process. As such, the onset and perpetuation of gut inflammation, characterizing inflammatory bowel diseases (IBD), namely Crohn's disease (CD) and ulcerative colitis (UC), are triggered by constitutive dysregulation of cytokine production [1]. Indeed, a wealth of data indicates the importance of genetic background in regulating the cytokine network in IBD; in fact, polymorphisms of cytokine/cytokine receptor genes have been shown to be associated with the

development of IBD [2,3,4]. For instance, several studies point out the associations of IBD with genetic polymorphisms involved in the signaling pathway of interleukin (IL)-1 family members, such as IL-1β [5], IL-1 receptor antagonist [6], and IL-18 [7,8,9].

IL-33 is a newly characterized cytokine belonging to the IL-1 family with the ability to induce Th2 cytokine production [10] and enhance both Th1 and Th2 [11], as well as Th17 immune responses [12,13] IL-33's effects are mediated through the binding of its receptor, IL-1 receptor like 1 (IL1RL1) or T1/ST2, and co-receptor, the IL-1 receptor accessory protein (IL1RAcP), both belonging to the Toll/IL-1 receptor (TIR) superfamily [14]. Several lines of evidence demonstrate the pathogenic role of IL-33 in numerous immune and inflammatory diseases, such as asthma [15], rheumatoid arthritis [12], multiple sclerosis [16] and

Table 1. Clinical and demographic characteristics of the study population.

	CD n=805		UC n=816	
Gender				
F	321	40%	344	42%
M	484	60%	472	58%
Duration of follow-up (yr)				
mean ± SD	8±7		9±7	
median ± SD	6 (1–37)		7 (1–41)	
Age at diagnosis (yr)				
mean ± SD	30±14		32±16	
median ± SD	28 (1–80)		30 (1–75)	
Early onset (<19 yrs)	155	20%	148	19%
Adult (≥19 yrs)	622	80%	640	81%
Missing	28		28	
≤16 (A1)	130	17%	125	16%
17–40 (A2)	483	62%	456	58%
>40 (A3)	164	21%	207	26%
Missing	28		28	
Disease localization CD, n				
Ileum (L1± L4)	256	36%		
Colon (L2± L4)	171	24%		
Ileo-colon (L3± L4)	286	40%		
Upper GI (L4)	6	1%		
Missing	86			
Disease extent UC, n				
Rectum (E1)			95	12%
Left colon (E2)			374	47%
Pancolitis (E3)			322	41%
Missing			25	
Disease behavior CD, n				
Inflammatory	475	61%		
Stricturing	209	27%		
Penetrating	94	12%		
Missing	27			
Perianal desease y/n	143/630	18%	20/765	3%
Missing	32		31	
Extra-intestinal manifestations y/n	327/446	42%	194/554	26%
Missing	32		68	
Family history of IBD y/n	55/725	7%	64/729	8%
Missing	25		23	
Smoking history				
Yes	229	30%	110	14%
No	402	53%	444	57%
Ex	127	17%	222	29%
Missing	47		40	
Surgery y/n	258/527	33%	77/711	10%
Missing	20		28	
Steroids y/n	510/295	63%	514/302	63%
*Refractory	73	14%	71	14%
*Responder+dependent	433	86%	438	86%

Table 1. Cont.

	CD n=805		UC n=816	
IMS (AZT/6MP, CICLO, MTX)				
Yes	302	38%	217	27%
No	503	62%	599	73%
Non Responder	17	15%	3	23%
Responder	96	85%	10	77%

*Steroids_Resp-DepvsRefrac.
CD: Crohn's disease, UC: ulcerative colitis, IMS: immunosuppressors.

anaphylaxis [17]. In addition, IL-33 may have dichotomous functions during inflammation, as it has been shown to be protective in a few inflammatory-related conditions, including atherosclerosis [18] and hepatitis [19]. Moreover, genetic dysregulation of the IL-33/IL1RL1 axis appears to be involved in conferring predisposition to several multifactorial diseases, such as Alzheimer's disease [20], asthma [21,22,23], nasal polyposis [24], allergic rhinitis [25], and atopic dermatitis [26].

Recently, several independent researchers have described marked alterations of IL-33 and IL1RL1 expression in IBD [27,28,29,30,31]. These studies, although focusing on different aspects, consistently demonstrated the upregulation of IL-33 in the inflamed colonic mucosa of IBD patients, with a greater prevalence in UC. Despite the aforementioned evidence suggesting involvement of the IL-33/IL1RL1 axis in the pathologic events leading to the development of IBD, no definitive data regarding the precise role of IL-33 during intestinal inflammation are available.

In the present study we aimed to establish the role of *IL-33* and *IL1RL1* genes in the risk of developing IBD in a well-characterized Italian cohort of adult and early onset IBD patients (805 CD and 816 UC), either by genotyping or by functional studies. Herein, we describe for the first time, the association between the rs3939286 *IL-33* polymorphism with both UC and CD, and between variants of *IL1RL1* with CD. Of note, the aforementioned SNP was also associated with specific clinical UC sub-phenotypes. Taken together, our data further suggest the involvement of IL-33 in the pathogenesis of IBD and provide insight into its possible role in the clinical features of chronic intestinal inflammation.

Materials and Methods

Ethics Statement

The study was approved by the Ethical Committee of "Casa Sollievo della Sofferenza" Hospital, San Giovanni Rotondo, and a voluntary written informed consent was obtained from all adult participants and related parents of patients under 19 years of age.

Patient Recruitment

Demographic and clinical of the Italian IBD patients and controls are shown in **Table 1**. The study group ($n = 2373$) consisted of 805 CD patients, 816 UC patients, and 752 healthy individuals as controls. 303 IBD patients had the initial diagnosis of IBD before their 19th year (155 CD and 148 UC).

Patients with diagnosis of CD or UC were included in the study based on clinical, endoscopic, and histologic findings according to the Montreal Classification [32]. All individuals were enrolled prospectively from the Gastroenterology Unit at the IRCCS "Casa Sollievo della Sofferenza" Hospital, San Giovanni Rotondo, from centers of the Italian Group of IBD (IG-IBD), and from pediatric centers of the Italian Society of Pediatric Gastroenterology, Hepatology and Nutrition (SIGENP). Clinical data for IBD patients were obtained retrospectively from clinical files. The control group consisted of blood donors and healthy individuals without history of immune-mediated diseases.

Biopsy Collection

Overall, 29 patients with active IBD, including 15 CD and 14 UC, were used in the present study. Mucosal colonic biopsies were obtained from adult patients undergoing routine colonoscopy at the IRCCS "Casa Sollievo della Sofferenza" Hospital, San Giovanni Rotondo. The activity of disease was evaluated by the Harvey-Bradshaw score (HBI) for CD, and the Mayo score for UC. After obtaining written informed consent, patients with an HBI >4 and a Mayo score >3 were enrolled. Biopsies were taken from inflamed and adjacent non-inflamed regions (10–15 cm distant from pathologic areas). Unaffected areas were defined as mucosal regions without any macroscopic/endoscopic signs of inflammation (e.g., discoloration, hemorrhagic appearance, edema, ulceration, or mucinous/fibrinous coating).

Selection of Tagging Single Nucleotide Polymorphisms (tSNPs) and Genotyping

The selection of SNPs for the present study was made considering previous association studies and the position of the SNPs in the IL-33 and IL1RL1 genes. IL-33 and IL1RL1 tSNPs were selected using genotypic data from the Caucasian (CEU) Phase II study, available from the HapMap project (http://www.hapmap.org) [33]. SNPs were identified using Haploview software version 4.2 [34] based on solid spine of linkage disequilibrium (LD) (r^2>0.8, haplotype frequency >5%, minor allele frequency >10%).

This process identified three SNPs for the IL-33 gene: rs3939286, rs7025417 and rs7044343 (**Figure S1**). The rs3939286 SNP was reported to be associated with nasal polyposis [24] and asthma [21]; the rs7025417 was chosen to tag haplotype block 2; the rs7044343 was selected based on its association with a decreased risk of developing Alzheimer's disease [20] and in high LD (r^2>0.8) with the tag SNP rs10975514 of the block 3. By contrast, the significant SNP identified in the CD and UC genome-wide meta-analysis [35,36,37] was rs10758669, located at 4.97 Mb on chromosome 9p24 encompassing the JAK2 gene, with a distance of 1.23 Mb from the selected rs3939286 (6.20 Mb) (**Figure S2**). The three selected SNPs for the IL1RL1 gene on chromosome 2q12 were rs2058660, rs2310173, and rs13015714 (**Figure S3, Figure S4**). The rs2058660 has already been found to be associated with CD [35]; and the rs2310173 was reported to be associated with UC [36]. In addition, the rs13015714 was found to be significantly associated with an increased risk for celiac disease (2q11–12, IL18RAP) [38].

Genomic DNA was extracted from whole blood samples by a standard non-enzymatic method, using the QIAamp DNA Blood Maxi Kit (Qiagen GmbH, Hilden, Germany). Samples were genotyped for the SNPs rs3939286, rs7025417, rs7044343, rs2058660, rs2310173, and rs13015714 using 5′exonuclease TaqMan genotyping assays on an ABI Prism 7900 Real-Time polymerase chain reaction (PCR) System, according to manufacturer's instructions (Applied Biosystems, Foster City, CA). The genotyping and data management were performed at the Research Laboratory of Gastroenterology Unit of the IRCCS 'Casa Sollievo della Sofferenza' Hospital, San Giovanni Rotondo, Italy.

IL-33 and IL1RL1 mRNA Quantification

Total RNA was extracted from biopsies using Trizol (Invitrogen, Paisley, UK) or RNeasy Mini Kit (Qiagen) according to the manufacturer's instructions. The amount of RNA was measured by NanoDrop ND-1000 spectrophotometer (NanoDrop Technologies Wilmington, Delaware, USA). The integrity and quality of isolated RNA was determined by Agilent Bioanalyzer 2100 (http://www.chem.agilent.com). In order to preserve the transcriptional profile of tissue specimens, the biopsies were rapidly transferred to RNAlater (Qiagen, Valencia, CA, USA) or snap-frozen in liquid nitrogen and stored until RNA extraction.

Microarray Data Analysis

Total RNA from biopsy specimens (29 IBD patients) was analyzed with the GeneChip Human Gene 1.0 ST Array System (www.affymetrix.com), which interrogates 28,869 well-annotated genes by using an average of 26 probes per gene. Each sample was processed according to the manufacturer's instructions. The Affymetrix raw data (.CEL file) were generated using the Affymetrix GeneChip Scanner 3000 7G and analyzed using Partek Genomic Suite Software v. 6.6 (Partek Inc., St. Louis, MO). Briefly, raw intensity values were imported by setting up robust multiarray analysis (RMA) background correction, quantile normalization, and log transformation. Principle component analysis (PCA) was performed as it is an excellent method for visualizing high-dimensional data and identifies outlier samples; mixed model ANOVA was performed in order to generate a comprehensive list of differentially-expressed genes by using a cutoff of P<0.05 for significance of gene-level expression.

For the purpose of this study, we selected the microarray data from all performed comparative analyses for the probe sets encoding the IL-33 and IL1RL1 genes.

Statistical Analysis

Statistical analysis was performed using SPSS software version 14.0 (SPSS, Chicago, IL, USA) and Haploview Software version 4.1 (http://www.broad.mit.edu/personal/mpg/haploview). The genotype frequencies for all investigated polymorphisms were tested for consistency with the Hardy-Weinberg equilibrium. Allelic and genotypic associations of SNPs were evaluated by Pearson's χ^2 test (or Fisher's when appropriate) followed by odds ratio and 95% CI. P-values of less than 0.05 were considered significant. Linkage disequilibrium between markers, haplotype structures and haplotype association analyses were also performed. Univariate and logistic regression analyses, on forward stepwise selection procedures, were carried out to correlate various clinical parameters with genotypes and to study pairwise interactions between SNPs of different genes using the number of risk alleles as predictor variables.

Results

Case–control Study

The allele and genotype frequencies of the six IL-33/IL1RL1 SNPs (IL-33: rs3939286, rs7025417, rs7044343; IL1RL1: rs2058660, rs2310173, rs13015714) were in accordance with the predicted Hardy-Weinberg equilibrium in all subgroups (CD, UC, and controls) (P>0.05).

The results for the whole study population are shown in **Tables 2,3**.

Association between IL-33 Polymorphisms and IBD

The rs3939286 variant of the IL-33 gene is associated with adult CD and UC patients. A significant allele and genotype association of SNP rs3939286 with CD [$P=0.004$, OR 1.27 (1.07–1.50); $P=0.035$, OR 1.24 (1.01–1.53), respectively] and with UC [$P=0.002$, OR 1.29 (1.09–1.52); $P=0.038$, OR 1.24 (1.01–1.52), respectively] was observed. After stratifying the CD and UC cohorts in different subgroups according to the age at diagnosis (<19 and ≥19 years), the distribution of allele and genotype frequencies of CD patients [$P=0.006$, OR 1.28 (1.07–1.53); $P=0.029$, OR 1.27 (1.02–1.58), respectively], and allelic frequencies of UC patients [$P=0.002$, OR 1.30 (1.09–1.56)], in comparison to that of control subjects, remained significant only for the adult population (**Tables 2,3**). All other *IL-33* SNPs investigated in both diseases did not show any significant differences in the allele and genotype frequencies in adult- and early-onset IBD.

Association between *IL1RL1* Polymorphisms and IBD

The rs13015714 and rs2058660 variants of the *IL1RL1* gene are associated with CD patients. A significant difference in allele and genotype frequencies of the rs13015714 SNP in CD population [$P=0.015$, OR 1.23 (1.04–1.46); $P=0.008$, OR 1.32 (1.07–1.62), respectively], adult-onset patients [$P=0.040$, OR 1.21 (1.00–1.45; $P=0.039$, OR 1.26 (1.01–1.57), respectively], and early-onset patients [$P=0.021$, OR 1.51 (1.06–2.16): genotype frequency], compared with controls, was observed. Analysis of frequency distribution of the rs2058660 variant revealed significant association with CD patients compared to controls [allelic $P=0.015$, OR 1.23 (1.04–1.46); genotypic $P=0.015$, OR 1.29 (1.05–1.58)]. The same genotype was also slightly increased in early-onset CD patients [$P=0.046$, OR 1.43 (1.00–2.03)], with a similar trend, not reaching statistical significance, in adult patients. Similarly, allele frequency was significantly different in CD adult patients [$P=3.45\times10^{-2}$, OR 1.21 (1.01–1.45)] (**Table 2**). No association was found between the *IL1RL1* polymorphisms and the risk of UC disease. However, at recessive model of inheritance, a significant decreased frequency of the rs230173 *IL1RL1* risk genotype [$P=0.033$, OR 0,77 (0.61–0.98)] was found compared with healthy controls. This association remained significant in the adult subgroup [$P=0.023$, OR 0,74 (0.58–0.96)] (**Table 3**).

Association between *IL-33* and *IL1RL1* Polymorphisms and Disease Phenotype

Analysis of genotype-phenotype was performed, interrogating, in each patient, the following clinical features: gender, age at diagnosis, IBD family history, smoking habit, severity and disease localization, presence of perianal fistulas, extraintestinal manifestations, previous abdominal surgery, use and response to medical therapy (mesalamine, corticosteroids, immunosuppressive drugs, azathioprine, 6-mercaptopurine, methotrexate, cyclosporine and infliximab). Patients were classified as responder or non-responder on the basis of a review of medical records as previously described [39].

An increased frequency of extensive colitis (E3vsE1) was observed in UC adult patients carrying the *IL-33* rs3939286 risk genotypes (AG+AA) (47% vs. 33%; $P=0.019$) compared with those carrying the GG wild-type genotype. Moreover, an increased frequency of the risk genotype in steroid-responsive, early-onset UC patients was also demonstrated (44% vs. 12%; $P=0.024$) (**Table 4**).

No other significant correlations of *IL-33* and *IL1RL1* genotypes with either clinical features of patients with UC or efficacy of medical therapy were found. In patients with CD, no significant association of either *IL-33* or *IL1RL1* polymorphisms with any clinical characteristics was demonstrated in both adult- and early-onset patient subgroups.

Table 2. Association of *IL33* and *IL1RL1* genes markers with Crohn's disease (CD); case-control study.

	Genotypes frequencies								Alleles frequencies								
	Case-Controls frequencies	Total CD		Adult CD		Early onset CD			Total CD		Adult CD		Early onset CD	
rs number		P value	OR (95% CI)	P value	OR (95% CI)	P value	OR (95% CI)		P value	OR (95% CI)	P value	OR (95% CI)	P value	OR (95% CI)
IL-33 Gene														
rs3939286	0.26–0.22	**0.035**	1.24 (1.01–1.53)	**0.029**	1.27 (1.02–1.58)	0.843	1.03 (0.72–1.48)		**0.004**	(1.27 1.07–1.50)	**0.006**	1.28 (1.07–1.53)	0.390	1.13 (0.84–1.52)
rs7025417	0.14–0.15	0.706	0.95 (0.74–1.21)	0.667	0.94 (0.73–1.23)	0.764	0.93 (0.62–1.43)		0.474	0.92 (0.7–1.17)	0.503	0.92 (0.74–1.14)	0.463	0.86 (0.59–1.27)
rs7044343	0.40–0.42	0.224	0.87 (0.71–1.08)	0.100	0.82 (0.66–1.04)	0.795	1.05 (0.72–1.52)		0.278	0.91 (0.78–1.06)	0.234	0.91 (0.79–1.06)	0.705	0.95 (0.74–1.22)
IL1RL1 Gene														
rs13015714	0.25–0.22	**0.008**	1.32 (1.07–1.62)	**0.039**	1.26 (1.01–1.57)	**0.021**	1.51 (1.06–2.16)		**0.015**	1.23 (1.04–1.46)	**0.040**	1.21 (1.00–1.45)	0.081	1.29 (0.96–1.72)
rs2058660	0.25–0.21	**0.015**	1.29 (1.05–1.58)	0.053	1.24 (0.99–1.54)	**0.046**	1.43 (1.00–2.03)		**0.015**	1.23 (1.04–1.46)	**0.034**	1.21 (1.01–1.45)	0.113	1.26 (0.94–1.68)
rs2310173	0.48–0.47	0.794	0.96 (0.75–1.23)	0.822	0.97 (0.74–1.26)	0.701	0.92 (0.60–1.40)		0.810	0.98 (0.85–1.13)	0.771	0.97 (0.84–1.13)	0.693	0.99 (0.77–1.27)

P value for genotype frequencies was obtained testing for differences between homo- and heterozygous carriers of risk allele *vs* non-carriers of risk allele. OR: corresponding odds ratio and 95% confidence intervals (95%CI). Significant P values (<0.05) are depicted in bold.

Table 3. Association of *IL-33* and *IL1RL1* genes markers with ulcerative colitis (UC); case-control study.

rs number	Case-Controls frequencies	Genotipes frequencies						Alleles frequencies					
		Total UC		Adult UC		Early onset UC		Total UC		Adult UC		Early onset UC	
		P value	OR (95% CI)	P value	OR (95% CI)	P value	OR (95% CI)	P value	OR (95% CI)	P value	OR (95% CI)	P value	OR (95% CI)
IL-33 Gene													
rs3939286	0.27-0.22	**0.038**	1.24 (1.012-1.52)	0.063	1.22 (0.98-1.52)	0.131	1.32 (0.92-1.89)	**0.002**	1.29 (1.09-1.52)	**0.002**	1.30 (1.09-1.56)	0.139	1.24 (0.93-1.67)
rs7025417	0.14-0.15	0.516	0.92(0.72-1.17)	0.304	0.87 (0.67-1.13)	0.580	1.12 (0.74-1.69)	0.410	0.91 (0.73-1.13)	0.260	0.87 (0.69-1.10)	0.724	1.06 (0.74-1.53)
rs7044343	0.40-0.42	0.055	0.81 (0.66-1.00)	0.062	0.81 (0.64-1.01)	0.393	0.85 (0.58-1.23)	0.352	0.93 (0.80-1.07)	0.434	0.94 (080-109)	0.698	0.95 (0.73-1.22)
IL1RL1 Gene													
rs13015714	0.22-0.22	0.239	1.13 (0.92-1.39)	0.245	1.14 (0.91-1.42)	0.172	1.28 (0.89-1.85)	0.675	1.03 (0.87-1.23)	0.714	1.03 (0.86-1.24)	0.250	1.19 (0.88-1.60)
rs2058660	0.22-0.21	0.140	1.16 (0.95-1.43)	0.117	1.19 (0.95-1.48)	0.293	1.21 (0.84-1.74)	0.426	1.07 (0.90-1.27)	0.411	1.07 (0.89-1.29)	0.330	1.16 (0.86-1.56)
rs2310173*	0.49-0.47	0.896	0.98 (0.78-1.23)	0.948	0.99 (0.78-1.26)	0.901	1.02 (0.68-1.53)	0.233	1.09 (0.94-1.25)	0.186	1.10 (0.95-1.28)	0.329	1.13 (0.88-1.45)
rs2310173*	(AA+Aavsaa)	**0.033**	0.77 (0.61-0.98)	**0.023**	0.74 (0.58-0.96)	0.125	0.72 (0.48-1.09)	0.233	0.91 (0.79-1.05)	0.186	0.90 (0.77-1.05)	0.329	0.88 (0.68-1.13)

P value for genotype frequencies was obtained testing for differences between homo- and heterozygous carriers of risk allele (Aa+aa) vs non-carriers of risk allele (AA). A = major allele; a = minor allele. OR: corresponding odds ratio and 95% confidence intervals (95%CI). Significant P values (<0.05) are depicted in bold.

IL-33 and *IL1RL1* Haplotype Analysis

No significant associations between either *IL-33* or *IL1RL1* haplotypes and disease risk was observed (**Table S1**).

IL-33 and *IL1RL1* Expression

IL-33 and IL1RL1 mRNA levels in colonic IBD biopsy samples revealed significant differences in UC and CD (**Figure S5**). In CD patients, IL-33 mRNA transcripts were 1.81-fold significantly increased in inflamed versus non-inflamed mucosa ($P = 0.0033$, FDR = 0.05); in contrast, no significant change in IL1RL1 mRNA expression was found. In UC patients, IL-33 and IL1RL1 mRNA levels showed a significant increase (1.69 fold, $P = 0.0012$, FDR = 0.03; 1.40-fold, $P = 0.0009$, FDR = 0.02, respectively) in inflamed compared to non-inflamed areas.

When comparing the allele dosage with mRNA expression profiles, no differences in IL-33 and IL1RL1 mRNA levels were found (data not shown).

Discussion

Although the precise etiology remains unknown, it is thought that IBD result from a dysregulated and aberrant immune response to intestinal flora in the context of a genetic predisposition. Moreover, an imbalance of pro- and anti-inflammatory mediators is a critical factor in IBD pathogenesis [40]. Cytokines are key regulators of the intestinal immune system and are known to participate in the disruption of the so-called normal state of controlled inflammation. Early, innate-type cytokines, primarily secreted by the intestinal epithelium as well as activated antigen presenting cells, including dendritic cells and macrophages, actively regulate the inflammatory response in UC and CD. These innate-type cytokines include members of the IL-1 family and have the ability to trigger and differentiate T cells, activating downstream adaptive immune responses. T cell dysregulation in IBD is characterized by aberrant clearance of overreactive and autoreactive cells and an imbalance of Treg/Th1, Th2 and Th17 cell populations. The lack of appropriate regulation from T cells, and/or an over-reactive response from effector T cells, contributes to the development and exacerbation of IBD [41].

Interleukin-33, a novel member of the IL-1 cytokine family [10], has been shown to elicit a Th2- like cytokine response in immunocompetent cells through binding and activation of the interleukin 1 receptor-like 1 [42]. The IL-33/IL1RL1 pathway plays an important role in host defense and in autoimmune, allergic, and chronic inflammatory disorders, such as asthma, dermatitis, rhinitis, arthritis, diabetes mellitus, atherosclerosis, and Alzheimer's disease [43]. Most recently, IL-33 has been associated with allergic airway inflammation and arthritis in experimental animal models [13,44]. Interestingly, blocking IL1RL1 receptor signaling has been shown to prevent arthritis development and airway inflammation [45,15].

The IL-33/IL1RL1 signaling axis has been implicated in IBD in several studies reporting IL1RL1 and IL-33 protein and mRNA expression in IBD patients [28]. An up-regulation of IL-33 in human biopsy specimens, particularly from active UC patients compared to controls was observed [27,28,29], identifying epithelial cells, myofibroblasts and macrophages as primary sources of IL-33 within the inflamed tissue of IBD patients. Similarly, an increase in IL1RL1 levels in the gut, mainly associated with the active state of UC, has been described, together with elevated circulating levels of IL1RL1 and IL-33 in IBD patients [28,29]; *Pastorelli et al.* also showed that anti-TNF therapy modulated IL1RL1 and IL-33 serum levels, increasing the

Table 4. Association between *IL-33* and rs3939286 polymorphism and disease phenotype.

Gene	SNP	Disease	Phenotype		No. of patients GG	No. of patients AG+AA	P value	OR (95% CI)
IL-33	rs3939286	UC adult	Localization (E3 vs E1)	Extensive UC (E3)	125 (53%)	112 (47%)	0.019	1.86 (1.10–3.14)
				Proctitis (E1)	56 (67%)	27 (33%)		
		UC early onset	Steroids	No	12 (32%)	26 (68%)	0.001	3.47 (1.57–7.64)
				Yes	64 (62%)	40 (38%)		
			Steroids	Refractory	14 (88%)	2 (12%)	0.024	5.32 (1.14–24.83)
				Responder+Dependent	50 (56%)	38 (44%)		

soluble isoform of IL1RL1, making more decoy receptors available, and reducing circulating IL-33 [29].

The research efforts of the IBD International Genetic Consortium, by means of hypothesis-free genome wide association studies (GWAs) [35,36,46] and Immunochip project [47], have led to the identification of 163 genomic loci. The majority of loci (67%) confer susceptibility to both Crohn's disease and ulcerative colitis, with only 30 loci thought to be specific for Crohn's disease and 23 specific for ulcerative colitis. For almost all of these new loci, the exact gene and/or causal variants remain to be determined. However, GWAs do not have perfect coverage, as about 30% of the common variants are not included on GWAs arrays, leaving gaps that need to be filled by targeted association studies. Moreover, the genetic susceptibility risk explained by GWAs loci to date, is not much higher than 20%, compared with an estimated overall genetic risk of about 40% (based on previous concordance studies in twins) [34,48]. Of particular relevance to the present study, IBD GWAs have identified genes related to innate immunity as a critical component in the pathogenesis of IBD [49–55]. In fact, several recent studies have attempted to document the genetic overlap between IBD and various auto-immune diseases, with approximately 51 IBD genes identified overlapping 23 different diseases, such as multiple sclerosis, rheumatoid arthritis, ankylosing spondylitis, psoriasis, asthma, SLE, and celiac disease [56], yielding significant insight into disease pathogenesis.

Thus, identification of the role of *IL-33* and *IL1RL1* in IBD susceptibility is in line with the recent concept of shared genetic determinants for clinically distinct disorders [57], and notwithstanding the number of IBD susceptibility genes that has increased dramatically over the last several years, genes associated with the IL-33 signaling pathway have not been reported to date. In the International IBD Genetics Consortium meta-analysis for CD and UC, no associated SNPs in *IL-33* were reported, while the rs10758669 variant (position 4971602) of *JAK2* was identified as a CD and UC risk locus (CD_{meta} $P=1.00\times10^{-13}$, UC_{meta} $P=8.52\times10^{-13}$) [36]. Our selected SNPs in *IL-33* are not in LD with the reported rs10758669 variant (**Figure S2**). Although the selected SNPs have not been reported in the meta-analysis, the significant association with the rs3939286 variant and both CD and UC, particularly in the adult population ($P=0.006$ and $P=0.002$, respectively), implicates *IL-33* as a novel IBD susceptibility gene. Interestingly, this genetic association was also found with the UC phenotype. Adult UC patient carriers of the rs3939286 variant were at a higher risk of developing extensive colitis compared to homozygous wild-type carriers (OR = 1.86). Moreover, early-onset patient carriers of the *IL33* rs3939286 risk

genotype were significantly more responsive to steroids (44%) compared with noncarriers (12%) (OR = 5.32).

Furthermore, we were able to confirm high levels of IL-33 expressed in the inflamed mucosa of both UC and CD patients, although the risk alleles did not influence the mRNA transcript levels. These data confirm that IL-33 mRNA expression is increased in UC and CD locally, within the colonic mucosa, and are indication of active inflammation.

At present, despite the wealth of data indicating the prominent alterations of IL-33/IL1RL1 expression in the inflamed mucosa of IBD patients, no definitive data have demonstrated the precise role of this axis during gut inflammatory conditions. Interestingly, experimental data obtained using different animal models of intestinal inflammation have produced conflicting results. In fact, IL-33 was shown to potently increase the production of pro-inflammatory cytokines, such as IL-5, IL-6 and IL-17, in SAMP1/YitFc mice, a mixed Th1/Th2 spontaneous model of chronic enteritis [30], whereas exogenous administration of IL-33 showed a protective effect in trinitrobenzene sulfonic acid (TNBS)-induced colitis, a chemically-induced model of colonic inflammation, mostly driven by a Th1 immune response [58]. In addition, three different groups demonstrated dichotomous functions of IL-33 in the setting of acute dextran sodium sulphate (DSS)-induced colitis [59–61]. Following epithelial barrier disruption caused by DSS administration, IL-33 appeared to worsen colitis, inducing the recruitment of neutrophils to the site of inflammation [59–61], whereas, during the recovery phase, IL-33 showed a prominent effect in promoting mucosal healing [59,61] and inducing goblet cell proliferation [60], eventually restoring epithelial barrier function.

The dichotomous role of the IL-33/IL1RL1 axis within the context of chronic intestinal inflammation has been previously proposed [62] and may explain the results obtained within the present study regarding the association of the rs3939286 polymorphism of *IL-33* with IBD and with specific UC phenotypes. The rs3939286 polymorphism has been previously shown to be associated with the development of Th2-driven pathologic conditions, such as nasal polyposis, asthma and systemic eosinophilia [21,22]. As such, it is likely that presence of the rs3939286 polymorphism confers greater bioactivity to IL-33, which is consistent with the exaggerated inflammatory response that characterizes IBD. Moreover, during the onset of UC, a disease mainly dominated by Th2 cytokines, the presence of the rs3939286 variant further promotes a pathogenic Th2 response and may push the phenotype towards a more extensive disease, such as pancolitis. On the other hand, during short term anti-inflammatory treatment, as in the case of steroid treatment, the production of pro-inflammatory cytokines is dampened; in this setting, the increased bioactivity of IL-33 may enhance the healing of mucosal damage, improving the restoration of epithelial barrier integrity, and favor the achievement of disease remission. Again, this may be consistent with the association of the rs3939286 polymorphism to a steroid responsive phenotype, as indicated by our results.

IL-33 exerts its biologic effects through binding of its receptor, the formerly orphaned receptor IL1RL1, also called T1 or ST2 [10]. Two different splice variants of ST2 have been described [63], leading to the synthesis of two different proteins: ST2L, a transmembrane receptor that activates downstream signaling upon IL-33 recognition, and sST2, a soluble molecule that likely serves as a decoy receptor, ultimately blocking IL-33's biologic effects. The *IL1RL1* gene is located on chromosome 2q12 and a number of IL1 family members, namely IL1R2, IL1R1, IL1RL2, IL18 receptor 1 (IL18R1), and IL18 receptor accessory protein (IL18RAP) reside in the immediate proximity of the *IL1RL1* gene. Interestingly, the *IL18RAP* gene was also recently shown to be associated with celiac disease, a chronic inflammatory disease of the small intestine with autoimmune features [38,64]. The region spans about 300 kb and is in high linkage disequilibrium. There is evidence for the involvement of genes surrounding *IL1RL1* in human and experimental disease, and therefore the causal locus responsible for genetic association signals from this region is difficult to determine. In fact, it is unclear at present whether the CD-associated (rs2058660) and UC-associated (rs2310173) SNPs in these regions tag two separate loci or one locus.

Our results demonstrate a significant difference in genotype frequencies of the rs2058660 (P = 0.015) and rs13015714 (P = 0.008) SNPs in the *IL1RL1* gene between CD patients and controls. The differences were still significant for the rs13015714 risk allele for both adult- (P = 0.039) and early-onset disease (P = 0.021). In addition, no significant changes in IL1RL1 mRNA expression levels were found in CD biopsy samples; conversely, a significant increase in IL1L1 mRNA transcripts from UC inflamed biopsies was observed (1.40-fold, P = 0.0009, FDR = 0.02), without influence of the allele dosage and the expression profiles.

Present literature does not provide robust hints about the functional significance of *IL1RL1* gene polymorphisms studied in the present paper (rs2058660, rs2310173, rs13015714); thus, it is not possible to speculate whether they lead to altered bioactivity of IL1RL1 isoforms. However, our results, showing an association of rs13015714 to CD, classically considered a Th1-driven disease, but not UC, may suggest that the presence of this specific polymorphism may impair the function of the IL-33/IL1RL1 axis. As a consequence, in the presence of a predisposing genetic background to IBD, the rs13015714 polymorphism may polarize the intestinal inflammation towards a Th1-dominated CD phenotype, rather than a Th2-dominated UC phenotype. Interestingly, it has been recently demonstrated that, while IL-33 promotes Th2 cytokine production through IL1RL1 binding, it is also capable of inducing non-polarized immune responses in an IL1RL1-independent manner, implicating the existence of a second IL-33 receptor or, more likely, the presence of IL-33's direct effect on DNA-transcription [65] through the DNA-binding domain possessed by this cytokine [66]. Therefore, it may be hypothesized that the rs13015714 polymorphism impairs the expression, or IL-33 binding capacity, of both IL1RL1 isoforms. As a consequence, IL-33 may be "free" from its decoy receptor and capable to exert its pro-inflammatory effects, eliciting a IL1RL1-independent inflammatory program and leading to susceptibility of a polarized Th1/Th17-mediated inflammatory condition, such as that observed in CD. In fact, recent evidence

suggests that IL-33 has the ability to polarize immune responses towards a Th17 profile in experimental models of arthritis [12,13].

Indeed, functional data regarding the effects of IL-33's rs3939286 and IL1RL1's rs13015714 polymorphisms on respective protein expression and bioactivity are needed to confirm these assumptions, solely based on disease and phenotype associations.

Taken together, our data suggest that risk variants in the IL-33/IL1RL1 system may influence IBD disease susceptibility, particularly in adult populations, and further support the importance of the IL-1 family of cytokines in the predisposition to both CD and UC. Moreover, a specific imbalance between IL-33 and IL1RL1 may play a pathogenic role in this process. The associations between the *IL-33* rs3939286 polymorphism and IBD, and between the *IL1RL1* rs13015714 and CD, further support the overlap in susceptibility loci/genes between IBD and other immune-mediated diseases. Of note, the aforementioned SNPs were reported to be associated with nasal polyposis [24], asthma [21] (rs3939286), and celiac disease [38] (rs13015714). Further investigation as well as targeted functional studies are needed to understand how IL-33 and IL1RL1 variants contribute to disease susceptibility in IBD, and whether presence of these polymorphic markers might have clinical therapeutic implications.

Supporting Information

Figure S1 View of the genomic region containing *IL-33* gene with the selected three single nucleotide polymorphisms.

Figure S2 Linkage disequilibrium plot of *IL-33* gene with genotyped polymorphisms (SNPs) and r² SNP map. The underlined SNP was selected from the International IBD Genetics Consortium meta-analysis [35].

Figure S3 Linkage disequilibrium in *IL1RL1* and surrounding genes on chromosome 2q12 with the selected two single nucleotide polymorphisms.

Figure S4 Block 1 and 2 of *IL1RL1* gene with the selected single nucleotide polymorphism.

Figure S5 Expression of *IL-33* and *IL1RL1* mRNA in intestinal biopsy samples from ulcerative colitis (UC) and Crohn's disease (CD) patients. mRNA levels were calculated as fold increased over respective adjacent noninflamed area (controls). The controls group fold change has value 1.

Table S1 Haplotype frequencies in Crohn's disease (CD) and ulcerative colitis (UC) patients compared with controls.

Acknowledgments

The authors thank dr. Biscaglia Giuseppe, Dr. Scimeca Daniela, Mrs Martino Giuseppina, Dr. Carella Massimo and Dr. Palumbo Orazio for their assistance with data collection and technical support. We are also grateful for the participation and support of the families and patients with IBD.

The following centers (physicians) contributed to the study by providing DNA samples and clinical information of their patients: SINGEP: S. Giovanni Rotondo (M. Pastore, M. D'Altilia); Roma (S.Cucchiara, A. Dilillo); Napoli (E. Berni, Canani, A.M. Staiano); Padova (G. Guariso, V. Lodde); Messina (C Romano, G. Vieni, C. Sferlazzas); Bari (V. Rutigliano, D. De Venuto); Parma (G.L. de Angelis); Palermo (S.Accomando, G.

Iacono); Foggia (A. Campanozzi); Napoli (F. Castiglione); Firenze (P. Lionetti); Genova (A. Barabino); Ancona (C. Catassi, S. Nobile); Pescara (G. Lombardi).

IG-IBD: Firenze (V. Annese, F. Tonelli); Padova (R. D'incà, G.C. Sturniolo, L. Oliva); Milano (M. Vecchi, S. Saibeni, S. Ardizzone); Bologna (P. Gionchetti, F. Rizzello); Roma (E. Corazziari, C. Prantera); Napoli (G. Riegler, S.Giaquinto); San Giovanni Rotondo (D. Scimeca, G. Biscaglia,

G. Martino).

Author Contributions

Conceived and designed the experiments: AL OP. Performed the experiments: GM BA TL GC. Analyzed the data: MRV. Contributed reagents/materials/analysis tools: MV FB AS RDI VA AA TTP LS. Wrote the paper: AL LP.

References

1. Kaser A, Zeissig S, Blumberg RS (2010) Inflammatory bowel disease. Annu Rev Immunol 28: 573–621.
2. Kim SW, Kim ES, Moon CM, Park JJ, Kim TI, et al. (2011) Genetic polymorphisms of IL-23R and IL-17A and novel insights into their associations with inflammatory bowel disease Gut 60: 1527–1536.
3. Andersen V, Ernst A, Christensen J, Østergaard M, Jacobsen BA, et al. (2010) The polymorphism rs3024505 proximal to IL-10 is associated with risk of ulcerative colitis and Crohns disease in a Danish case-control study. BMC Med Genet 11: 82.
4. Palmieri O, Latiano A, Salvatori E, Valvano MR, Bossa F, et al. (2010) The - A2518G polymorphism of monocyte chemoattractant protein-1 is associated with Crohn's disease. Am J Gastroentero 105: 1586–1594.
5. Nemetz A, Nosti-Escanilla MP, Molnár T, Köpe A, Kovács A, et al. (1999) IL1B gene polymorphisms influence the course and severity of inflammatory bowel disease. Immunogenetics 49: 527–531.
6. Stokkers PC, van Aken BE, Basoski N, Reitsma PH, Tytgat GN, et al. (1998) Five genetic markers in the interleukin 1 family in relation to inflammatory bowel disease. Gut 43: 33–39.
7. Tamura K, Fukuda Y, Sashio H, Takeda N, Bamba H, et al. (2002) IL18 polymorphism is associated with an increased risk of Crohn's disease. J Gastroenterol 37 Suppl 14: 111–116.
8. Aizawa Y, Sutoh S, Matsuoka M, Negishi M, Torii A, et al. (2005) Association of interleukin-18 gene single-nucleotide polymorphisms with susceptibility to inflammatory bowel disease. Tissue Antigens 65: 88–92.
9. Glas J, Török HP, Tonenchi L, Kapser J, Schiemann U, et al. (2005) Association of polymorphisms in the interleukin-18 gene in patients with Crohn's disease depending on the CARD15/NOD2 genotype. Inflamm Bowel Dis 11: 1031–1037.
10. Schmitz J, Owyang A, Oldham E, Song Y, Murphy E, et al. (2005) IL- 33, an interleukin-1 cytokine that signals via the IL-1 receptor-related protein ST2 and induces T helper type 2-associated cytokines. Immunity 23: 479–490.
11. Smithgall MD, Comeau MR, Yoon BR, Kaufman D, Armitage R, Smith DE (2008) IL-33 amplifies both Th1- and Th2-type responses through its activity on human basophils, allergen-reactive Th2 cells, iNKT and NK cells. Int Immunol 20: 1019–1030.
12. Xu D, Jiang HR, Kewin P, Li Y, Mu R, et al. (2008) IL-33 exacerbates antigen-induced arthritis by activating mast cells. Proc Natl Acad Sci U S A 105: 10913–10918.
13. Palmer G, Talabot-Ayer D, Lamacchia C Toy D, Seemayer CA, et al. (2009) Inhibition of interleukin-33 signaling attenuates the severity of experimental arthritis. Arthritis Rheum 60: 738–749.
14. Chackerian AA, Oldham ER, Murphy EE, Schmitz J, Pflanz S, Kastelein RA (2007) IL-1 receptor accessory protein and ST2 comprise the IL-33 receptor complex. J Immunol 179: 2551–2555.
15. Hayakawa H, Hayakawa M, Kume A, Tominaga S (2007) Soluble ST2 blocks interleukin-33 signaling in allergic airway inflammation. J Biol Chem 282: 26369–26380.
16. Li M, Li Y, Liu X, Gao X, Wang Y (2012) IL-33 blockade suppresses the development of experimental autoimmune encephalomyelitis in C57BL/6 mice. J Neuroimmunol 247: 25–31.
17. Pushparaj PN, Tay HK, H'ng SC, Pitman N, Xu D, et al. (2009) The cytokine interleukin-33 mediates anaphylactic shock. Proc Natl Acad Sci U S A 106: 9773–9778.
18. Miller AM, Xu D, Asquith DL, Denby L, Li Y, et al. (2008) IL-33 reduces the development of atherosclerosis. J Exp Med 205: 339–346.
19. Volarevic V, Mitrovic M, Milovanovic M, Zelen I, Nikolic I, et al. (2012) Protective role of IL-33/ST2 axis in Con A-induced hepatitis. J Hepatol 56: 26–33.
20. Chapuis J, Hot D, Hansmannel F, Kerdraon O, Ferreira S, et al. (2009) Transcriptomic and genetic studies identify IL-33 as a candidate gene for Alzheimer's disease. Mol Psychiatry 14: 1004–1016.
21. Gudbjartsson DF, Bjornsdottir US, Halapi E, Helgadottir A, Sulem P, et al. (2009) Sequence variants affecting eosinophil numbers associate with asthma and myocardial infarction. Nat Genet 41: 342–347.
22. Bossé Y, Lemire M, Poon AH, Daley D, He JQ, et al. (2009) Asthma and genes encoding components of the vitamin D pathway. Respir Res 10: 98.
23. Wu H, Romieu I, Shi M, Hancock DB, Li H, et al. (2010) Evaluation of candidate genes in a genome-wide association study of childhood asthma in Mexicans. J Allergy Clin Immunol 125: 321–327.
24. Buysschaert ID, Grulois V, Eloy P, Jorissen M, Rombaux P, et al. (2010) Genetic evidence for a role of IL33 in nasal polyposis. Allergy 65: 616–622.
25. Castano R, Bossé Y, Endam LM, Desrosiers M (2009) Evidence of association of interleukin-1 receptor-like 1 gene polymorphisms with chronic rhinosinusitis. Am J Rhinol Allergy 23: 377–384.
26. Shimizu M, Matsuda A, Yanagisawa K, Hirota T, Akahoshi M, et al. (2005) Functional SNPs in the distal promoter of the ST2 gene are associated with atopic dermatitis. Hum Mol Genet 14: 2919–2927.
27. Seidelin JB, Bjerrum JT, Coskun M, Widjaya B, Vainer B, Nielsen OH (2010) IL-33 is upregulated in colonocytes of ulcerative colitis. Immunol Lett 128: 80–85.
28. Beltrán CJ, Núñez LE, Díaz-Jiménez D, Farfan N, Candia E, et al. (2010) Characterization of the novel ST2/IL-33 system in patients with inflammatory bowel disease. Inflamm Bowel Dis 16: 1097–1107.
29. Pastorelli L, Garg RR, Hoang SB, Spina L, Mattioli B, et al. (2010) Epithelial-derived IL-33 and its receptor ST2 are dysregulated in ulcerative colitis and in experimental Th1/Th2 driven enteritis. Proc Natl Acad Sci U S A 107: 8017–8022.
30. Kobori A, Yagi Y, Imaeda H, Ban H, Bamba S, et al. (2010) Interleukin-33 expression is specifically enhanced in inflamed mucosa of ulcerative colitis. J Gastroenterol 45: 999–1007.
31. Sponheim J, Pollheimer J, Olsen T, Balogh J, Hammarström C, et al. (2010) Inflammatory bowel disease-associated interleukin-33 is preferentially expressed in ulceration-associated myofibroblasts. Am J Pathol 177: 2804–2815.
32. Silverberg MS, Satsangi J, Ahmad T, Arnott ID, Bernstein CN, et al. (2005) Toward an integrated clinical, molecular and serological classification of inflammatory bowel disease: Report of a Working Party of the 2005 Montreal World Congress of Gastroenterology. Can J Gastroenterol 19 (suppl A): 5–36.
33. International HapMap Project. Database of genes associated with human disease and response to pharmaceuticals [HapMap web site]. Available from: www.hapmap.org.
34. Barrett JC, Fry B, Maller J, Daly MJ (2005) Haploview: analysis and visualization of LD and haplotype maps. Bioinformatics 21: 263–265.
35. Franke A, McGovern DPB, Barrett JC, Wang K, Radford-Smith GL et al. (2010) Genome-wide metaanalysis increases to 71 the number of confirmed Crohn's disease susceptibility loci. Nat Genet 42: 1118–1125.
36. Anderson CA, Boucher G, Lees CW, Franke A, D'Amato M, et al. (2011) Meta-analysis identifies 29 additional ulcerative colitis risk loci, increasing the number of confirmed associations to 47. Nat Genet 43: 246–452.
37. McGovern DP, Gardet A, Törkvist L, Goyette P, Essers J, et al. (2010) Genome-wide association identifies multiple ulcerative colitis susceptibility loci. Nat Genet 42: 332–337.
38. Koskinen LL, Einarsdottir E, Dukes E, Heap GA, Dubois P et al. (2009) Association study of the IL18RAP locus in three European populations with celiac disease. Hum Mol Genet 18: 1148–1155.
39. Cucchiara S, Latiano A, Palmieri O, Canani RB, D'Incà R, et al. (2007) Polymorphisms of tumor necrosis factor-alpha but not MDR1 influence response to medical therapy in pediatric-onset inflammatory bowel disease. J Pediatr Gastroenterol Nutr 44: 171–179.
40. Cominelli F (2004) Cytokine-based therapies for Crohn's disease–new paradigms. N Engl J Med 351: 2045–2048.
41. Strober W, Fuss I, Mannon P (2007) The fundamental basis of inflammatory bowel disease. J Clin Invest 117: 514–521.
42. Mitcham JL, Parnet P, Bonnert TP, Garka KE, Gerhart MJ, et al. (1996) T1/ST2 signaling establishes it as a member of an expanding interleukin-1 receptor family. J. Biol. Chem 271: 5777–5783.
43. Oboki K, Ohno T, Kajiwara N, Saito H, Nakae S (2010) IL-33 and IL-33 receptors in host defense and diseases. Allergol Int 59: 143–160.
44. Kearley J, Buckland KF, Mathie SA, Lloyd CM (2009) Resolution of allergic inflammation and airway hyperreactivity is dependent upon disruption of the T1/ST2-IL-33 pathway. Am J Respir Crit Care Med 179: 772–781.
45. Iikura M, Suto H, Kajiwara N, Oboki K, Ohno T, et al. (2007) IL-33 can promote survival, adhesion and cytokine production in human mast cells. Lab Invest 87: 971–978.
46. Imielinski M, Baldassano RN, Griffiths A, Russell RK, Annese V, et al. (2009) Common variants at five new loci associated with early-onset inflammatory bowel disease. Nat Genet 41: 1335–1340.
47. Jostins L, Ripke S, Weersma RK, Duerr RH, McGovern DP, et al. (2012) Host-microbe interactions have shaped the genetic architecture of inflammatory bowel disease. Nature 491: 119–124.
48. Van Limbergen J, Wilson DC, Satsangi J (2009) The genetics of Crohn's disease. Annu Rev Genomics Human Genet 10: 89–116.

49. Smith AM, Rahman FZ, Hayee B, Graham SJ, Marks DJ, et al. (2009) Disordered macrophage cytokine secretion underlies impaired acute inflammation and bacterial clearance in Crohn's disease. J Exp Med 206: 1883–1897.

50. Ogura Y, Bonen DK, Inohara N, Nicolae DL, Chen FF, et al. (2001) A frameshift mutation in NOD2 associated with susceptibility to Crohn's disease. Nature 411: 603–606.

51. Hampe J, Franke A, Rosenstiel P, Till A, Teuber M, et al. (2007) A genome-wide association scan of nonsynonymous SNPs identifies a susceptibility variant for Crohn disease in ATG16L1. Nat Genet 39: 207–211.

52. Rioux JD, Xavier RJ, Taylor KD, Silverberg MS, Goyette P, et al. (2007) Genome-wide association study identifies new susceptibility loci for Crohn disease and implicates autophagy in disease pathogenesis. Nat Genet 39: 596–604.

53. Villani AC, Lemire M, Fortin G, Louis E, Silverberg MS, et al. (2009) Common variants in the NLRP3 region contribute to Crohn's disease susceptibility. Nat Genet 41: 71–76.

54. Hugot JP, Chamaillard M, Zouali H, Lesage S, Cézard JP, et al. (2001) Association of NOD2 leucine-rich repeat variants with susceptibility to Crohn's disease. Nature 411: 599–603.

55. Parkes M, Barrett JC, Prescott NJ, Tremelling M, Anderson CA et al. (2007) Sequence variants in the autophagy gene IRGM and multiple other replicating loci contribute to Crohn's disease susceptibility. Nat Genet 39: 830–832.

56. Lees CW, Barrett JC, Parkes M Satsangi J (2011) New IBD genetics: common pathways with other diseases. Gut 60: 1739–1753.

57. Seldin MF, Amos CI (2009) Shared susceptibility variations in autoimmune diseases: a brief perspective on common issues. Genes Immun 10: 1–4.

58. Duan L, Chen J, Zhang H, Yang H, Zhu P, et al. (2012) IL-33 ameliorates experimental colitis through promoting Th2/Foxp3(+) Treg responses in mice. Mol Med Mar 12. Epub ahead of print.

59. Oboki K, Ohno T, Kajiwara N, Arae K, Morita H, et al. (2010) IL-33 is a crucial amplifier of innate rather than acquired immunity. Proc Natl Acad Sci U S A 107: 18581–18586.

60. Imaeda H, Andoh A, Aomatsu T, Uchiyama K, Bamba S, et al. (2011) Interleukin-33 suppresses Notch ligand expression and prevents goblet cell depletion in dextran sulfate sodium-induced colitis. Int J Mol Med 28: 573–578.

61. Groβ P, Doser K, Falk W, Obermeier F, Hofmann C (2012) IL-33 attenuates development and perpetuation of chronic intestinal inflammation. Inflamm Bowel Dis Apr 16. Epub ahead of print.

62. Pastorelli L, De Salvo C, Cominelli MA, Vecchi M, Pizarro TT (2011) Novel cytokine signaling pathways in inflammatory bowel disease: insight into the dichotomous functions of IL-33 during chronic intestinal inflammation. Therap Adv Gastroenterol 4: 311–323.

63. Oshikawa K, Yanagisawa K, Tominaga S, Sugiyama Y (2002) Expression and function of the ST2 gene in a murine model of allergic airway inflammation. Clin Exp Allergy 32: 1520–1526.

64. Plaza-Izurieta L, Castellanos-Rubio A, Irastorza I, Fernández-Jimenez N, Gutierrez G, et al. (2011) Revisiting genome wide association studies (GWAS) in coeliac disease: replication study in Spanish population and expression analysis of candidate genes. J Med Genet 48: 493–496.

65. Luzina IG, Pickering EM, Kopach P, Kang PH, Lockatell V, et al. (2012) Full-Length IL-33 Promotes Inflammation but not Th2 Response In Vivo in an ST2-Independent Fashion. J Immunol 189: 403–410.

66. Carriere V, Roussel L, Ortega N, Lacorre DA, Americh L, et al. (2007) IL-33, the IL-1-like cytokine ligand for ST2 receptor, is a chromatin-associated nuclear factor in vivo. Proc Natl Acad Sci U S A 104: 282–287.

13

Analysis of *IL12B* Gene Variants in Inflammatory Bowel Disease

Jürgen Glas[1,2,3,9], Julia Seiderer[1,9], Johanna Wagner[1,2], Torsten Olszak[1,4], Christoph Fries[1,2], Cornelia Tillack[1], Matthias Friedrich[1,2], Florian Beigel[1], Johannes Stallhofer[1], Christian Steib[1], Martin Wetzke[1,2,5], Burkhard Göke[1], Thomas Ochsenkühn[1], Julia Diegelmann[1,2*], Darina Czamara[6], Stephan Brand[1*]

1 Department of Medicine II - Grosshadern, Ludwig-Maximilians-University (LMU), Munich, Germany, 2 Department of Preventive Dentistry and Periodontology, LMU, Munich, Germany, 3 Department of Human Genetics, Rheinisch-Westfälische Technische Hochschule (RWTH), Aachen, Germany, 4 Division of Gastroenterology, Brigham & Women's Hospital, Harvard Medical School, Boston, United States of America, 5 Department of Pediatrics, Hannover Medical School, Hannover, Germany, 6 Max-Planck-Institute of Psychiatry, Munich, Germany

Abstract

Background: *IL12B* encodes the p40 subunit of IL-12, which is also part of IL-23. Recent genome-wide association studies identified *IL12B* and *IL23R* as susceptibility genes for inflammatory bowel disease (IBD). However, the phenotypic effects and potential gene-gene interactions of *IL12B* variants are largely unknown.

Methodology/Principal Findings: We analyzed *IL12B* gene variants regarding association with Crohn's disease (CD) and ulcerative colitis (UC). Genomic DNA from 2196 individuals including 913 CD patients, 318 UC patients and 965 healthy, unrelated controls was analyzed for four SNPs in the *IL12B* gene region (rs3212227, rs17860508, rs10045431, rs6887695). Our analysis revealed an association of the *IL12B* SNP rs6887695 with susceptibility to IBD ($p = 0.035$; OR 1.15 [95% CI 1.01–1.31] including a trend for rs6887695 for association with CD (OR 1.41; [0.99–1.31], $p = 0.066$) and UC (OR 1.18 [0.97–1.43], $p = 0.092$). CD patients, who were homozygous C/C carriers of this SNP, had significantly more often non-stricturing, non-penetrating disease than carriers of the G allele ($p = 6.8 \times 10^{-5}$; OR = 2.84, 95% CI 1.66–4.84), while C/C homozygous UC patients had less often extensive colitis than G allele carriers ($p = 0.029$; OR = 0.36, 95% CI 0.14–0.92). *In silico* analysis predicted stronger binding of the minor C allele of rs6887695 to the transcription factor RORα which is involved in Th17 differentiation. Differences regarding the binding to the major and minor allele sequence of rs6887695 were also predicted for the transcription factors HSF1, HSF2, MZF1 and Oct-1. Epistasis analysis revealed weak epistasis of the *IL12B* SNP rs6887695 with several SNPs (rs11889341, rs7574865, rs7568275, rs8179673, rs10181656, rs7582694) in the *STAT4* gene which encodes the major IL-12 downstream transcription factor STAT4 ($p < 0.05$) but there was no epistasis between *IL23R* and *IL12B* variants.

Conclusions/Significance: The *IL12B* SNP rs6887695 modulates the susceptibility and the phenotype of IBD, although the effect on IBD susceptibilty is less pronounced than that of *IL23R* gene variants.

Editor: Giovambattista Pani, Catholic University Medical School, Italy

Funding: J. Glas was supported by a grant from the Broad Medical Foundation (IBD-0126R2). J. Seiderer and J. Diegelmann were supported by grants from the Ludwig-Maximilians-University Munich (FöFoLe Nr. 422; Habilitationsstipendium, LMUExcellent to J.S. and Promotionsstipendium to J.D.); J. Seiderer was also supported by the Robert-Bosch-Foundation and the Else Kröner-Fresenius-Stiftung (81/08//EKMS08/01). S. Brand was supported by grants from the DFG (BR 1912/6-1), the Else Kröner-Fresenius-Stiftung (Else Kröner Exzellenzstipendium 2010; 2010_EKES.32), and by grants of Ludwig-Maximilians-University Munich (Excellence Initiative, Investment Funds 2008 and FöFoLe program). J. Wagner was supported by a grant from the Ludwig-Maximilians-University Munich (FöFoLe). The funders had no role in study design, data collection and analysis, decision to publish, or preparation of the manuscript.

Competing Interests: The authors have declared that no competing interests exist.

* E-mail: stephan.brand@med.uni-muenchen.de (SB); julia.diegelmann@med.uni-muenchen.de (JD)

9 These authors contributed equally to this work.

Introduction

The identification of the IL-23/Th17 pathway as a key regulator of intestinal immune homeostasis and proinflammatory responses in defense to microbial infection has elucidated new potential therapeutic targets in inflammatory bowel diseases (IBD) [1,2,3,4]. Genome-wide association studies (GWAS) and large cohort studies demonstrated that *IL23R* [3,5,6,7] and additional genes involved in Th17 differentiation (e.g., *IL12B*, *JAK2*, *TYK2*, *STAT3*, *CCR6*, *IL2/IL21* and *TNFSF15*) are associated with the susceptibility to Crohn's disease (CD) and partly also to ulcerative colitis (UC) [5,8,9,10,11]. Moreover, a pathway analysis using data from the Wellcome Trust Case Control Consortium (WTCCC) uncovered significant associations of CD and IL-12/IL-23 pathway components, harbouring 20 genes such as *IL12B*, *JAK2*, *STAT3* and *CCR6* [12]. Functionally, the proinflammatory cytokines IL-12 and IL-23 play critical and unique roles in bridging the innate and adaptive immune systems in IBD [4,13] and are produced primarily by activated dendritic cells (DCs) and macrophages in response to microbial stimulation. IL-12 promotes the differentiation of naive CD4+ T cells into mature interferon-γ (IFN-γ)-producing Th1 effector cells and is a potent stimulus of natural killer and CD8+ T cells [14,15]. In contrast, IL-23, a heterodimeric cytokine composed of a p19 subunit and a p40 subunit of which the latter is shared with IL-12, is required for the generation of memory T cells and drives differentiation of Th17 cells [16,17]. Th17 cytokines such as IL-17A, IL-17F, IL-21, IL-22, IL-26 and the Th17 chemokine CCL20 have been particularly implicated as key cytokines involved in the intestinal inflammation of CD [1,18,19,20,21,22,23].

On the genetic level, *IL12B* encodes the IL-12 p40 subunit shared by IL-12 and IL-23 cytokines while *IL23R* encodes one of the two subunits of the IL-23 receptor [24]. Antibody therapy directed against the IL-12/IL-23 p40 subunit demonstrated some clinical efficacy in CD patients [25]. Since the first identification of *IL23R* as susceptibility gene in IBD by Duerr *et al.* [3], various GWAS and cohort studies have confirmed *IL23R* not only as a major susceptibility gene in IBD but also in the pathogenesis of other autoimmune diseases such as psoriasis [26,27] and ankylosing spondylitis [28], implicating common proinflammatory pathways. Genetic variants in the *IL12B* region have also been associated with the susceptibility to psoriasis, ankylosing spondylitis, and infectious diseases such as leprosy and tuberculosis [29,30,31,32,33]. In contrast, data on *IL12B* variants and their role in asthma [34,35], rheumatoid arthritis [36] or multiple sclerosis [37] remain controversial. While recent GWAS meta-analyses by Barrett *et al.* [5], Franke *et al.* [9], and Anderson *et al.* [10] established *IL12B* as IBD susceptibility gene, smaller studies showed inconsistent results [38,39]. Cohort studies in the Spanish [38] and Japanese [39] population demonstrated an association of *IL12B* SNPs with the susceptibility to IBD; however with different results, reporting associations with CD susceptibility in the Japanese cohort (rs6887695) [39] and to UC (rs6887695) but not to CD susceptibility in the Spanish cohort [38]. Moreover, the phenotypic effects of *IL12B* and potential gene-gene interactions contributing to IBD susceptibility are largely unknown.

Since the exact role of *IL12B* for IBD susceptibility in the German population and IBD phenotype behaviour remains unclear, we aimed to perform a detailed genotype-phenotype analysis in a large IBD cohort and an analysis for potential epistatic interactions with other gene variants involved in IL-12 and IL-23 signaling and implicated in IBD susceptibility such as *IL23R* and *STAT4* [3,40] which encodes the major IL-12-induced downstream transcription factor STAT4.

Methods

Ethics statement

The study was approved by the Ethics committee of the Medical Faculty of Ludwig-Maximilians-University Munich and written, informed consent was obtained from all patients prior to the study. Study protocols adhered to the ethical principles for medical research involving human subjects of the Helsinki Declaration (as detailed under: http://www.wma.net/en/30publications/10policies/b3/index.html).

Study population and IBD phenotype assessment

Overall, the study population (n = 2196) consisted of 1231 IBD patients including 913 patients with CD, 318 patients with UC, and 965 healthy, unrelated controls, all of Caucasian origin. The demographic and clinical data (behaviour and location of IBD, disease-related complications, immunosuppressive therapy and

history of previous surgeries) of the patients were recorded by analysis of patient charts and a detailed questionnaire including an interview at time of enrolment. The diagnosis of CD or UC was determined according to established guidelines based on endoscopic, radiological, and histopathological criteria. Patients with CD were assessed following the Montreal classification based on the age at diagnosis (A), location (L), and behaviour (B) of the disease [41]. In patients with UC, anatomic location was also based on the Montreal classification using the criteria ulcerative proctitis (E1), left-sided UC (distal UC; E2), and extensive UC (pancolitis; E3). Patients with indeterminate colitis were excluded from the study. The demographic characteristics of the IBD study population were collected blind to the results of the genotype analyses and are summarized in Table 1.

DNA extraction and genotyping of the IL12B variants

From all study participants, blood samples were taken and genomic DNA was isolated from peripheral blood leukocytes using the DNA blood mini kit from Qiagen (Hilden, Germany) according to the manufacturer's guidelines. Four *IL12B* SNPs (rs3212227, rs17860508, rs10045431 and rs6887695) were genotyped by PCR and melting curve analysis using a pair of fluorescence resonance energy transfer (FRET) probes in a LightCycler® 480 Instrument (Roche Diagnostics, Mannheim, Germany) as described in previous studies [6,40,42,43]. These *IL12B* SNPs were selected based on previous studies showing associations with CD or other autoimmune diseases such as psoriasis. Specifically, the SNPs rs3212227 and rs6887695 were selected from the study of Cargill and co-workers [29], while rs6887695 was also investigated in the study of Parkes *et al.* [8]. The SNP rs10045431 was selected from the study of Barrett and co-workers [5]. Additionally, the SNP rs17860508 located within the promoter of *IL12B* was included because of its potential functional relevance regarding gene expression [44]. The total

Table 1. Demographic characteristics of the IBD study population.

	Crohn's disease n = 913	Ulcerative colitis n = 318	Controls n = 965
Gender			
Male (%)	48.9	52.2	63.5
Female (%)	51.1	47.8	36.5
Age (yrs)			
Mean ± SD	40.9±13.2	44.2±14.8	46.0±10.3
Range	15–83	17–88	19–68
Body mass index			
Mean ± SD	23.0±4.2	23.9±4.5	
Range	13–41	15–54	
Age at diagnosis (yrs)			
Mean ± SD	26.1±12.3	28.9±14.5	
Range	1–78	2–81	
Disease duration (yrs)			
Mean ± SD	13.4±8.9	12.2±8.3	
Range	0–47	1–50	
Positive family history of IBD (%)	16.8	17.4	

volume of the PCR was 5 μl containing 25 ng of genomic DNA, 1× Light Cycler 480 Genotyping Master Mix (Roche Diagnostics), 2.5 pmol of each primer and 0.75 pmol of each FRET probe (TIB MOLBIOL, Berlin, Germany). In the case of rs3212227 and rs10045431, the concentrations of the forward primers and in the case of rs17860508 the concentration of the reverse primer was reduced to 0.5 pmol. In the case of rs6887695 the concentration of the reverse primer was reduced to 1.25 pmol and in the case of rs744166 the concentration of the forward primer was reduced to 0.75 pmol, respectively. Two SNPs were analyzed in a multiplex reaction, the combinations were rs3212227+rs17860508 and rs10045431+rs6887695. The PCR comprised an initial denaturation step (95°C for 10 min) and 45 cycles (95°C for 10°C sec, 60 for 10 sec, 72°C for 15 sec). The melting curve analysis comprised an initial denaturation step (95°C for 1 min), a step rapidly lowering the temperature to 40°C and holding for 2 min, and a heating step slowly (1 acquisition/°C) increasing the temperature up to 95°C and continuously measuring the fluorescence intensity. The results of the melting curve analysis were confirmed by analyzing two patient samples for each possible genotype using sequence analysis. For sequencing, the total volume of the PCR was 100 μl containing 250 ng of genomic DNA, 1× PCR-buffer (Qiagen, Hilden, Germany), a final MgCl$_2$ concentration of 2 mM, 0.5 mM of a dNTP mix (Sigma, Steinheim, Germany), 2.5 units of HotStar Plus Taq^{TM} DNA polymerase (Qiagen) and 10 pmol of each primer (TIB MOLBIOL). The PCR comprised an initial denaturation step (95°C for 5 min), 35 cycles (denaturation at 94°C for 30 sec, primer annealing at 65°C for 30 sec, extension at 72°C for 30 sec) and a final extension step (72°C for 10 min). The PCR products were purified using the QIAquick PCR Purification Kit (Qiagen) and sequenced by a commercial sequencing company (Sequiserve, Vaterstetten, Germany). All sequences of primers and FRET probes and primer annealing temperatures used for genotyping and for sequence analysis, respectively, are given in Supplementary Tables S1 and S2.

STAT4 and IL23R genotyping

For analysis of epistatic interactions, seven *STAT4* SNPs (rs11889341, rs7574865, rs7568275, rs8179673, rs10181656, rs7582694, rs10174238) and 10 *IL23R* SNPs (rs1004819, rs7517847, rs10489629, rs2201841, rs11465804, rs11209026 = p.Arg381Gln, rs1343151, rs10889677, rs11209032, rs1495965) were genotyped by PCR and melting curve analysis using a pair of fluorescence resonance energy transfer (FRET) probes in a LightCycler® 480 Instrument (Roche Diagnostics, Mannheim, Germany) as described previously [6,40]. The majority of *IL23R* and *STAT4* genotype data were available from previous studies [6,40].

In silico analysis of transcription factor binding sites

SNPs rs3212227, rs17860508, rs10045431 and rs6887695 were analyzed for potential transcription factor binding sites applying the online tool TFSEARCH (http://www.cbrc.jp/research/db/TFSEARCH.html). It is based on the TRANSFAC database developed at GBF Braunschweig, Germany [45]. The threshold score for binding sites was set to 75.0 (score = 100.0 * ('weighted sum'−min)/(max−min); max. score = 100). For each SNP, major and minor alleles including the flanking sequences 15 bp upstream and downstream were analyzed. Only human transcription factors were included in the analysis.

Statistical analyses

Power calculation was performed using the Genetic Power Calculator (http://pngu.mgh.harvard.edu/~purcell/gpc/). Each genetic marker was tested for Hardy-Weinberg equilibrium in the control population. For data evaluation, we used PLINK (http://pngu.mgh.harvard.edu/~purcell/plink/) and R-2.13.1. (http://cran.r-project.org). Haplotypes tests were performed in a sliding-window approach including up to 4 markers. Epistasis between different SNPs was tested using the −epistasis option on PLINK. Genotype-phenotype associations were assessed using logistic regression.

Results

The IL12B polymorphisms rs6887695 is associated with increased IBD susceptibility

In all three subgroups (CD, UC, and controls), the allele frequencies of the *IL12B* SNPs (rs3212227, rs17860508, rs10045431, rs6887695) were in accordance with the predicted Hardy-Weinberg equilibrium (Table 2). The *IL12B* SNP rs6887695 showed an association with increased IBD susceptibility (p = 0.035; OR 1.15 [95% CI 1.01–1.31]). In addition, there was a trend for rs6887695 for association with CD (OR 1.41 [95% CI 0.99–1.31], p = 0.066) and UC (OR 1.18 [95% CI 0.97–1.43], p = 0.092) and a trend for association of rs10045431 with UC (OR 0.83 [95% 0.68–1.02], p = 0.083; Table 2).

IL12B haplotype analysis

We next performed a detailed haplotype analysis in our IBD cohort. As shown in Tables 3 and 4, we could not demonstrate significant associations of *IL12B* haplotypes with CD and UC susceptibility. A haplotype of all four investigated SNPs (rs3212227-rs17860508-rs10045431-rs6887695) showed a trend for association with CD (p = 0.053); however, this potential association signal did not reach statistical significance and was uncorrected for multiple testing.

Genotype-phenotype analysis: C/C homozygosity for the SNP rs6887695 is associated with non-stricturing, non-penetrating Crohn's disease

The majority of previous GWAS meta-analyses showing an association with *IL12B* were performed in CD patients with predominant ileal involvement [5,9]. To exclude that only a certain IBD subphenotype such as ileal CD is associated with *IL12B*, we further investigated potential associations of *IL12B* SNPs with the anatomic location in IBD patients Genotype-phenotype analysis showed a weak association of rs3212227 with colonic CD (p = 0.04) but not with ileal involvement. In addition, we analyzed the *IL12B* SNP rs6887695, for which we found a trend for association with CD and UC, regarding potential phenotypic consequences in CD and UC. CD patients, who were homozygous C/C carriers of this SNP, had significantly more often a non-stricturing, non-penetrating disease phenotype than carriers of the G allele (= combined group of heterozygous C/G and wildtype G/G carriers; p = 6.8×10^{-5} (Table 5). This strong association remained significant following Bonferroni correction for multiple testing. C/C homozygous carriers of the *IL12B* SNP rs6887695 had also less stenoses than G carriers (p = 0.038) and there was a trend towards less penetrating disease (p = 0.062), less fistulas (p = 0.085), and less surgery (p = 0.063; Table 5). In UC, homozygous C/C carriers of the *IL12B* SNP rs6887695 had significantly more often left-sided UC (p = 0.006) but less often extensive UC (p = 0.029) than the combined group of heterozygous C/G and wildtype G/G carriers (Table 6).

Table 2. Associations of *IL12B* gene markers in CD and UC case-control association studies.

SNP	Minor allele	Crohn's disease n=913			Ulcerative colitis n=318			Inflammatory bowel disease n=1231			Controls n=965
		MAF	p value	OR [95% CI]	MAF	p value	OR [95% CI]	MAF	p value	OR [95% CI]	MAF
rs3212227	G	0.209	0.684	0.97 [0.82-1.13]	0.214	0.777	1.03 [0.83-1.29]	0.206	0.820	0.98 [0.85-1.14]	0.209
rs17860508	TTAGAG	0.485	0.974	1.00 [0.88-1.14]	0.489	0.854	1.02 [0.85-1.22]	0.486	0.903	1.01 [0.89-1.14]	0.484
rs10045431	A	0.271	0.258	0.92 [0.80-1.06]	0.252	0.083	0.83 [0.68-1.02]	0.266	0.109	0.90 [0.78-1.02]	0.288
rs6887695	C	0.329	0.066	1.41 [0.99-1.31]	0.336	0.092	1.18 [0.97-1.43]	0.330	**0.035**	1.15 [1.01-1.31]	0.300

The category "Inflammatory bowel disease" represents the combined CD and UC cohort. Minor allele frequencies (MAF), allelic test *P*-values, and odds ratios (OR, shown for the minor allele) with 95% confidence intervals (CI) are depicted for both the CD and UC case-control cohorts. Significant associations (p<0.05) are highlighted in **bold fonts**, suggestive associations (p<0.10) are depicted in *Italic fonts*.

Table 3. Haplotypes of *IL12B* SNPs in the CD case-control sample and omnibus p-values for association with CD susceptibility.

Haplotype combination	Omnibus p-value
rs3212227-rs17860508	0.957
rs17860508-rs10045431	0.333
rs10045431-rs6887695	0.168
rs3212227-rs17860508-rs10045431	0.219
rs17860508-rs10045431-rs6887695	0.202
rs3212227-rs17860508-rs10045431-rs6887695	*0.053*

P-values showing a trend towards significance are depicted in *Italic fonts*.

Analysis for epistasis of IL12B with IL23R and STAT4 gene variants regarding susceptibility to Crohn's disease

Next, we analyzed potential evidence for epistasis of *IL12B* variants with other CD susceptibility genes involved in IL-12 and Th17 signaling, including CD-associated variants in the *IL23R* and *STAT4* gene [3,6,40]. Analysis for gene-gene interaction revealed weak epistasis of *IL12B* SNP rs6887695 with 7 out of the 8 analyzed *STAT4* gene variants (p<0.05) regarding CD susceptibility (Table 7). However, following Bonferroni correction, none of these associations remained significant. In addition, there was no evidence for epistasis between *IL23R* and *IL12B* variants (Table 7).

In silico analysis of IL12B SNPs identifies potential differences in transcription factor binding to major and minor alleles

To analyze if SNPs in the *IL12B* region modify the binding of transcription factors to DNA and thereby modulating gene expression, we analyzed SNPs rs3212227, rs17860508, rs10045431 and rs6887695 including the surrounding sequences for potential binding sites as described in the methods section. The results are shown in table 8. Interestingly, the highest differences in binding scores for the major and the minor alleles was found for rs6887695, the only SNP that was associated with overall IBD susceptibility in our study cohort. Moreover, in homozygous carriers of the minor allele of rs6887695, there were significant associations with specific CD and UC phenotypes. While the transcription factors HSF1, HSF2, MZF1 and Oct-1 were predicted to bind with very high probability to the sequence comprising the major G allele, predicted

Table 4. Haplotypes of *IL12B* SNPs in the UC case-control sample and omnibus p-values for association with UC susceptibility.

Haplotype combination	Omnibus p-value
rs3212227-rs17860508	0.614
rs17860508-rs10045431	0.319
rs10045431-rs6887695	0.126
rs3212227-rs17860508-rs10045431	0.288
rs17860508-rs10045431-rs6887695	0.206
rs3212227-rs17860508-rs10045431-rs6887695	0.300

Table 5. Genotype-phenotype-analysis of SNP rs6887695 in patients with Crohn's disease (CD).

IL12B	(1) CC	(2) CG	(3) GG	P_{CC}	OR_{CC}
rs6887695	n = 100	n = 394	n = 409		[95% CI]
Location					
(n = 768)	n = 80	n = 331	n = 357		
Terminal ileum	11	55	46	1.000	0.92
(L1)	(13.8%)	(16.6%)	(12.9%)		[0.45–1.88]
Colon	6	43	49	0.158	0.53
(L2)	(7.5%)	(13.0%)	(13.7%)		[0.20–1.30]
Ileocolon	60	230	258	0.514	1.23
(L3)	(75.0%)	(69.5%)	(72.3%)		[0.70–2.17]
Upper GI	3	3	4	0.076	3.79
(L4)	(3.8%)	(0.9%)	(1.1%)		[0.76–16.69]
Behaviour[1]					
(n = 690)	n = 72	n = 293	n = 325		
Non-stricturing & Non-penetrating	31	65	75	**6.8×10⁻⁵***	2.84
(B1)	(43.1%)	(22.2%)	(23.1%)		[1.66–4.84]
Stricturing	14	87	85	0.160	0.63
(B2)	(19.4%)	(29.7%)	(26.2%)		[0.32–1.19]
Penetrating	27	141	165	0.062	0.61
(B3)	(37.5%)	(48.1%)	(50.8%)		[0.36–1.04]
					0.36
				9.5×10⁻⁵*	[0.21–0.62]
				(B2+B3)	(B2+B3)
Use of immuno-suppressive agents[2]	50	202	225	0.604	0.84
(n = 477/583)	(79.7%)	(82.1%)	(82.1%)		[0.42–1.69]
Surgery because of CD[3]	35	188	200	0.063	0.63
(n = 423/808)	(42.2%)	(52.9%)	(54.2%)		[0.39–1.027]
Fistulas	33	172	193	0.085	0.67
(n = 398/825)	(39.3%)	(47.8%)	(50.7%)		[0.41–1.08]
Stenosis	42	221	225	**0.038**	0.62
(n = 488/827)	(48.3%)	(61.1%)	(59.5%)		[0.39–0.98]

P_{CC}: P-value for testing for differences between homozygous carriers of the C allele (C/C) and heterozygous and non-carriers of the C allele. OR_{CC}: corresponding odds ratios and 95% confidence intervals (95% CI). Significant P-values (<0.05) are depicted in **bold**, P-values showing a trend towards significance are depicted in *Italic fonts*. P-values marked with an asterisk * remained significant after Bonferroni correction.
[1]Disease behaviour was defined according to the Montreal classification. A stricturing disease phenotype was defined as presence of stenosis without penetrating disease. The diagnosis of stenosis was made surgically, endoscopically, or radiologically (using MRI enteroclysis).
[2]Immunosuppressive agents included azathioprine, 6-mercaptopurine, 6-thioguanin, methotrexate, infliximab and/or adalimumab.
[3]Only surgery related to CD-specific problems (e.g. fistulectomy, colectomy, ileostomy) was included.

binding to the minor C allele was substantially lower (Table 8). On the other hand, the binding score for the transcription factor RORα was higher for the minor C allele (Table 8). Therefore, differential DNA binding of transcription factors in this genomic region followed by differential gene transcription might be one reason for the disease-modifying abilities of this SNP that we observed in our genotype-phenotype analysis.

Discussion

This study presents a detailed genotype-phenotype analysis investigating *IL12B* SNPs as potential susceptibility gene variants in a large Caucasian IBD cohort. A major focus of this study was the analysis of potential epistatic interactions with key gene variants of the IL-12 and IL-23/Th17 pathway such as *IL23R* and *STAT4*. We demonstrated that the *IL12B* variant rs6887695 is

weakly associated with overall IBD susceptibility (p = 0.035), with trends for association with both CD and UC susceptibility. Moreover, a haplotype block formed by the four investigated *IL12B* SNPs showed a trend for association with CD (p = 0.05). Considering our findings and the strong association signal for this gene in the recent GWAS [9,10], *IL12B* can be regarded as established IBD susceptibility gene. In contrast to the very large IBD GWAS, our sample size (n = 2196) was smaller, resulting in limited power, particularly for the UC cohort. For example, a power calculation, which assumed an OR of 1.2 and an allele frequency of 0.20 for the rarest *IL12B* variant rs3212227, demonstrated that our study had 63.1% power to detect a nominal significant finding (alpha = 0.05) in the CD cohort but had only a power of 38.2% in the UC cohort. However, based on the results of this study, the strength of a potential association of *IL12B* with IBD is several log-fold weaker than that shown for

Table 6. Genotype-phenotype-analysis of SNP rs6887695 in patients with ulcerative colitis (UC) for which detailed phenotypic data based on the Montreal classification was available.

IL12B	(1) CC	(2) CG	(3) GG	P_CC	OR_CC
rs6887695	n = 34	n = 145	n = 138		**[95% CI]**
Location					
(n = 193)	n = 25	n = 94	n = 74		
Proctitis (E1)	3	10	11	1.000	0.96
	(12.0%)	(10.6%)	(14.9%)		[0.21–3.78]
				0.030	[1.07–7.03]
				(E1+E2)	(E1+E2)
Left-sided UC (E2)	9	10	11	**0.006***	3.94
	(36.0%)	(10.6%)	(14.9%)		[1.40–11.02]
Extensive UC (E3)	13	74	52	**0.029**	0.36
	(52.0%)	(78.7%)	(70.3%)		[0.14–0.92]
Extra-intestinal manifestations	3	26	24	0.747	0.66
(n = 53/149)	(27.3%)	(35.1%)	(37.5%)		[0.13–2.91]
Use of immunosuppressive agents	22	97	82	0.818	1.23
(n = 201/267)	(78.6%)	(77.6%)	(71.9%)		[0.45–3.57]
Abscesses	2	6	4	0.365	1.77
(n = 12/240)	(7.7%)	(5.4%)	(3.9%)		[0.25–9.41]

For each variable, the number of patients included is given. P_{CC} P-value for testing for differences between homozygous carriers of the C allele and heterozygous/non-carriers of the C allele. OR_{CC}: corresponding odds ratios and 95% confidence intervals (95% CI). Significant P-values (<0.05) are depicted in **bold fonts**. P-values marked with an asterisk remained significant following Bonferroni correction.

Table 7. Analysis for gene-gene interaction of *IL12B* with *IL23R* and *STAT4* variants, respectively, regarding susceptibility to Crohn's disease (CD).

IL12B SNPs	rs3212227	rs17860508	rs10045431	rs6887695
IL23R SNPs				
rs1004819	0.408	0.731	0.474	0.450
rs7517847	0.902	0.895	0.743	0.956
rs10489629	0.577	0.284	0.757	0.561
rs2201841	0.497	0.428	0.080	0.189
rs11465804	0.793	0.852	0.819	0.110
rs11209026 = p.Arg381Gln	0.280	0.752	0.929	0.181
rs1343151	0.970	0.745	0.874	0.971
rs10889677	0.485	0.688	0.108	0.120
rs11209032	0.311	0.473	0.890	0.427
rs1495965	0.641	0.640	0.518	0.624
STAT4 SNPs				
rs11889341	0.732	0.092	0.160	**0.025**
rs7574865	0.845	0.069	0.223	**0.031**
rs7568275	0.725	0.115	0.229	**0.045**
rs8179673	0.659	0.120	0.160	**0.035**
rs10181656	0.618	0.115	0.230	**0.040**
rs7582694	0.818	0.085	0.162	**0.021**
rs10174238	0.354	0.200	0.625	0.247

Significant associations are highlighted in **bold fonts**. None of the associations remained significant following Bonferroni correction.

IL23R in our cohort [6] and other major CD susceptibility genes such as *NOD2* and *ATG16L1* (Supplemental Table S3), suggesting a more important role for IL-23R than IL-12/23 p40 in the genetic susceptibility to IBD. This is in agreement with the recent IBD meta-analyses [9,10], which showed much stronger IBD association signals for *IL23R* than for *IL12B*. Similarly, smaller studies failed to show an association of *IL12B* SNPs with IBD or showed only weak associations with CD or UC [46,47,48] (see Supplemental Table S4 for an overview on published studies on *IL12B* in IBD). Even large studies such as the study by Festen et al., which included 1,455 UC patients and 1,902 controls, was unable to show an association of *IL12B* with UC [49], further demonstrating that very large patient cohorts are necessary to show convincing associations with this gene locus. Therefore, *IL23R* is a more important genetic modifier of IBD susceptibility than *IL12B*, suggesting a more important pathogenic role of Th17 cells, which express IL-23R, than Th1 cells, which develop under the control of IL-12.

Currently, there are limited data on how *IL12B* may functionally influence IBD susceptibility in humans. A very recent study in mice demonstrated that a polymorphism in the coding region of murine *Il12b* promotes IL-12p70 and IL-23 heterodimer formation [50]. The authors hypothesized that the high synthesis rate of IL-12/23 cytokines resulting from efficient binding may lead to rapid proinflammatory skewing of immune responses and disturbance of the homeostatic balance resulting in higher susceptibility for IBD [50]. Other gene variants may also modulate IL-12 expression as recently demonstrated by our group showing increased basal levels of IL-12p40 in CD patients with two mutated *NOD2* alleles [51]. Currently, it is unclear which *IL12B* SNP is the "true" disease-causing variant. We therefore performed a detailed *in silico* analysis of *IL12B* regarding potential transcription factor binding sites and demonstrated for

Table 8. Overview of potential transcription factor binding sites in the genomic regions harboring the analyzed *IL12B* SNPs rs6887695, rs10045431, rs17860508, and rs3212227.

IL12B SNP	Factor	Consensus sequence[‡]	position relative to SNP (5′ to 3′)	Binding score major allele	Binding score minor allele
rs6887695 (approx. 65 kb upstream of *IL12B*):					
GTGTAGTGTAGTGGT[*C/G*]AATAGTCTGGATTTA					
	HSF2	NGAANNWTCK	−1 to +8	*85.9*	*68.6*
	AML-1a	TGCGGT	−6 to −1	85.4	85.4
	MZF1	NGNGGGGA	−6 to +1	*84.3*	*67.0*
	Oct-1	NNGAATATKCANNNN	−5 to +9	*82.5*	*70.6*
	AML-1a	TGCGGT	−14 to −9	81.4	81.4
	AML-1a	TGCGGT	−9 to −4	81.4	81.4
	Th1/E4	NNNNGNRTCTGGMWTT	−1 to +14	80.4	80.8
	HSF1	RGAANRTTCN	−1 to +8	*79.0*	*62.7*
	RORα	NWAWNNAGGTCAN	−10 to +2	*64.4*	*75.9*
rs10045431 (approx. 57 kb upstream of *IL12B*):					
GCAGGCACAGCCCAG[*A/C*]ATTAAACTCTCAAAT					
	Oct-1	CWNAWTKWSATRYN	−2 to +11	79.6	75.5
	SRY	AAACWAM	+4 to +10	77.3	77.3
	Pbx-1	ANCAATCAW	−2 to +6	**75.5**	**69.6**
	Sp1	GRGGCRGGGW	−11 to −2	75.3	75.3
	Tst-1/Oct-6	NNKGAWTWANANTKN	−4 to +10	*70.8*	*81.2*
rs17860508* (approx. 2.7 kb upstream of *IL12B*):					
AATGTGGGGGCCACA[*-/G/GC/TTAGA/TTAGAG*]CCTCTCTCGGAGACA					
	GATA-3[&]	NNGATARGN	0 to +9	**82.5**	**74.1**
	AML-1a	TGCGGT	−6 to −1	83.7	83.7
	AML-1a	TGCGGT	−13 to −8	82.7	82.7
	MZF1	NGNGGGGA	−13 to −6	80.9	80.9
	Oct1[§]	NNRTAATNANNN	−6 to +1	79.3	77.5
	Sp1[#]	GRGGCRGGGW	−7 to +3	*75.3*	*61.6*
rs3212227 (3′-UTR of *IL12B*):					
TGTATTTGTATAGTT[*A/C*]GATGCTAAATGCTCA					
	C/EBP	NNTKTGGWNANNN	−13 to −1	87.7	87.7
	Brn-2/Oct-3	NNCATNSRWAATNMRN	−1 to +16	85.1	83.2
	TATA	NCTATAAAAR	−11 to −2	84.7	84.7
	SRY	AAACWAM	−10 to −4	80.9	80.9
	Oct-1	TNTATGNTAATT	−1 to +10	80.2	79.6
	Tst-1/Oct-6	NNKGAWTWANANTKN	0 to +14	79.2	77.1
	CDP CR	NATYGATSSS	−3 to +6	**78.5**	**73.1**
	Oct-1	CWNAWTKWSATRYN	−7 to +6	**77.6**	**83.7**
	SRY	AAACWAM	−15 to −9	77.3	77.3
	C/EBP	NNTKTGGWNANNN	−1 to +10	76.2	76.9
	CDP CR	NATYGATSSS	−5 to +4	75.3	73.1
	SRY	NWWAACAAWANN	−9 to +2	71.8	76.2

Binding scores differing more than 5 points between major and minor alleles are depicted in **bold**. Scores differing more than 10 points are depicted in ***bold italic***. The binding score threshold for each allele was set to 75.0.
‡Different consensus sequences for the same transcription factor are caused by the deduction of the sequences from different matrices in the TRANSFAC database [45].
*For rs17860508, more than two alleles exist. For the major allele, the score comprises the highest score from all four non-minor alleles (-, G, GC, TTAGA). & = score for the GC allele; # = score for the (-) allele; § = score for the TTAGA allele.
UTR = untranslated region;
Nucleotide codes: K = G or T, M = A or C, R = A or G, S = C or G, W = A or T, N = A, G, C or T.

rs6887695 (out of the four analyzed *IL12B* SNPs) the highest likelihood of changes in transcription factor binding. This is consistent with the results of our genotype analysis in which only rs6887695 was associated with overall IBD susceptibility and potential epistasis with *STAT4* SNPs.

For rs6887695, the *in silico* analysis predicted changes in the binding of the transcription factors HSF1, HSF2, MZF1, Oct-1 and RORα. HSF1 plays a role in protecting against DSS-induced colitis [52]. MZF1 and Oct-1 are transcriptional regulators of SERPINA3 [53,54] which has been implicated as one of the epithelium-derived genes involved in the antibacterial defense [55]. In addition, our *in silico* analysis predicted for the transcription factor RORα stronger binding to the minor C allele. Interestingly, RORα plays together with RORγt a key role in the development of Th17 cells which are involved in the pathogenesis of CD and UC [1] and may explain the association of rs6887695 with increased IBD susceptibility found in our study. Although Th17 cells are recognized as proinflammatory T cell population, their major effector cytokines IL-17A and IL-22 may have also protective functions under certain circumstances [19,56,57,58,59]. Similarly, studies indicated for RORα not only proinflammatory effects but also a role as negative regulator of inflammatory responses [60]. For example, RORα inhibits TNF-α-induced IL-6, IL-8 and COX-2 expression in human primary smooth-muscle cells by negatively interfering with the NF-κB signaling pathway and reducing p65 translocation [60]. This may correlate with our genotype-phenotype analysis which demonstrated a less severe disease phenotype for homozygous C/C carriers of the *IL12B* SNP rs6887695. CD patients, who were homozygous C/C carriers of this SNP, had significantly more often non-stricturing, non-penetrating disease than carriers of the G allele ($p = 6.8 \times 10^{-5}$), while C/C homozygous UC patients had less often extensive colitis than G allele carriers ($p = 0.029$).

IL12B is another example for a common susceptibility gene for CD and UC which is supported by the results of our study showing a trend for rs6887695 for association with both CD and UC. Out of 99 currently known IBD susceptibility gene loci (71 in CD and 47 in UC), at least 28 susceptibility loci are shared between CD and UC [9,10]. Remarkably, the strongest cluster of common CD and UC susceptibility genes is formed by genes related to the IL-23/Th17 pathway including *IL12B* [61]. Similar to *IL23R*, *IL12B* is also a shared susceptibility gene with other IBD-associated diseases such as psoriasis [29] and ankylosing spondylitis [28], providing an explanation of the increased incidence of these extraintestinal manifestations in IBD patients.

The initial GWAS focused on CD patients with ileal CD. To exclude that the associations found in recent GWAS meta-analysis are based only on certain IBD subphenotypes, we performed a detailed genotype-phenotype analysis focusing also on the anatomic disease localization. Interestingly, genotype-phenotype analysis showed an association of *IL12B* rs3212227 with colonic CD but not with ileal CD. It is likely that many of the susceptibility loci, which are shared by CD and UC, may predispose to a common phenotype such as colonic (and not ileal) IBD. This is supported by the association of the *IL12B* SNP rs3212227 with colonic CD and the trend for an association signal of rs6887695 with both CD and UC susceptibility found in our study. Similarly, in another study from New Zealand, carriers of the minor C allele of the *IL12B* SNP rs6887695 had a decreased risk of ileal disease [48]. A recent study analyzing the same SNP (rs6887695) suggested additional environmental triggers regarding the risk of this *IL12B* SNP on CD susceptibility. Analyzing differences in associated genes between smoking and non-smoking CD patients,

it implicated a complex gene-environment interaction demonstrating an association of *IL12B* SNP rs6887695 in non-smoking, but not in smoking patients [62].

In addition, our analysis of potential gene-gene interactions revealed weak epistasis of *IL12B* SNP rs6887695 with 7 out of 8 analyzed *STAT4* gene variants (p<0.05). This is highly interesting, given that STAT4 is the major downstream transcription factor of IL-12. However, considering our limited sample size and the borderline significance of this interaction, which was lost after Bonferroni correction, this potential gene-gene interaction needs further analysis in very large cohorts or GWAS meta-analyses. However, in contrast to our hypothesis-driven study, which analyzed SNPs in the *IL12B* gene encoding IL-12 p40 and the gene *STAT4* encoding the major IL-12 downstream transcription factor STAT4, GWAS are limited by the problem of multiple testing to a much greater extent than our study. Given the large number of SNPs analyzed in GWAS, the correction factor (to correct for multiple testing) is much higher than in our study, which may result in the elimination of potentially true gene-gene interactions. Moreover, in the study by Anderson et al. no formal testing for epistasis has been performed [10]. In addition, in the manuscript by Franke et al. [9], only epistasis between the 71 significantly associated CD loci, which did not include *STAT4*, was analyzed.

In summary, in contrast to Th17 cell-modifying and strongly IBD-associated *IL23R* gene variants, *IL12B* variants have a lesser role in the susceptibility to CD and UC in the German population, suggesting a more important role of IL-23R-expressing Th17 cells than Th1 cells in the CD pathogenesis. This observation is supported by similar results of large GWAS [5,9,10], in which *IL23R* showed stronger associations with IBD susceptibility than *IL12B*, although these GWAS clearly established *IL12B* as IBD susceptibility gene. Our *IL12B in silico* analysis and the results of our genotype analysis suggest rs6887695 as likely disease-causing *IL12B* variant. Homozygous C/C carriers of this SNP were protected against stricturing and penetrating CD and showed less often extensive UC which may be related to the alteration of the binding of certain transcription factors such as RORα as predicted by our *in silico* analysis. We demonstrated for rs688769 potential epistasis with *STAT4*, encoding the major downstream transcription factor of IL-12 which would link IL-12 and STAT4 for the first time on a genetic level. Moreover, similar to an association of the *STAT4* SNP rs7574865 with colonic CD [40], we found an association of the *IL12B* SNP rs3212227 with an increased risk for colonic CD. Based on the gene-gene interaction found for *IL12B* and *STAT4* in this study, large meta-analyses (e.g., by the International IBD Genetics Consortium), which may include our data should further investigate potential epistasis between the main IBD susceptibility genes as major pathomechanism in the disease pathogenesis. Further fine mapping and functional studies are required to clarify the "true" disease-causing *IL12B* variant and its pathogenic role in IBD susceptibility.

Supporting Information

Table S1 Primer sequences (F: forward primer, R: reverse Primer), FRET probe sequences, and primer annealing temperatures used for genotyping of *IL12B* variants. Note: FL: Fluorescein, LC610: LightCycler-Red 610; LC640: LightCycler-Red 640; LC670: LightCycler-Red 670. The polymorphic position within the sensor probe is underlined. A phosphate is linked to the 3′-end of the acceptor probe to prevent elongation by the DNA polymerase in the PCR given based on a median split.

Table S2 Primer sequences used for the sequence analysis of the *IL12B* variants.

Table S3 Comparison of the association signals of *IL12B* with the association signals of the three most strongly CD-associated genes *NOD2*, *IL23R* and *ATG16L1* in the Munich IBD case-control cohort. Minor allele frequencies (MAF), allelic test *P*-values, and odds ratios (OR, shown for the minor allele) with 95% confidence intervals (CI) are depicted for both the CD and UC case-control cohorts. Details on the analyses of *NOD2*, *IL23R* and *ATG16L1* gene variants were published in previous studies.

Table S4 Overview of published studies on *IL12B* in patients with inflammatory bowel diseases. CD: Crohn's disease; UC: ulcerative colitis.

Author Contributions

Conceived and designed the experiments: SB JG. Performed the experiments: JW MW MF CF JD. Analyzed the data: DC JG SB. Contributed reagents/materials/analysis tools: JG SB CS J. Stallhofer BG DC T. Ochsenkühn T. Olszak. Wrote the paper: J. Seiderer SB JG JD. Recruited, interviewed and treated the participating patients: CT FB J. Seiderer J. Stallhofer T. Ochsenkühn T. Olszak SB. Provided funding for the study: SB JG J. Seiderer BG.

References

1. Brand S (2009) Crohn's disease: Th1, Th17 or both? The change of a paradigm: new immunological and genetic insights implicate Th17 cells in the pathogenesis of Crohn's disease. Gut 58: 1152–1167.
2. Neurath MF (2007) IL-23: a master regulator in Crohn disease. Nat Med 13: 26–28.
3. Duerr RH, Taylor KD, Brant SR, Rioux JD, Silverberg MS, et al. (2006) A genome-wide association study identifies IL23R as an inflammatory bowel disease gene. Science 314: 1461–1463.
4. Abraham C, Cho J (2009) Interleukin-23/Th17 pathways and inflammatory bowel disease. Inflamm Bowel Dis 15: 1090–1100.
5. Barrett JC, Hansoul S, Nicolae DL, Cho JH, Duerr RH, et al. (2008) Genome-wide association defines more than 30 distinct susceptibility loci for Crohn's disease. Nat Genet 40: 955–962.
6. Glas J, Seiderer J, Wetzke M, Konrad A, Torok HP, et al. (2007) rs1004819 is the main disease-associated IL23R variant in German Crohn's disease patients: combined analysis of IL23R, CARD15, and OCTN1/2 variants. PLoS ONE 2: e819.
7. Rioux JD, Xavier RJ, Taylor KD, Silverberg MS, Goyette P, et al. (2007) Genome-wide association study identifies new susceptibility loci for Crohn disease and implicates autophagy in disease pathogenesis. Nat Genet 39: 596–604.
8. Parkes M, Barrett JC, Prescott NJ, Tremelling M, Anderson CA, et al. (2007) Sequence variants in the autophagy gene IRGM and multiple other replicating loci contribute to Crohn's disease susceptibility. Nat Genet 39: 830–832.
9. Franke A, McGovern DP, Barrett JC, Wang K, Radford-Smith GL, et al. (2010) Genome-wide meta-analysis increases to 71 the number of confirmed Crohn's disease susceptibility loci. Nat Genet 42: 1118–1125.
10. Anderson CA, Boucher G, Lees CW, Franke A, D'Amato M, et al. (2011) Meta-analysis identifies 29 additional ulcerative colitis risk loci, increasing the number of confirmed associations to 47. Nat Genet 43: 246–252.
11. Glas J, Stallhofer J, Ripke S, Wetzke M, Pfennig S, et al. (2009) Novel genetic risk markers for ulcerative colitis in the IL2/IL21 region are in epistasis with IL23R and suggest a common genetic background for ulcerative colitis and celiac disease. Am J Gastroenterol 104: 1737–1744.
12. Wang K, Zhang H, Kugathasan S, Annese V, Bradfield JP, et al. (2009) Diverse genome-wide association studies associate the IL12/IL23 pathway with Crohn Disease. Am J Hum Genet 84: 399–405.
13. Langrish CL, McKenzie BS, Wilson NJ, de Waal Malefyt R, Kastelein RA, et al. (2004) IL-12 and IL-23: master regulators of innate and adaptive immunity. Immunol Rev 202: 96–105.
14. Chan SH, Perussia B, Gupta JW, Kobayashi M, Pospisil M, et al. (1991) Induction of interferon gamma production by natural killer cell stimulatory factor: characterization of the responder cells and synergy with other inducers. J Exp Med 173: 869–879.
15. Parronchi P, Romagnani P, Annunziato F, Sampognaro S, Becchio A, et al. (1997) Type 1 T-helper cell predominance and interleukin-12 expression in the gut of patients with Crohn's disease. Am J Pathol 150: 823–832.
16. Oppmann B, Lesley R, Blom B, Timans JC, Xu Y, et al. (2000) Novel p19 protein engages IL-12p40 to form a cytokine, IL-23, with biological activities similar as well as distinct from IL-12. Immunity 13: 715–725.
17. Ciric B, El-behi M, Cabrera R, Zhang GX, Rostami A (2009) IL-23 drives pathogenic IL-17-producing CD8+ T cells. J Immunol 182: 5296–5305.
18. Seiderer J, Elben I, Diegelmann J, Glas J, Stallhofer J, et al. (2008) Role of the novel Th17 cytokine IL-17F in inflammatory bowel disease (IBD): upregulated colonic IL-17F expression in active Crohn's disease and analysis of the IL17F p.His161Arg polymorphism in IBD. Inflamm Bowel Dis 14: 437–445.
19. Brand S, Beigel F, Olszak T, Zitzmann K, Eichhorst ST, et al. (2006) IL-22 is increased in active Crohn's disease and promotes proinflammatory gene expression and intestinal epithelial cell migration. Am J Physiol Gastrointest Liver Physiol 290: G827–838.
20. Dambacher J, Beigel F, Zitzmann K, De Toni EN, Goke B, et al. (2009) The role of the novel Th17 cytokine IL-26 in intestinal inflammation. Gut 58: 1207–1217.
21. Brand S, Olszak T, Beigel F, Diebold J, Otte JM, et al. (2006) Cell differentiation dependent expressed CCR6 mediates ERK-1/2, SAPK/JNK, and Akt signaling resulting in proliferation and migration of colorectal cancer cells. J Cell Biochem 97: 709–723.
22. Fujino S, Andoh A, Bamba S, Ogawa A, Hata K, et al. (2003) Increased expression of interleukin 17 in inflammatory bowel disease. Gut 52: 65–70.
23. Monteleone G, Monteleone I, Fina D, Vavassori P, Del Vecchio Blanco G, et al. (2005) Interleukin-21 enhances T-helper cell type I signaling and interferon-gamma production in Crohn's disease. Gastroenterology 128: 687–694.
24. Parham C, Chirica M, Timans J, Vaisberg E, Travis M, et al. (2002) A receptor for the heterodimeric cytokine IL-23 is composed of IL-12Rbeta1 and a novel cytokine receptor subunit, IL-23R. J Immunol 168: 5699–5708.
25. Sandborn WJ, Feagan BG, Fedorak RN, Scherl E, Fleisher MR, et al. (2008) A randomized trial of Ustekinumab, a human interleukin-12/23 monoclonal antibody, in patients with moderate-to-severe Crohn's disease. Gastroenterology 135: 1130–1141.
26. Huffmeier U, Lascorz J, Bohm B, Lohmann J, Wendler J, et al. (2009) Genetic variants of the IL-23R pathway: association with psoriatic arthritis and psoriasis vulgaris, but no specific risk factor for arthritis. J Invest Dermatol 129: 355–358.
27. Smith RL, Warren RB, Eyre S, Ho P, Ke X, et al. (2008) Polymorphisms in the IL-12beta and IL-23R genes are associated with psoriasis of early onset in a UK cohort. J Invest Dermatol 128: 1325–1327.
28. Burton PR, Clayton DG, Cardon LR, Craddock N, Deloukas P, et al. (2007) Association scan of 14,500 nonsynonymous SNPs in four diseases identifies autoimmunity variants. Nat Genet 39: 1329–1337.
29. Cargill M, Schrodi SJ, Chang M, Garcia VE, Brandon R, et al. (2007) A large-scale genetic association study confirms IL12B and leads to the identification of IL23R as psoriasis-risk genes. Am J Hum Genet 80: 273–290.
30. Danoy P, Pryce K, Hadler J, Bradbury LA, Farrar C, et al. (2010) Association of variants at 1q32 and STAT3 with ankylosing spondylitis suggests genetic overlap with Crohn's disease. PLoS Genet 6: e1001195.
31. Filer C, Ho P, Smith RL, Griffiths C, Young HS, et al. (2008) Investigation of association of the IL12B and IL23R genes with psoriatic arthritis. Arthritis Rheum 58: 3705–3709.
32. Nair RP, Ruether A, Stuart PE, Jenisch S, Tejasvi T, et al. (2008) Polymorphisms of the IL12B and IL23R genes are associated with psoriasis. J Invest Dermatol 128: 1653–1661.
33. Morahan G, Kaur G, Singh M, Rapthap CC, Kumar N, et al. (2007) Association of variants in the IL12B gene with leprosy and tuberculosis. Tissue Antigens 69 Suppl 1: 234–236.
34. Hirota T, Suzuki Y, Hasegawa K, Obara K, Matsuda A, et al. (2005) Functional haplotypes of IL-12B are associated with childhood atopic asthma. J Allergy Clin Immunol 116: 789–795.
35. Tug E, Ozbey U, Tug T, Yuce H (2009) Relationship between the IL-12B promoter polymorphism and allergic rhinitis, familial asthma, serum total IgE, and eosinophil level in asthma patients. J Investig Allergol Clin Immunol 19: 21–26.
36. Chang M, Saiki RK, Cantanese JJ, Lew D, van der Helm-van Mil AH, et al. (2008) The inflammatory disease-associated variants in IL12B and IL23R are not associated with rheumatoid arthritis. Arthritis Rheum 58: 1877–1881.
37. Begovich AB, Chang M, Caillier SJ, Lew D, Catanese JJ, et al. (2007) The autoimmune disease-associated IL12B and IL23R polymorphisms in multiple sclerosis. Hum Immunol 68: 934–937.
38. Marquez A, Mendoza JL, Taxonera C, Diaz-Rubio M, De La Concha EG, et al. (2008) IL23R and IL12B polymorphisms in Spanish IBD patients: no evidence of interaction. Inflamm Bowel Dis 14: 1192–1196.
39. Yamazaki K, Takahashi A, Takazoe M, Kubo M, Onouchi Y, et al. (2009) Positive association of genetic variants in the upstream region of NKX2-3 with Crohn's disease in Japanese patients. Gut 58: 228–232.
40. Glas J, Seiderer J, Nagy M, Fries C, Beigel F, et al. (2010) Evidence for STAT4 as a common autoimmune gene: rs7574865 is associated with colonic Crohn's disease and early disease onset. PLoS ONE 5: e10373.
41. Silverberg MS, Satsangi J, Ahmad T, Arnott ID, Bernstein CN, et al. (2005) Toward an integrated clinical, molecular and serological classification of

inflammatory bowel disease: Report of a Working Party of the 2005 Montreal World Congress of Gastroenterology. Can J Gastroenterol 19 Suppl A: 5–36.

42. Glas J, Konrad A, Schmechel S, Dambacher J, Seiderer J, et al. (2008) The ATG16L1 gene variants rs2241879 and rs2241880 (T300A) are strongly associated with susceptibility to Crohn's disease in the German population. Am J Gastroenterol 103: 682–691.

43. Glas J, Seiderer J, Fries C, Tillack C, Pfennig S, et al. (2011) CEACAM6 gene variants in inflammatory bowel disease. PLoS ONE 6: e19319.

44. Muller-Berghaus J, Kern K, Paschen A, Nguyen XD, Kluter H, et al. (2004) Deficient IL-12p70 secretion by dendritic cells based on IL12B promoter genotype. Genes Immun 5: 431–434.

45. Heinemeyer T, Wingender E, Reuter I, Hermjakob H, Kel AE, et al. (1998) Databases on transcriptional regulation: TRANSFAC, TRRD and COMPEL. Nucleic Acids Res 26: 362–367.

46. Torkvist L, Halfvarson J, Ong RT, Lordal M, Sjoqvist U, et al. (2010) Analysis of 39 Crohn's disease risk loci in Swedish inflammatory bowel disease patients. Inflamm Bowel Dis 16: 907–909.

47. Peter I, Mitchell AA, Ozelius L, Erazo M, Hu J, et al. (2011) Evaluation of 22 genetic variants with Crohn's disease risk in the Ashkenazi Jewish population: a case-control study. BMC Med Genet 12: 63.

48. Ferguson LR, Han DY, Fraser AG, Huebner C, Lam WJ, et al. (2010) IL23R and IL12B SNPs and Haplotypes Strongly Associate with Crohn's Disease Risk in a New Zealand Population. Gastroenterol Res Pract 2010: 539461.

49. Festen EA, Stokkers PC, van Diemen CC, van Bodegraven AA, Boezen HM, et al. (2010) Genetic analysis in a Dutch study sample identifies more ulcerative colitis susceptibility loci and shows their additive role in disease risk. Am J Gastroenterol 105: 395–402.

50. Zwiers A, Fuss IJ, Seegers D, Konijn T, Garcia-Vallejo JJ, et al. (2011) A polymorphism in the coding region of Il12b promotes IL-12p70 and IL-23 heterodimer formation. J Immunol 186: 3572–3580.

51. Beynon V, Cotofana S, Brand S, Lohse P, Mair A, et al. (2008) NOD2/CARD15 genotype influences MDP-induced cytokine release and basal IL-12p40 levels in primary isolated peripheral blood monocytes. Inflamm Bowel Dis 14: 1033–1040.

52. Tanaka K, Namba T, Arai Y, Fujimoto M, Adachi H, et al. (2007) Genetic evidence for a protective role for heat shock factor 1 and heat shock protein 70 against colitis. J Biol Chem 282: 23240–23252.

53. Chelbi ST, Wilson ML, Veillard AC, Ingles S, Zhang J, et al. (2012) Genetic and epigenetic mechanisms collaborate to control SERPINA3 expression and its association with placental diseases. Hum Mol Genet. 2012 Jan 31. [Epub ahead of print].

54. Morgan K, Kalsheker NA (1997) Regulation of the serine proteinase inhibitor (SERPIN) gene alpha 1-antitrypsin: a paradigm for other SERPINs. Int J Biochem Cell Biol 29: 1501–1511.

55. Flach CF, Qadri F, Bhuiyan TR, Alam NH, Jennische E, et al. (2007) Broad up-regulation of innate defense factors during acute cholera. Infect Immun 75: 2343–2350.

56. O'Connor W, Jr., Kamanaka M, Booth CJ, Town T, Nakae S, et al. (2009) A protective function for interleukin 17A in T cell-mediated intestinal inflammation. Nat Immunol 10: 603–609.

57. Sugimoto K, Ogawa A, Mizoguchi E, Shimomura Y, Andoh A, et al. (2008) IL-22 ameliorates intestinal inflammation in a mouse model of ulcerative colitis. J Clin Invest 118: 534–544.

58. Zenewicz LA, Yancopoulos GD, Valenzuela DM, Murphy AJ, Stevens S, et al. (2008) Innate and adaptive interleukin-22 protects mice from inflammatory bowel disease. Immunity 29: 947–957.

59. Glas J, Seiderer J, Bayrle C, Wetzke M, Fries C, et al. (2011) The role of osteopontin (OPN/SPP1) haplotypes in the susceptibility to Crohn's disease. PLoS One 6: e29309.

60. Delerive P, Monte D, Dubois G, Trottein F, Fruchart-Najib J, et al. (2001) The orphan nuclear receptor ROR alpha is a negative regulator of the inflammatory response. EMBO Rep 2: 42–48.

61. Lees CW, Barrett JC, Parkes M, Satsangi J (2011) New IBD genetics: common pathways with other diseases. Gut 60: 1739–1753.

62. van der Heide F, Nolte IM, Kleibeuker JH, Wijmenga C, Dijkstra G, et al. (2010) Differences in genetic background between active smokers, passive smokers, and non-smokers with Crohn's disease. Am J Gastroenterol 105: 1165–1172.

14

CEACAM6 Gene Variants in Inflammatory Bowel Disease

Jürgen Glas[1,2,3◊], Julia Seiderer[1◊], Christoph Fries[1,2], Cornelia Tillack[1], Simone Pfennig[1], Maria Weidinger[1], Florian Beigel[1], Torsten Olszak[1,4], Ulrich Lass[5], Burkhard Göke[1], Thomas Ochsenkühn[1], Christiane Wolf[6], Peter Lohse[7], Bertram Müller-Myhsok[6], Julia Diegelmann[1,2], Darina Czamara[6], Stephan Brand[1]*

1 Department of Medicine II - Grosshadern, Ludwig-Maximilians-University, Munich, Germany, 2 Department of Preventive Dentistry and Periodontology, Ludwig-Maximilians-University, Munich, Germany, 3 Department of Human Genetics, Rheinisch-Westfälische Technische Hochschule, Aachen, Germany, 4 Division of Gastroenterology, Hepatology and Endoscopy, Brigham and Women's Hospital, Harvard Medical School, Boston, Massachusetts, United States of America, 5 TIB MOLBIOL Syntheselabor GmbH, Berlin, Germany, 6 Max-Planck-Institute of Psychiatry, Munich, Germany, 7 Department of Clinical Chemistry, Ludwig-Maximilians-University, Munich, Germany

Abstract

Background: The carcinoembryonic antigen-related cell adhesion molecule 6 (CEACAM6) acts as a receptor for adherent-invasive *E. coli* (AIEC) and its ileal expression is increased in patients with Crohn's disease (CD). Given its contribution to the pathogenesis of CD, we aimed to investigate the role of genetic variants in the *CEACAM6* region in patients with inflammatory bowel diseases (IBD).

Methodology: In this study, a total of 2,683 genomic DNA samples (including DNA from 858 CD patients, 475 patients with ulcerative colitis (UC), and 1,350 healthy, unrelated controls) was analyzed for eight *CEACAM6* SNPs (rs10415946, rs1805223 = p.Pro42Pro, rs4803507, rs4803508, rs11548735 = p.Gly239Val, rs7246116 = pHis260His, rs2701, rs10416839). In addition, a detailed haplotype analysis and genotype-phenotype analysis were performed. Overall, our genotype analysis did not reveal any significant association of the investigated *CEACAM6* SNPs and haplotypes with CD or UC susceptibility, although certain *CEACAM6* SNPs modulated CEACAM6 expression in intestinal epithelial cell lines. Despite its function as receptor of AIEC in ileal CD, we found no association of the *CEACAM6* SNPs with ileal or ileocolonic CD. Moreover, there was no evidence of epistasis between the analyzed *CEACAM6* variants and the main CD-associated *NOD2, IL23R* and *ATG16L1* variants.

Conclusions: This study represents the first detailed analysis of *CEACAM6* variants in IBD patients. Despite its important role in bacterial attachment in ileal CD, we could not demonstrate a role for *CEACAM6* variants in IBD susceptibility or regarding an ileal CD phenotype. Further functional studies are required to analyze if these gene variants modulate ileal bacterial attachment.

Editor: Jörg Hermann Fritz, McGill University, Canada

Funding: J. Glas was supported by a grant from the Broad Medical Foundation (IBD-0126R2). J. Seiderer and J. Diegelmann were supported by grants from the Ludwig-Maximilians-University Munich (FoeFoLe Nr. 422; Habilitationsstipendium, LMUExcellent to J.S. and Promotionsstipendium to J.D.); J. Seiderer was also supported by the Robert-Bosch-Foundation and the Else Kroener-Fresenius-Stiftung (81/08//EKMS08/01). S. Brand was supported by grants from the DFG (BR 1912/5-1), the Else Kroener-Fresenius-Stiftung (Else Kroener Fresenius Memorial Stipendium 2005; P50/05/EKMS05/62), by the Ludwig-Demling Grant 2007 from DCCV e.V., and by grants of Ludwig-Maximilians-University Munich (Excellence Initiative, Investment Funds 2008 and FFoLe program). U. Lass is a employee of TIB MOLBIOL Syntheselabor GmbH. The funders had no role in study design, data collection and analysis, decision to publish, or preparation of the manuscript. TIB MOLBIOL Syntheselabor GmbH provided help with designing the FRET probes but had no role in study design, data collection and analysis, decision to publish, or preparation of the manuscript.

Competing Interests: U. Lass is an employee of TIB MOLBIOL Syntheselabor GmbH, which is marketing FRET probes for genotyping. However, TIB MOLBIOL Syntheselabor GmbH had no role in study design, data collection and analysis, decision to publish, or preparation of the manuscript.

* E-mail: stephan.brand@med.uni-muenchen.de

◊ These authors contributed equally to this work.

Introduction

Crohn's disease (CD) and ulcerative colitis (UC) are chronic inflammatory bowel diseases (IBD), characterized by an aberrant mucosal immune response to bacteria-derived antigens in the gut of genetically susceptible hosts [1,2]. Although the exact pathogenesis of IBD still remains unsolved, current evidence indicates that defective T-cell apoptosis [3] and autophagy [4,5,6,7] as well as an impairment of intestinal epithelial barrier function [8,9] play important roles. This

hypothesis is strengthened by data from genetic association studies identifying CD susceptibility genes involved in innate immunity and bacterial recognition (*NOD2/CARD15*) [10,11], and from genome-wide association studies (GWAS), which identified susceptibility genes involved in autophagy (*ATG16L1, IRGM*) [4,5] and the proinflammatory IL-23/Th17 pathway [12].

While a specific causative pathogen in IBD has not been found so far [13,14], investigations of the regulatory mechanisms operating at the mucosal level suggest that regulatory cells reactive to the commensal intestinal microflora might play a role in cross-reactive protection toward different bacterial antigens [15]. Moreover, there is raising evidence for a major role of certain bacteria such as adherent-invasive *E. coli* (AIEC) in ileal CD [16,17,18]. Interestingly, the carcinoembryonic antigen-related cell adhesion molecule 6 (CEACAM6) has recently shown to act as a receptor for AIEC, supporting ileal bacterial colonization as a major pathomechanism in CD [19]. The carcinoembryonic antigen (CEA) family consists of two subfamilies, the CEACAM subgroup and the pregnancy specific glycoprotein (PSG) subgroup [20,21]. CEACAM family members were found to be expressed in epithelial, endothelial, and hematopoietic cells, including T-lymphocytes, natural killer (NK) cells, dendritic cells (DC) and neutrophils. They may also be useful as biomarkers in cancer since they are often over-expressed in ovarian, endometrial, breast, lung, and colon carcinomas [21,22,23]. Depending on the tissue involved, CEACAMs are transmitting signals that result in a variety of effects including regulation of the cell cycle, tumor suppression, angiogenesis, lymphocyte activation and adhesion [22,23,24,25,26,27,28,29]. CEACAM1, CEACAM5, and CEACAM6 represent three of the CEACAM subfamily members expressed in intestinal epithelial cells. There is increased expression of CEACAM5 and CEACAM6 at the apical surface of the ileal epithelium in CD patients [19]. Moreover, ileal lesions in CD patients were found to be colonized by pathogenic AIEC [19], strengthening the hypothesis that an abnormal intestinal expression of CEACAM6 in CD patients is associated with an increased colonization of AIEC via type 1 pili expression inducing gut inflammation [18]. AIEC adhere to and invade intestinal epithelial cells [30] resulting in AIEC accumulation in macrophages leading to high amounts of TNF-α [31], thereby perpetuating intestinal inflammation.

Given the potential implication of dysfunctional CEACAM6 expression in the pathogenesis of IBD, we aimed to analyze the role of *CEACAM6* SNPs in IBD susceptibility. A total of eight single nucleotide polymorphisms (SNPs) were analyzed in a large German cohort of CD and UC patients. Five SNPs in the *CEACAM6* region (rs10415946, rs4803507, rs4803508, rs2701, rs10416839) were selected from the data of the international HapMap project covering the *CEACAM6* gene plus 10 kB flanking the centromeric and telomeric end of the gene, respectively. Additional selection criteria for the SNPs were a minor allele frequency of at least 5% and a r^2 of 1. The SNPs rs4803507 and rs4803508 are localized in intron 2, rs2701 is localized within exon 6 encoding the 3'-untranslated region, while the SNPs rs10415946 and rs10416839 are within the 5'- and the 3'-flanking region, respectively. Additionally, the coding variants rs1805223 = p.Pro42Pro (exon 2), rs11548735 = p.Gly239Val and rs7246116 = pHis260His (exon 4) were investigated for which allele frequencies are published und which display a minor allele frequency of at least 5% in the Caucasian population. The structure of the *CEACAM6* gene and the

localization of the SNPs investigated in the presented study are shown in figure 1. Considering the abnormal expression of CEACAM6 in the ileal epithelium of CD patients and its role as receptor for ileal AIEC [19], we also analyzed for a potential association with an ileal CD phenotype and investigated potential gene-gene interactions with the *NOD2* gene, which has been shown to be a strong predictor of ileal CD, as well as with other CD susceptibility genes such as *IL23R* and *ATG16L1*.

Materials and Methods

Ethics statement

The study was approved by the local Ethics committee of the Ludwig-Maximilians-University of Munich (Department of Medicine) and adhered to the ethical principles for medical research involving human subjects of the Helsinki Declaration. Prior to the study, we obtained written, informed consent from all patients included.

Study population and characterization of disease phenotype

The study population comprised 858 patients with CD, 475 patients with UC, and 1350 healthy, unrelated controls of Caucasian origin. The study was approved by the local Ethics committee of the Ludwig-Maximilians-University of Munich (Department of Medicine) and adhered to the ethical principles for medical research involving human subjects of the Helsinki Declaration. Prior to the study, we obtained written, informed consent from all patients included. The phenotypic assessment was performed blind to the results of the genotypic data and included demographic data and clinical parameters (behaviour and anatomic location of IBD, disease-related complications, previous surgery or immunosuppressive therapy) which were recorded by investigation of patient charts and a detailed questionnaire. The diagnosis of CD or UC was based on established international guidelines including endoscopic, radiological, and histopathological criteria [32,33]. Patients with CD were assessed according to the Montreal classification [33] based on age at diagnosis (A), location (L), and behaviour (B) of disease. In patients with UC, anatomic location was also assessed in accordance to the Montreal classification [33], using the criteria ulcerative proctitis (E1), left-sided UC (distal UC; E2), and extensive UC (pancolitis; E3). Patients with indeterminate colitis were excluded from the study. The demographic and phenotypic data of the IBD study population are summarized in Table 1.

DNA extraction and genotyping of the *CEACAM6* variants

Blood samples were taken from all participants of the study and genomic DNA was isolated from peripheral blood leukocytes using the DNA blood mini kit from Qiagen (Hilden, Germany)

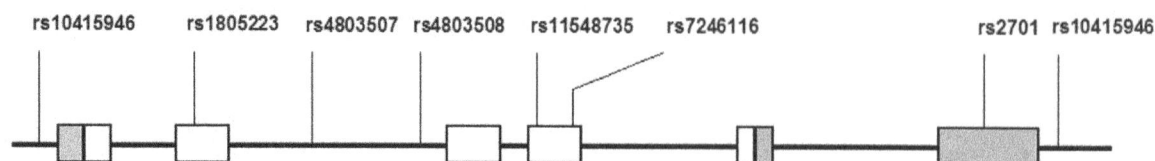

Figure 1. Exon-intron structure of the *CEACAM6* gene and relative positions of single nucleotide polymorphisms (SNPs) investigated in the presented study. This figure represents the genomic structure of the *CEACAM6* gene consisting of 6 exons and indicates the positions of the *CEACAM6* SNPs studied. The SNPs rs4803507 and rs4803508 are localized in intron 2, rs2701 is localized in exon 6 encoding the 3'-untranslated region, while the SNPs rs10415946 and rs10416839 are within the 5'- and the 3'-flanking region, respectively. The coding variant rs1805223 = p.Pro42Pro is located in exon 2, while rs11548735 = p.Gly239Val and rs7246116 = pHis260His are located in exon 4. The grey part of exons 1 represents the 5' untranslated region, the grey part of exons 5 and exon 6 represent the 3' untranslated region.

Table 1. Demographic and phenotypic disease characteristics of the study population.

	Crohn's disease *n = 858*	Ulcerative colitis *n = 475*	Controls *n = 1350*
Gender			
Male (%)	45.3	47.9	62.6
Female (%)	54.7	52.5	37.4
Age (yrs)			
Mean ± SD	40.2±13.2	42.4±14.4	45.8±10.7
Range	11–81	7–86	18–71
Body mass index			
Mean ± SD	23.1±4.2	23.9±4.1	
Range	13–40	15–41	
Age at diagnosis (yrs)			
Mean ± SD	27.7±11.8	32.0±13.3	
Range	1–78	9–81	
Disease duration (yrs)			
Mean ± SD	11.9±8.6	10.5±7.7	
Range	0–44	1–40	
Positive family history of IBD (%)	16.0	16.1	
Disease localization (Crohn's disease)			
*n = 764**			
L1 (ileal)	113		
L2 (colonic)	97		
L3 (ileocolonic)	554		
+ L4 (upper GI)**	88		
Disease behaviour (Crohn's disease)			
*n = 754**			
B1 (non-stricturing, non-penetrating)	187		
B2 (stricturing)	208		
B3 (penetrating)	359		
Disease extent (Ulcerative colitis)			
*n = 260**			
E1 (proctitis)		24	
E2 (left-sided UC)		96	
E3 (pancolitis)		140	

Disease localization and disease behaviour for Crohn's disease and the disease extent in ulcerative colitis are given according to the Montreal classification of inflammatory bowel diseases.
*Given is the number of patients for which the corresponding disease phenotype information was available.
**Additional upper GI involvement.

according to the manufacturer's guidelines. Eight *CEACAM6* SNPs (rs10415946, rs1805223 = p.Pro42Pro, rs4803507, rs4803508, rs11548735 = p.Gly239Val, rs7246116 = pHis260His, rs2701, rs10416839) were genotyped by PCR and melting curve analysis using a pair of fluorescence resonance energy transfer (FRET) probes in a LightCycler® 480 Instrument (Roche Diagnostics, Mannheim, Germany) as described in previous studies [34,35,36]. The total volume of the PCR was 5 µl containing 25 ng of genomic DNA, 1× Light Cycler 480 Genotyping Master Mix (Roche Diagnostics), 2.5 pmol of each primer and 0.75 pmol of each FRET probe (TIB MOLBIOL, Berlin, Germany). In the case of rs1805223, rs4803507 and rs4803508, the concentration of the forward primer, and in the case of rs10415946 and rs2701, the concentration of the reverse primer, were reduced to 1.25 pmol.

Two SNPs were analyzed in a multiplex reaction, the combinations were: rs10415946+rs4803508, rs1805223+rs4803507, rs11548735+rs7246116 and rs2701+rs10416839. For the combination rs11548735+rs7246116 only one primer pair was used. The PCR comprised an initial denaturation step (95°C for 10 min) and 45 cycles (95°C for 10°C sec, 60 for 10 sec, 72°C for 15 sec). Details on the melting curve analysis and on the PCR used for sequencing were published in previous studies [34,35,36]. The PCR products were purified using the QIAquick PCR Purification Kit (Qiagen) and sequenced by a commercial sequencing company (Sequiserve, Vaterstetten, Germany). All sequences of primers and FRET probes and primer annealing temperatures used for genotyping and for sequence analysis are given in Tables 2 and 3.

Table 2. Primer sequences (F: forward primer, R: reverse Primer) and FRET probe sequences used for genotyping of *CEACAM6* variants.

Polymorphism	Primer sequences	FRET probe sequences
rs10415946	F: AGCCCTGGATGTGTCCAC A: AGTCCCTGGGGTCCTCAA	TGGATTTACCCCCAGCAAG-FL LC670-AGGTCACAGAGATGTTTGGGGTCCTAG
rs1805223 = p.Pro42Pro	F: CCACCCTAATGCATAGGTCC A: CGATTCTGTGGCAGGTTGT	GAATCCACGCCATTCAATG-FL LC670-CGCAGAGGGGAAGGAGGTTCTTC
rs4803507	F: GCATCGTTCCTTCCTTTATGTA A: TTTTTCCATAAGTGGAGATCGTT	GAATTCACAACACACCTAAACC-FL LC640-AGTATGTTATCAAGAAAAATACTACTTCCAGCCC
rs4803508	F: CCTGTCCCCCTCACTGTCT A: TTTTTCCATAAGTGGAGATCGTT	CTGCTGAAAGATCCAATCCC-FL LC610-GCCAGGCTGCACAGTATCCTTGGG
rs11548735 = p.Gly239Val	F: TGGTTGAGACTTCAGGGTTGT A: TATGGGCTTGGCACATATAGG	CCCAGATGTCCCCACCAT-FL LC610-TCCCCCTCAAAGGCCAATTACCGTC
rs7246116 = pHis260His	F: TGGTTGAGACTTCAGGGTTGT A: TATGGGCTTGGCACATATAGG	CCTGCCACGCAGCCTCTA-FL LC670-CCCACCTGCACAGTACTCTTGGTTTATCAA
rs2701	F: AAGATGTCAAAACAAGACTCCTCA A: AAGTCCAACTCTGAAAAGGACC	CAAGATAGATCTGACACTCTGTTAAGT-FL LC610-ACCCTCTGAAGCTACTTCTTGTGAAATACT
rs10416839	F: CTTTCAGTTATATGTTGGCTCACTT A: AAAAACACAGCATTATAGATCAACAG	CCAGTGGCAGTTTCCTCTG-FL LC640-TGTAGTCTGAATCAGGTGTACAACTGAGCC

Note: FL: Fluorescein, LC610: LightCycler-Red 610; LC640: LightCycler-Red 640. The polymorphic position within the sensor probe is underlined. A phosphate is linked to the 3'-end of the acceptor probe to prevent elongation by the DNA polymerase in the PCR.

Genotyping data of the three main CD-associated *NOD2* variants p.Arg702Trp (rs2066844), p.Gly908Arg (rs2066845), and p.Leu1007fsX1008 (rs2066847) were available from previous studies [34,37]. Similarly, for epistasis analysis genotype data for the main CD-associated *IL23R* variants (rs1004819, rs7517847, rs10489629, rs2201841, rs11465804, rs11209026 (p.Arg381Gln), rs1343151, rs10889677, rs11209032, rs1495965) and *ATG16L1* SNPs (rs13412102, rs12471449, rs6431660, rs1441090, rs2289472, rs2241880 (p.Thr300Ala), rs2241879, rs3792106, rs4663396) were available from previous studies [34–36].

RNA isolation and quantitative PCR

Total RNA was isolated from five intestinal epithelial cell (IEC) lines (DLD-1, HCT116, HT-29, SW480, T84) as indicated with the Qiagen RNeasy Kit and was reverse transcribed using Roche Transcriptor First Strand cDNA Synthesis Kit. Quantitative PCR was performed with SYBR Green PCR Master Mix from Roche on a LightCycler480 instrument. The following primers were used for amplification: *CEACAM6* forward 5'-CACAACCTGCCCCA-GAATCGTAT-3'; *CEACAM6* reverse 5'-TTGGGCAGCT-CCGGGTATACATG-3'; *β-actin* forward 5'-GCCAACCGCGA-GAAGATGA-3'; *β-actin* reverse 5'-CATCACGATGCCAG-TGGTA-3'. β-actin expression was used to normalize gene expression in the respective samples.

Statistical analyses

Each genetic marker was tested for Hardy-Weinberg equilibrium in the three subgroups of the study population. Fisher's exact test was used for comparison between categorical variables, while Student's t test was applied for quantitative variables. Single-marker allelic tests were performed with Pearson's χ^2 test. All tests were two-tailed, considering p-values<0.05 as significant. Odds ratios were calculated for the minor allele at each SNP. For multiple comparisons, Bonferroni correction was applied where

Table 3. Primer sequences used for the sequence analysis of the *CEACAM6* variants.

Polymorphism	Primer sequences
rs10415946	TGCAGAAAGAACAATTCAGAATCTTA CTTGGGTCTGTCAGCACC
rs1805223 = p.Pro42Pro	GGGTGAAGAGACCTGCTCAG CGCCTTTGTACCAGCTGTAAC
rs4803507	ACGTTGCTTCTAATTTGGCA GAAAAGTTTGTCAGGAGTTTAGACC
rs4803508	CCTGTCCCCCTCACTGTCT ATGGGTGATGATGGGACTTC
rs11548735 = p.Gly239Val, rs7246116 = pHis260His	TGGTTGAGACTTCAGGGTTGT TATGGGCTTGGCACATATAGG
rs2701	AAGATGTCAAAACAAGACTCCTCA AGAACAGGTGAGTCTAGAAGTCCA
rs10416839	CTTTCAGTTATATGTTGGCTCACTT AAAAACACAGCATTATAGATCAACAG

Table 4. Associations of *CEACAM6* gene markers in the case-control association studies.

SNP	Minor allele	Crohn's disease *n = 858*			Ulcerative colitis *n = 475*			Controls *n = 1350*	HapMap-CEU** *n = 120*
		MAF/HWE	p value	OR [95% CI]	MAF/HWE	p value	OR [95% CI]	MAF/HWE	MAF
rs10415946	G	0.383/0.506	0.21	1.08 [0.96–1.23]	0.338/0.113	0.16	0.89 [0.76–1.04]	0.364/0.906	0.440
rs1805223 = p.Pro42Pro	A	0.309/0.679	0.21	1.09 [0.95–1.24]	0.264/0.235	0.12	0.87 [0.74–1.03]	0.291/0.262	0.342
rs4803507	A	0.307/0.803	0.24	1.08 [0.96–1.24]	0.269/0.454	0.26	0.90 [0.76–1.06]	0.290/0.234	0.280
rs4803508	A	0.377/0.266	0.25	0.95 [0.84–1.08]	0.406/0.622	0.35	1.07 [0.92–1.25]	0.389/0.606	0.358
rs11548735 = p.Gly239Val	T	0.399/0.885	0.62	0.97 [0.86–1.10]	0.422/1	0.44	1.06 [0.92–1.24]	0.407/0.612	0.422
rs7246116 = pHis260His	T	0/*	1.00	-	0.001/1	0.26	-	0/*	unknown
rs2701	G	0.401/0.942	0.62	0.97 [0.85–1.09]	0.423/0.903	0.47	1.06 [0.91–1.23]	0.409/0.778	0.408
rs10416839	T	0.359/0.653	0.24	1.08 [0.95–1.23]	0.371/1	0.11	1.14 [0.97–1.32]	0.341/0.545	0.292

Minor allele frequencies (MAF), p-value for deviation from Hardy-Weinberg equilibrium (HWE), allelic test *P*-values, and odds ratios (OR, shown for the minor allele) with 95% confidence intervals (CI) are depicted for both the CD and UC case-control cohorts. Measurements for linkage disequilibrium (LD) are provided in Tables 11, 12 and 13.
*monomorphic SNP.
**The MAFs in the HapMap-CEU population (= Utah residents with Northern and Western European ancestry) are derived from the NCBI SNP database (available under http://www.ncbi.nlm.nih.gov/snp).

Table 5. Haplotypes of *CEACAM6* SNPs in Crohn's disease (CD) case-control sample and omnibus p-values for association with CD susceptibility.

Haplotype combination	omnibus p-value
rs10415946-rs1805223	0.46
rs1805223-rs4803507	0.40
rs4803507-rs4803508	0.84
rs4803508-rs11548735	0.63
rs11548735-rs7246116	0.85
rs7246116-rs2701	0.78
rs2701-rs10416839	0.36
rs10415946-rs1805223-rs4803507	0.40
rs1805223-rs4803507-rs4803508	0.58
rs4803507-rs4803508-rs11548735	0.74
rs4803508-rs11548735-rs7246116	0.63
rs11548735-rs7246116-rs2701	0.74
rs7246116-rs2701-rs10416839	0.36
rs10415946-rs1805223-rs4803507-rs4803508	0.48
rs1805223-rs4803507-rs4803508-rs11548735	0.67
rs4803507-rs4803508-rs11548735-rs7246116	0.75
rs4803508-rs11548735-rs7246116-rs2701	0.39
rs11548735-rs7246116-rs2701-rs10416839	0.38
rs10415946-rs1805223-rs4803507-rs4803508-rs11548735	0.70
rs1805223-rs4803507-rs4803508-rs11548735-rs7246116	0.67
rs4803507-rs4803508-rs11548735-rs7246116-rs2701	0.59
rs4803508-rs11548735-rs7246116-rs2701-rs10416839	0.21
rs10415946-rs1805223-rs4803507-rs4803508-rs11548735-rs7246116	0.70
rs1805223-rs4803507-rs4803508-rs11548735-rs7246116-rs2701	0.66
rs4803507-rs4803508-rs11548735-rs7246116-rs2701-rs10416839	0.39
rs10415946-rs1805223-rs4803507-rs4803508-rs11548735-rs7246116-rs2701	0.77
rs1805223-rs4803507-rs4803508-rs11548735-rs7246116-rs2701-rs10416839	0.41
rs10415946-rs1805223-rs4803507-rs4803508-rs11548735-rs7246116-rs2701-rs10416839	0.39

Given are the omnibus p-values for the *CEACAM6* haplotype combinations regarding CD susceptibility.

Table 6. Haplotypes of *CEACAM6* SNPs in ulcerative colitis (UC) case-control sample and omnibus p-values for association with UC susceptibility.

Haplotype combination	omnibus p-value
rs10415946-rs1805223	0.50
rs1805223-rs4803507	0.60
rs4803507-rs4803508	0.73
rs4803508-rs11548735	0.50
rs11548735-rs7246116	0.65
rs7246116-rs2701	0.55
rs2701-rs10416839	0.60
rs10415946-rs1805223-rs4803507	0.50
rs1805223-rs4803507-rs4803508	0.82
rs4803507-rs4803508-rs11548735	0.73
rs4803508-rs11548735-rs7246116	0.37
rs11548735-rs7246116-rs2701	0.69
rs7246116-rs2701-rs10416839	0.60
rs10415946-rs1805223-rs4803507-rs4803508	0.81
rs1805223-rs4803507-rs4803508-rs11548735	0.83
rs4803507-rs4803508-rs11548735-rs7246116	0.58
rs4803508-rs11548735-rs7246116-rs2701	0.50
rs11548735-rs7246116-rs2701-rs10416839	0.54
rs10415946-rs1805223-rs4803507-rs4803508-rs11548735	0.87
rs1805223-rs4803507-rs4803508-rs11548735-rs7246116	0.76
rs4803507-rs4803508-rs11548735-rs7246116-rs2701	0.55
rs4803508-rs11548735-rs7246116-rs2701-rs10416839	0.39
rs10415946-rs1805223-rs4803507-rs4803508-rs11548735-rs7246116	0.87
rs1805223-rs4803507-rs4803508-rs11548735-rs7246116-rs2701	0.75
rs4803507-rs4803508-rs11548735-rs7246116-rs2701-rs10416839	0.48
rs10415946-rs1805223-rs4803507-rs4803508-rs11548735-rs7246116-rs2701	0.87
rs1805223-rs4803507-rs4803508-rs11548735-rs7246116-rs2701-rs10416839	0.49
rs10415946-rs1805223-rs4803507-rs4803508-rs11548735-rs7246116-rs2701-rs10416839	0.82

Given are the omnibus p-values for the *CEACAM6* haplotype combinations regarding UC susceptibility.

Table 7. Associations of *CEACAM6* gene markers with the anatomic location of Crohn's disease (CD) according to the Montreal classification [33].

Anatomic location	rs10415946	rs1805223 = p.Pro42Pro	rs4803507	rs4803508	rs11548735 = p.Gly239Val	rs7246116 = pHis260His	rs2701	rs10416839
L1 (ileal) n = 113	0.320	0.321	0.559	0.876	0.961	*	0.997	0.566
L2 (colonic) n = 97	0.854	0.988	0.970	0.611	0.751	*	0.684	0.580
L3 (ileocolonic) n = 554	0.451	0.759	0.803	0.425	0.684	*	0.691	0.114
Any ileal involvement (L1+L3) n = 667	0.373	0.586	0.689	0.620	0.771	*	0.744	0.117

P-values are depicted for the CD case-control cohorts.
*There were no carriers of the minor allele of rs7146116 in the CD and control cohort.

Table 8. Analysis for gene-gene interactions between *CEACAM6* and *NOD2* variants regarding susceptibility to Crohn's disease (CD).

CEACAM6 SNPs NOD2 SNPs	rs10415946	rs1805223	rs4803507	rs4803508	rs11548735	rs7246116	rs2701	rs10416839
rs2066844 p.Arg702Trp	0.56	0.37	0.39	0.31	0.62	*	0.65	0.77
rs2066845 p.Gly908Arg	0.06	0.28	0.28	0.54	0.35	*	0.43	0.58
rs2066847 p.Leu1007fsX1008	0.93	0.80	0.97	0.51	0.71	*	0.56	0.82

p-values for epistasis analysis between *CEACAM6* and *NOD2* SNPs in the CD case-control sample.
*There were no carriers of the minor allele of rs7146116 in the CD and control cohort.

indicated. Interactions between different polymorphisms were tested using logistic regression in R using the number of minor alleles as predictor variable, therefore implementing an Armitage test of trend. Data were evaluated by using the SPSS 13.0 software (SPSS Inc., Chicago, IL, USA) and R-2.4.1. (http://cran.r-project.org). For haplotype analysis, PLINK v 1.06 (http://pngu.mgh.harvard.edu/~purcell/plink/) was used running a sliding window approach with variation of the window size from 2 to 8 included markers and using the option "hap-logistic". Linkage disequilibrium (LD) was also analyzed using PLINK.

Results

CEACAM6 variants are not associated with IBD susceptibility

The genotyping success rates were at least 99% for all eight SNPs tested and were comparable between the controls and the CD and UC patients groups. In all three subgroups (CD, UC, and controls), the allele frequencies of the *CEACAM6* SNPs rs10415946, rs1805223 = p.Pro42Pro, rs4803507, rs4803508, rs11548735 = p.Gly239Val, rs7246116 = p.His260His, rs2701, rs10416839 were in accordance with the predicted Hardy-Weinberg equilibrium (Table 4). Overall, we observed no significant differences in the frequencies of the investigated *CEACAM6* SNPs in CD and UC patients compared to healthy

controls (Table 4) implicating no significant association of *CEACAM6* variants and IBD susceptibility. Only two patients (both with UC) were minor allele carriers of the rare *CEACAM6* SNP rs7246116 = p.His260His, therefore not allowing a comparative analysis of this SNP regarding CD susceptibility.

CEACAM6 haplotypes are not associated with CD and UC susceptibility

Considering recent evidence showing that certain *CEACAM6* haplotypes modulate susceptibility to bacterial infections [38], we next performed a detailed haplotype analysis in our IBD cohort. However, as shown in Tables 5 and 6, we could not demonstrated significant associations of *CEACAM6* haplotypes with CD and UC susceptibility.

The CEACAM6 variants are not associated with an ileal disease phenotype in CD patients

Since CEACAM6 has recently shown to act as a receptor for AIEC, thereby promoting bacterial colonization in ileal CD [19], we further investigated whether *CEACAM6* SNPs are associated with ileal disease in CD patients. Based on a phenotype analysis according to the Montreal classification of IBD [33], the detailed phenotypic data available from a subcohort of 667 CD patients was analyzed for disease localization. None of the investigated *CEACAM6* SNPs was associated with ileal or ileocolonic CD

Table 9. Analysis for gene-gene interaction with *CEACAM6*.and *IL23R* variants regarding susceptibility to Crohn's disease (CD).

CEACAM6 SNPs IL23R SNPs	rs10415946	rs1805223	rs4803507	rs4803508	rs11548735	rs7246116	rs2701	rs10416839
rs1004819	0.13	0.31	0.29	0.50	0.46	*	0.52	0.95
rs7517847	0.67	0.20	0.31	0.17	0.23	*	0.27	0.81
rs10489629	0.64	0.09	0.11	0.97	0.79	*	0.71	0.98
rs2201841	0.52	0.42	0.40	0.61	0.50	*	0.46	0.63
rs11465804	0.20	0.13	0.19	0.59	0.26	*	0.32	0.76
rs11209026	0.08	0.05	0.08	0.35	0.28	*	0.35	0.91
rs1343151	0.35	**0.04**	0.06	0.83	0.57	*	0.60	0.64
rs10889677	0.55	0.48	0.44	0.77	0.66	*	0.62	0.51
rs11209032	0.43	0.52	0.53	0.87	0.99	*	0.89	0.19
rs1495965	0.47	0.66	0.58	0.73	0.61	*	0.84	0.32

p-values for epistasis between *CEACAM6*.and *IL23R* SNPs in the CD case-control sample. After Bonferroni correction, the association highlighted in bold did not remain significant.
*There were no carriers of the minor allele of rs7146116 in the CD and control cohort.

Table 10. Analysis for gene-gene interaction between *CEACAM6* and *ATGT16L1* variants regarding susceptibility to Crohn's disease (CD).

CEACAM6 SNPs *ATG16L1* SNPs	rs10415946	rs1805223	rs4803507	rs4803508	rs11548735	rs7246116	rs2701	rs10416839
rs13412102	0.89	0.89	0.72	0.89	0.55	*	0.55	0.79
rs12471449	0.49	0.44	0.40	0.74	0.58	*	0.56	**0.04**
rs6431660	0.53	0.66	0.50	0.87	0.98	*	0.93	0.66
rs1441090	0.56	0.32	0.26	0.78	0.89	*	0.95	0.27
rs2289472	0.67	0.65	0.49	0.67	0.86	*	0.83	0.57
rs2241880	0.84	0.74	0.57	0.64	0.81	*	0.83	0.58
rs2241879	0.93	0.81	0.68	0.74	0.73	*	0.72	0.56
rs3792106	0.67	0.52	0.44	0.50	0.69	*	0.73	0.83
rs4663396	0.81	0.93	0.80	0.56	0.85	*	0.90	0.15

p-values for epistasis between *CEACAM6* and *ATGT16L1* SNPs in the CD case-control sample. After Bonferroni correction, the association highlighted in bold did not remain significant.
*There were no carriers of the minor allele of rs7146116 in the CD and control cohort.

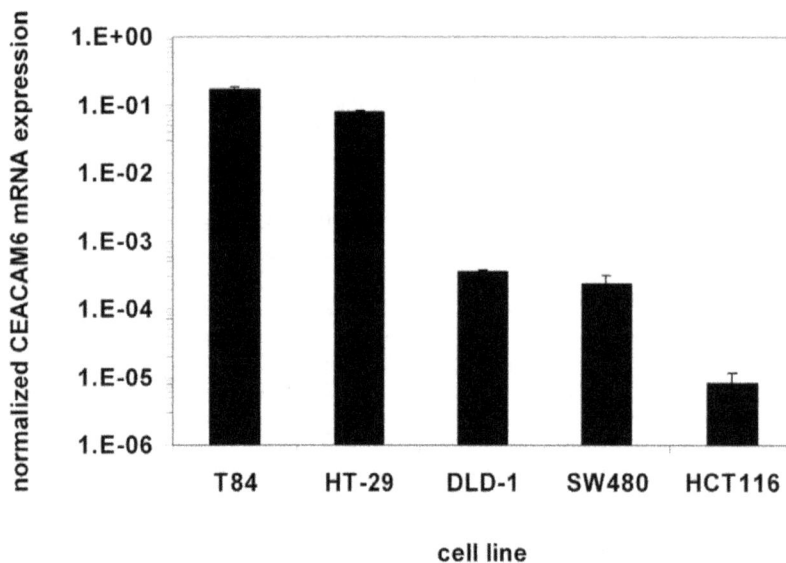

cell line SNP	T84	HT-29	DLD-1	SW480	HCT116
rs10415946	*AG*	AA	AA	AA	AA
rs1805223	*GG*	AG	AG	AG	AG
rs4803507	GG	GG	GG	GG	GG
rs4803508	AA	GG	AA	AA	GG
rs11548735	GT	GT	TT	TT	*GG*
rs7246116	GG	GG	GG	GG	GG
rs2701	AG	AG	GG	GG	*AA*
rs10416839	GT	GT	GG	GG	*TT*

Figure 2. Analysis of CEACAM6 gene expression and *CEACAM6* gene variants in intestinal epithelial cell (IEC) lines. (A) Total RNA isolated from IEC lines as indicated was reverse transcribed and was analyzed for CEACAM6 gene expression by quantitative PCR. T84 cells express CEACAM6 at the highest level followed by HT-29 cells, and intermediate CEACAM6 expression was found in SW480 and DLD-1 cells. CEACAM6 expression was close to the detection limit after 40 PCR cycles in HCT116 cells (note the logarithmic scale on the y-axis). CEACAM6 expression was normalized to β-actin expression in the respective cDNA samples. (B) Genomic DNA was isolated from IEC lines and 8 SNPs in *CEACAM6* were analyzed as indicated by DNA sequencing. The respective alleles for these SNPs in each cell line are depicted in the table. This analysis revealed that T84, the cell line with the highest CEACAM6 expression, and HCT116 cells, the cell line with the lowest CEACAM6 expression, are the only IEC lines with unique genotypes for certain *CEACAM6* SNPs (depicted in bold italic). DLD-1 and SW480 cells have identical genotypes for all SNPs analyzed and nearly identical CEACAM6 expression levels.

(Table 7). However, we have to acknowledge that the sample size has limited power to detect weak disease associations. For example, based on 667 patients with a L1/L3 disease phenotype, a minor allele frequency of 0.40 and an OR of 1.1, the power is 28.88% to detect an effect on a significance level of 5% (Genetic Power Calculator, http://pngu.mgh.harvard.edu/~purcell/gpc/).

Analysis for gene-gene interaction with CD-associated *NOD2*, *IL23R* and *ATG16L1* variants

Given the raising evidence for a key role of CEACAM6 in the complex interaction of the mucosal immune system and intestinal bacteria, we next analyzed for potential epistasis between *CEACAM6* SNPs (rs10415946, rs1805223 = p.Pro42Pro, rs4803507, rs4803508, rs11548735 = p.Gly239Val, rs7246116 = pHis260His, rs2701, rs10-416839) and the three main CD-associated *NOD2/CARD15* variants p.Arg702Trp (rs2066844), p.Gly908Arg (rs2066845), and p.Leu1007fsX1008 (rs2066847) which have previously shown to be strongly associated with CD and ileal disease localization. However, there was no evidence for epistasis between the *CEACAM6* SNPs and the three analyzed *NOD2/CARD15* variants (Table 8).

Recently, we demonstrated an association of the *IL23R* SNP rs1004819 (TT homozygous carriers) with ileal CD [34]. Therefore, we also analyzed for potential gene-gene interaction between *CEACAM6* SNPs and the major CD-associated *IL23R* variants. However, we did not find evidence for epistasis between *CEACAM6* and *IL23R* regarding CD susceptibility (Table 9).

In addition, novel findings indicate a major role for *ATG16L1* in Paneth cell development in the terminal ileum. Therefore, we also analyzed for potential epistasis between the *CEACAM6* SNPs and the major CD-associated *ATG16L1* SNPs. However, we were also unable to demonstrate evidence for epistasis between these two genes (Table 10).

p-values for epistasis between *CEACAM6* and *ATGT16L1* SNPs in the CD case-control sample. After Bonferroni correction, the association highlighted in bold did not remain significant.

*There were no carriers of the minor allele of rs7146116 in the CD and control cohort.

CEACAM6 genotypes modulate CEACAM6 expression in intestinal epithelial cell lines

To analyze a potential influence of *CEACAM6* gene variants on CEACAM6 gene expression, we determined CEACAM6 mRNA levels in five intestinal epithelial cell (IEC) lines DLD-1, HCT116, HT-29, SW480 and T84 by quantitative PCR. This analysis revealed considerable differences in CEACAM6 expression depending on the cell line. While T84 cells showed the highest expression, the expression in HCT116 cells was four orders of magnitude smaller and close to the detection limit (Fig. 2A).

Table 11. Analysis for linkage disequilibrium between *CEACAM6* SNPs in patients with Crohn's disease.

	rs10415946	rs4803507	rs4803508	rs2701	rs10416839
rs10415946	*	*	*	*	*
rs4803507	0.65/0.96	*	*	*	*
rs4803508	0.12/0.58	0.09/0.59	*	*	*
rs2701	0.12/0.53	0.10/0.57	0.80/0.95	*	*
rs10416839	<0.01/0.03	<0.01/0.13	0.25/0.85	0.31/0.90	*

Values are given as r²/D'-measurements.

Table 12. Analysis for linkage disequilibrium between *CEACAM6* SNPs in patients with ulcerative colitis.

	rs10415946	rs4803507	rs4803508	rs2701	rs10416839
rs10415946	*	*	*	*	*
rs4803507	0.70/0.98	*	*	*	*
rs4803508	0.15/0.65	0.11/0.67	*	*	*
rs2701	0.14/0.61	0.10/0.60	0.87/0.97	*	*
rs10416839	<0.01/0.09	<0.01/0.11	0.29/0.89	0.33/0.91	*

Values are given as r²/D'-measurements.

SW480 and DLD-1 cells showed similar, intermediate expression (Fig. 2A). Interestingly, when these cell lines were analyzed for *CEACAM6* gene variants, only T84 and HCT116 cells, the two cell lines with the highest and lowest CEACAM6 expression, respectively, had unique genotype variants when compared with the other cell lines (Fig. 2B). While T84 cells were the only cells that had a unique genotype for rs10415946 and rs1805223 = p.Pro42Pro, HCT116 had a unique genotype in SNPs rs11548735 = p.Gly239Val, rs2701 and rs10416839. SW480 and DLD-1 cells had identical *CEACAM6* genotypes and their CEACAM6 expression was nearly identical (Fig. 2A and 2B). A detailed analysis regarding linkage disequilibrium between the investigated *CEACAM6* SNPs stratified for CD, UC and controls is given in Tables 11, 12 and 13.

Discussion

In summary, our study represents the first detailed analysis of *CEACAM6* SNPs regarding disease susceptibility and phenotypic consequences in IBD patients. Compared to previous GWAS, our study had a more complete coverage of the *CEACAM6* gene region (see details in Table 14). Overall, we did not observe a significant influence of the investigated *CEACAM6* SNPs on CD and UC susceptibility. Moreover, a detailed haplotype analysis did not reveal significant associations with IBD susceptibility. CEACAM6 has recently shown to act as a receptor for AIEC suggesting an important role in bacterial colonization of the ileal mucosa in CD patients [19]. However, none of the investigated *CEACAM6* SNPs was associated with ileal or ileocolonic CD.

Interestingly, a recent study demonstrated that the defect in CEACAM family members in intestinal epithelial cells isolated from CD patients appears to be related to the aberrant nuclear localization of the transcription factor SOX9 [39] which regulates cell proliferation and is required for Paneth cell differentiation in

Table 13. Analysis for linkage disequilibrium between *CEACAM6* SNPs in controls.

	rs10415946	rs4803507	rs4803508	rs2701	rs10416839
rs10415946	*	*	*	*	*
rs4803507	0.68/0.98	*	*	*	*
rs4803508	0.15/0.63	0.09/0.60	*	*	*
rs2701	0.14/0.60	0.09/0.57	0.81/0.94	*	*
rs10416839	0.01/0.12	<0.01/0.06	0.23/0.84	0.29/0.90	*

Values are given as r²/D'-measurements.

Table 14. Coverage of the *CEACAM6* gene region by the Illumina Hap300 chip and the Affymetrix 500 k chip utilized in previous genome-wide association studies (GWAS).

Chromosomal position (bp) of the *CEACAM6* SNP	Position in the *CEACAM6** gene	*CEACAM6* SNPs analyzed in our study	*CEACAM6* SNPs covered by the Illumina Hap300 chip	*CEACAM6* SNPs covered by the Affymetrix 500k chip
46,948,446	upstream		rs3764577	
46,950,899	upstream	rs10415946		
46,952,409	intragenic	rs1805223 = P42P		
46,953,560	intragenic			rs3795018
46,954,095	intragenic			rs11669653
46,954,731	intragenic		rs3795020	
46,955,390	intragenic	rs4803507		
46,956,489	intragenic	rs4803508		
46,957,729	intragenic	rs11548735 = G239V		
46,957,793	intragenic	rs7246116 = H260H		
46,962,846	intragenic		rs10413359	
46,966,939	intragenic	rs2701		rs2701
46,970,128	downstream			rs6508997
46,972,172	downstream	rs10416839	rs10416839	

*Position of the *CEACAM6* gene on chromosome 19: 46,951,341 bp to 46,967,953 bp.

the intestinal epithelium [40,41]. However, ileal CD is characterized by a specific decrease in Paneth cell alpha-defensins and defective Paneth cell-mediated host defense [42] which has been linked to the *NOD2* genotype [43], although this finding is opposed by the results of a recent study [44], and additional modifiers of Paneth cell function such as XBP1 are involved [45]. Therefore, one might speculate whether the role of CEACAM6 in ileal bacterial colonization is regulated via SOX9 expression implicating defective Paneth cell function in patients with small bowel CD. Given the association of defensin secretion with the *NOD2* genotype [43] and the findings of numerous previous studies including studies from our IBD center demonstrating ileal disease localization in CD patients with *NOD2* mutations [37,46,47], we also tested for potential gene-gene interaction of *CEACAM6* and *NOD2*. However, we found no evidence for epistasis between these two genes regarding CD susceptibility. Further functional studies analyzing the complex interaction of intestinal CEACAM6 expression and bacterial adherence in the gut particularly of CD patients carrying *CEACAM6* variants will therefore be required. Given the important role of *ATG16L1* in Paneth cell development of the terminal ileum and the role of *IL23R* in the development of proinflammatory Th17 cells, we also analyzed for epistasis of these two genes with *CEACAM6* but were unable to find evidence for significant epistasis of these genes regarding CD susceptibility.

Interestingly, a recent study indicated that *CEACAM6* and a regulatory element near the 3′ end of *CEACAM3* are associated with disease severity in patients with cystic fibrosis [48]. However, a previous study in IBD patients suggested that heterozygous carriers of the ΔF508 mutation in the *CFTR* gene, the main susceptibility gene for patients with cystic fibrosis, might exert a protective effect in CD [49], suggesting opposing effects of genetic risk loci for cystic fibrosis and IBD.

In the meta-analysis of Barrett et al. [50], a SNP (rs4807569) within the chromosomal region 19q13, in which the *CEACAM6* gene is located, was weakly associated with CD, but this association could not be confirmed in a replication cohort. In the recent meta-analysis of Franke et al. [51], two SNPs (rs

736289 and rs281376) within this region were strongly associated with CD. However, the distance between these SNPs and the *CEACAM6* gene is 9 and 7 megabases, respectively, and thus, the disease causing variant within this region remains to be identified.

CEACAM6 is also a major target gene for Smad3-mediated TGF-β signaling [52]. Since Smad3 differentially regulates the induction of regulatory and inflammatory Th17 cell differentiation [53], which are key players in the IBD pathogenesis [54], further investigations analyzing Th17 cell differentiation in IBD patients carrying *CEACAM6* variants might also be of high interest. Moreover, very recent evidence from studies in mice demonstrated that colonization of the small intestine with a single commensal microbe, segmented filamentous bacterium (SFB), is sufficient to induce Th17 cells in the lamina propria [55]. These SFB adhere tightly to the surface of epithelial cells in the terminal ileum of mice with Th17 cells but are absent from mice that have few Th17 cells [55]. Further studies will have to characterize if SFB adherence is mediated (similar to AIEC adherence) by CEACAM family members.

In summary, we performed the first systemic analysis of *CEACAM6* gene variants in IBD patients. Despite the great importance of CEACAM6 as receptor for AIEC on the ileal mucosa of CD patients, we were unable to demonstrate a specific role of *CEACAM6* variants in IBD susceptibility. Furthermore, there was no evidence for an association with ileal CD or for epistasis with *NOD2*, *IL23R*, and *ATG16L1* variants in CD susceptibility. Further functional studies will be necessary to elucidate how *CEACAM6* gene variants may modulate bacterial colonization in IBD patients. Even if this study was unable to find a role for *CEACAM6* gene variants in IBD susceptibility, the CEACAM6 protein is likely to be an important mediator of the pathogenesis of CD [56].

Acknowledgments

This work contains parts of the unpublished degree theses of C. Fries.

Author Contributions

Conceived and designed the experiments: JG JD SB. Performed the experiments: JG CF JD. Analyzed the data: JG SP CW BM-M JD DC SB. Contributed reagents/materials/analysis tools: JG JS CF CT SP MW FB

TOlszak UL BG TOchsenkühn CW PL BM-M JD DC SB. Wrote the paper: JS JG DC JD SB. Organized the collaboration between the research institutions: SB.

References

1. Xavier RJ, Podolsky DK (2007) Unravelling the pathogenesis of inflammatory bowel disease. Nature 448: 427–434.
2. Podolsky DK (2002) Inflammatory bowel disease. N Engl J Med 347: 417–429.
3. Mudter J, Neurath MF (2007) Apoptosis of T cells and the control of inflammatory bowel disease: therapeutic implications. Gut 56: 293–303.
4. Parkes M, Barrett JC, Prescott NJ, Tremelling M, Anderson CA, et al. (2007) Sequence variants in the autophagy gene IRGM and multiple other replicating loci contribute to Crohn's disease susceptibility. Nat Genet 39: 830–832.
5. Hampe J, Franke A, Rosenstiel P, Till A, Teuber M, et al. (2007) A genome-wide association scan of nonsynonymous SNPs identifies a susceptibility variant for Crohn disease in ATG16L1. Nat Genet 39: 207–211.
6. Cooney R, Baker J, Brain O, Danis B, Pichulik T, et al. (2010) NOD2 stimulation induces autophagy in dendritic cells influencing bacterial handling and antigen presentation. Nat Med 16: 90–97.
7. Travassos LH, Carneiro LA, Ramjeet M, Hussey S, Kim YG, et al. (2010) Nod1 and Nod2 direct autophagy by recruiting ATG16L1 to the plasma membrane at the site of bacterial entry. Nat Immunol 11: 55–62.
8. Sydora BC, Macfarlane SM, Walker JW, Dmytrash AL, Churchill TA, et al. (2007) Epithelial barrier disruption allows nondisease-causing bacteria to initiate and sustain IBD in the IL-10 gene-deficient mouse. Inflamm Bowel Dis 13: 947–954.
9. Silva MA (2009) Intestinal dendritic cells and epithelial barrier dysfunction in Crohn's disease. Inflamm Bowel Dis 15: 436–453.
10. Hugot JP, Chamaillard M, Zouali H, Lesage S, Cezard JP, et al. (2001) Association of NOD2 leucine-rich repeat variants with susceptibility to Crohn's disease. Nature 411: 599–603.
11. Ogura Y, Bonen DK, Inohara N, Nicolae DL, Chen FF, et al. (2001) A frameshift mutation in NOD2 associated with susceptibility to Crohn's disease. Nature 411: 603–606.
12. Duerr RH, Taylor KD, Brant SR, Rioux JD, Silverberg MS, et al. (2006) A genome-wide association study identifies IL23R as an inflammatory bowel disease gene. Science 314: 1461–1463.
13. Pineton de Chambrun G, Colombel JF, Poulain D, Darfeuille-Michaud A (2008) Pathogenic agents in inflammatory bowel diseases. Curr Opin Gastroenterol 24: 440–447.
14. Sokol H, Lay C, Seksik P, Tannock GW (2008) Analysis of bacterial bowel communities of IBD patients: what has it revealed? Inflamm Bowel Dis 14: 858–867.
15. Cario E, Podolsky DK (2006) Toll-like receptor signaling and its relevance to intestinal inflammation. Ann N Y Acad Sci 1072: 332–338.
16. Rhodes JM (2007) The role of Escherichia coli in inflammatory bowel disease. Gut 56: 610–612.
17. Rolhion N, Darfeuille-Michaud A (2007) Adherent-invasive Escherichia coli in inflammatory bowel disease. Inflamm Bowel Dis 13: 1277–1283.
18. Carvalho FA, Barnich N, Sivignon A, Darcha C, Chan CH, et al. (2009) Crohn's disease adherent-invasive Escherichia coli colonize and induce strong gut inflammation in transgenic mice expressing human CEACAM. J Exp Med 206: 2179–2189.
19. Barnich N, Carvalho FA, Glasser AL, Darcha C, Jantscheff P, et al. (2007) CEACAM6 acts as a receptor for adherent-invasive E. coli, supporting ileal mucosa colonization in Crohn disease. J Clin Invest 117: 1566–1574.
20. Khan WN, Frangsmyr L, Teglund S, Israelsson A, Bremer K, et al. (1992) Identification of three new genes and estimation of the size of the carcinoembryonic antigen family. Genomics 14: 384–390.
21. Obrink B (1997) CEA adhesion molecules: multifunctional proteins with signal-regulatory properties. Curr Opin Cell Biol 9: 616–626.
22. Kuespert K, Pils S, Hauck CR (2006) CEACAMs: their role in physiology and pathophysiology. Curr Opin Cell Biol 18: 565–571.
23. Thom I, Schult-Kronefeld O, Burkholder I, Schuch G, Andritzky B, et al. (2009) Expression of CEACAM-1 in pulmonary adenocarcinomas and their metastases. Anticancer Res 29: 249–254.
24. Greicius G, Severinson E, Beauchemin N, Obrink B, Singer BB (2003) CEACAM1 is a potent regulator of B cell receptor complex-induced activation. J Leukoc Biol 74: 126–134.
25. Muenzner P, Rohde M, Kneitz S, Hauck CR (2005) CEACAM engagement by human pathogens enhances cell adhesion and counteracts bacteria-induced detachment of epithelial cells. J Cell Biol 170: 825–836.
26. Nagaishi T, Iijima H, Nakajima A, Chen D, Blumberg RS (2006) Role of CEACAM1 as a regulator of T cells. Ann N Y Acad Sci 1072: 155–175.
27. Dango S, Sienel W, Schreiber M, Stremmel C, Kirschbaum A, et al. (2008) Elevated expression of carcinoembryonic antigen-related cell adhesion molecule 1 (CEACAM-1) is associated with increased angiogenic potential in non-small-cell lung cancer. Lung Cancer 60: 426–433.
28. Nagaishi T, Pao L, Lin SH, Iijima H, Kaser A, et al. (2006) SHP1 phosphatase-dependent T cell inhibition by CEACAM1 adhesion molecule isoforms. Immunity 25: 769–781.
29. Gray-Owen SD, Blumberg RS (2006) CEACAM1: contact-dependent control of immunity. Nat Rev Immunol 6: 433–446.
30. Boudeau J, Glasser AL, Masseret E, Joly B, Darfeuille-Michaud A (1999) Invasive ability of an Escherichia coli strain isolated from the ileal mucosa of a patient with Crohn's disease. Infect Immun 67: 4499–4509.
31. Glasser AL, Boudeau J, Barnich N, Perruchot MH, Colombel JF, et al. (2001) Adherent invasive Escherichia coli strains from patients with Crohn's disease survive and replicate within macrophages without inducing host cell death. Infect Immun 69: 5529–5537.
32. Lennard-Jones JE (1989) Classification of inflammatory bowel disease. Scand J Gastroenterol Suppl 170: 2–6; discussion 16–19.
33. Silverberg MS, Satsangi J, Ahmad T, Arnott ID, Bernstein CN, et al. (2005) Toward an integrated clinical, molecular and serological classification of inflammatory bowel disease: Report of a Working Party of the 2005 Montreal World Congress of Gastroenterology. Can J Gastroenterol 19 Suppl A: 5–36.
34. Glas J, Seiderer J, Wetzke M, Konrad A, Torok HP, et al. (2007) rs1004819 is the main disease-associated IL23R variant in German Crohn's disease patients: combined analysis of IL23R, CARD15, and OCTN1/2 variants. PLoS ONE 2: e819.
35. Glas J, Stallhofer J, Ripke S, Wetzke M, Pfennig S, et al. (2009) Novel genetic risk markers for ulcerative colitis in the IL2/IL21 region are in epistasis with IL23R and suggest a common genetic background for ulcerative colitis and celiac disease. Am J Gastroenterol 104: 1737–1744.
36. Glas J, Seiderer J, Pasciuto G, Tillack C, Diegelmann J, et al. (2009) rs224136 on chromosome 10q21.1 and variants in PHOX2B, NCF4, and FAM92B are not major genetic risk factors for susceptibility to Crohn's disease in the German population. Am J Gastroenterol 104: 665–672.
37. Seiderer J, Schnitzler F, Brand S, Staudinger T, Pfennig S, et al. (2006) Homozygosity for the CARD15 frameshift mutation 1007fs is predictive of early onset of Crohn's disease with ileal stenosis, entero-enteral fistulas, and frequent need for surgical intervention with high risk of re-stenosis. Scand J Gastroenterol 41: 1421–1432.
38. Callaghan MJ, Rockett K, Banner C, Haralambous E, Betts H, et al. (2008) Haplotypic diversity in human CEACAM genes: effects on susceptibility to meningococcal disease. Genes Immun 9: 30–37.
39. Roda G, Dahan S, Mezzanotte L, Caponi A, Roth-Walter F, et al. (2009) Defect in CEACAM family member expression in Crohn's disease IECs is regulated by the transcription factor SOX9. Inflamm Bowel Dis 15: 1775–1783.
40. Bastide P, Darido C, Pannequin J, Kist R, Robine S, et al. (2007) Sox9 regulates cell proliferation and is required for Paneth cell differentiation in the intestinal epithelium. J Cell Biol 178: 635–648.
41. Mori-Akiyama Y, van den Born M, van Es JH, Hamilton SR, Adams HP, et al. (2007) SOX9 is required for the differentiation of paneth cells in the intestinal epithelium. Gastroenterology 133: 539–546.
42. Wehkamp J, Salzman NH, Porter E, Nuding S, Weichenthal M, et al. (2005) Reduced Paneth cell alpha-defensins in ileal Crohn's disease. Proc Natl Acad Sci U S A 102: 18129–18134.
43. Wehkamp J, Harder J, Weichenthal M, Schwab M, Schaffeler E, et al. (2004) NOD2 (CARD15) mutations in Crohn's disease are associated with diminished mucosal alpha-defensin expression. Gut 53: 1658–1664.
44. Simms LA, Doecke JD, Walsh MD, Huang N, Fowler EV, et al. (2008) Reduced alpha-defensin expression is associated with inflammation and not NOD2 mutation status in ileal Crohn's disease. Gut 57: 903–910.
45. Kaser A, Lee AH, Franke A, Glickman JN, Zeissig S, et al. (2008) XBP1 links ER stress to intestinal inflammation and confers genetic risk for human inflammatory bowel disease. Cell 134: 743–756.
46. Seiderer J, Brand S, Herrmann KA, Schnitzler F, Hatz R, et al. (2006) Predictive value of the CARD15 variant 1007fs for the diagnosis of intestinal stenoses and the need for surgery in Crohn's disease in clinical practice: results of a prospective study. Inflamm Bowel Dis 12: 1114–1121.
47. Schnitzler F, Brand S, Staudinger T, Pfennig S, Hofbauer K, et al. (2006) Eight novel CARD15 variants detected by DNA sequence analysis of the CARD15 gene in 111 patients with inflammatory bowel disease. Immunogenetics 58: 99–106.
48. Stanke F, Becker T, Hedtfeld S, Tamm S, Wienker TF, et al. (2010) Hierarchical fine mapping of the cystic fibrosis modifier locus on 19q13 identifies an association with two elements near the genes CEACAM3 and CEACAM6. Hum Genet 127: 383–394.
49. Bresso F, Askling J, Astegiano M, Demarchi B, Sapone N, et al. (2007) Potential role for the common cystic fibrosis DeltaF508 mutation in Crohn's disease. Inflamm Bowel Dis 13: 531–536.

50. Barrett JC, Hansoul S, Nicolae DL, Cho JH, Duerr RH, et al. (2008) Genome-wide association defines more than 30 distinct susceptibility loci for Crohn's disease. Nat Genet 40: 955–962.

51. Franke A, McGovern DPB, Barrett JC, Wang K, Radford-Smith GL, et al. (2010) Genome-wide meta-analysis increases to 71 the number of confirmed Crohn's disease susceptibility loci. Nat Genet 42: 1118–1121.

52. Han SU, Kwak TH, Her KH, Cho YH, Choi C, et al. (2008) CEACAM5 and CEACAM6 are major target genes for Smad3-mediated TGF-beta signaling. Oncogene 27: 675–683.

53. Martinez GJ, Zhang Z, Chung Y, Reynolds JM, Lin X, et al. (2009) Smad3 differentially regulates the induction of regulatory and inflammatory T cell differentiation. J Biol Chem 284: 35283–35286.

54. Brand S (2009) Crohn's disease: Th1, Th17 or both? The change of a paradigm: new immunological and genetic insights implicate Th17 cells in the pathogenesis of Crohn's disease. Gut 58: 1152–1167.

55. Ivanov II, Atarashi K, Manel N, Brodie EL, Shima T, et al. (2009) Induction of intestinal Th17 cells by segmented filamentous bacteria. Cell 139: 485–498.

56. Abraham C, Cho JH (2007) Bugging of the intestinal mucosa. N Engl J Med 357: 708–710.

15

A Low Dose of Fermented Soy Germ Alleviates Gut Barrier Injury, Hyperalgesia and Faecal Protease Activity in a Rat Model of Inflammatory Bowel Disease

Lara Moussa[1,2], Valérie Bézirard[1], Christel Salvador-Cartier[1], Valérie Bacquié[1], Corinne Lencina[1], Mathilde Lévêque[1], Viorica Braniste[1], Sandrine Ménard[1], Vassilia Théodorou[1⑨], Eric Houdeau[1*⑨]

1 Neuro-Gastroenterology and Nutrition, Institut National de la Recherche Agronomique, UMR1331 Toxalim, INRA/INPT/UPS, Toulouse, France, 2 GENIBIO, Lorp-Sentaraille, France

Abstract

Pro-inflammatory cytokines like macrophage migration inhibitory factor (MIF), IL-1β and TNF-α predominate in inflammatory bowel diseases (IBD) and TNBS colitis. Increased levels of serine proteases activating protease-activated receptor 2 (PAR-2) are found in the lumen and colonic tissue of IBD patients. PAR-2 activity and pro-inflammatory cytokines impair epithelial barrier, facilitating the uptake of luminal aggressors that perpetuate inflammation and visceral pain. Soy extracts contain phytoestrogens (isoflavones) and serine protease inhibitors namely Bowman-Birk Inhibitors (BBI). Since estrogens exhibit anti-inflammatory and epithelial barrier enhancing properties, and that a BBI concentrate improves ulcerative colitis, we aimed to evaluate if a fermented soy germ extract (FSG) with standardized isoflavone profile and stable BBI content exert cumulative or synergistic protection based on protease inhibition and estrogen receptor (ER)-ligand activity in colitic rats. Female rats received orally for 15 d either vehicle or FSG with or without an ER antagonist ICI 182.780 before TNBS intracolonic instillation. Macroscopic and microscopic damages, myeloperoxidase activity, cytokine levels, intestinal paracellular permeability, visceral sensitivity, faecal proteolytic activity and PAR-2 expression were assessed 24 h, 3 d and 5 d post-TNBS. FSG treatment improved the severity of colitis, by decreasing the TNBS-induced rise in gut permeability, visceral sensitivity, faecal proteolytic activity and PAR-2 expression at all post-TNBS points. All FSG effects were reversed by the ICI 182.780 except the decrease in faecal proteolytic activity and PAR-2 expression. In conclusion, the anti-inflammatory properties of FSG treatment result from two distinct but synergic pathways i.e an ER-ligand and a PAR-2 mediated pathway, providing rationale for potential use as adjuvant therapy in IBD.

Editor: Benoit Foligne, Institut Pasteur de Lille, France

Funding: This work was funded by GENIBIO, Midi Pyrenees Region, ANRT (Association Nationale de Recherche et de Technologie). The funders had no role in study design, data collection and analysis, decision to publish, or preparation of the manuscript.

Competing Interests: The authors have the following interests. This work was partly funded by GENIBIO, the employer of Lara Moussa. The fermented soy germ ingredient (FSG) used in the study was industrially processed as ground powder under the trademark Primasoy® by GENIBIO. There are no further patents, products in development or marketed products to declare.

* E-mail: Eric.Houdeau@toulouse.inra.fr

⑨ These authors contributed equally to this work.

Introduction

Inflammatory bowel diseases (IBD), namely Crohn's disease (CD) and ulcerative colitis (UC), are chronic and relapsing inflammatory conditions characterized by an abnormal immune response to microbiota, impaired epithelial barrier function, tissue damage, and abdominal pain [1,2,3]. In both disorders, mucosal immune cells produce large amounts of chemokines and cytokines, including macrophage migration inhibitory factor (MIF), IL-1β and TNF-α, both orchestrating the immuno-inflammatory process leading to epithelial barrier defect, tissue damage [3]. On the other hand, proteases originated from various cell populations such as tryptase, trypsin, thrombin and cathepsin G may act as inflammatory mediators [4,5] by cleaving and activating protease-activated receptors (PARs) which represent novel members of the G-protein-coupled receptor family. Among the PARs family, PAR-2 has been largely studied in the context of inflammation.

Interestingly, the levels of potential activators of PAR-2 such as serine-proteases are increased in the colonic tissue of IBD patients [4,5,6]. Both PAR-2 activity and proinflammatory cytokines impair epithelial barrier by decreasing tight junction (TJ) protein expression [3,4], hence facilitate the entry of luminal aggressors perpetuating inflammation and pain [7].

A variety of medical therapies have been used for treatment of IBD patients. Among them immunosuppressive medications are prominent [8], with benefits observed in both clinical remission and mucosal healing. However, beside these conventional therapies, patients with IBD often question clinicians about dietary suggestions to improve their symptoms and quality of life [9]. During the last decade, soy extracts have attracted attention because of their anti-inflammatory properties in animal models of IBD [10] partly due to a reduced expression of inflammatory mediators [11]. Soy extracts are mainly characterized by the presence of isoflavones and their content of a family of serine protease (trypsin-like) inhibitors known as Bowman-Birk Inhibitors (BBI) [12]. However, the isoflavone profile and concentration as well as the BBI content vary according to the extract considered. A beneficial effect in terms of rates of remission and clinical response has been observed in patients with UC treated with a concentrate of BBI [13]. Soy isoflavones such as genistein, daidzein and its metabolite equol exhibit estrogen-like activity [14]. In the colon, estrogen receptors (ERs) signalling enhance expression of trans-membrane TJ proteins in non-inflamed conditions [15], and decrease proinflammatory cytokine production in experimental colitis [16,17]. Soy isoflavones have been shown to enhance intestinal tight junction (TJ) barrier integrity [18] although the precise mechanism underlying amelioration of TJ barrier remains unclear. If recent attention has been made on the beneficial properties of purified genistein or isoflavone-enriched diet in colitis [10,19], the estrogenic potential of isoflavones to enhance TJ barrier integrity in inflamed tissues remains to be investigated. This study was conducted using a fermented soy-germ (FSG) extract containing daidzein, glycitein and genistein present in aglycone forms resulting from fermentation [20], which represent the gut absorbable isoflavone forms [21], as well as stable levels of BBI.

Regarding the composition of the FSG extract used in this study, we aimed to evaluate whether this compound may exert cumulative or synergistic protection based on protease inhibition and ER-ligand activity in a model of experimental colitis in rats.

Materials and Methods

Ethics statement
All experimental protocols were approved by the Local Animal Care and Use Committee of Institut National de la Recherche Agronomique.

Animals and sexual cycle stage determination
Female Wistar rats (Janvier SA, Le Genest St Isle, France) were housed under controlled conditions of temperature ($21\pm1°C$) and illumination (12 h light, 12 h dark) with free access to water and fed standard pellets (UAR pellets, Epinay, France). Estrous cycle stages were assessed through vaginal smears as previously described [15].

Fermented soy germ ingredient
The FSG was industrially processed as ground powder under the trademark Primasoy® by GENIBIO (Lorp-Sentaraille, France). This compound had an average content of isoflavones of 34.7 μmol/g of product (55% daidzein, 30% glycitein and 15% genistein in aglycone forms). Bowman-Birk protease inhibitors were quantified in chymotrypsin inhibitory (CI) units, where 1 CI is the amount needed to inhibit 1 mg of bovine pancreatic chymotrypsin [20].

FSG was diluted in water and prepared daily in order to administer in 1 ml volume, 0.45 mg isoflavone aglycone forms equivalent/d/rat and 1 BBI CI/d/rat as described previously [22].

Induction of experimental colitis
Colitis was induced by an intra-colonic (IC) administration of TNBS (2,4,6-trinitrobenzene sulphonic acid) at a dose of 80 mg/kg in 50% ethanol. TNBS was infused through a silicone catheter introduced 7 cm into the anus under acepromazine–ketamine anaesthesia, as previously described [23].

Macroscopic damage scores
Immediately after sacrifice, the colon was removed and rinsed with saline. Intestinal damage was scored according to a modified scale of Wallace et al [24]. Briefly, the presence of mucosal hyperemia and bowel wall thickening, the severity and extent of ulceration and necrosis, the tissue adhesion, and the occurrence of diarrhea were rated according to a macroscopic damage score (MDS) ranging from 0 (normal appearance) to 13 (severe lesions).

Microscopic damages
To evaluate microscopic damages (MD), samples of the distal colon were fixed in Duboscq-brazil solution during 24 h, dehydrated and embedded in paraffin. Samples were then cut into 5 μm thick transversal sections, mounted on glass slides, stained with hematoxylin and eosin, then observed with a light microscope (Nikon 90i, Nikon, France). The MD were assessed according to a modified histological grading scale described by Fabia and al [25]. Several parameters were observed as ulceration, mucus cell depletion, oedema, inflammatory cell infiltration and vessel dilatation. Each parameter estimated was graded 0–3 depending on the severity of the changes found: (0) no change, (1) mild, (2) moderated or (3) severe changes. MD were calculated by adding the scores of all parameters cited above.

Myeloperoxidase activity assay
The activity of the enzyme myeloperoxidase (MPO), a marker of polymorphonuclear primary granules, was determined in the colon. Immediately after sacrifice, a distal colonic segment (1 cm long) was taken off, suspended in potassium phosphate buffer (KH_2PO_4 44 mM, K_2HPO_4 6 mM, pH 6.0), homogenized on ice with Polytron (PCU-2, Kinematica GmbH, Lucerne, Switzerland) and submitted to three cycles of freezing and thawing. Homogenates were then centrifuged at 10000 rpm for 15 min at 4°C. The pellets were resuspended in hexadecyl trimethylammonium bromide buffer (0.5% (wt/vol) in potassium phosphate buffer) to release MPO from polymorphonuclear neutrophil primary granules. These suspensions were sonicated (Büchi, Flawil, Switzerland) on ice and centrifuged at 10000 rpm for 15 min at 4°C. Supernatant fractions were diluted in potassium phosphate buffer containing 0.167 mg O-dianisidine dihydrochloride/ml and 0.00005% (vol/vol) H_2O_2. MPO from human neutrophils (Sigma, Saint Quentin Fallavier, France; 0.1 U/ml) was used as a standard. Changes in absorbance at 450 nm were recorded with a spectrophotometer (mc2UV, Safas, Monaco) every 10 s over 2 min. One unit of MPO activity was defined as the quantity of MPO degrading 1 μmol H_2O_2 min^{-1} ml^{-1} at 25°C. Protein concentrations (mg/ml) were determined using a modified method of Lowry (Detergent Compatible Assay, BioRad, Ivry/Seine, France) and MPO activity was expressed as MPO units/g protein.

Tissue protein extraction and ELISA
Tissue proteins were extracted with RIPA buffer (1% Igepal, 0.5% deoxycholic acid, and 0.1% sodium dodecyl sulfate in Tris-buffered saline 1x; pH 7.4) with protease inhibitor cocktail (Roche Diagnostics, Mannheim, Germany). Clear lysates were prepared by centrifugation at 10000 g for 10 min, and protein concentrations were assessed using the BC Assay Uptima kit (Interchim). Samples were then processed for ELISA using commercial kits to determine colonic contents of IL-1β, and IL-10 (ELISA kits, Duoset R&D Systems, Lille, France). Data were expressed as concentration per mg of total proteins.

MIF expression by Western blot

Briefly, tissue proteins were extracted with RIPA buffer as above, and equal protein amounts of each extract were separated in 15% SDS-polyacrylamide gel and transferred onto 0.45 μm nitrocellulose membranes (Whatman, Dominique Deutscher, Brumath, France). Membranes were blocked with Odyssey blocking buffer (Rockland, Tebu-bio, France), then incubated overnight at 4°C with the rabbit anti-MIF antibody (Torrey Pines Biolabs; 1/1000) or anti-GAPDH antibody (Cell signaling Technology, Ozyme, St Quentin-en Yvelines, France; 1/1000) used as internal standard. After washing, fluorescent CF770 anti-rabbit antibody (Biotium, Hayward, CA; 1/1000) was added for 1 hour at room temperature and protected from light. Membranes were scanned and the intensity of bands was analysed on infrared imaging system Odyssey (Li-Cor, Lincoln, NE). MIF expression was assessed relative to GAPDH for each sample analysed.

Faecal proteolytic activity assay

Supernatants of faecal homogenates (25 μl) were incubated with 1 ml of reaction buffer (0.15 M/L NaCl and 20 mmol/L Tris-HCl, pH 8.5) and 1 ml of 0.5% (w/v) azocasein (Sigma, St.Quentin Fallavier, France) at 37°C. The reaction was stopped after 20 min with 1 ml of 10% (v/v) trichloroacetic acid (Sigma). Following centrifugation, absorption of the clear supernatant was measured at 366 nm. Proteolytic activity of the supernatants was normalized to protein content.

PAR-2 immunohistochemistry

Colonic tissue samples were fixed in 4% formalin and incubated for 24 h in 30% of sucrose at 4°C. Samples were embedded in Tissue Tek medium (Euromedex, Souffelweyesheim, France) and frozen in isopentane at −45°C. Cryostat sections (7 μm) were post-fixed with acetone (10 min, −20°C) and hydrated in phosphate-buffered saline (PBS)-milk (0.1%). After incubation in blocking solution (PBS-0.25% Triton X100-0.1% BSA), sections were incubated overnight at 4°C with primary goat polyclonal antibody for PAR-2 (1/1000) (SantaCruz, California, USA). Sections were then washed in PBS-milk (0.1%) and incubated for 1 h at room temperature with biotinylated donkey anti-goat secondary antibody (1/1000) (Interchim, Montluçon, France), then 45 min at room temperature with FITC-avidine (1/500) (Clinisciences, Montrouge, France). Sections were mounted in Vectashield Hard set mounting medium (Clinisciences, Montrouge, France) and examined under a Nikon 90i fluorescence microscope (Nikon, Champigny-sur-Marne, France). PAR-2 area fraction per μm^2 of epithelium was quantified using Nikon-Elements-Ar software.

Intestinal paracellular permeability

Intestinal paracellular permeability (IPP) was performed using ^{51}Cr-EDTA (Perkin–Elmer Life Sciences, Paris, France) as a marker of tight junctions paracellular permeation. ^{51}Cr-EDTA (0.7 μCi) was diluted in 500 μl of saline and administered *per os* 24 h, 3 d or 5 d after induction of colitis. Animals were placed in metabolic cages, and faeces and urine were collected separately during 24 h. The radioactivity in urine was measured on a gamma counter (Cobra II, Packard Meriden, CT, USA). Permeability to ^{51}Cr-EDTA was expressed as percentage of administered radio-activity recovered in 24 h urines.

Surgical procedure

Animals were surgically prepared for abdominal striated muscle electromyography according to a previously described technique [23]. Briefly, rats were equipped with three groups of three NiCr wire electrodes (60 cm in length, 80 μm in diameter) implanted into the abdominal external oblique musculature. Electrodes were exteriorized on the back of the neck and protected by a glass tube attached to the skin.

Distension procedure and electromyographic recordings

Rats were accustomed to be in polypropylene tunnels (6 cm diameter, 25 cm length) for 2 d before colorectal distension (CRD). A balloon (2 mm diameter; 4 cm length) consisting of a latex condom was introduced into the anus, fixed at the base of the tail and connected to a computerized barostat INRA [26]. The balloon was inflated progressively in steps of 15 mmHg, each step of inflation lasting 5 min. Colorectal pressure and balloon volume (referring to the intestinal compliance) were continuously monitored on a potentiometric recorder (L6517; Linseis, Selb, Germany) with a paper speed of 1 cm.min^{-1}. The striated muscle spike bursts, related to abdominal cramps, were recorded on an electroencephalograph machine (Mini VIII; Alvar, Paris, France) from implanted electrodes. Differential amplification, using a short time constant (0.03s), allow us to detect high frequency spike bursts corresponding to abdominal cramps.

Experimental protocol

Female Wistar rats were divided into 11 groups (n = 10 per group) and received orally for 15 d either vehicle (Ve; 1 ml of water) or FSG, with or without the ER antagonist ICI 182.780 (2 mg/kg/day, s.c) administered from day 11 until 15 of the treatment. Colitis was induced by IC instillation of TNBS/ethanol (80 mg/kg) on day 15 of the treatment. Non-inflamed rats received IC instillation of sterile saline solution. Body weight was evaluated every 2 days from the beginning of the treatment until 5 d post-TNBS. In a first series, animals were sacrificed 24 h, 3 d and 5 d post-colitis. MDS were determined at all time points post-TNBS. Colonic samples were taken for (i) MD and MPO activity assessments, (ii) IL-1β, IL-10 level measurements, (iii) MIF and PAR-2 expression. Faecal pellets were collected for proteolytic activity assessment. In a second series, IPP to oral ^{51}Cr-EDTA was measured 24 h, 3 d and 5 d post-TNBS in 24 h urines. Finally, in a last series at 5 d post-TNBS, visceral sensitivity in response to CRD was evaluated in animals previously equipped with NiCr electrodes implanted in the abdominal muscle.

Two additional sets of experiments were also conducted. In the first one, a group of 10 male Wistar rats received orally for 15 d the FSG treatment. On day 15, TNBS colitis was induced as described above, and MPO activity was evaluated 24 h and 3 d post-TNBS. In the second one, to test curative effects of FSG treatment, 10 female Wistar rats were orally given FSG starting the day of TNBS instillation until 5 days post-TNBS. MPO activity was evaluated on days 1, 3 and 5 post-TNBS.

Table 1. Body weight loss (g) in Ve or FSG-treated colitic rats.

Days post-TNBS	Ve-treated group	FSG-treated group
1	13±1.7	10±1.3
3	39±3.6**	35+2.7**
5	33±4.1*	29±3.5*

Values are presented as means ± SEM.
*p<0.05 *vs* body weight before TNBS administration,
**p<0.01 *vs* body weight before TNBS administration.
(One way-ANOVA followed by Tukey test).

A

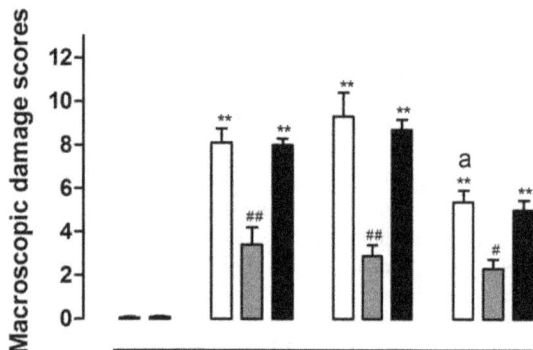

B

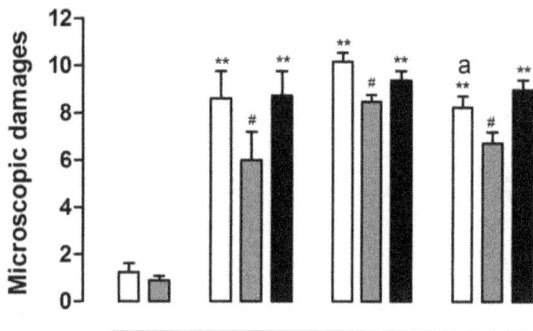

C

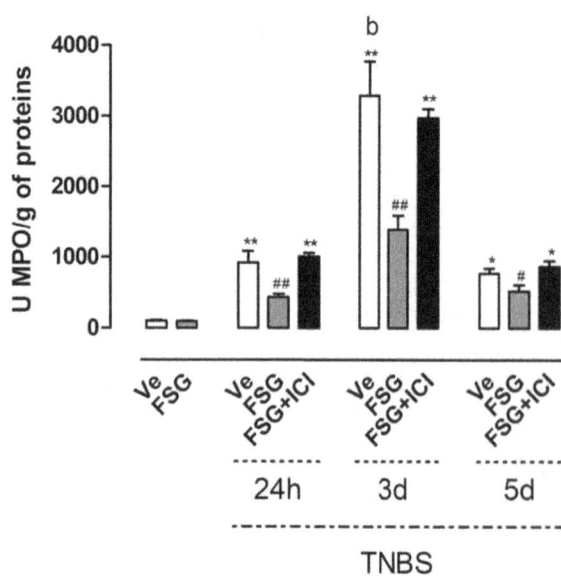

Figure 1. Effects of FSG treatment on the severity of TNBS-induced colitis. (A) MDS, (B) MD, (C) MPO activity were evaluated in presence or absence of the ER antagonist ICI 182.780. Values are presented as means ± SEM. Statistical analysis were performed by One way-ANOVA with post hoc comparison by Tukey test. *p<0.05 vs noninflamed group, **p<0.01 vs noninflamed group, #p<0.05 vs inflamed vehicle, ##p<0.01 vs inflamed vehicle, ap<0.05 vs Ve-treated rats 3 d post-TNBS, bp<0.05 vs Ve-treated rats 24 h and 5 d post-TNBS.

Statistical analysis

All data are presented as means±SEM. Statistical analysis were performed using Graph Pad Prism 4.0 (GraphPad, San Diego, CA). One-way ANOVA followed by Tukey's post-test was used to examine the effects of FSG treatment on TNBS-evoked IBD-like symptoms. Statistical significance was set at p<0.05.

Results

Effects of FSG on body weight

After 15 days of treatment with FSG, animals did not show any difference in body weight compared with control rats orally treated with Ve (data not shown). Body weight loss started 24 h after TNBS induction of colitis, to reach ~13% on day 3 post-TNBS compared to non-inflamed rats, then started increasing (~3%) 5 d after TNBS administration. Rats treated with FSG showed similar body weight loss after TNBS administration compared to Ve-treated colitic rats (Table 1).

FSG treatment attenuates the severity of TNBS-induced colitis

TNBS administration resulted in colon inflammation associated with hyperemia, ulceration and bowel wall thickening, leading to a significant increase (p<0.01) in MDS 24 h, 3 d and 5 d after colitis induction compared with non colitic animals (Figure 1A). Oral FSG treatment significantly decreased MDS from days 1 to 5 after TNBS (p<0.05) (Figure 1A).

Microscopic damage evaluation by histology has shown that colitic rats exhibited disruption of the epithelial barrier, oedema, vessel dilatation and a marked infiltration of inflammatory cells on days 1, 3 and 5 post-TNBS, corroborating MDS (Figure 1B). FSG-treated rats revealed a pronounced reduction in MD (p<0.05) compared with TNBS rats (Figure 1B). Colonic inflammation was also associated with increased mucosal neutrophil infiltration since colitic rats displayed an increase in MPO activity 24 h, 3 d and 5 d post-TNBS when compared to control non-inflamed rats (p<0.05). However, this increase was significantly higher (p<0.05) on day 3 post-TNBS vs 24 h and 5 d post-TNBS (Figure 1C). The oral treatment by FSG significantly reduced TNBS-induced increase in colonic MPO activity at all time points after induction of colitis (p<0.05) (Figure 1C). However, the effects of FSG treatment on MDS, MD and MPO activity did not reflect a total inhibition since values obtained for these parameters remained higher than in rats without colitis (Figure 1). All FSG effects on TNBS-induced colitis were blocked in the presence of the ER antagonist ICI 182.780 (Figure 1). Of note, FSG treatment in non-colitic rats had no effect per se on all inflammatory parameters evaluated compared with Ve-treated rats without TNBS colitis (Figure 1).

In a distinct series of experiments conducted in male rats, the preventive treatment with FSG decreased MPO activity at 24 h (p<0.05) and 3 d (p<0.01) post-TNBS when compared to corresponding Ve-treated colitic rats (see Figure S1). In addition, FSG given in a curative way in female rats (from TNBS administration until 5 days post-TNBS) decreased MPO activity on days 3 (p<0.01) and 5 (p<0.05) after induction of colitis (see Figure S2).

FSG treatment affects cytokine profile in TNBS-colitic rats

In this set of experiments, we investigated the effects of oral treatment with FSG on the expression or release of the pro-inflammatory cytokines MIF and IL-1β, as well as the anti-inflammatory cytokine IL-10 in colonic tissues. MIF was significantly over-expressed only 24 h after TNBS administration ($p < 0.05$) (Figure 2A) while colonic levels of IL-1β were markedly increased at 24 h, 3 d and 5 d after TNBS-induced colitis ($p < 0.01$) (Figure 2B). FSG treatment did not affect colonic concentrations of MIF and IL-1β in non-colitic rats (Figures 2A, B). In contrast, the oral FSG treatment significantly decreased MIF expression 24 h after colitis ($p < 0.05$) and IL-1β levels on days 1 and 3 post-TNBS ($p < 0.05$; $p < 0.01$ respectively) compared to corresponding values obtained in colitic rats (Figures 2A, B). The effects of FSG on MIF expression and IL-1β release were reversed in the presence of ICI 182.780 (Figures 2A, B). Interestingly, in non-colitic rats, as well as in colitic animals at 24 h, 3 d and 5 d post-TNBS, the FSG treatment significantly increased IL-10 release ($p < 0.05$) (Figure 2C). The FSG-induced effects on IL-10 colonic levels were reversed following ICI 182.780 (Figure 2C).

FSG prevents TNBS-induced increase in intestinal paracellular permeability

Further, we assessed whether FSG treatment could improve TNBS-induced rise in intestinal permeability. TNBS administration significantly increased the IPP during the whole post-colitis period evaluated (Figure 3). This effect was more pronounced at 24 h and 3 d post-TNBS ($p < 0.01$) than at 5 d ($p < 0.05$). Moreover, no difference in TNBS-induced IPP changes was observed in colitic rats according to the phase of the sexual cycle (data no shown). FSG oral treatment strongly reduced the TNBS-induced increase of intestinal permeability ($p < 0.01$) at all time points post-TNBS (Figure 3). The FSG effect on IPP in colitic rats was reversed by the ICI 182.780 administration (Figure 3).

FSG prevents TNBS-induced visceral hypersensitivity

In a final set of experiments, we investigated the ability of FSG treatment to prevent the inflammation-associated visceral hypersensitivity. Five days after TNBS administration, the number of abdominal contractions at applied pressures of 30, 45 and 60 mmHg was significantly increased ($p < 0.01$) in comparison with Ve-treated non-colitic group of rats (Figure 4A). FSG treatment strongly decreased ($p < 0.05$) the TNBS-induced hypersensitivity to CRD (Figure 4A), while concomitant treatment with ICI 182.780 reversed this effect of FSG (Figure 4A). As expected, TNBS administration resulted in a decrease of colonic compliance ($p < 0.05$) when compared to Ve-treated non colitic group (Figure 4B). FSG treatment did not affect colonic compliance in basal conditions (i.e. non-inflamed rats) in comparison with the Ve-treated non-colitic group (Figure 4B). Similarly, colonic compliance remained unchanged in FSG-treated vs Ve-treated colitic rats, indicating that the effect of FSG treatment on visceral sensitivity did not result from changes in muscle compliance.

FSG treatment prevents TNBS-induced increase of faecal proteolytic activity and colonic PAR-2 over-expression

Taking into account the BBI content of the FSG, we investigated its influence on intestinal proteolytic activity. Faecal proteolytic activity was significantly increased in colitic rats ($p < 0.05$) from 24 h to 5 d post-TNBS (Figure 5). FSG treatment fully prevented this effect at all time-points post-TNBS (Figure 5). ICI 182.780 administration failed to reverse this FSG effect

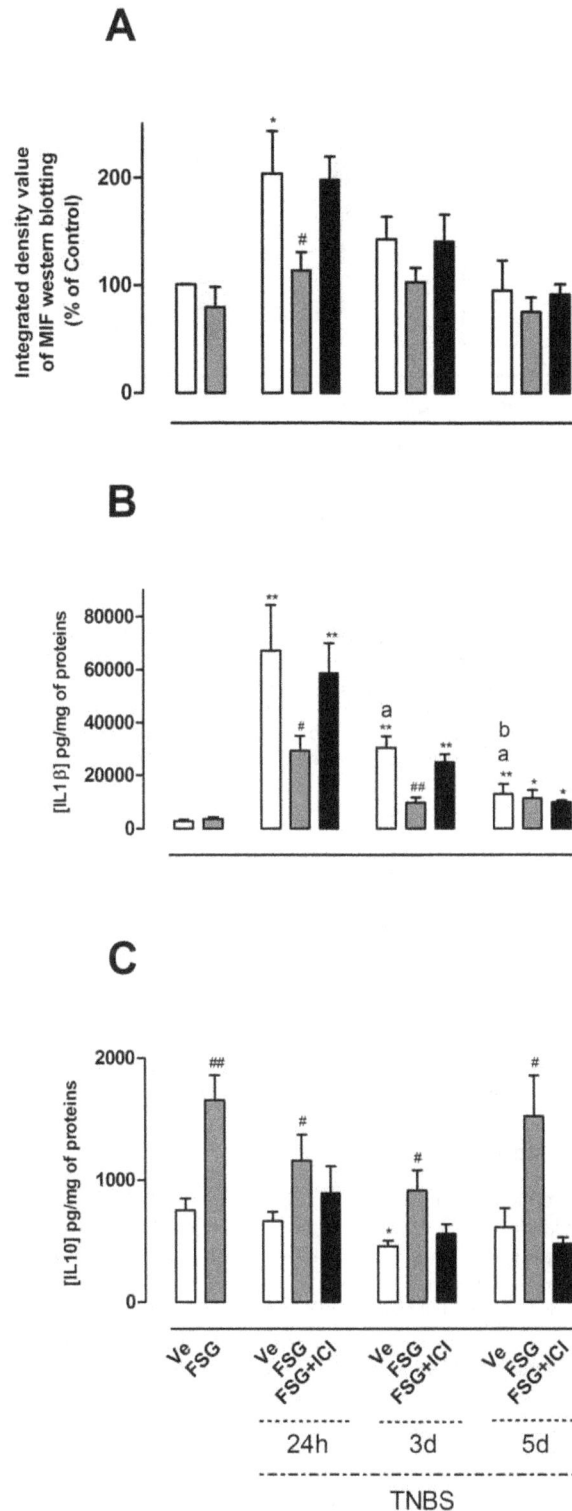

Figure 2. Effects of FSG treatment on cytokine profile after TNBS colitis. Effects of FSG on (A) MIF expression, (B) IL-1β, (C) IL-10 levels were evaluated in non inflamed colon and 24 h, 3 d, 5 d after TNBS-induced colitis in presence or absence of the ER antagonist ICI 182.780. Values are presented as means ± SEM. Statistical analysis were performed by One way-ANOVA with post hoc comparison by Tukey test. *$p < 0.05$ vs non inflamed group, **$p < 0.01$ vs non inflamed group, #$p < 0.05$ vs inflamed vehicle, ##$p < 0.01$ vs inflamed vehicle, [a]$p < 0.05$ vs Ve-treated rats 24 h post-TNBS, [b]$p < 0.05$ vs Ve-treated rats 3 d post-TNBS.

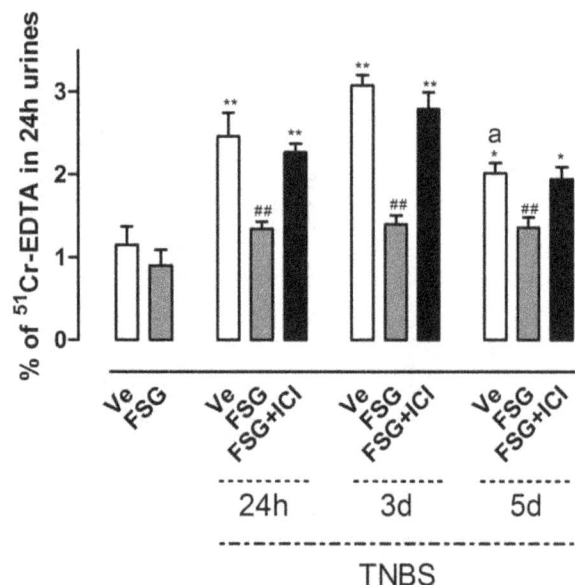

Figure 3. Effects of FSG treatment on TNBS-induced changes in intestinal paracellular permeability ± ER antagonist ICI182.780. Values are presented as means ± SEM. Statistical analysis were performed by One way-ANOVA with post hoc comparison by Tukey test. *$p < 0.05$ vs non inflamed group, **$p < 0.01$ vs non inflamed group, ##$p < 0.01$ vs inflamed vehicle, [a]$p < 0.05$ vs Ve-treated rats 3 d post-TNBS.

(Figure 5). Further, in basal conditions (i.e. non-colitic rats), a 15 d oral treatment by FSG did not affect faecal proteolytic activity since values obtained were similar to those obtained in Ve-treated non colitic rats (Figure 5). PAR-2 expression was increased in TNBS treated rats as reflected by immunochemistry from 24 h to 5 d post-TNBS (Figure 6). In basal conditions, FSG treatment did not affect PAR-2 expression in comparison to controls, whereas this treatment significantly reduced the TNBS-induced PAR-2 over-expression at all time-points post-TNBS evaluated (Figure 6).

Discussion

Inflammatory bowel diseases, including CD and UC, are chronic inflammatory gastrointestinal conditions characterized by an inappropriate innate and adaptive immune systems response [2], increased luminal protease activity [6], over-expression of PAR-2 [27], epithelial barrier defects [3] and abdominal pain [1]. In this study, we show that an oral treatment with a fermented soy germ ingredient (FSG) reduces inflammatory response, intestinal permeability and visceral hypersensitivity in a rat model of colitis through two distinct pathways. These protective effects occurred partly through a phytoestrogen-derived ER-signalling in the gut, able to reduce pro-inflammatory cytokine profile and to enhance epithelial barrier function. Additionally, the protease inhibitor activity of the FSG compound prevented the increase of luminal protease activity, and decreased colonic epithelial PAR-2 over-expression in colitic rats, independently of ER-ligand activity. Overall, these preventive effects occurred with a daily-administered dose of isoflavones equivalent aglycone forms (0.45 mg per day/rat) close to the authorized isoflavone daily intake in humans according to the European safety guidelines (1 mg/kg BW/day).

TNBS intracolonically administered to rats induces immunologic responses and gut barrier defects reproducing symptoms characterising chronic and relapsing IBD conditions [28]. For

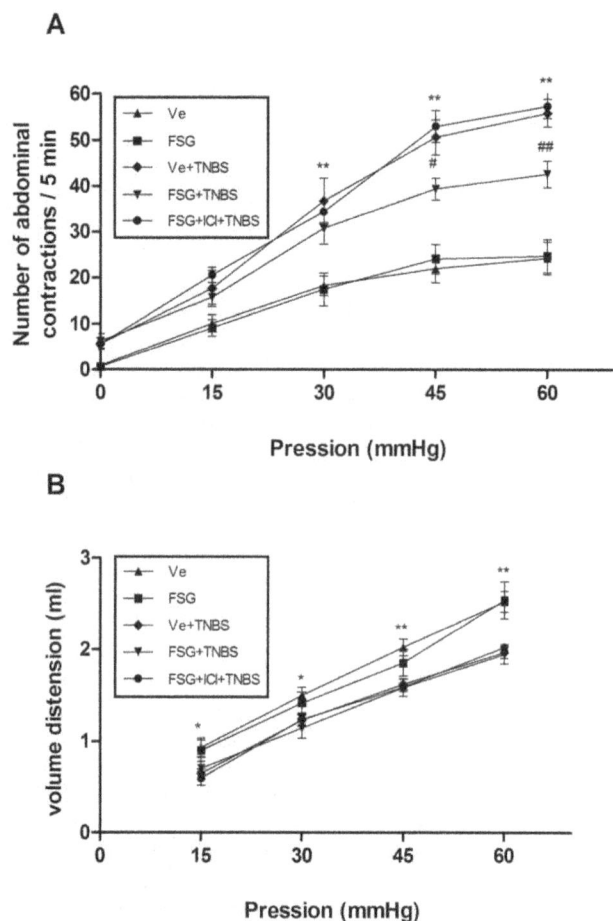

Figure 4. Effects of FSG treatment on (A) TNBS-induced visceral hypersensitivity in response CRD (B) colonic compliance. Abdominal response and colonic compliance were determined on 5th day post-TNBS in presence or absence of the ER antagonist ICI 182.780. Values are presented as means ± SEM. Statistical analysis were performed by One way-ANOVA with post hoc comparison by Tukey test. *$p < 0.05$ vs non inflamed group, **$p < 0.01$ vs non inflamed group, #$p < 0.05$ vs inflamed vehicle, ##$p < 0.01$ vs inflamed vehicle.

example, pro-inflammatory cytokines including IL-1β, TNF-α or IL-6 are consistently elevated in IBD [29], and high serum levels of MIF are detected in patients with active CD [30]. MIF stimulates the T Helper (TH) 1 cytokine network (mainly IL-1β and TNF-α) involved in the acute inflammatory response and its maintenance [30,31]. Similarly, these cytokines are produced in TNBS colitis [16]. In addition, transmural infiltration of neutrophils is a pathological feature of IBD [32]. TNBS colitis also increases MPO activity in the colonic mucosa, an index of neutrophil infiltration. Our study shows that FSG treatment prevented the colitis-induced increase in IL-1β and MIF in the rat colon. Concomitantly, the preventive FSG treatment prevented the increase in MPO activity in female and male rats, indicating inhibition of neutrophil influx in inflamed tissues. Since both MIF and IL-1β induce neutrophil recruitement [33,34], and that blockade of MIF activity down-regulates IL-1β [31,35], it is likely that the decrease of neutrophil influx and IL-1β release in the inflamed areas would result from FSG-mediated inhibition of MIF production in the acute phase of colitis. In addition, increased IL-10 limits TH1 immune responses [36], and deficiency in human IL-10 function related to IL-10 or its receptor IL-10R mutations was reported in the IBD patho-

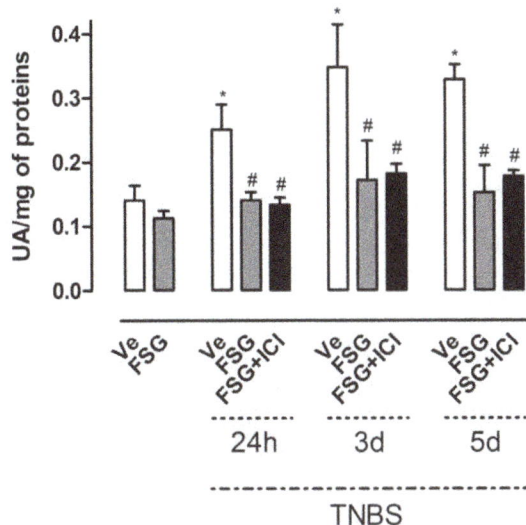

Figure 5. Effects of FSG treatment on TNBS-induced changes in faecal proteolytic activity ± ER antagonist ICI182.780. Data are expressed as means ± SEM. One way-ANOVA with post hoc comparison by Tukey test was used to analyse the data. *p<0.05 *vs* non inflamed group, #p<0.01 *vs* inflamed vehicle.

genesis [37]. FSG treatment increased basal IL-10 release and this effect was maintained in colitic rats. Since IL-10 production can inhibit pro-inflammatory cytokines release [38], we suggest that this mechanism also contributes to the preventive properties of FSG treatment, through downstream modulation of the TNBS-induced TH1 immune response. Interestingly, a reduction in the severity of TNBS colitis was also observed after curative treatment with FSG. Indeed, oral administration of FSG starting from the day of TNBS instillation to 5 days later resulted to a significant decrease in MPO activity on days 3 and 5 post-colitis (see Figure S2). This finding highlights that the anti-inflammatory effect exerted by the FSG treatment is mainly linked to early inflammatory cascade prevention in the colonic mucosa above reported in TNBS colitis.

In IBD as well as in experimental colitis models, oxidative stress has been incriminated in the inflammatory response. One may hypothesize that the antioxidant activity of FSG may contribute to alleviate TNBS injury. However, previous studies report that prevention of colonic inflammation through reduction of the reactive oxygen species (ROS) depends on the severity of colitis. Indeed, transgenic mice overproducing an antioxidant enzyme (CuZn-SOD) exhibit fewer lesions when submitted to mild, but not severe colitis [39]. The TNBS colitis used in the current study is considered as severe regarding the massive mucosal insult observed, mimicking acute IBD. In a study comparing the protective effects of different flavonoids against photo-oxidative stress, isoflavones demonstrate amplification of the photodamage, probably linked to their weak ability to scavenge ROS [40]. This is in agreement with previous literature showing that the structure of isoflavones confers weaker antioxidant properties when compared with other flavonoids [41]. Taken together, these data suggest that the anti-inflammatory effect of the FSG treatment reported herein is unlikely to be linked to its antioxidant properties.

Several studies report that estrogens have anti-inflammatory activity in colitis [16,17,42], partly occurring through ER-dependent down-regulation of MIF production by epithelial cells and macrophages [16]. ERs are widely expressed in the gut with marked expression of ERβ in colonic epithelial cells [43]. An ERβ agonist, ERB-041 displayed anti-inflammatory activity in the HLA-B27 transgenic rat model of IBD [42]. Of note, isoflavones such as genistein and daidzein act primarily through ERβ [14], and the aglycone forms are the gut absorbable forms [21]. Interestingly, the FSG compound tested, contains 85% of these phyotestrogens present in aglycone forms. Oral genistein displayed curative properties in TNBS colitic rats [10]. In this study, we show that the FSG anti-inflammatory effects as well as the increase on basal IL-10 release were blocked by the ER antagonist ICI 182.780, demonstrating that these properties are linked to ER-ligand activity.

Intestinal paracellular permeability (IPP) is increased in TNBS colitic rats, a situation that mimics epithelial barrier defect in IBD [3,44]. IPP is mainly regulated by tight junction (TJ) proteins [45]. In IBD, the release of pro-inflammatory cytokines increases intestinal permeability [46,47], partly through reduced expression of TJ proteins and/or disassembly of TJ protein complex [48]. We

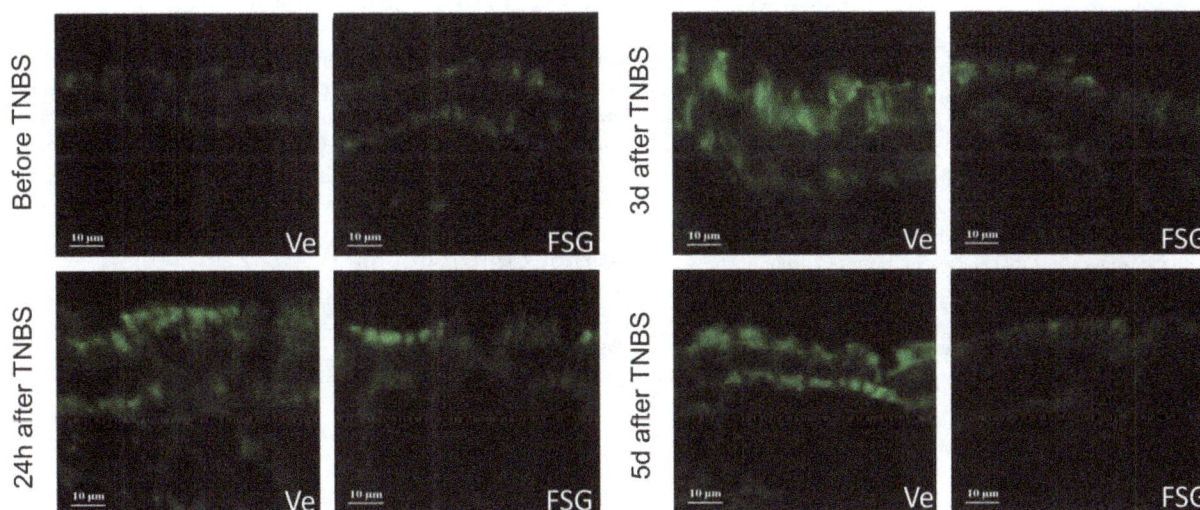

Figure 6. Immunohistochemical staining of longitudinal colonic section for PAR-2 expression. PAR-2 expression was evaluated in colonic epithelial cells in non inflamed colon and 24 h, 3 d, 5 d after TNBS-induced colitis in vehicle (Ve) or FSG treated rats.

found that the FSG treatment limits the TNBS-induced increase of gut permeability, and this effect was blocked by ICI 182.780, highlighting involvement of an ER-ligand signalling pathway. These data are consistent with studies showing a protective role of isoflavones on intestinal TJ barrier [18]. ERβ signalling pathways in the colon decrease intestinal permeability through up-regulation of TJ protein expression, *in vivo* and in *vitro* [15]. Interestingly, estrogenic activity of FSG has been shown to counteract increased gut permeability by enhancing TJ protein expression in a stress rat model [22]. On the other hand, down-regulation of IL-10 contributes to increased intestinal permeability in colitis [49]. We suggest that FSG may enhance junctional complexes leading to prevention of IPP.

In addition to estrogenic properties, FSG contains BBI (a highly heat stable protease inhibitors) that may contribute to the anti-inflammatory activity. This characteristic (which is absent in phytoestrogen-enriched diets or a simple mixture of isolated isoflavones) is of importance since BBI have been reported to inhibit activated tissue proteases in colitic rats [50], and a concentrate of BBI exerts beneficial effects in UC patients [13]. In UC patients, increased faecal serine protease and colonic PAR-2 expression have been reported [27]. Herein, we show for the first time that TNBS exacerbates the PAR-2 expression in the rat colon during the whole post-TNBS period. This is in agreement with previous animal studies showing that PAR-2 deficiency protects from the development of inflammation induced by three different models of colitis, including TNBS [51]. In our study, we report that anti-inflammatory properties of FSG are also linked to blockade of PAR-2 over-expression in the inflamed rat colon, whereas this treatment did not change PAR-2 expression in basal conditions. Since PAR-2 activation by PAR agonists leads to increased intestinal permeability in rodents [4], we suggest that the FSG ability to inhibit protease activity and PAR-2 expression pattern in colitic rats contributes in synergy with the ER-ligand activity pathway to its anti-inflammatory properties.

Abdominal pain and spasms are common symptoms in IBD. In UC patients as well as in experimental colitis, rectal hypersensitivity and lowering of pain thresholds have been observed [1,23]. We show that FSG treatment prevents TNBS-induced hypersensitivity to CRD without changes in colonic compliance, indicating that this antinociceptive effect did not result from changes in colonic muscular tone. Further, FSG treatment prevents TNBS-induced visceral hypersensitivity through an ER-ligand activity pathway since this effect was reversed by ICI 182.780. This result contrasts with previous data showing that in ovariectomized (OVX) colitic rats, estradiol replacement enhances visceral signal processing following colonic inflammation [52]. A possible explanation to this discrepancy may be attributed to (i) the hormonal status of animals, i.e OVX *vs* cyclic female rats used herein or (ii) the route of administration, i.e subcutaneous injection *vs* chronic oral treatment. For instance, chronic FSG or estradiol oral treatment in stressed cyclic rats prevents stress-induced hypersensitivity, suggesting that these compounds orally absorbed did not influence the already primed nociceptive pathway by endogenous sexual steroids [22]. In our study, the FSG-induced decrease in pain sensitivity may be linked to its anti-inflammatory

properties as well as its ability to decrease TNBS-induced rise in intestinal permeability. Indeed, FSG treatment decreases IL-1β release in colitic rats, a cytokine able to sensitize the capsaicin receptor TRPV1 involved in inflammatory hyperalgesia [53]. Additionally, serine proteases such as cathepsins released during colitis, activate nociceptors to induce visceral pain via PAR-2 [54], and FSG may limit this pathway. Overall, the FSG-mediated improvement of epithelial barrier integrity restricts the passage of luminal agents, thus the release of pro-inflammatory mediators able to sensitize nerve afferences, thus leading to downstream visceral pain.

In conclusion, the anti-inflammatory properties of FSG treatment result from two distinct but synergic pathways linked to its composition. The phytoestrogenic property activates the ER-ligand activity related pathway, whereas the presence of BBI involves a PAR-2 mediated pathway. Highlighting these mechanisms of action provide rationale for potential use of this compound as adjuvant therapy in IBD.

Supporting Information

Figure S1 Effects of FSG treatment on the severity of TNBS-induced colitis in male rats. Male Wistar rats were given orally for 15 d either vehicle or FSG treatment. Induction of TNBS colitis was performed on day 15 of the treatment as reported in females (see Materials and Methods section). Rats were sacrificed 24 h and 3 d post-colitis. Colon samples were taken for myeloperoxidase activity (MPO) assessments as described in Materials and Methods. Colonic MPO level showed significant neutrophil infiltration 24 h and 3 d post-TNBS in comparison to non-inflamed male rats ($p < 0.01$). As observed in females (Figure 1C), FSG pretreatment resulted in decreased MPO activity ($p < 0.05$) at 24 h and 3 d post-colitis compared to Ve-treated animals. Values are means ± SEM. [**]$p < 0.01$ *vs* basal, [##]$p < 0.01$, [#]$p < 0.05$ *vs* corresponding Ve group, [a]$p < 0.05$ *vs* Ve group of rats at 24 h post-TNBS.

Figure S2 Curative effect of FSG treatment in female rats submitted to TNBS colitis. Female Wistar rats were orally given daily either vehicle or FSG from the day of TNBS colonic instillation until sacrifice at 24 h, 3 d and 5 d post-colitis. TNBS administration induced a significant increase in MPO activity at 24 h, 3 d and 5 d post-colitis ($p < 0.01$). Interestingly, a daily oral treatment with FSG beginning the day of TNBS administration induced a drop of colonic MPO levels at 3 and 5 d post-TNBS in comparison to Ve control rats ($p < 0.05$). Values are means ± SEM. [**]$p < 0.01$ *vs* basal, [##]$p < 0.01$, [#]$p < 0.05$ *vs* corresponding Ve group, [a]$p < 0.05$ *vs* Ve group of rats at 3 d post-TNBS.

Author Contributions

Conceived and designed the experiments: LM VT EH. Performed the experiments: LM V. Bézirard CS-C V. Bacquié CL ML V. Braniste SM. Analyzed the data: LM. Wrote the paper: LM VT EH.

References

1. Drewes AM, Frokjaer JB, Larsen E, Reddy H, Arendt-Nielsen L, et al. (2006) Pain and mechanical properties of the rectum in patients with active ulcerative colitis. Inflamm Bowel Dis 12: 294–303.

2. Shih DQ, Targan SR (2008) Immunopathogenesis of inflammatory bowel disease. World J Gastroenterol 14: 390–400.

3. Soderholm JD, Streutker C, Yang PC, Paterson C, Singh PK, et al. (2004) Increased epithelial uptake of protein antigens in the ileum of Crohn's disease mediated by tumour necrosis factor alpha. Gut 53: 1817–1824.

4. Cenac N, Garcia-Villar R, Ferrier L, Larauche M, Vergnolle N, et al. (2003) Proteinase-activated receptor-2-induced colonic inflammation in mice: possible involvement of afferent neurons, nitric oxide, and paracellular permeability. J Immunol 170: 4296–4300.

5. Raithel M, Winterkamp S, Pacurar A, Ulrich P, Hochberger J, et al. (2001) Release of mast cell tryptase from human colorectal mucosa in inflammatory bowel disease. Scand J Gastroenterol 36: 174–179.

6. Roka R, Rosztoczy A, Leveque M, Izbeki F, Nagy F, et al. (2007) A pilot study of fecal serine-protease activity: a pathophysiologic factor in diarrhea-predominant irritable bowel syndrome. Clin Gastroenterol Hepatol 5: 550–555.

7. Bueno L, Fioramonti J, Garcia-Villar R (2000) Pathobiology of visceral pain: molecular mechanisms and therapeutic implications. III. Visceral afferent pathways: a source of new therapeutic targets for abdominal pain. Am J Physiol Gastrointest Liver Physiol 278: G670–676.

8. Baumgart DC, Sandborn WJ (2007) Inflammatory bowel disease: clinical aspects and established and evolving therapies. Lancet 369: 1641–1657.

9. Brown AC, Rampertab SD, Mullin GE (2011) Existing dietary guidelines for Crohn's disease and ulcerative colitis. Expert Rev Gastroenterol Hepatol 5: 411–425.

10. Seibel J, Molzberger AF, Hertrampf T, Laudenbach-Leschowski U, Diel P (2009) Oral treatment with genistein reduces the expression of molecular and biochemical markers of inflammation in a rat model of chronic TNBS-induced colitis. Eur J Nutr.

11. Young D, Ibuki M, Nakamori T, Fan M, Mine Y (2012) Soy-derived di- and tripeptides alleviate colon and ileum inflammation in pigs with dextran sodium sulfate-induced colitis. J Nutr 142: 363–368.

12. Birk Y (1985) The Bowman-Birk inhibitor. Trypsin- and chymotrypsin-inhibitor from soybeans. Int J Pept Protein Res 25: 113–131.

13. Lichtenstein GR, Deren JJ, Katz S, Lewis JD, Kennedy AR, et al. (2008) Bowman-Birk inhibitor concentrate: a novel therapeutic agent for patients with active ulcerative colitis. Dig Dis Sci 53: 175–180.

14. Kuiper GG, Lemmen JG, Carlsson B, Corton JC, Safe SH, et al. (1998) Interaction of estrogenic chemicals and phytoestrogens with estrogen receptor beta. Endocrinology 139: 4252–4263.

15. Braniste V, Leveque M, Buisson-Brenac C, Bueno L, Fioramonti J, et al. (2009) Oestradiol decreases colonic permeability through oestrogen receptor beta-mediated up-regulation of occludin and junctional adhesion molecule-A in epithelial cells. J Physiol 587: 3317–3328.

16. Houdeau E, Moriez R, Leveque M, Salvador-Cartier C, Waget A, et al. (2007) Sex steroid regulation of macrophage migration inhibitory factor in normal and inflamed colon in the female rat. Gastroenterology 132: 982–993.

17. Verdu EF, Deng Y, Bercik P, Collins SM (2002) Modulatory effects of estrogen in two murine models of experimental colitis. Am J Physiol Gastrointest Liver Physiol 283: G27–36.

18. Suzuki T, Hara H (2011) Role of flavonoids in intestinal tight junction regulation. J Nutr Biochem 22: 401–408.

19. Morimoto M, Watanabe T, Yamori M, Takebe M, Wakatsuki Y (2009) Isoflavones regulate innate immunity and inhibit experimental colitis. J Gastroenterol Hepatol.

20. Hubert J, Berger M, Nepveu F, Paul F, Daydé J (2008) Effects of fermentation on the phytochemical composition and antioxidant properties of soy germ. Food Chem 109: 709–721.

21. Setchell KD, Brown NM, Zimmer-Nechemias L, Brashear WT, Wolfe BE, et al. (2002) Evidence for lack of absorption of soy isoflavone glycosides in humans, supporting the crucial role of intestinal metabolism for bioavailability. Am J Clin Nutr 76: 447–453.

22. Moussa L, Bezirard V, Salvador-Cartier C, Bacquie V, Houdeau E, et al. (2012) A new soy germ fermented ingredient displays estrogenic and protease inhibitor activities able to prevent irritable bowel syndrome-like symptoms in stressed female rats. Clin Nutr.

23. Morteau O, Hachet T, Caussette M, Bueno L (1994) Experimental colitis alters visceromotor response to colorectal distension in awake rats. Dig Dis Sci 39: 1239–1248.

24. Wallace JL, Keenan CM, Cucala M, Mugridge KG, Parente L (1992) Mechanisms underlying the protective effects of interleukin 1 in experimental nonsteroidal anti-inflammatory drug gastropathy. Gastroenterology 102: 1176–1185.

25. Fabia R, Ar'Rajab A, Johansson ML, Andersson R, Willen R, et al. (1993) Impairment of bacterial flora in human ulcerative colitis and experimental colitis in the rat. Digestion 54: 248–255.

26. Hachet T, Caussette M (1993) A multifunction and programmable computer-ized barostat. Gastroenterol Clin Biol 17: 347–351.

27. Kim JA, Choi SC, Yun KJ, Kim DK, Han MK, et al. (2003) Expression of protease-activated receptor 2 in ulcerative colitis. Inflamm Bowel Dis 9: 224–229.

28. Appleyard CB, Wallace JL (1995) Reactivation of hapten-induced colitis and its prevention by anti-inflammatory drugs. Am J Physiol 269: G119–125.

29. Reinecker HC, Steffen M, Witthoeft T, Pflueger I, Schreiber S, et al. (1993) Enhanced secretion of tumour necrosis factor-alpha, IL-6, and IL-1 beta by isolated lamina propria mononuclear cells from patients with ulcerative colitis and Crohn's disease. Clin Exp Immunol 94: 174–181.

30. de Jong YP, Abadia-Molina AC, Satoskar AR, Clarke K, Rietdijk ST, et al. (2001) Development of chronic colitis is dependent on the cytokine MIF. Nat Immunol 2: 1061–1066.

31. Murakami H, Akbar SM, Matsui H, Horiike N, Onji M (2002) Macrophage migration inhibitory factor activates antigen-presenting dendritic cells and induces inflammatory cytokines in ulcerative colitis. Clin Exp Immunol 128: 504–510.

32. Alzoghaibi MA (2005) Neutrophil expression and infiltration into Crohn's intestine. Saudi J Gastroenterol 11: 63–72.

33. Arai Y, Takanashi H, Kitagawa H, Okayasu I (1998) Involvement of interleukin-1 in the development of ulcerative colitis induced by dextran sulfate sodium in mice. Cytokine 10: 890–896.

34. Makita H, Nishimura M, Miyamoto K, Nakano T, Tanino Y, et al. (1998) Effect of anti-macrophage migration inhibitory factor antibody on lipopolysaccharide-induced pulmonary neutrophil accumulation. Am J Respir Crit Care Med 158: 573–579.

35. Ohkawara T, Nishihira J, Takeda H, Hige S, Kato M, et al. (2002) Amelioration of dextran sulfate sodium-induced colitis by anti-macrophage migration inhibitory factor antibody in mice. Gastroenterology 123: 256–270.

36. Moore KW, de Waal Malefyt R, Coffman RL, O'Garra A (2001) Interleukin-10 and the interleukin-10 receptor. Annu Rev Immunol 19: 683–765.

37. Glocker EO, Kotlarz D, Boztug K, Gertz EM, Schaffer AA, et al. (2009) Inflammatory bowel disease and mutations affecting the interleukin-10 receptor. N Engl J Med 361: 2033–2045.

38. Paul G, Khare V, Gasche C (2012) Inflamed gut mucosa: downstream of interleukin-10. Eur J Clin Invest 42: 95–109.

39. Kruidenier L, van Meeteren ME, Kuiper I, Jaarsma D, Lamers CB, et al. (2003) Attenuated mild colonic inflammation and improved survival from severe DSS-colitis of transgenic Cu/Zn-SOD mice. Free Radic Biol Med 34: 753–765.

40. Filipe P, Silva JN, Haigle J, Freitas JP, Fernandes A, et al. (2005) Contrasting action of flavonoids on phototoxic effects induced in human skin fibroblasts by UVA alone or UVA plus cyamemazine, a phototoxic neuroleptic. Photochem Photobiol Sci 4: 420–428.

41. Manach C, Williamson G, Morand C, Scalbert A, Remesy C (2005) Bioavailability and bioefficacy of polyphenols in humans. I. Review of 97 bioavailability studies. Am J Clin Nutr 81: 230S–242S.

42. Harnish DC, Albert LM, Leathurby Y, Eckert AM, Ciarletta A, et al. (2004) Beneficial effects of estrogen treatment in the HLA-B27 transgenic rat model of inflammatory bowel disease. Am J Physiol Gastrointest Liver Physiol 286: G118–125.

43. Konstantinopoulos PA, Kominea A, Vandoros G, Sykiotis GP, Andricopoulos P, et al. (2003) Oestrogen receptor beta (ERbeta) is abundantly expressed in normal colonic mucosa, but declines in colon adenocarcinoma paralleling the tumour's dedifferentiation. Eur J Cancer 39: 1251–1258.

44. Hering NA, Fromm M, Schulzke JD (2012) Determinants of colonic barrier function in inflammatory bowel disease and potential therapeutics. J Physiol 590: 1035–1044.

45. Turner JR (2006) Molecular basis of epithelial barrier regulation: from basic mechanisms to clinical application. Am J Pathol 169: 1901–1909.

46. Adams RB, Planchon SM, Roche JK (1993) IFN-gamma modulation of epithelial barrier function. Time course, reversibility, and site of cytokine binding. J Immunol 150: 2356–2363.

47. Wang F, Graham WV, Wang Y, Witkowski ED, Schwarz BT, et al. (2005) Interferon-gamma and tumor necrosis factor-alpha synergize to induce intestinal epithelial barrier dysfunction by up-regulating myosin light chain kinase expression. Am J Pathol 166: 409–419.

48. Weber CR, Turner JR (2007) Inflammatory bowel disease: is it really just another break in the wall? Gut 56: 6–8.

49. Madsen KL, Malfair D, Gray D, Doyle JS, Jewell LD, et al. (1999) Interleukin-10 gene-deficient mice develop a primary intestinal permeability defect in response to enteric microflora. Inflamm Bowel Dis 5: 262–270.

50. Hawkins JV, Emmel EL, Feuer JJ, Nedelman MA, Harvey CJ, et al. (1997) Protease activity in a hapten-induced model of ulcerative colitis in rats. Dig Dis Sci 47: 1969–1980.

51. Hyun E, Andrade-Gordon P, Steinhoff M, Vergnolle N (2008) Protease-activated receptor-2 activation: a major actor in intestinal inflammation. Gut 57: 1222–1229.

52. Ji Y, Tang B, Traub RJ (2005) Modulatory effects of estrogen and progesterone on colorectal hyperalgesia in the rat. Pain 117: 433–442.

53. Eijkelkamp N, Heijnen CJ, Elsenbruch S, Holtmann G, Schedlowski M, et al. (2009) G protein-coupled receptor kinase 6 controls post-inflammatory visceral hyperalgesia. Brain Behav Immun 23: 18–26.

54. Cattaruzza F, Lyo V, Jones E, Pham D, Hawkins J, et al. (2011) Cathepsin S is activated during colitis and causes visceral hyperalgesia by a PAR2-dependent mechanism in mice. Gastroenterology 141: 1864–1874 e1861–1863.

16

Investigation of Multiple Susceptibility Loci for Inflammatory Bowel Disease in an Italian Cohort of Patients

Anna Latiano[1]*, **Orazio Palmieri**[1], **Tiziana Latiano**[1], **Giuseppe Corritore**[1], **Fabrizio Bossa**[1], **Giuseppina Martino**[1], **Giuseppe Biscaglia**[1], **Daniela Scimeca**[1], **Maria Rosa Valvano**[1], **Maria Pastore**[2], **Antonio Marseglia**[2], **Renata D'Incà**[3], **Angelo Andriulli**[1], **Vito Annese**[4]

1 Gastroenterology Unit, IRCCS "Casa Sollievo della Sofferenza," San Giovanni Rotondo, Italy, **2** Division of Paediatrics, IRCCS "Casa Sollievo della Sofferenza," San Giovanni Rotondo, Italy, **3** Department of Surgical and Gastroenterological Sciences, University of Padua, Padua, Italy, **4** Division of Gastroenterology, University Hospital Careggi, Florence, Italy

Abstract

Background: Recent GWAs and meta-analyses have outlined about 100 susceptibility genes/loci for inflammatory bowel diseases (IBD). In this study we aimed to investigate the influence of SNPs tagging the genes/loci PTGER4, TNFSF15, NKX2-3, ZNF365, IFNG, PTPN2, PSMG1, and HLA in a large pediatric- and adult-onset IBD Italian cohort.

Methods: Eight SNPs were assessed in 1,070 Crohn's disease (CD), 1,213 ulcerative colitis (UC), 557 of whom being diagnosed at the age of ≤16 years, and 789 healthy controls. Correlations with sub-phenotypes and major variants of NOD2 gene were investigated.

Results: The SNPs tagging the TNFSF15, NKX2-3, ZNF365, and PTPN2 genes were associated with CD (P values ranging from 0.037 to 7×10^{-6}). The SNPs tagging the PTGER4, NKX2-3, ZNF365, IFNG, PSMG1, and HLA area were associated with UC (P values 0.047 to 4×10^{-5}). In the pediatric cohort the associations of TNFSF15, NKX2-3 with CD, and PTGER4, NKX2-3, ZNF365, IFNG, PSMG1 with UC, were confirmed. Association with TNFSF15 and pediatric UC was also reported. A correlation with NKX2-3 and need for surgery ($P = 0.038$), and with HLA and steroid-responsiveness ($P = 0.024$) in UC patients was observed. Moreover, significant association in our CD cohort with TNFSF15 SNP and colonic involvement ($P = 0.021$), and with ZNF365 and ileal location ($P = 0.024$) was demonstrated.

Conclusions: We confirmed in a large Italian cohort the associations with CD and UC of newly identified genes, both in adult and pediatric cohort of patients, with some influence on sub-phenotypes.

Editor: Jan-Hendrik Niess, Ulm University, Germany

Funding: The study was supported by a grant from the Italian Minister of the Health (RC0902GA33). The funders had no role in study design, data collection and analysis, decision to publish, or preparation of the manuscript.

Competing Interests: The authors have declared that no competing interests exist.

* E-mail: a.latiano @operapadrepio.it

Introduction

The pathogenesis of inflammatory bowel diseases (IBD), namely Crohn's disease (CD) and ulcerative colitis (UC), is still incompletely understood, but it is widely accepted that the two conditions result from an inappropriate and exaggerated mucosal immune response to constituents of the intestinal flora in a genetically susceptible host [1,2]. In the past year, genome-wide association (GWA) studies have identified several genes involved in the pathogenesis of IBD and, subsequently GWAS meta-analysis has led to confirmation of more than 70 genes or loci that confer susceptibility to CD and 47 to UC, mostly in adult populations [3,4,5]. In particular, GWA and replications studies identified gene variants, including protein tyrosine phosphatase nonreceptor type 2 (PTPN2), NK2 transcription factor related locus 3 (NKX2-3), and tumor necrosis factor superfamily member 15

(TNFSF15) [6,7,8]. A subsequent North American GWA study identified two additional loci for UC located on chromosome 1p36 and 12q15, each of them harboring multiple genes, including several with a definite role in inflammation and immunity, like group II secreted phospholipase A2 (PLA2G2E), interferon gamma (IFNG), interleukin 26 (IL26) and interleukin 22 (IL22). In addition, combined genome-wide significant evidence for association was found at two additional loci, namely HLA on chromosome 6p21 and IL23R (interleukin-23 receptor) on chromosome 1p31 [9]. Finally, a GWA study carried out in pediatric-onset IBD patients identified two novel IBD loci located on chromosome 20q13 and 21q22, close to the tumor necrosis factor receptor superfamily member 6B (TNFRSF6B) and proteasome-assembling chaperone 1 (PSMG1) genes [10].

In the present study, we investigated whether potential loci reported in the meta-analysis and GWA studies on chromosomes

5p13 (*PTGER4*), 12q15 (*IFNG*, *IL22*, *IL26*), 6p21 (*HLA*), 21q22 (*PSMG1*), and *PTPN2*, *NKX2-3*, *TNFSF15*, were associated in a large and phenotypically well-characterized Italian cohort of IBD patients, and we also attempted to elucidate their involvement in early onset disease. In addition, we tested the potential epistasis between these variants and IBD-associated *NOD2/CARD15* SNPs, as well as possible genotype-phenotype correlations.

Materials and Methods

Ethics statement

The IBD cohort and unaffected controls were recruited from adult individuals referred the IRCCS, "Casa Sollievo della Sofferenza " Hospital in San Giovanni Rotondo, and from pediatric centers of the Italian Society of Pediatric Gastroenterology, Hepatology and Nutrition (SIGENP). Written informed consent was obtained from all adult participants and, for patients under age of 19 years, from related parents. Ethical approval was acquired from the Ethics Review Board of "Casa Sollievo della Sofferenza" Hospital, San Giovanni Rotondo, and each participating center approved the recruitment protocol. The study was supported by a grant from the Italian Minister of the Health (RC0902GA33).

Extensive clinical characterization was available for all patients. The diagnosis of CD or UC was established by conventional clinical, radiological, endoscopic, and histological findings [11]. The CD phenotype was classified based on age at disease onset (A), maximal extent of disease (L), and behavior (B) according to the Montreal classification [12,13]. In patients with UC the colon location was also classified according to the Montreal classification, by distinguishing ulcerative proctitis (E1), left-side colitis (E2), and extensive colitis (E3). For all IBD patients further clinical characteristics were analyzed, namely the occurrence of previous resective surgery, IBD family history, smoking habits, extra-intestinal manifestations and response to medical therapy. More specifically the need for use of corticosteroids, immunosuppressors (thiopurines and methotrexate) and anti-TNF agents were evaluated. In addition, on the basis of review of medical records, patients with the use of corticosteroid (CS) were classified as CS-responder (at least one course of systemic steroids with clinical remission reported in the medical history), or CS-refractory (when an unsuccessful clinical response was achieved leading to alternative therapies like surgery, use of anti-TNF or other immunosuppressors drugs) [14,15]. Patients with incomplete or unclear information were excluded from this analysis.

SNPs analysis and genotyping

We selected 8 polymorphisms for genotyping: three of them (rs4613763, rs4263839, rs11190140) identified by the CD GWA study meta-analysis [3], two (rs10761659, rs2542151) by the WTCCC [6] as showing the strongest association signals, two (rs2395185, rs1558744) by the first UC GWA study [9], and one (rs2836878) by a GWA analysis for early-onset IBD [10]. The genotypic variants in the *NOD2/CARD15* gene (rs2066844, rs2066845, rs2066847) had already been analyzed for all patients and controls. Genomic DNA was extracted from peripheral blood leukocytes by standard procedures using the DNA blood maxi kit from Qiagen (Hilden, Germany) in accordance with the manufacturer's instructions. All of the genotyping was performed at the Molecular Laboratory of the Gastroenterology Unit at the San Giovanni Rotondo Hospital, Italy. Genotyping was performed using Custom Taqman® SNP assay (Applied Biosystems, Foster City, CA), following manufacturer's instructions. The overall success rate of the genotyping assay was over 98%.

Statistical analysis

Statistical analysis was performed using Haploview Software version 4.1 (http://www.broad.mit.edu/personal/mpg/haploview) and SPSS software version 13.0 (Chicago, IL, USA). Hardy-Weinberg Equilibrium (HWE) tests were performed for all investigated polymorphisms independently among cases and controls. For the case-control analysis, comparisons of genotypes and allele frequencies was performed using X^2 or Fisher's exact test, where appropriate. Genotype-phenotype associations were first analyzed by means of univariate analysis and subsequently expressed as Odds Ratios (OR) with 95% confidence intervals (95% CI) by means of stepwise logistic regression analysis. For detecting gene-gene interactions we used a logistic regression based on forward stepwise selection procedures using the number of risk alleles as predictor variable. P values of less than 0.05 were considered significant.

Results

Case-control analysis with IBD patients

A total of 2283 individuals with IBD, including 1070 with CD and 1213 with UC, was analyzed. The control group consisted of 789 individuals from the same ethnicity who did not have IBD (neither CD nor UC). Clinical and demographic features of the IBD cases are listed in **Table 1**. There were 296 CD patients and 261 UC patients with the initial diagnosis before their 16th birthday. The adult cohort was constituted of 774 patients with CD and 952 with UC.

We compared single-marker allele frequencies using χ^2 statistics (**Tables 2–3**). Frequencies were in accordance with the Hardy-Weinberg equilibrium. In the overall cohort of IBD patients, four markers were above the threshold for significance for CD: the *TNFSF15* (rs4263839, P = 7.183×10^{-6}), *NKX2-3* (rs11190140, P = 0.003), *ZNF365* (rs10761659, P = 0.007), and *PTPN2* (rs2542151, P = 0.037). Of these four markers, two, namely, rs11190140 (P = 4×10^{-5}), and rs10761659 (P = 4×10^{-5}), were also associated with UC. In this latter subset of patients, four more markers, *PTGER4* rs4613763 (P = 0.012), *HLA-BTNL2* rs2395185 (P = 0.001), *IFNG-IL22-IL26* rs1558744 (P = 0.007), and *PSMG1* rs2836878 (P = 0.047) were exclusively associated.

To determine whether the previously identified variants were shared by both adult and pediatric individuals, we stratified all IBD patients according to their age at initial diagnosis. For the adult subset, associations were confirmed for all SNPs for either CD and UC with two remarkable exceptions: the rs4613763 variant, which was associated with CD (P = 0.031)(**Table 4**), and the rs2836878 variant which lost the association for UC (**Table 5**). Concerning childhood-onset cohort, the genotype frequencies of all considered polymorphisms remained significantly associated for UC, with the exception of the rs2395185 variant (**Table 5**). In CD pediatric patients the association was confirmed for rs4263839 (P = 0.008) and rs11190140 (P = 0.007) variants (**Table 4**).

Genotype association with IBD phenotypes

We also assessed whether the investigated SNPs could bear an influence on specific disease phenotypes, such as gender, disease location and behavior, resective surgery, family history, smoking habit, extra-intestinal manifestations, and medical therapies. At logistic regression analysis (**Table 6**), using a custom/stepwise model (forward entry) and after correction for all other covariates (age at diagnosis, disease localization, duration of follow-up, smoking status, etc), a significant association with the rs2395185 variant of the *HLA* gene and steroid-response (P = 0.024, OR =

Table 1. Clinical and demographic characteristics of the study population.

	CD	UC
	n = 1070	n = 1213
Gender		
F	468 (44)	511 (42)
M	602 (56)	702 (58)
Duration of follow-up (yr)		
mean ± SD	8±7	9±7
median (range)	6 (1–37)	7 (1–41)
Age at diagnosis (yr)		
mean ± SD	27±15	31±16
median (range)	25 (1–79)	28 (1–83)
≤16 (A1)	296 (28)	261 (21)
17–40 (A2)	586 (55)	642 (53)
> 40 (A3)	188 (17)	310 (26)
Disease location CD, n (%)		
Ileum (L1±L4)	331 (31)	
Colon (L2±L4)	265 (25)	
Ieo-colon (L3±L4)	465 (43)	
Upper GI (L4)	9 (1)	
Disease extent UC, n (%)		
Rectum (E1)		139 (11)
Left colon (E2)		554 (46)
Pancolitis (E3)		520 (43)
Disease behavior CD, n (%)		
Inflammatory	677 (63)	
Stricturing	279 (26)	
Penetrating	114 (11)	
Perianal Disease		
No	882 (82)	
yes	188 (18)	
EIM		
No	651 (61)	908 (75)
yes	419 (39)	305 (25)
Family history		
No	959 (90)	1107 (91)
yes	111 (10)	106 (9)
Smoker		
Yes	292 (32)	164 (15)
No	490 (53)	622 (57)
Ex	140 (15)	311 (28)
Resection		
No	749 (70)	1082 (89)
yes	321 (30)	131 (11)
Steroids		
Refractory	83 (13)	101(13)
Responder	569 (87)	673 (87)
IMS (AZT/6MP, Ciclo, MTX)		
No	676 (42)	927(58)
Yes	394 (58)	286 (42)
Infliximab		

Table 1. Cont.

	CD	UC
	n = 1070	n = 1213
No	914 (85)	1168 (96)
Yes	156 (15)	45 (4)

CD: Crohn's disease; UC: ulcerative colitis; EIM: extra-intestinal manifestations. IMS: immunosuppressors.
*For 148 CD and 116 UC patients the information is missing.

2.07, CI 95% 1.10–3.89), and positive family history (P < 0.01, OR = 3.68, CI 95% 1.93–7.04) in UC patients was observed. In the CD cohort, the *ZNF365* (rs10761659) SNP was associated with ileal location (L1) compared to patients with colonic (L2) involvement (81.2% vs 72.1%, P = 0.024, OR = 1.67, CI 95%, 1.06–2.62). Moreover, colon involvement in CD was significantly more frequent (45%) in patients carrying the minor variant (AA+Aa) of *TNFSF15* (rs4263839) SNP vs a 35% frequency observed in those with only ileal involvement (P = 0.021, OR = 1.54, 5% CI, 1.06–2.22). A negative association was found for the minor allele of the *NKX2-3* (rs11190140) gene in UC patients with needs for surgery (P = 0.038, OR = 0.64, 95% CI, 0.42–0.97). In CD, the same variant prevailed in patients with smoking habit (P = 0.018, OR = 1.46, CI 95%, 1.06–2.00). There was no effect of the other four SNPs (*PTGER4*-rs4613763, *PTPN2*-rs2542151, *IFNG*-rs1558744, *PSMG1*-rs2836878) on all the evaluated sub-phenotypes (data not shown).

We asked whether the identified genotype/phenotype associations would differ after stratifying the IBD population in respect to age at diagnosis. For the *HLA*-rs2395185 SNP the association persisted both in the adult- (P = 0.003) and in the pediatric-onset subset of patients (P = 0.006) with a positive family history (**Table 6**). Despite the large number of pediatric-onset IBD patients investigated, a trend was found for the genotype/phenotype frequencies of rs10761659, rs4263839, and rs11190140 SNPs, but did not reach statistical significance.

Gene-gene interactions

The possible interactions of tested variants (rs4613763, rs2395185, rs4263839, rs11190140, rs10761659, rs1558744, rs2542151, and rs2836878) with polymorphisms in the established susceptibility gene *NOD2/CARD15* (the three main polymorphisms rs2066844, rs2066845, and rs2066847: at least 1 variant against wild type) were evaluated. After correction for multiple testing, there was no significant evidence for interaction among the considered SNPs (P > 0.05) (data not shown), thus implying that each gene independently contributes to the disease risk.

Discussion

Recent GWA studies have enhanced our understanding of the complex genetic architecture of IBD. Most associations appear to be common to both types of IBD, while some genes/loci may be specific to adult- or pediatric-onset, and the factors that determine age of onset are unknown at present.

The major aim of our study was to examine recently described potential association of genes involved in the immune response and inflammation (*PTGER4*, *HLA*, *TNFSF15*, *NKX2-3*, *ZNF365*, *IFNG*, *PTPN2*, and *PSMG1*) in adult and pediatric-onset IBD in an Italian population.

Table 2. Genotype distribution of associated SNPs in Crohn's disease (CD) patients and healthy controls.

Gene(s) or locus	SNP	No. of CD genotyped			No. of control genotyped			P value	OR (95% CI)
		AA*	Aa	aa	AA*	Aa	aa		
PTGER4	rs4613763	7 (1.1%)	127 (19.3%)	523 (79.6%)	2 (0.4%)	86 (15.7%)	460 (83.9%)	0.0531	1.34 (0.99–1.80)
HLA, BTNL2	rs2395185	-	-	-	22 (5.1%)	154 (35.7%)	256 (59.2%)	-	-
TNFSF15	rs4263839	57 (6.3%)	322 (35.2%)	535 (58.5%)	74 (9.4%)	339 (43.0%)	376 (47.6%)	7.183E-06	0.65 (0.53–0.78)
NKX2-3	rs11190140	163 (18.8%)	437 (50.2%)	270 (31.0%)	176 (22.5%)	414 (52.9%)	193 (24.6%)	0.0039	0.73 (0.58–0.90)
ZNF365	rs10761659	240 (30.2%)	379 (47.7%)	175 (22.1%)	131 (24.3%)	255 (47.2%)	154 (28.5%)	0.0070	1.41 (1.09–1.81)
IFNG, IL22, IL26	rs1558744	-	-	-	77 (13.9%)	262 (47.4%)	214 (38.7%)	-	-
PTPN2	rs2542151	21 (2.4%)	229 (26.3%)	622 (71.3%)	10 (1.3%)	178 (22.8%)	591 (75.9%)	0.0371	1.26 (1.01-1.57)
PSMG1	rs2836878	10 (3.4%)	113 (38.3%)	172 (58.3%)	43 (7.6%)	203 (35.9%)	320 (56.5%)	ns	ns

A* denotes a risk allele.
OR: odds ratio; CI: confidence interval.
SNP: single nucleotide polymorphism.

Using a case-control design, we were able to replicate associations between GWA reported SNPs with CD (*TNFSF15* rs4263839, P = 7.183×10^{-6}; *NKX2-3* rs11190140, P = 0.003; *ZNF365* rs10761659, P = 0.007; *PTPN2* rs2542151, P = 0.037), and UC (*NKX2-3* rs11190140, P = 4×10^{-5}; *ZNF365* rs10761659, P = 4×10^{-5}; *PTGER4* rs4613763, P = 0.012; *HLA-BTNL2* rs2395185, P = 0.001; *IFNG-IL22-IL26* rs1558744, P = 0.007; *PSMG1* rs2836878, P = 0.047).

In addition, our analysis reveals significant association with pediatric UC cohort for six out the eight investigated variants, each of them with a P value < 0.016 (*PTGER4, TNFSF15, NKX2-3, ZNF365, IFNG,* and *PSMG1*): this finding suggests that these genes may also be involved in susceptibility to UC pediatric-onset.

To date, no studies on the tested polymorphisms have indicated associations with specific sub-phenotype. We were able to demonstrate, by stepwise logistic regression analysis, a correlation with, *NKX2-3* and need for surgery (P = 0.038), and with *HLA* and steroid-responsiveness (P = 0.024), and a positive family history in UC patients. Moreover, significant association in our CD cohort with *TNFSF15* SNP and colonic involvement (P = 0.021), and with *ZNF365* and ileal location (P = 0.024) was demonstrated.

The clinical significance of these associations, if any, remains to be investigated.

A summary of previously described allelic distributions of SNPs of genes/loci analyzed is depicted in Supplementary Table S1.

Kugathasan *et al* [10] carried out a GWA analysis in a pediatric-onset IBD and identified a significant association of both CD and UC with an intergenic SNP, rs2836878, located on chromosome 21q22 in a small region of linkage disequilibrium that harbors no genes but is close to the *PSMG1* gene. The association was also reiterated by the largest GWA study conducted so far in early-onset IBD (UC: $P = 2.65 \times 10^{-9}$)[16]. In keeping with previous finding is the contribution of the *PSMG1* locus to disease susceptibility in adult UC [17]. McGovern *et al* [18] confirmed the association after combining data from two new GWA studies and performing a meta-analysis with a published study. A trend for similar associations at rs2836878 variant was observed in CD Canadian cohort but did not achieve statistical significance [19](Table S1). Our results confirm the association in particular with pediatric-onset UC, pinpointing to a significant relevance of the 21q22 for UC. Larger studies that include functional data on the *PSMG1* gene will be required to confirm association at this locus.

Table 3. Genotype distribution of associated SNPs in ulcerative colitis (UC) patients and healthy controls.

Gene(s) or locus	SNP	No. of UC genotyped			No. of control genotyped			P value	OR (95% CI)
		AA*	Aa	aa	AA*	Aa	aa		
PTGER4	rs4613763	8 (1.2%)	142 (20.5%)	542 (78.3%)	2 (0.4%)	86 (15.7%)	460 (83.9%)	0.0126	1.45 (1.08–1.93)
HLA, BTNL2	rs2395185	29 (3.7%)	221 (28.1%)	537 (68.2%)	22 (5.1%)	154 (35.7%)	256 (59.2%)	0.0017	0.68 (0.53–0.86)
TNFSF15	rs4263839	66. (7.3%)	375 (41.6%)	460 (51.1%)	74 (9.4%)	339 (43.0%)	376 (47.6%)	ns	ns
NKX2-3	rs11190140	162 (17.9%)	438 (48.3%)	306 (33.8%)	176 (22.5%)	414 (52.9%)	193 (24.6%)	4E-05	0.64 (0.52–0.79)
ZNF365	rs10761659	168 (28.8%)	309 (53.0%)	106 (18.2%)	131 (24.3%)	255 (47.2%)	154 (28.5%)	4E-05	1.79 (1.36–2.38)
IFNG, IL22, IL26	rs1558744	167 (20.1%)	401 (48.2%)	264 (31.7%)	77 (13.9%)	262 (47.4%)	214 (38.7%)	0.0076	1.36 (1.08–1.70)
PTPN2	rs2542151	10 (1.1%)	232 (25.4%)	672 (73.5%)	10 (1.3%)	178 (22.8%)	591 (75.9%)	ns	ns
PSMG1	rs2836878	32 (3.7%)	302 (34.5%)	540 (61.8%)	43 (7.6%)	203 (35.9%)	320 (56.5%)	0.0473	0.80 (0.65–0.99)

A* denotes a risk allele.
OR: odds ratio; CI: confidence interval.
SNP: single nucleotide polymorphism.

Table 4. Genotype distribution of associated SNPs in adult- and childhood-onset Crohn's disease (CD) cohort.

SNP	No. of Adult CD genotyped			No. of Pediatric CD genotyped				P value	OR (95% CI)
	AA	Aa	aa	AA	Aa	aa			
rs4613763	6 (1.2%)	99 (20.0%)	389 (78.8%)	1 (0.6%)	28 (17.2%)	134 (82.2%)	Adult	0.0310	1.41 (1.03–1.93)
							Pediatric	ns	ns
rs2395185	-	-	-	-	-	-	Adult	-	-
							Pediatric	-	-
rs4263839	35 (5.5%)	223 (35.2%)	376 (59.3%)	22 (7.8%)	99 (35.4%)	159 (56.8%)	Adult	<0.001	0.62 (0.51–0.77)
							Pediatric	0.0087	0.69 (0.52–0.91)
rs11190140	116 (19.4%)	301 (50.4%)	180 (30.2%)	47 (17.2%)	136 (49.8%)	90 (33.0%)	Adult	0.0258	0.84 (0.72–0.98)
							Pediatric	0.0075	0.66 (0.49–0.89)
rs10761659	187 (30.4%)	301 (48.8%)	128 (20.8%)	53 (29.8%)	78 (43.8%)	47 (26.4%)	Adult	0.0022	1.52 (1.16–1.99)
							Pediatric	ns	ns
rs1558744	-	-	-	-	-	-	Adult	-	-
							Pediatric	-	-
rs2542151	13 (2.1%)	169 (27.8%)	426 (70.1%)	8 (3.0%)	60 (22.8%)	196 (74.2%)	Adult	0.0153	1.34 (1.06–1.70)
							Pediatric	ns	ns
rs2836878	-	-	-	-	-	-	Adult	-	-
							Pediatric	-	-

A significant association of genetic variants of the *TNFSF15* (*TL1A*) gene on chromosome 9q33 with CD was observed in a large cohort of Japanese patients, in several European cohorts [8,20,21], in US Jewish patients [22], in the combined data from the NIDDK IBD Consortium and the WTCCC [3], in Koreans patients [23], and in UC GWA study [7]. The *TNFSF15* is the only gene that has been associated in either Asiatic and European IBD patients [8,19](Table S1). *TNFSF15* is a member of tumor necrosis factor (TNF) superfamily that binds to death domain receptor 3 (DR3, TNFRSF25) and is expressed in endothelial cells, lymphocytes, plasma cells, monocytes, and dendritic cells [24,25]. Our analysis confirms the TNFSF15 as a susceptibility locus in CD both in adult and pediatric population (P = < 0.001, and P = 0.008 respectively), and shows an association also with early onset UC (P = 0.016).

The WTCCC [6] reported on CD cases a novel association involving a cluster of SNPs around the rs10883365 variant on chromosome 10q24.2, which maps within *NKX2-3* (NK2 transcription factor related, locus 3) gene, a member of the NKX family of homeodomain-containing transcription factors. The results of Parkes *et al* [26] supported this findings with an independent set of CD cases and controls of European descent. In addition, a large-scale meta-analysis [3] on CD cohort and replication study on IBD samples [7] found association with rs11190140 polymorphism in complete linkage disequilibrium with the risk allele at the SNP rs10883365 from the WTCCC study (r^2 = 1.0). In addition, a modest association was also reported with UC in a nonsynonymous SNP scan [27], in GWA scan for UC [17], and in the UC GWA meta-analysis and

Table 5. Genotype distribution of associated SNPs in adult- and childhood-onset ulcerative colitis (UC) cohort.

SNP	No. of Adult UC genotyped			No. of Pediatric UC genotyped				P value	OR (95% CI)
	AA	Aa	aa	AA	Aa	aa			
rs4613763	5 (5.2%)	78 (18.4%)	341 (80.42%)	3 (1.1%)	64 (23.9%)	201 (75.0%)	Adult	ns	ns
							Pediatric	0.0022	1.74 (1.21–2.49)
rs2395185	19 (3.1%)	176 (28.4%)	425 (68.5%)	10 (6.0%)	45 (26.9%)	112 (67.1%)	Adult	0.0019	0.67 (0.52–0.86)
							Pediatric	ns	ns
rs4263839	50 (7.5%)	289 (43.4%)	327 (49.1%)	16 (6.8%)	86(36.6%)	133 (56.6%)	Adult	ns	ns
							Pediatric	0.0161	0.69 (0.52–0.94)
rs11190140	132 (19.8%)	313 (46.9%)	222 (33.3%)	30 (12.6%)	125 (52.3%)	84 (35.1%)	Adult	0.0003	0.66 (0.52–0.82)
							Pediatric	0.0014	0.60 (0.44–0.82)
rs10761659	121 (27.7%)	235 (53.8%)	81 (18.5%)	47 (32.2%)	74 (50.7%)	25 (17.1%)	Adult	0.0003	1.75 (1.29–2.38)
							Pediatric	0.0054	1.93 (1.21–3.09)
rs1558744	127 (18.7%)	329 (48.5%)	223 (32.8%)	40 (26.1%)	72 (47.1%)	41 (26.8%)	Adult	0.0326	1.29 (1.02–1.63)
							Pediatric	0.0067	1.72 (1.16–2.56)
rs2542151	8 (1.2%)	169 (24.9%)	500 (73.9%)	2 (0.8%)	63 (26.6%)	172 (72.6%)	Adult	ns	ns
							Pediatric	ns	ns
rs2836878	30 (4.2%)	252 (35.6%)	426 (60.2%)	2 (1.2%)	50 (30.1%)	114 (68.7%)	Adult	ns	ns
							Pediatric	0.0051	0.59 (0.41–0.86)

Table 6. Correlation between risk alleles and clinical characteristics in Crohn's disease (CD) and ulcerative colitis (UC) patients at Multivariate Analysis.

	CD		UC	
	Adult *n = 728*	**Pediatric** *n = 342*	**Adult** *n = 952*	**Pediatric** *n = 261*
HLA rs2395185			*steroid-responsive* P = 0.024 OR 2.07 CI 95% (1.10–3.89)	
			family history P<0.01 OR 3.68 CI 95% (1.93–7.04)	
			Adult P = 0.003 OR 4.16 CI 95% (1.62–10.71)	*Pediatric* P = 0.006 OR 3.81 CI 95%(1.45–9.97)
ZNF365 rs10761659	*colon vs ileum* P = 0.024 OR 1.67 CI 95% (1.06–2.62)			
TNFSF15 rs4263839	*colon vs ileum* P = 0.021 OR 1.54 CI 95% (1.06–2.22)			
NKX2-3 rs11190140	*smoking* P = 0.018 OR 1.46 CI 95% (1.06–2.00)		*surgery* P = 0.038 OR 0.64 CI 95% (0.42–0.97)	

replication studies [18](Table S1). Similarly, in the present study the rs11190140 variant was associated with an increased risk for both CD and UC (P = 0.003 and P = 4×10^{-5} respectively), both in the adult and early-onset cohort. Abnormal expression of NKX2-3 may alter gut migration of antigen-responsive lymphocytes and influence the intestinal inflammatory response. NKX2-3-deficient mice develop splenic and gut-associated lymphoid tissue abnormalities with disordered segregation of T and B cells [28].

A highly attractive candidate gene for IBD, owing to its anti-inflammatory function and involvement in type 1 diabetes susceptibility and rheumatoid arthritis [29], is the *PTPN2* (protein tyrosine phosphatase, non-receptor type 2) located on chromosome 18p11, which encodes for a tyrosine phosphatase expressed in T cells, a negative regulator of inflammation. A novel association at rs2542151 of the *PTPN2* gene and CD was identified [6], replicated [26,30] and confirmed [3]. In contrast, Franke *et al* [7] observed this association with UC, a finding replicated in the recent GWA on UC [17]. In addition, associations with CD pediatric was also demonstrated [16,31](Table S1). In the present investigation the association was observed only in adult CD (P = 0.015) confirming its role as an adult-susceptibility gene.

The UC GWAS in European ancestry samples [9] indentified loci on chromosomes 1p36 and 12q15 where are genes involved in inflammation and immunity, such as *PLA2GIIE* (phospholipase A2, group IIE), *IFNG* (interferon-γ), *IL22* (interleukin-22), and *IL26* (interleukin-26); previous associations were replicated in GWA meta-analysis [18](Table S1). We were able to replicate the association between the rs1558744 SNP on chromosome 12q15 and UC (P = 0.007), and interestingly after stratifying the cohort with respect to age at diagnosis, the association was observed also in the pediatric-onset patients (adult P = 0.03; pediatric P = 0.006).

Several independent genome-wide scans in inflammatory bowel disease have shown evidence of linkage to the MHC region [32,33], which is characterized by extensive LD blocks (up to 3 Mb) and several genes (250 genes), mainly involved in immune-related functions. Recent genome-wide association studies in UC confirmed the association with the HLA with the maximal association signal at rs2395185, in a region spanning *BTNL2* to *HLA-DQB1* genes [9,18]. Recently, SNP and the HLA data

convincingly show that the main signal is located in a narrow genomic window containing the *HLA-DRB1* gene and strongly suggest that the more common *HLA-DRB1*1101* allele plays a primary role in both UC and CD susceptibility [34]. This association to the *DRB1* locus is consistent with other published GWAs in UC [9,35,36], also in Japanese population [37]. The same region was identified in the meta-analysis of CD genome-wide association studies [3]. Recent genome-wide association study in early-onset IBD [16] validated this known adult-onset IBD locus in their CD, UC, and IBD dataset, further supporting the importance of this region in IBD risk (Table S1). Allelic and genotype association analysis in our cohort showed that the polymorphism was significantly associated with overall susceptibility to UC (P = 0.001), and in particular with adult subset (P = 0.001).

In the study of Libioulle *et al* [38] a region on chromosome 5p13.1 contributing to CD susceptibility was identified. The disease-associated alleles were found to correlate with expression levels of the prostaglandin receptor EP4, which binds prostaglandin E2 (PGE2) and is encoded by *PTGER4*. In the same region the meta-analysis of three GWAS [3] identified rs4613763 as the most strongly associated SNP. No highly significant association of the *PTGER4* region was documented in the studies of the NIDDK [39] and the WTCCC [6]. Recently GWAS showed significant evidence for association also with UC [18] (Table S1). Similarly, our data indicated significant association with adult CD (P = 0.031), and early-onset UC (P = 0.002).

In the WTCCC GWA [6], a locus at chromosome 10q21 around rs10761659, a non-coding intergenic SNP mapping 14-kb telomeric to a zinc finger gene known as *ZNF365*, was detected. The locus was replicated both in pediatric CD and UC [16,31], and adult-onset CD [3,40] (Table S1). We were able to confirm this association with CD (P = 0.007), and UC (P = 4×10^{-5}), and after stratifying the cohort with respect to age at diagnosis the association was confirmed in adult CD (P = 0.002), and either adult (P = 0.0002), and in pediatric UC patients (P = 0.005).

In conclusion, our study has confirmed recently described associations, in particular between the *PTGER4*, *HLA*, *TNFSF15*, *NKX2-3*, *ZNF365*, *IFNG*, *PTPN2*, and *PSMG1* genes and IBD in adults and in some cases for the first time also in children. Furthermore, we were able to identify the influence of the investigated genes on clinical expression and localization on CD and UC patients, but the clinical significance of these associations remains to be investigated and replicated. Further characterization, fine mapping, and functional studies of these genetic regions are needed to discover the pathogenetic role of these newly identified genes/loci.

Acknowledgments

The authors wish to thank all the patients and families that participated in this study. The following physicians of the SIGENP* and adult Gastrointestinal Units contributed to the study by providing DNA samples and clinical information of their patients: *Ancona: Catassi, Nobile S; *Bari: Rutigliano V, De Venuto D; *Foggia: Campanozzi A; *Messina: Vieni G, Sferlazzas C; Milano: Bianchi Porro G, Vecchi M, Saibeni S; Napoli: Riegler G, *Napoli: Berni Canani E, Staiano AM; Padova: D'incà R, Sturniolo GC; *Padova: Guariso G, Lodde V; *Palermo: Accomando S; *Parma: de Angelis GL; *Pescara: Lombardi G; *Reggio Calabria: Romano C; *Roma: Cucchiara S, Borrelli O, Bascietto C; S. Giovanni Rotondo: *Firenze: Lionetti P; *Genova: Barabino A; *S. Giovanni Rotondo: D'Altilia M.

Author Contributions

Conceived and designed the experiments: LA PO AV. Performed the experiments: LT CG. Analyzed the data: VMR. Contributed reagents/materials/analysis tools: BF MG BG SD PM MA DIR. Wrote the paper: LA. Supervised manuscript preparation and patient recruitment: AA AV. Supervised writing of the manuscript: AA.

References

1. Xavier RJ, Podolsky DK (2007) Unravelling the pathogenesis of inflammatory bowel disease. Nature 448: 427–434.
2. Sartor RB (2008) Microbial influences in inflammatory bowel diseases. Gastroenterology 134: 577–594.
3. Barrett JC, Hansoul S, Nicolae DL, Cho JH, Duerr RH, et al. (2008) Genome-wide association defines more than 30 distinct susceptibility loci for Crohn's disease. Nat Genet 40: 955–26.
4. Anderson CA, Boucher G, Lees CW, Franke A, D'Amato M, et al. (2011) Meta-analysis identifies 29 additional ulcerative colitis risk loci, increasing the number of confirmed associations to 47. Nat Genet 43: 246–52.
5. Franke A, McGovern DP, Barrett JC, Wang K, Radford-Smith GL, et al. (2010) Genome-wide meta-analysis increases to 71 the number of confirmed Crohn's disease susceptibility loci. Nat Genet 42: 1118–25.
6. Wellcome Trust Case Control Consortium (2007) Genome-wide association study of 14,000 cases of seven common diseases and 3,000 shared controls. Nature 47: 61–87.
7. Franke A, Balschun T, Karlsen TH, Hedderich J, May S, et al. (2008) Replication of signals from recent studies of Crohn's disease identifies previously unknown disease loci for ulcerative colitis. Nat Genet 40: 713–5.
8. Thiébaut R, Kotti S, Jung C, Merlin F, Colombel JF, et al. (2009) TNFSF15 polymorphisms are associated with susceptibility to inflammatory bowel disease in a new European cohort. Am J Gastroenterol 104: 384–91.
9. Silverberg MS, Cho JH, Rioux JD, McGovern DP, Wu J, et al. (2009) Ulcerative colitis-risk loci on chromosomes 1p36 and 12q15 found by genome-wide association study. Nat Genet 41: 216–20.
10. Kugathasan S, Baldassano RN, Bradfield JP, Sleiman PM, Imielinski M, et al. (2008) Loci on 20q13 and 21q22 are associated with pediatric-onset inflammatory bowel disease. Nat Genet 40: 1211–1215.
11. Podolsky DK (2002) Inflammatory bowel disease. N Engl J Med 347: 417–29.
12. Silverberg MS, Satsangi J, Ahmad T, Arnott ID, Bernstein CN, et al. (2005) Toward an integrated clinical, molecular and serological classification of inflammatory bowel disease: Report of a Working Party of the 2005 Montreal World Congress of Gastroenterology. Can J Gastroenterol 19(Suppl A): 5–36.
13. IBD Working Group of the European Society for Paediatric Gastroenterology, Hepatology and Nutrition (2005) Inflammatory bowel disease in children and adolescents: recommendations for diagnosis–the Porto criteria. J Pediatr Gastroenterol Nutr 41: 1–7.
14. Munkholm P, Langholz E, Davidsen M, Binder V (1994) Frequency of glucocorticoid resistance and dependency in Crohn's disease. Gut 35: 360–2.
15. Faubion WA, Jr., Loftus EV, Jr., Harmsen WS, Zinsmeister AR, Sandborn WJ (2001) The natural history of corticosteroid therapy for inflammatory bowel disease: a population-based study. Gastroenterology 121: 255–60.
16. Imielinski M, Baldassano RN, Griffiths A, Russell RK, Annese V, et al. (2009) Common variants at five new loci associated with early-onset inflammatory bowel disease. Nat Genet 41: 1335–1340.
17. The UK IBD Genetics Consortium, the Wellcome Trust Case Control Consortium 2 (2009) Genome-wide association study of ulcerative colitis identifies three new susceptibility loci, including the HNF4A region. Nat Genet 12: 1330–1334.
18. McGovern DP, Gardet A, Törkvist L, Goyette P, Essers J, et al. (2010) Genome-wide association identifies multiple ulcerative colitis susceptibility loci. Nat Genet 42: 332–7.
19. Amre DK, Mack DR, Morgan K, Fujiwara M, Israel D, et al. (2009) Investigation of Reported Associations Between the 20q13 and 21q22 Loci and Pediatric-Onset Crohn's Disease in Canadian Children. Am J Gastroenterol 104: 2824–8.
20. Yamazaki K, McGovern D, Ragoussis J, Paolucci M, Butler H, et al. (2005) Single nucleotide polymorphisms in TNFSF15 confer susceptibility to Crohn's disease. Hum Mol Genet 14: 3499–3506.
21. Tremelling M, Berzuini C, Massey D, Bredin F, Price C, et al. (2008) Contribution of TNFSF15 gene variants to Crohn's disease susceptibility confirmed in UK population. Inflamm Bowel Dis 14: 733–7.
22. Picornell Y, Mei L, Taylor K, Yang H, Targan SR, et al. (2007) TNFSF15 is an ethnic-specific IBD gene. Inflamm Bowel Dis 13: 1333–1338.
23. Yang SK, Lim J, Chang HS, Lee I, Li Y, et al. (2008) Association of TNFSF15 with Crohn's disease in Koreans. Am J Gastroenterol 103: 1437–42.
24. Migone TS, Zhang J, Luo X, Zhuang L, Chen C, et al. (2002) TL1A is a TNF-like ligand for DR3 and TR6/DcR3 and functions as a T cell costimulator. Immunity 16: 479–92.
25. Prehn JL, Mehdizadeh S, Landers CJ, Luo X, Cha SC, et al. (2004) Potential role for TL1A, the new TNF-family member and potent costimulator of IFN-gamma, in mucosal inflammation. Clin Immunol 112: 66–77.
26. Parkes M, Barrett JC, Prescott NJ, Tremelling M, Anderson CA, et al. (2007) Sequence variants in the autophagy gene IRGM and multiple other replicating loci contribute to Crohn's disease susceptibility. Nat Genet 39: 830–2.
27. Fisher SA, Tremelling M, Anderson CA, Gwilliam R, Bumpstead S, et al. (2008) Genetic determinants of ulcerative colitis include the ECM1 locus and five loci implicated in Crohn's disease. Nat Genet 40: 710–2.
28. Pabst O, Förster R, Lipp M, Engel H, Arnold HH (2000) NKX2.3 is required for MAdCAM-1 expression and homing of lymphocytes in spleen and mucosa-associated lymphoid tissue. EMBO J 2: 2015–23.
29. Todd JA, Walker NM, Cooper JD, Smyth DJ, Downes K, et al. (2007) Robust associations of four new chromosome regions from genome-wide analyses of type 1 diabetes. Nat Genet 7: 857–64.
30. Weersma RK, Stokkers PC, Cleynen I, Wolfkamp SC, Henckaerts L, et al. (2009) Confirmation of multiple Crohn's disease susceptibility loci in a large Dutch-Belgian cohort. Am J Gastroenterol 104: 630–8.
31. Amre DK, Mack DR, Morgan K, Israel D, Deslandres C, et al. (2010) Susceptibility loci reported in genome-wide association studies are associated with Crohn's disease in Canadian children. Aliment Pharmacol Ther 31: 1186–91.
32. Satsangi J, Welsh KI, Bunce M, Julier C, Farrant JM, et al. (1996) Contribution of genes of the major histocompatibility complex to susceptibility and disease phenotype in inflammatory bowel disease. Lancet 4: 1212–7.
33. Rioux JD, Silverberg MS, Daly MJ, Steinhart AH, McLeod RS, et al. (2000) Genomewide search in Canadian families with inflammatory bowel disease reveals two novel susceptibility loci. Am J Hum Genet 66: 1863–70.
34. International MHC and Autoimmunity Genetics Network, Rioux JD, Goyette P, Vyse TJ, Hammarström L, et al. (2009) Mapping of multiple susceptibility variants within the MHC region for 7 immune-mediated diseases. Proc Natl Acad Sci U S A 106: 18680–5.
35. Fisher SA, Tremelling M, Anderson CA, Gwilliam R, Bumpstead S, et al. (2008) Genetic determinants of ulcerative colitis include the ECM1 locus and five loci implicated in Crohn's disease. Nat Genet 40: 710–2.
36. Franke A, Balschun T, Karlsen TH, Sventoraityte J, Nikolaus S, et al. (2008) Sequence variants in IL10, ARPC2 and multiple other loci contribute to ulcerative colitis susceptibility. Nat Genet 40: 1319–23.
37. Asano K, Matsushita T, Umeno J, Hosono N, Takahashi A, et al. (2009) A genome-wide association study identifies three new susceptibility loci for ulcerative colitis in the Japanese population. Nat Genet 41: 1325–9.
38. Libioulle C, Louis E, Hansoul S, Sandor C, Farnir F, et al. (2007) Novel Crohn disease locus identified by genome-wide association maps to a gene desert on 5p13.1 and modulates expression of PTGER4. PLoS Genet 3: e58.
39. Rioux JD, Xavier RJ, Taylor KD, Silverberg MS, Goyette P, et al. (2007) Genome-wide association study identifies new susceptibility loci for Crohn disease and implicates autophagy in disease pathogenesis. Nat Genet 39: 596–604.
40. Essers JB, Lee JJ, Kugathasan S, Stevens CR, Grand RJ, et al. (2009) Established genetic risk factors do not distinguish early and later onset Crohn's disease. Inflamm Bowel Dis 15: 1508–14.

17

Characterization of Human CD39⁺ Th17 Cells with Suppressor Activity and Modulation in Inflammatory Bowel Disease

Maria Serena Longhi[1,2]*, Alan Moss[1], Aiping Bai[1], Yan Wu[1], Huang Huang[1], Adam Cheifetz[1], Francisco J. Quintana[3], Simon C. Robson[1]*

1 Division of Gastroenterology, Department of Medicine, Beth Israel Deaconess Medical Center, Harvard University, Boston, United States of America, **2** Institute of Liver Studies, King's College London School of Medicine at King's College Hospital, London, United Kingdom, **3** Center for Neurologic Diseases, Brigham and Women's Hospital, Harvard Medical School, Boston, United States of America

Abstract

Induced regulatory T-cells (iT-reg) and T helper type 17 (Th17) in the mouse share common CD4 progenitor cells and exhibit overlapping phenotypic and functional features. Here, we show that human Th17 cells endowed with suppressor activity (supTh17) can be derived following exposure of iT-reg populations to Th17 polarizing conditions. In contrast to "pathogenic" Th17, supTh17 display immune suppressive function and express high levels of CD39, an ectonucleotidase that catalyzes the conversion of pro-inflammatory extracellular nucleotides ultimately generating nucleosides. Accordingly, supTh17 exhibit nucleoside triphosphate diphosphohydrolase activity, as demonstrated by the efficient generation of extracellular AMP, adenosine and other purine derivatives. In addition supTh17 cells are resistant to the effects of adenosine as result of the low expression of the A2A receptor and accelerated adenosine catalysis by adenosine deaminase (ADA). These supTh17 can be detected in the blood and in the lamina propria of healthy subjects. However, these supTh17 cells are diminished in patients with Crohn's disease. In summary, we describe a human Th17 subpopulation with suppressor activity, which expresses high levels of CD39 and consequently produces extracellular adenosine. As these uniquely suppressive CD39⁺ Th17 cells are decreased in patients with inflammatory bowel disease, our findings might have implications for the development of novel anti-inflammatory therapeutic approaches in these and potentially other immune disorders.

Editor: Simon Patrick Hogan, Cincinnati Children's Hospital Medical Center, University of Cincinnati College of Medicine, United States of America

Funding: Dr Maria Serena Longhi is supported by a Clinician Scientist Fellowship from the Medical Research Council and by a Sheila Sherlock Travel Fellowship from the Royal College of Physicians (London, UK). The study was supported by funds from the National Institute of Health to Prof Simon C Robson - R01HL094400, P01HL107152, P01HL087203 and P01AI045897. The funders had no role in study design, data collection and analysis, decision to publish, or preparation of the manuscript.

Competing Interests: The authors have declared that no competing interests exist.

* E-mail: srobson@bidmc.harvard.edu (SR); maria.longhi@kcl.ac.uk (ML)

Introduction

CD4⁺CD25^high^FOXP3⁺ regulatory T-cells (T-reg) are central to the maintenance of immune homeostasis [1–4]. T-reg prevent or even reverse experimental autoimmunity, and T-reg cellular defects have been observed in association with various autoimmune disorders, such as those associated with vascular thrombophilia as in inflammatory bowel disease [1–3]. T-reg exert suppressive function by releasing inhibitory cytokines, such as IL-10 [5,6], TGF-β [7,8] and IL-35 [9]; by cytolysis, mainly mediated by granzyme B [10]; by modulating the maturation and the antigen presenting ability of dendritic cells [11]; or by metabolic disruption either by depriving of IL-2 effector cells [12] or by hydrolyzing pro-inflammatory ATP into immunomodulatory adenosine, secondary to the specific co-expression of CD39 and CD73 ectonucleotidases by such cells [13,14].

In contrast, T helper type 17 lymphocytes (Th17) are an effector subset that develops independently of Th1 and Th2 cell lineages. Th17 cells drive inflammatory and autoimmune conditions in both mice and humans and have been linked to intestinal inflammation [15,16]. CD4⁺ T-cells can be differentiated into Th17 cells when

exposed to TGF-β in combination with IL-6 or IL-21 in mice and to IL-6, TGF-β and IL-1β in humans, or into induced (i)T-reg under the influence of TGF-β [15,16]. Additional studies have shown that, in addition to TGF-β, other factors including IL-2 [17,18] and anti-CD3/anti-CD28 [19] play a role in iT-reg generation, even after a short stimulation period [19]. iT-reg and Th17 cells, however, may not be terminally differentiated and iT-reg in particular show phenotypic and functional plasticity [20].

Using genetic lineage tracing of Foxp3 T-reg, Zhou and colleagues observed that a significant proportion of Foxp3⁺ cells undergo down-regulation and in some cases loss of Foxp3 expression is noted [21]. These 'ex-Foxp3' cells display an effector memory cell phenotype, produce pro-inflammatory cytokines and are numerically increased in experimental autoimmune diabetes [21]. Moreover, exposure of T-reg to IL-6 can down-regulate both Foxp3 and IL-17 expression, suggesting that T-reg may be 'subverted' to Th17-like cells [22]. In addition, it has been reported that T-reg can further acquire effector properties - i.e. IFNγ production - when cultured in the presence of IL-12 [23]. These 'Th1-like' T-reg show diminished suppressive activity that can be only partially reversed by blockade of IFNγ or IL-12 removal [23].

The stimulation of naïve T-cells with TGF-β and IL-6 triggers IL-17 production but it also induces the expression of IL-10, limiting the pathogenic potential of these cells [24]. Indeed, additional studies have reported that IL-17[+] T-cells can limit tissue damage during inflammation [25,26]. In experimental murine tumor settings, it has been demonstrated that CD39 and CD73 expressed by 'suppressor' Th17 cells (supTh17) suppress tumor-specific immunity [27]. Whether comparable human supTh17 cells exist has been unexplored to date.

CD39 hydrolyses ATP and ADP into AMP, which is then converted into adenosine by CD73. The regulatory properties of CD39 were initially noted in studies conducted on CD39[null] mice in which an enhanced production of IFNγ, IL-1β, IL-6 and TNF-α was found [28,29]. CD39 and CD73 expression on murine T-reg is required for the suppressive function of these cells, which results from the production of adenosine [4]. Accordingly, T-reg isolated from CD39[null] mice are unable to block allograft rejection in adoptive transfer studies [13].

Expression of CD39 has been reported on human T-reg in parallel to FOXP3 and low levels of CD127 [30,31]. Human T-reg do not co-express high levels of CD73 with CD39 in contrast to murine counterparts. Thus AMP conversion to adenosine by human CD39[+] T-reg is thought to result from paracrine mechanisms by the presence of CD73 on target or neighboring cells [31]. Regardless of the molecular mechanism involved, it has been shown that human CD39[+] T-reg exert preferential suppression on CD4 target cell IL-17 production [32].

Defective numbers of CD39[+] T-reg have been reported in patients with multiple sclerosis, autoimmune hepatitis [33] and CD39 polymorphisms linked to low-level CD39 expression have also been described in Crohn's disease [30,32,34]. Recent studies have shown that in addition to T-reg, CD39 is also expressed on a subset of memory cells with effector function [35]. Although this expression of CD39 by human T-reg has been reported and putative roles dissected, the demonstration and relevance of specific CD39 expression by human Th17 cells has been unexplored to date.

We describe here a population of human supTh17 cells that in contrast to prototypic pathogenic Th17 display high levels of both CD39 and FOXP3 and exhibit immune suppressive properties. Our new observations also provide mechanistic insights into the development of supTh17 and indicate the role of CD39 and purinergic immunomodulation. The pathophysiological relevance of these cells is supported by the detection of decreased frequencies of CD39[+] supTh17 cells in both peripheral blood and lamina propria of patients with Crohn's disease, an illness characterized by manifestations of unfettered intestinal inflammation.

Materials and Methods

Subjects

Peripheral blood mononuclear cells (PBMCs) were isolated from platelet-depleted blood (leukofilters) obtained from 68 healthy blood donors (Blood Donor Center at Children's Hospital, Boston, MA). PBMCs were also obtained from 25 patients with Crohn's disease, recruited from the Gastroenterology Division, Beth Israel Deaconess Medical Center (BIDMC), Boston MA. Of these patients, 11 were studied during active disease (median Harvey Bradshaw Index, HBI: 8, range 2 to 25) while 14 were in remission (median HBI: 0, range 0–12). At the time of investigations, 11 patients were receiving infliximab, 2 were on steroids and 2 on immunomodulatory drugs.

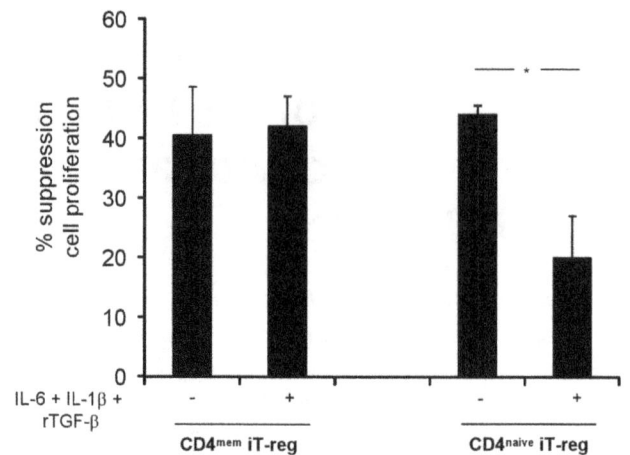

Figure 1. Suppressor ability of iT-reg derived from CD4[+]CD45RO[+] memory (CD4[mem]) and from CD4[+]CD45RA[+] naïve (CD4[naïve]) cells. The ability of iT-reg obtained from CD4[mem] and CD[naïve]-derived Th17 cells was evaluated after 4-day co-culture by ^{3}H-thymidine incorporation in 5 healthy subjects. Mean (+SEM) percentage suppression of CD4 effectors by CD4[mem] or CD4[naïve] iT-reg before and after exposure to IL-6, IL-1β and rTGF-β. CD4[mem] but not CD4[naïve] iT-reg maintain their suppressor ability after exposure to Th17 driving cytokines. *$P \leq 0.05$.

Ethics Statement

The study was approved by BIDMC Institutional Review Committee. Written consent was obtained from all study participants.

Cell Purification

PBMCs were obtained by density gradient centrifugation on Ficoll-Paque (GE Healthcare, Uppsala, Sweden). Cell viability, determined by Trypan Blue exclusion, exceeded 98%. Lamina propria mononuclear cells (LPMCs) were isolated from freshly biopsied colonic tissue. The tissue was initially washed with PBS, cut into small sections and incubated in calcium and magnesium-free HBSS containing 4 mM EDTA and 1 mM dithiothreitol at 37°C for 15 min. Epithelia were removed by discarding the supernatants. This procedure was repeated three times. The tissue was then minced, resuspended in RPMI 1640 containing 10% FCS, 400 U/ml collagenase D and 0.01 mg/ml DNase I, and then incubated at 37°C for 1.5 hour with pipetting every 30 min. The digested tissue was filtered and centrifuged at 600×g for 7 min. Collected cells were pelleted, resuspended in PBS 1% FCS and stained as indicated below.

Cell Sorting and Culture

CD4[mem] and CD4[naïve] cells were sorted as CD4[+]CD45RO[+] and CD4[+]CD45RA[+] from PBMCs using a BD FACSAria (BD Biosciences, San José, CA) (purity higher than 98%). Cells were cultured in complete RPMI 1640 medium (Invitrogen, Carlsbad, CA) supplemented with 2 mM L-glutamine, 100 U/ml penicillin, 100 μg/ml streptomycin, 1% non-essential amino acids and 10% FCS and exposed for 3 days to Th17 polarizing conditions (Figure S1), i.e. IL-6 (50 ng/ml)+IL-1β (10 ng/ml)+TGF-β (3 ng/ml) [36–38] and anti-CD3/anti-CD28 T-cell expander (bead/cell ratio: 1/50) (Dynal Invitrogen). In some experiments cells were exposed to additional Th17 polarizing conditions, namely IL-6+IL-1β+IL-23 (20 ng/ml) or IL-6+IL-1β+IL-23+TGF-β. All cytokines were from R&D Systems (Minneapolis, MN). Cells were then stimulated for

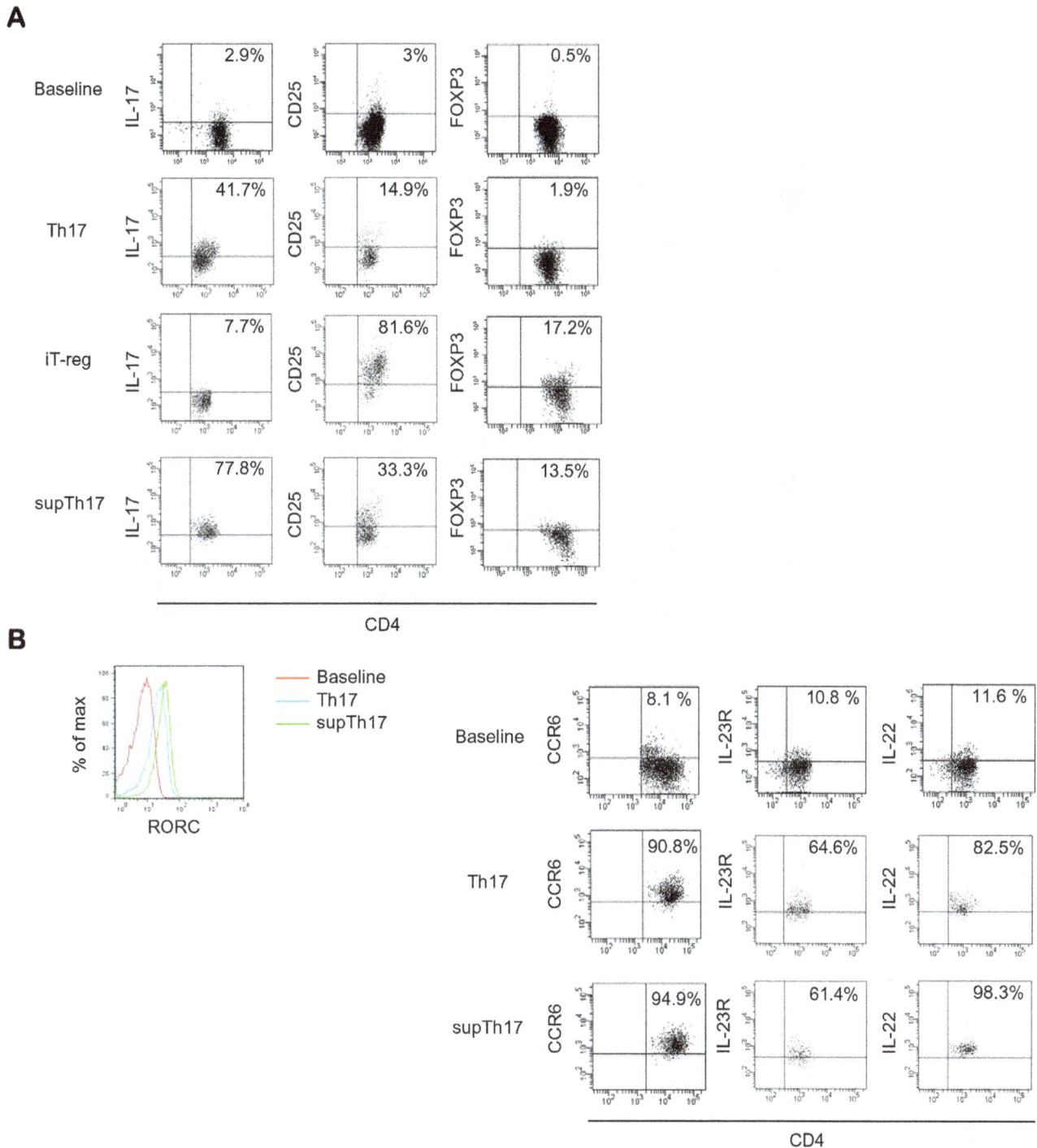

Figure 2. Phenotypic properties of supTh17. Phenotype of CD4^{mem} at baseline and of Th17, obtained from CD4^{mem} after 3-day exposure to IL-6+IL-1β+rTGF-β; iT-reg, obtained following exposure of Th17 to high concentration IL-2 and T-cell expander; and supTh17, obtained upon iT-reg exposure to IL-6+IL-1β+rTGF-β. Cell phenotype was determined in 12 healthy subjects. (A) Representative flow cytometry plots of CD4 (X axis) and IL-17, CD25 and FOXP3 (Y axis) fluorescence. (B) Representative histogram depicting RORC fluorescence in CD4^{mem} at baseline, Th17 and supTh17; representative flow cytometry plots of CD4 (X axis) and CCR6, IL-23R and IL-22 (Y axis) fluorescence. Compared to prototypic Th17, supTh17 display higher frequencies of IL-17^{+}, FOXP3^{+} and IL-22^{+} lymphocytes, express similar levels of RORC and contain comparable numbers of CCR6^{+} cells.

4 days in the presence of iT-reg polarizing conditions consisting of high concentration IL-2 (300 U/ml) and T-cell expander (bead/cell ratio: 1/2) [39,40] and then re-exposed to the same Th17 polarizing conditions indicated above for additional 3 days (Figure S1). Cells obtained after exposure to Th17 and iT-reg polarizing conditions are referred to as Th17 and iT-reg; cells obtained after iT-reg exposure to Th17 driving conditions are indicated as supTh17 (Figure S1). Functional properties of Th17, iT-reg and supTh17 are described in the 'Results' section.

A

B

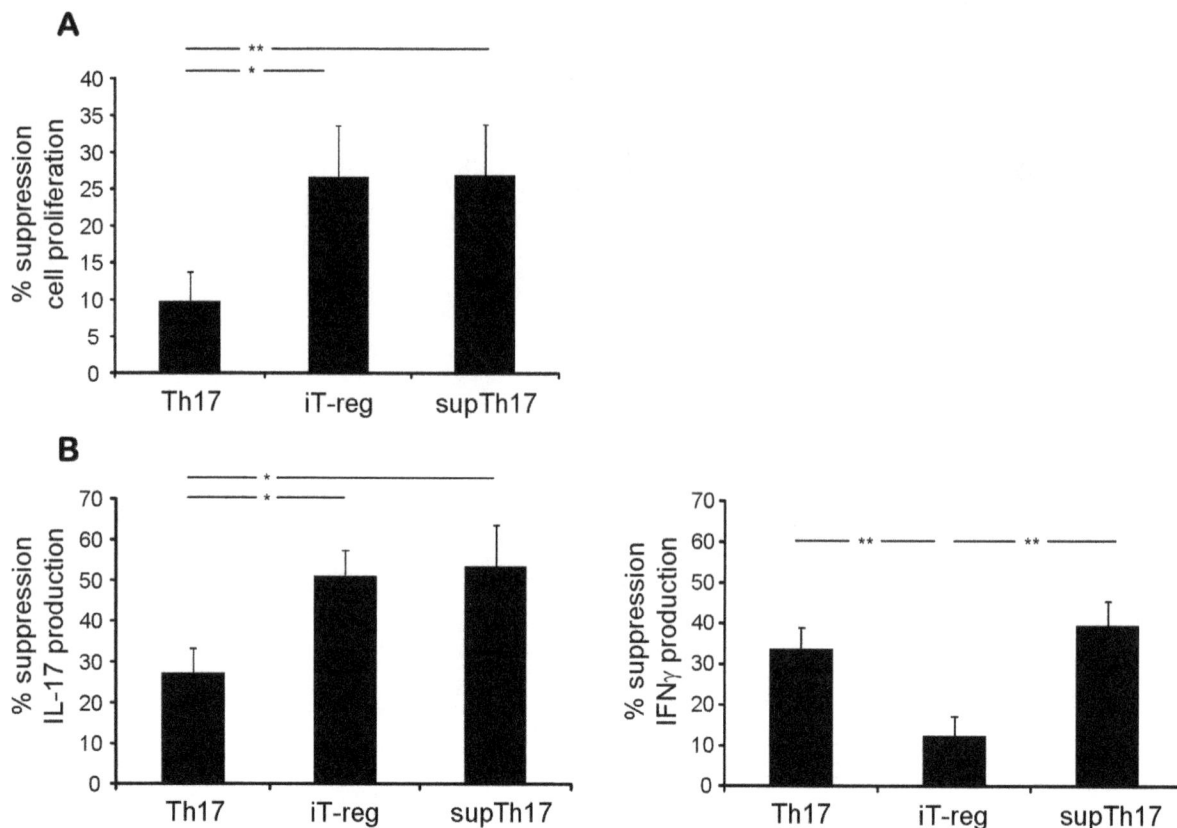

Figure 3. supTh17 suppressive ability. The ability of Th17, iT-reg and supTh17 cells to control CD4 target cell proliferation was evaluated after 4-day co-culture by ^{3}H-thymidine incorporation in 10 healthy subjects. (A) Mean (+SEM) percentage inhibition of CD4 effector cell proliferation by Th17, iT-reg and supTh17 cells. (B) The ability of Th17, iT-reg and supTh17 cells to control CD4 target cell IL-17 and IFNγ production was evaluated after 4-day co-culture by intracellular cytokine staining in 10 healthy subjects. Mean (+SEM) percentage inhibition of CD4 effector cell IL-17 and IFNγ production by Th17, iT-reg and supTh17 cells. Compared to prototypic Th17, supTh17 exerted more effective control over CD4 cell proliferation and pro-inflammatory cytokine production. *$P \le 0.05$; **$P \le 0.01$.

Flow Cytometry

Cell phenotype was assessed by 6-colour flow cytometry following cell incubation with FITC, PE, PE-Cy7, Pacific blue (PB), APC and APC-Cy7-conjugated anti-human antibodies to: CD4 (clone#: OKT4), CD45RO (clone#: UCHL1), CD45RA (clone#: HI100), CD25 (clone#: BC96), CD26 (clone#: BA5b), CD39 (clone#: A1), CD73 (clone#: AD2), CCR6 (clone#: G034E3) (all from Biolegend, San Diego, CA) and IL-23R (R&D Systems, clone#: 218213). Frequency of FOXP3, RORC and Stat-3 positive cells was assessed by intracellular staining following cell fixation and permeabilization with Cytofix/Cytoperm (BD Biosciences) and incubation with PB, APC and PE-conjugated anti-human FOXP3 (Biolegend, clone#: 206D), RORC (eBioscience, San Diego, CA; clone#: AFKJS-9) and Stat-3 (BD Bioscience, clone #: 49/p-Stat-3). Frequency of cytokine-producing cells was determined after exposure to phorbol 12-myristate 13-acetate (PMA, 10 ng/ml, Sigma-Aldrich) and Ionomycin (500 ng/ml) for 60 minutes and to Brefeldin A (20 μg/ml, Sigma-Aldrich) for additional 5 hours. Staining was carried out using PE, PB, and APC-conjugated anti-human antibodies to IFNγ (Biolegend, clone#: 45.B3), IL-17A (Biolegend, clone#: BL168), IL-10 (BD Biosciences, clone#: JES3-19F1), IL-2 (BD Bioscience, clone#: MQ1-17H12) and IL-22 (eBioscience, clone#: IL22JOP). Isotype controls were from BD Biosciences. Cells were acquired on a BD LSRII (BD Biosciences) and analyzed using BD FACSDiva software. 3–5×10^4 events were acquired for

each sample. Positively stained cell populations were gated based on unstained, single stained and isotype stained controls. Effect of adenosine (Sigma-Aldrich, St. Louis, MO) on Th17, iT-reg and supTh17 phenotype was assessed in parallel experiments. Adenosine was added at 50 μM to memory CD4 cells at baseline; after 3 days when exposing cells to iT-reg polarizing conditions; and after additional 4 days when re-stimulating cells in the presence of Th17 skewing conditions. Controls consisted of cultures in the absence of adenosine.

In vitro Suppression Assay

The ability of Th17, iT-reg and supTh17 to control target cell proliferation and effector cytokine production was evaluated following 4-day co-culture with CD4 responder cells. Following 24 hour resting in cytokine and bead-free medium, Th17, iT-reg and supTh17 were added at 1/8 ratio to autologous CD4 target cells (2.5×10^4 cells/well) previously exposed to IL-2 (30 U/ml) and T-cell expander (bead/cell ratio: 1:2) for 5 to 7 days. The 1:8 ratio was selected because capable of exerting a detectable regulatory function in preliminary experiments where ratios of 1:16, 1:8, 1:4 and 1:2 were compared as these putatively reflect pathophysiological proportions between suppressor and effector lymphocytes. Parallel cultures of CD4 responder cells and of Th17, iT-reg and supTh17 on their own were performed under identical conditions. All experiments were performed in duplicates. After 4 days, cultures were pulsed with 0.25 μCi/well ^{3}H-

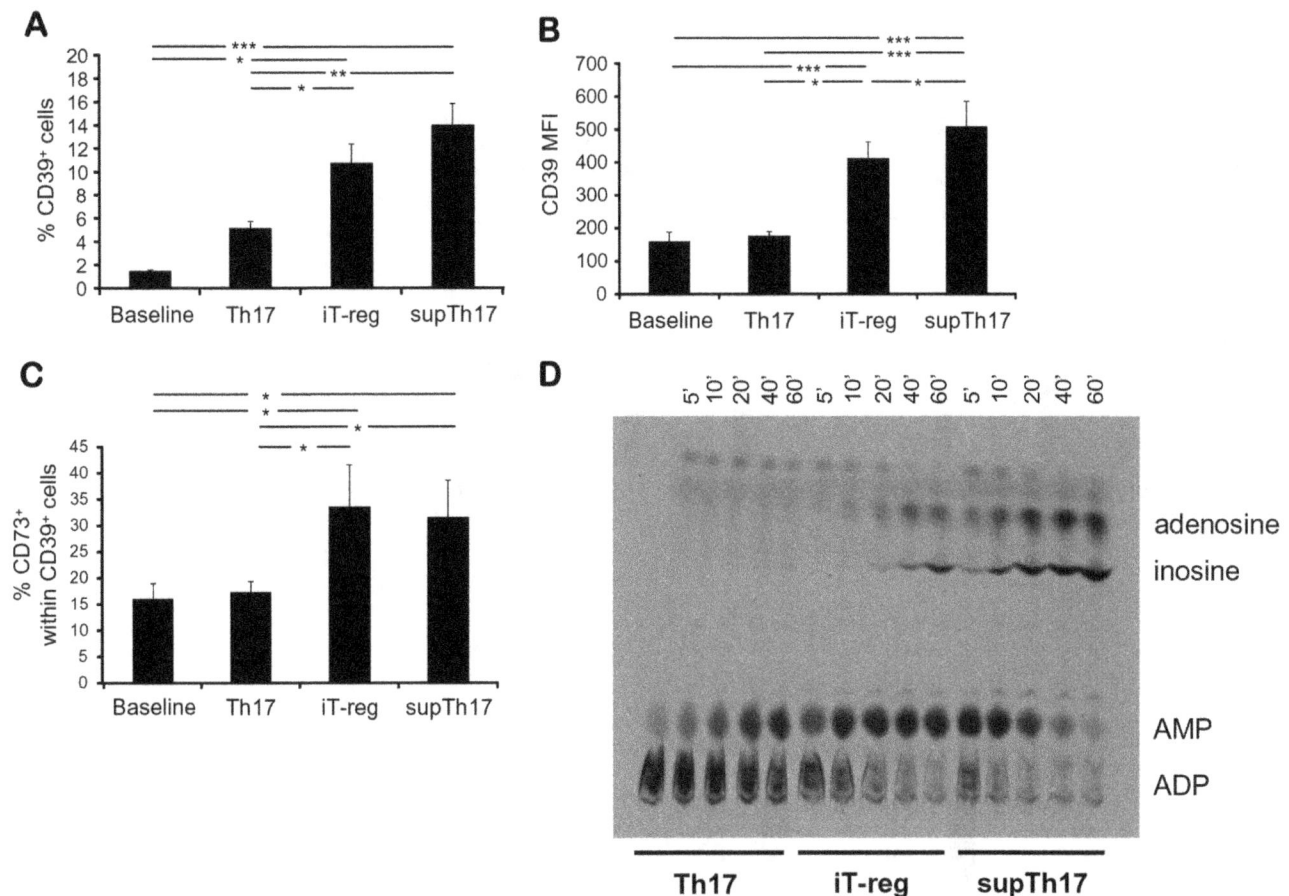

Figure 4. Expression of CD39 and CD73 ectonucleotidases and associated ectoenzymatic activity. (A) Mean (+SEM) frequency of (A) CD39+ cells, (B) CD39 mean fluorescence intensity (MFI) and of (C) CD39+CD73+ cells within CD4mem at baseline and within Th17, iT-reg and supTh17. Results from 12 healthy subjects are shown. *$P \leq 0.05$; **$P \leq 0.01$; ***$P \leq 0.001$. (D) CD39 ADPase enzymatic activity was assessed by TLC following incubation of Th17, iT-reg and supTh17 with [14C] radiolabeled ADP substrates. A representative of 3 independent experiments is shown. In accordance with high levels of CD39 and CD73, supTh17 generate AMP, adenosine and its derivative inosine.

thymidine and harvested 18 hours later using a cell harvester (Tomtec, Hamden, CT). Incorporated thymidine was measured by liquid scintillation spectroscopy. In preliminary experiments, inhibition of CD4 target cell proliferation in the absence and presence of suppressor cells was also analyzed using carboxy fluorescein succinimidyl ester (CFSE) staining. As CFSE- and ³H-thymidine-based assays gave comparable results, given the requirement for fewer cells, ³H-thymidine was used to measure proliferation in subsequent experiments. The ability of Th17, iT-reg and supTh17 cells to control the production of IFNγ and IL-17 by target cells was determined by intracellular cytokine staining after 4-day co-culture as detailed above. The effect of adenosine on Th17, iT-reg and supTh17 ability to suppress was tested in parallel experiments.

Quantitative Real-time PCR

Expression of A1, A2A, A2B and A3 adenosine receptors, and of phosphodiesterases (PDE) 4A and PDE4B was determined by real-time PCR. Total RNA was extracted from $2–3 \times 10^5$ cells using TRIzol reagent (Invitrogen) and mRNA was reverse transcribed using iScript cDNA Synthesis kit (Bio-Rad Laboratories, Hercules, CA) according to the manufacturer's instructions. Sequences of adenosine receptors were as previously described [41]. PDE primer sequences were as follows:

PDE4A: Forward 5′ ACACAGCAGTGACGCTAATCCAGA 3′

Reverse 5′ ATTCACTGGAGGAGGTGGCTCAAA 3′

PDE4B: Forward 5′ ACAGCCTGATGCTCAGGACATTCT 3′

Reverse 5′ AAACTTCTCCATCAGACCCTGGCA 3′

PCR amplification conditions were as previously reported [41]. Samples were run on a Stratagene MX3005P (Agilent Technologies, Santa Clara, CA) and results were analyzed by matched software and expressed as relative quantification. Relative gene expression was determined by normalizing to human β-actin (primer sequence as previously reported [41]).

Immunoblot Analysis

5×10^5 cells were lysed in ice-cold RIPA buffer, containing 1% NP-40, 0.25% sodium deoxycolate, 50 mM Tris-HCl and 150 mM NaCl and supplemented with Complete Proteinase Inhibitor Cocktails (Roche Diagnostics, Indianapolis, IN) and Phosphatase Inhibitor Cocktails (Sigma-Aldrich). Following 30 minutes incubation on ice, samples were spun at $14,000 \times g$ for 30 minutes. Supernatants (containing total cell lysates) were collected and total protein concentration determined using Bio-Rad *Dc* protein assay reagent (Bio-Rad Laboratories) using bovine serum albumin as standard. Following protein denaturation with SDS,

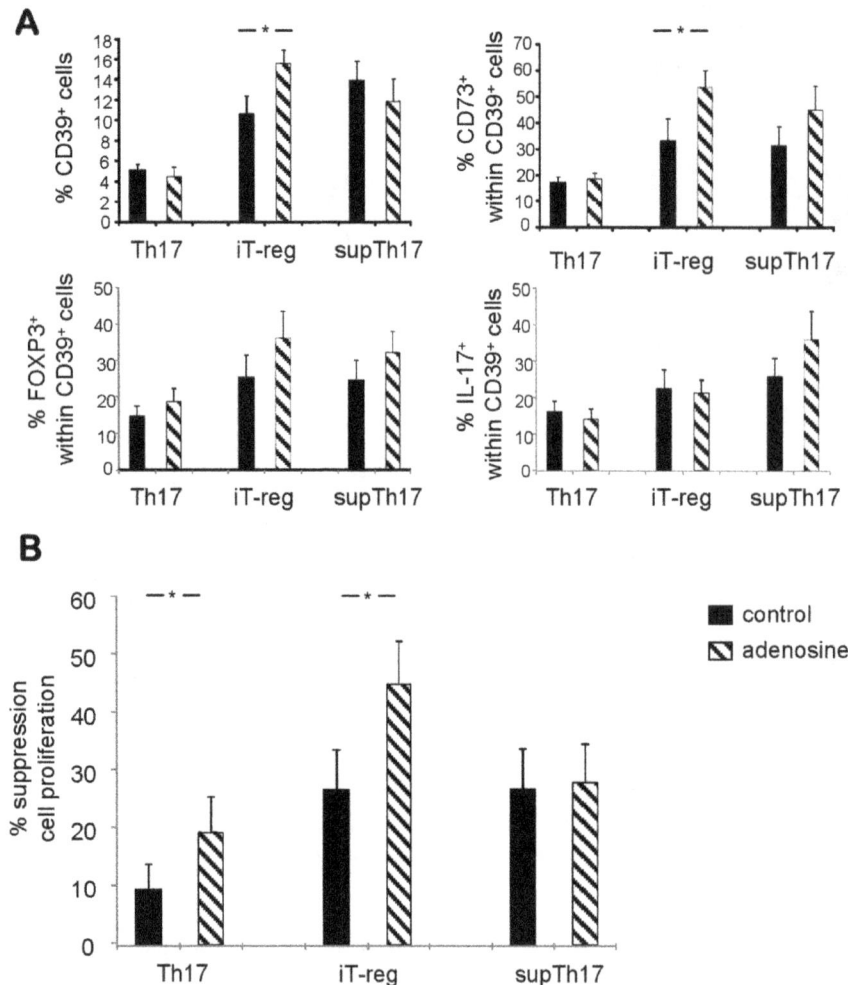

Figure 5. Adenosinergic effects on cell immune phenotype and function. (A) Mean (+SEM) frequency of CD39$^+$ cells and of CD73$^+$, FOXP3$^+$ and IL-17$^+$ lymphocytes within them in CD4^{mem} at baseline, Th17, iT-reg and supTh17. Results from n = 12 healthy subjects. (B) Mean (+SEM) inhibition of CD4 T-cell proliferation by Th17, iT-reg and supTh17 in the absence or presence of adenosine. Adenosine boosts expression of CD39 and CD73 and enhances the suppressor properties of iT-reg, while not having any effect on supTh17. *$P \leq 0.05$.

cell lysates were separated on a 4–12% Criterion XT Bis-Tris SDS-PAGE (Bio-Rad Laboratories). 10 μg of protein were loaded per lane. Gels were run for 20 minutes at 80 V and then at 110 V for additional 80 minutes. Proteins were then transferred onto PVDF membranes (Immobilon-P, Millipore, Billerica, MA) by semi-dry electroblotting and subsequently incubated in blocking buffer containing 2.5% skimmed milk. Following 60 minutes, mouse anti-adenosine deaminase (ADA) antibody (Abcam, Cambridge, MA) was applied at 1 μg/ml. Following overnight incubation membranes were incubated for 60 minutes with HRP-labeled goat anti-mouse (Thermo Scientific, Rockford, IL) at 1/50,000. Bands were visualized using SuperSignal West Femto Maximum Sensitivity Substrate (Thermo Scientific) according to the manufacturer's instructions. For immunoblot normalization, the same membranes were stripped (using a buffer containing 15 g glycine, 1 g SDS and 10 ml Tween20) and re-probed with mouse anti-human β-actin (Abcam) at 1/20,000 and subsequently with a HRP-labeled goat anti-mouse polyclonal antibody at 1/20,000. ADA band density was determined using Scion Image Processing Program (Release Beta 4.0.2).

Ectonucleotidase Enzymatic Activity Analysis

Thin layer chromatography (TLC) was performed as previously described [13,42]. 3×10^5 Th17, iT-reg and supTh17 were incubated with 2 mCi/ml [C^{14}]ADP (GE Healthcare Life Sciences) in 10 mM Ca^{2+} and 5 mM Mg^{2+}. Then, 5 μl aliquots, collected at 5, 10, 20, 40 and 60 minutes, were analyzed for the presence of [C^{14}]ADP hydrolysis products by TLC and applied onto silica gel matrix plates (Sigma-Aldrich). [C^{14}]ADP and the radiolabeled derivatives were separated using an appropriate solvent mixture as previously described [43].

Statistical Analysis

Results are expressed as mean±SEM (obtained from at least 5 subjects per group and from at least 3 independent *in vitro* experiments). Smirnov goodness of fit test was performed to test the normality of variable distribution. Paired and unpaired Student's *t* test were used for comparing normally distributed data; Wilcoxon's rank sum test and Mann Whitney test were used for non-normally distributed data. ANOVA repeated measures or one-way ANOVA, followed by Tukey's multiple comparisons test, was used to compare the means of multiple samples. For all

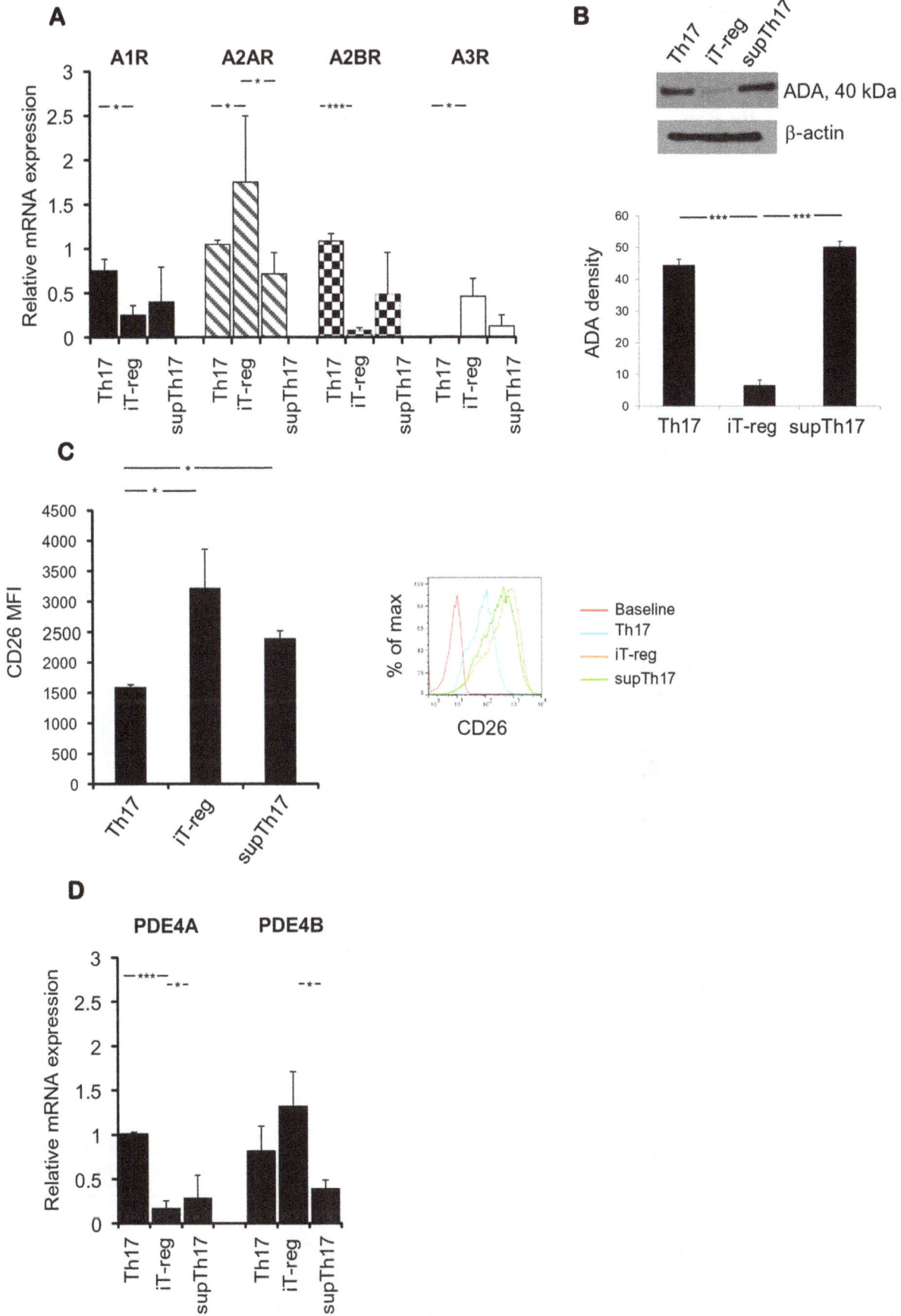

Figure 6. Purinergic molecular signatures of supTh17 cells. (A) Relative mRNA expression of A1, A2A, A2B, A3 receptors by Th17, iT-reg and supTh17 was determined by quantitative real-time PCR in 10 healthy subjects. Results are expressed as mean+SEM. (B) Expression of ADA was determined by immunoblot analysis. One representative of 3 independent experiments is shown. Mean (+SEM) ADA densities noted in Th17, iT-reg and supTh17 cells are also shown. (C) Mean (+SEM) CD26 MFI in Th17, iT-reg and supTh17 cells obtained from 5 healthy subjects was evaluated by flow cytometry. A representative histogram of CD26 fluorescence in CD4^{mem} at baseline, Th17, iT-reg and supTh17 is shown. (D) Mean (+SEM) relative mRNA expression of PDE4A and PDE4B was determined by quantitative real-time PCR in 10 healthy subjects. supTh17 uniquely express low levels of A2A adenosine receptor, exhibit ADA activity associated with CD26 but do not substantially up-regulate levels of PDE. *$P \leq 0.05$; ***$P \leq 0.001$.

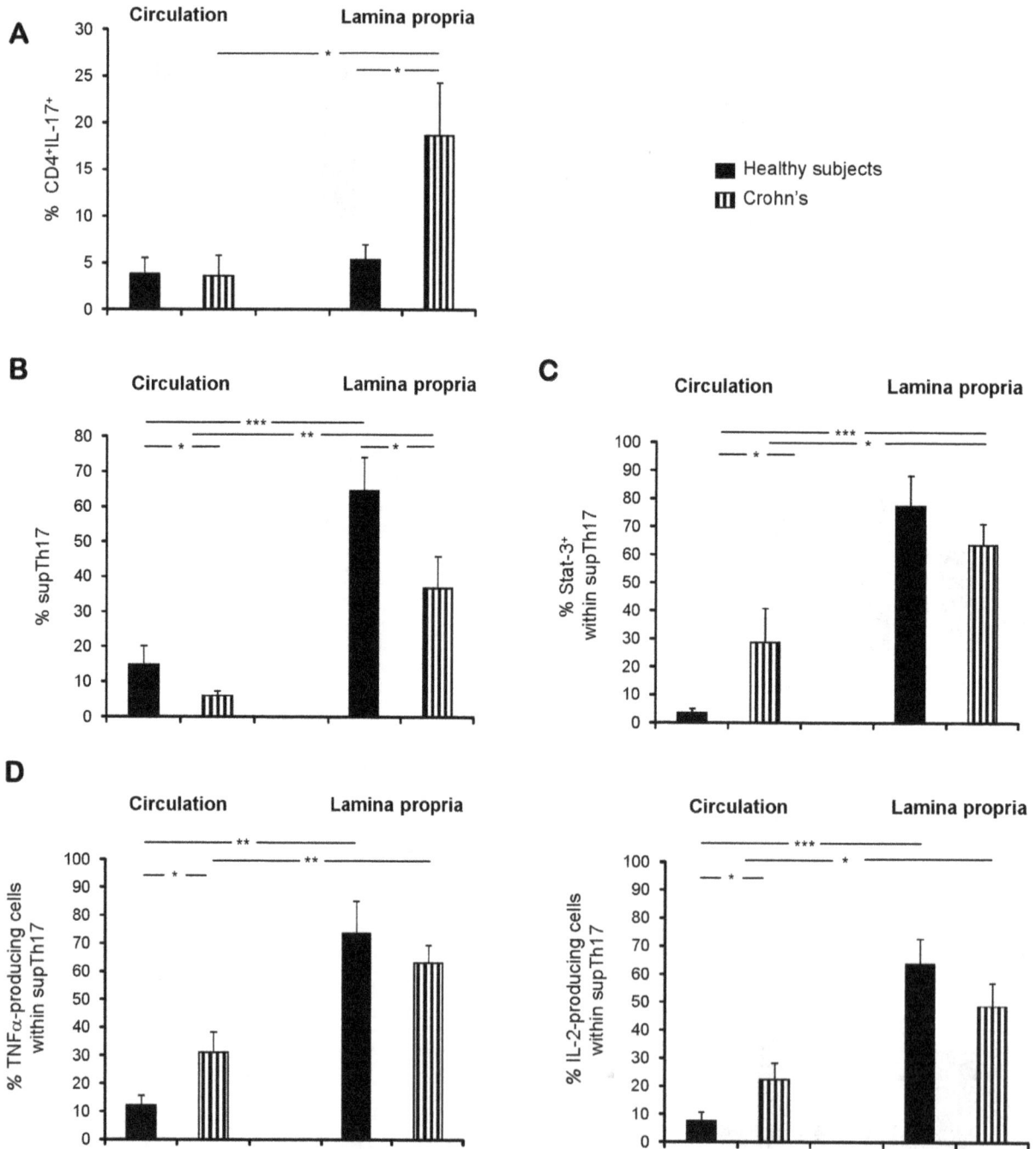

Figure 7. Demonstration of supTh17 cells in healthy subjects and associated decreases in Crohn's disease. The frequency of CD4$^+$IL-17$^+$ and of supTh17 was determined in PBMCs and LPMCs by flow cytometry. supTh17 were identified by initially gating CD4$^+$CD45RO$^+$ cells within PBMCs or LPMCs and then by determining the proportion of CD39$^+$IL-17$^+$ and FOXP3$^+$ within them. Mean (+SEM) frequency of (A) CD4$^+$IL-17$^+$ and of (B) supTh17 cells in the circulation and in the lamina propria. Mean (+SEM) frequency of supTh17 positive for (C) Stat-3 and for (D) TNF-α and IL-2 in the circulation and in the lamina propria. Healthy subjects: n = 17; Crohn's: n = 25; *$P \leq 0.05$; **$P \leq 0.01$; ***$P \leq 0.001$.

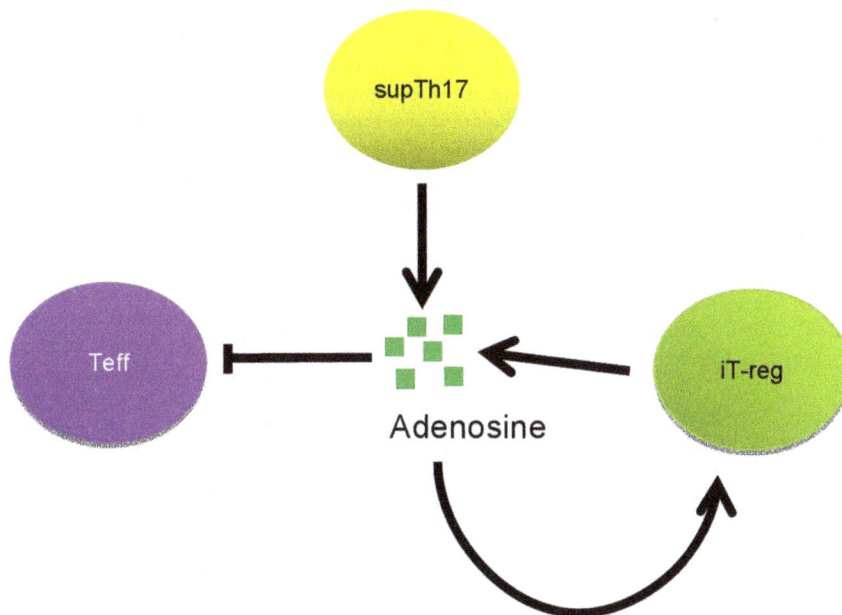

Figure 8. SupTh17, iT-reg and purinergic control of T-cell immune responses. Both supTh17 and iT-reg cells have the capacity to suppress effector T-cells (Teff) by generating adenosine. In a manner distinct from iT-reg which are anergic, however, supTh17 express low levels of A2A receptor and exhibit nucleoside scavenging ecto-enzymatic activity. These properties confer on supTh17 an important intrinsic resistance to suppressive effects of adenosine, which may develop in parallel with prolonged cellular activation in accordance with memory T-cell status. These differences suggest that supTh17 might undergo conversion and be recruited as suppressor-type cells in the later evolution of immune responses where these cells may persist at sites of resolving injury.

comparisons a *P* value ≤0.05 was considered significant. Statistical analysis was performed using SPSS version 19.0.

Results

supTh17 are Phenotypically Different from Prototypic Th17 Cells and Display Regulatory Function

In order to first investigate whether human Th17 cells can acquire regulatory functions per se, we activated CD4+CD45RO+ memory (CD4mem) and CD4+CD45RA+ naïve (CD4naïve) T-cells under Th17 polarizing conditions. Next, we exposed these cells to iT-reg polarizing conditions. Finally, to evaluate the stability of the polarized T-cells, we re-activated them in the presence of Th17 skewing conditions, as detailed in Methods (see also Figure S1). In these studies, Th17 polarizing conditions consisted of 3-day exposure to IL-6, IL-1β and TGF-β, a cytokine cocktail previously shown to result in the efficient differentiation of IL-17 producing cells in humans [36–38,44], and to low dose anti-CD3/anti-CD28. Further, iT-reg polarizing conditions consisted of 4-day stimulation in the presence of high concentration IL-2 and anti-CD3/anti-CD28, shown to be particularly effective at inducing high numbers of effective iT-reg [39,40,44].

We found that iT-reg obtained from CD4mem-derived Th17 cells had persistent and stable suppressor activity following "re-activation" in the setting of Th17 polarizing conditions (Figure 1). In contrast, iT-reg obtained from CD4naïve-derived Th17 cells, had lost most of their suppressive ability once re-activated in the presence of Th17 polarizing conditions (Figure 1). Therefore, we focused consequent studies on iT-reg derived from CD4mem.

Figures 2 and S2 illustrate the phenotype of CD4mem cells at baseline; after 3-day exposure to Th17 polarizing conditions; after further 4-day stimulation in the presence of iT-reg polarizing conditions; and then after 3-day re-exposure to Th17 driving

cytokines. CD4mem cells at baseline contained low frequencies of IL-17-producing, CD25+ and FOXP3+ lymphocytes (Figures 2A and S2A–C). Following 3-day exposure to IL-6, IL-1β and TGF-β, CD4mem cells displayed higher numbers of IL-17-producing cells, while maintaining low frequencies of CD25+ and FOXP3+ lymphocytes (Figures 2A and S2A–C).

Cells obtained following Th17 exposure to iT-reg polarizing conditions displayed a decrease in the number of IL-17+ lymphocytes and an increase in the frequency of CD25+ and FOXP3+ cells (Figures 2A and S2A–C). These cells contained minimal proportions of effector cytokines like IFNγ or IL-2 (Figure S3). After iT-reg exposure to Th17 polarizing conditions, we noted marked increases in the number of cells producing IL-17, decreases in lymphocytes positive for CD25 and frequencies of FOXP3+ lymphocytes that were similar to iT-reg although higher than Th17 cells (Figures 2A and S2A–C). When contrasted to prototypic Th17, these supTh17 cells displayed higher expression of RORC, higher numbers of IL-22+ lymphocytes and similar proportions of cells positive for CCR6 and IL-23 receptor (IL-23R) (Figure 2B).

When next considering suppressive functions (Figures 3A and S4A), we observed that supTh17 controlled CD4 target cell proliferation in a comparable manner to iT-reg, and more effectively than did prototypic Th17 cells. With regard to suppression of pro-inflammatory cytokine production (Figures 3B and S4B–C), supTh17 effectively controlled IL-17 and IFNγ cytokine production by CD4 effector cells. In contrast, iT-reg, while effectively inhibiting production of IL-17, exerted only weak control over CD4 T-cell IFNγ production.

In summary, supTh17 can be obtained following exposure of CD4mem-derived iT-reg to Th17 polarizing conditions. In contrast to prototypic Th17, these cells contain higher frequencies of IL-17 producing and FOXP3$^+$ lymphocytes and furthermore display effective and stable suppressive function.

The supTh17 Cells Express both CD39 and CD73 thereby Generating Adenosine and other Nucleoside Derivatives

Given the regulatory properties displayed by supTh17 and the association between CD39 and immunoregulation [13,32], we determined the expression of CD39 in supTh17 and compared it with that of CD4^{mem} cells at baseline, Th17 and iT-reg. As shown in Figure 4A and 4B, supTh17 contained the highest frequencies of CD39$^+$ cells and displayed the highest CD39 MFI, being therefore clearly distinguishable from prototypic Th17 cells that displayed low numbers of CD39$^+$ lymphocytes and low CD39 MFI.

To evaluate whether different Th17 polarizing conditions influence CD39 expression, we obtained Th17 and supTh17 cells upon exposure to IL-6, IL-1β and IL-23 or IL-6, IL-1β, IL-23 and TGF-β. As depicted in Figure S5A, no differences were observed in the frequency of CD39$^+$ cells in the presence of different Th17-inducing cytokine cocktails.

We next evaluated the phenotypic properties of CD39$^+$ cells within supTh17 and compared with those of CD39$^+$ cells within CD4^{mem} at baseline, Th17 and iT-reg (Figures 4C, S5B and S6A–C). supTh17 cells contained proportions of cells positive for CD73 - the ectonucleotidase working in tandem with CD39 to generate adenosine - and for FOXP3 comparable to iT-reg and higher than Th17 cells and CD4^{mem} cells at baseline (Figures 4C, S5B and S6A). No significant differences in the frequencies of IL-10$^+$ and RORC$^+$ cells were noted between supTh17 and the other cell subsets (Figure S6B–C).

Given the concomitant expression of CD39 and CD73 by both supTh17 and iT-reg, we determined the ability of these cells to generate adenosine. Cell ectoenzymatic activity was assessed by thin layer chromatography (TLC) following cell incubation with [C^{14}] radiolabeled ADP. As depicted in Figure 4D, supTh17 and iT-reg were both able to generate adenosine that supTh17 cells further effectively degraded into inosine. In contrast, Th17 cells were capable of hydrolyzing ADP into AMP but did not generate extracellular adenosine, in accordance with low levels of CD39 and CD73 expression. In keeping with concomitant CD39 and CD73 expression, supTh17 are therefore competent in generating adenosine, which is then effectively degraded into inosine.

Effects of Adenosinergic Signaling on Cell Phenotype and Function

We then tested the effect of adenosine exposure on supTh17 and compared with that in iT-reg and Th17 cells. Adenosine increased the frequency of CD39$^+$ and CD73$^+$ cells among iT-reg while not having any effect on the frequency of these cells among Th17 and supTh17 cells (Figures 5A and S7 and data not shown). Exposure to exogenous adenosine did not affect the proportion of FOXP3$^+$ and IL-17$^+$ cells in any of the three cell subsets (Figure 5A). With regard to suppressive function, adenosine enhanced the ability of iT-reg and, though to a lesser extent, Th17 cells to control CD4 target cell proliferation while not having any effect on the suppression exerted by supTh17 (Figure 5B). The above data show that adenosine boosts the phenotypic and functional properties of iT-reg while not having any effect on supTh17.

We then examined possible mechanisms that could further account for resistance of supTh17 to exogenous adenosine. We considered that resistance to adenosine may result from low expression levels of adenosine receptors, from high levels of

adenosine deaminase (ADA), which degrades adenosine into inosine, and/or high expression of phosphodiesterases (PDE) - the enzymes degrading the phosphodiester bond of cAMP. Thus, we determined the expression of A1, A2A, A2B and A3 adenosine receptors by quantitative real-time PCR. The expression of A2A receptor, known to be involved in down-regulation of inflammation and protection from tissue damage [45], was decreased at mRNA levels in supTh17, when compared to Th17 and iT-reg (Figure 6A).

In order to test whether adenosine resistance of supTh17 was the result of enhanced adenosine clearance, we first assessed the expression of ADA. We observed expression of ADA in Th17 and supTh17 (Figure 6B), indicating that both these cell types have the ability to deaminate adenosine. In contrast, ADA was only weakly expressed in iT-reg (Figure 6B). ADA is completely functional at the cell surface (known as ecto-ADA), where it directly interacts with the dipeptidylpeptidase IV (CD26) and regulates adenosine receptors. ADA activity depends on CD26, the expression of which has been recently reported to be increased on human Th17 [46]. We therefore assessed the expression of CD26 and found that the CD26 MFI was higher in iT-reg and supTh17 compared to Th17 (Figure 6C). These data indicate that the effective degradation of adenosine into inosine displayed by supTh17 relies on the co-expression of both ADA and CD26. In contrast Th17 and iT-reg, which express either ADA (Th17) or CD26 (iT-reg), do not display effective deamination activity (Figure 6C).

We next determined the expression of PDE4A and PDE4B. We found that both enzymes are expressed by Th17, iT-reg and supTh17 (Figure 6D). The supTh17, however, did not overexpress any of the PDE, ruling out the possibility that the adenosine resistance noted in these cells result from high levels of cAMP clearance. We therefore conclude that supTh17 resistance to exogenous adenosine is associated with low A2A adenosine receptor expression and enhanced scavenging of nucleosides by ecto-adenosine deaminase.

Demonstration of supTh17 in Healthy Subjects and in Patients with Crohn's Disease

To investigate the biological relevance of supTh17, the frequency of CD4$^+$IL-17$^+$ and that of supTh17 was determined in PBMCs and LPMCs obtained from healthy subjects and Crohn's patients. These supTh17 were identified by initially gating CD4$^+$CD45RO$^+$ cells within PBMCs or LPMCs and then by determining the proportion of CD39$^+$IL-17$^+$ and FOXP3$^+$ within this population.

While the proportion of CD4$^+$IL-17$^+$ in PBMCs cells was similar in the two groups, that of CD4$^+$IL-17$^+$ lymphocytes obtained from the lamina propria was higher in Crohn's patients than in healthy subjects (Figure 7A). In patients, the frequency of CD4$^+$IL-17$^+$ cells was markedly higher in the lamina propria compared to the circulation (Figure 7A). We then determined the frequency of supTh17 in both compartments. These supTh17 were decreased in Crohn's patients, when compared to healthy subjects, both within PBMC and LPMC populations (Figures 7B and S8). In both groups, supTh17 were increased in the lamina propria compared to the circulation (Figures 7B and S8). When analyzed for expression of Stat-3 known to modulate Th17 immunosuppressive activity through up-regulation of CD39 [27] - circulating supTh17 from Crohn's patients displayed higher proportion of cells positive for this marker than did comparably prepared cells from healthy subjects (Figure 7C) [27]. In both groups, supTh17 from the lamina propria contained higher proportions of lymphocytes that were positive for Stat-3 (Figure 7C). Analysis of cytokine profiles show that supTh17 from

Crohn's disease patients had higher frequencies of TNF-α^+ and IL-2$^+$ cells - pro-inflammatory cytokines previously reported to be decreased in populations of Th17 cells with suppressive properties isolated from the small intestine [47], than the respective supTh17 from healthy subjects in the circulation (albeit not in the lamina propria; Figure 7D). In both groups, supTh17 in the lamina propria contained higher proportions of TNF-α^+ and IL-2$^+$ cells than did the counterparts in the circulation (Figure 7D). No differences in the frequencies of supTh17 and of TNF-α^+ and IL-2$^+$ cells within them were noted between patients with either active or inactive disease. The above data indicate that supTh17 are highly represented in the lamina propria and that the frequencies of these cells are lower in the periphery in Crohn's disease, where in contrast these cells also express increased levels of pro-inflammatory cytokines.

Discussion

We have shown that a population of human supTh17 cells can be derived following the exposure of iT-reg to Th17 polarizing conditions *in vitro*. These putative supTh17 display phenotypic features of both effector Th17 (i.e. production of IL-17 and expression of CCR6, IL-22 and IL-23R) and iT-reg (expression of FOXP3) and importantly control effector cell function by inhibiting CD4 cell proliferation as well as production of IFNγ and IL-17. It is not clear whether these cells might be representative of a late stage in Th17 differentiation, in which the effector potential of prototypic Th17 cells is attenuated or rather constitute unique cell subsets in which overlapping regulatory and effector features coexist.

The robust *in vitro* system used in the present study enabled us to observe changes in T-cell phenotype and function upon stimulation in the presence of Th17 and iT-reg polarizing conditions. Previous studies have documented differentiation of CD4 cells into Th17 or iT-reg following short- and medium-term cell culture *in vitro* [17,18,48,49]. These and our studies may be of particular relevance to disease settings, in which antigen-primed CD4 memory cells may be sequentially exposed to different cytokine milieus and undergo modulation accordingly, during either inflammatory or remission phases.

Given the putative importance of CD39 in immunoregulation, particularly concerning purinergic mechanisms governing the suppressive function of iT-reg, we studied whether supTh17 expressed this ectonucleotidase. Our data show that, in contrast to prototypic Th17 cells, supTh17 display high levels of CD39. Furthermore, supTh17 cells also co-express ecto-5'-ectonucleotidase CD73, which is pivotal in the generation of adenosine from AMP. These supTh17, in contrast to prototypic Th17, have the potential to generate adenosine in a manner comparable to iT-reg, which can be noted by standard biochemical tests (Figure 4D). However, in a manner distinct from iT-reg, the extracellular adenosine that is generated by supTh17 undergoes further degradation, given the concomitant expression of adenosine deaminase and CD26 by these cells. In accordance with the low CD73 levels expressed, prototypic Th17 cells were unable to generate adenosine.

When we examined the effect of exogenous adenosine on supTh17 phenotypic and functional properties, we could observe that these cells were resistant to the effect of this mediator. Curiously, these cells did not undergo upregulation of CD39 expression nor did these cells exhibit amelioration of suppressive function, in the manner observed in anergic type iT-reg.

Adenosine resistance in supTh17 cells is likely to be conferred by low levels of A2A adenosine receptor and by higher levels of adenosine catalysis. The A2A adenosine receptor is primarily known to mediate anti-inflammatory effects: lymphocytes from A2A receptor $(-/-)$ mice show higher rates of cell proliferation and produce high IFNγ levels upon stimulation [50]. A2A receptor stimulation has established inhibitory effects on Th1 and Th17 effector cell generation and, in contrast, favors generation of FOXP3$^+$ and LAG-3$^+$ regulatory T-cells [51]. Our data suggest that the most likely mechanisms for supTh17 resistance to adenosine are linked to low A2A receptor levels and enhanced levels of adenosine catalysis, enabled by ADA and CD26 co-expression. We have observed that iT-reg display marked decreases in mRNA levels of the A2B adenosine receptor. This observation might have relevance for the differential effects of A2B versus A2A signaling by these cells. Furthermore, Moriyama and Sitkovsky have demonstrated in studies of A2AR versus A2BR expression in transfected cells that substantive proportions of A2BR are preferentially degraded by the proteasome, a mechanism that might be also operative here in differentiating Th17 cells from iT-reg [52].

The observation that supTh17 are resistant to adenosinergic modulation implies that these cells are not conventional suppressors, nor are these cells anergic. The supTh17 cells might adapt their own intrinsic ability to regulate or inflict damage according to the immunological context in which they operate. Given that in these cells, both regulatory (i.e. adenosine generation, suppressive function) and pro-inflammatory (i.e. low levels of A2A and inosine generation) features co-exist, it is plausible to suggest that supTh17 might reside in a form of 'purinergic limbo' and unresponsiveness until a crucial time where this balance may be perturbed. This temporal 'status' would enable supTh17 cells to influence extrinsic homeostatic properties of target cells via suppression mediated through generation of adenosine while maintaining intrinsic resistance to this immune suppressive molecule. In contrast, iT-reg exert suppression via production of adenosine, while being also wholly susceptible to the nucleoside modulatory effects that might stabilize their immune suppressive phenotype (Figure 8; [4,31]). At variance with iT-reg, supTh17 are not subjected to this autocrine loop, suggesting that these cells, in contrast, may play roles as both regulators of late stage immune responses and in the maintenance of T-cell memory functionality.

Another important finding of this investigation is that supTh17 could be enumerated in both circulation and lamina propria of healthy subjects and patients with Crohn's disease. These cells appear to preferentially home to the intestine, as demonstrated by their high percentages in the lamina propria, suggesting that the intestine may be the compartment where Th17 cells undergo regulation. Our data indicate there are higher percentages of supTh17 cells expressing Stat-3 in the lamina propria indicating that this transcription factor may have a role in the expression of CD39 and induction of supTh17 in the colon [27]. In agreement with these data, in mouse models of colitis, pathogenic Th17 cells are also considered to undergo regulation in the intestine where these cells acquire phenotypic and functional T-reg-like properties [47].

Importantly, supTh17 numbers are markedly decreased in Crohn's patients. This decrease might theoretically result in disease exacerbation and perpetuation because of the decreased ability of effector Th17 to undergo regulation. Previous clinical studies demonstrated impaired immunoregulation and particularly numerically defective and dysfunctional T-reg in these same disease settings [53,54].

Hence, the increased numbers of effector Th17 cells, also shown here may originate from defective control usually operated by active immune suppression - i.e. primarily defective T-reg, or alternatively be the result of decreased Th17 autoregulation. Interestingly, supTh17 from Crohn's patients appear skewed towards a pro-inflammatory phenotype as these cells contain higher frequencies of TNF-α and IL-2 pro-inflammatory cytokines than those noted in healthy controls.

In conclusion, we have shown that human supTh17 can be obtained upon exposure of iT-reg to Th17 driving conditions *in vitro*.

High levels of CD39 expression distinguish these immune suppressive cells from effector pathogenic Th17 cells. We propose that these fundamental alterations in purinergic signaling might control tissue damage while limiting cellular pathogenicity in local and systemic inflammatory illnesses, such as in Crohn's disease. Promoting the local expansion of supTh17 cells and the maintenance of these should boost local immune suppressive activities and augment diminished T-reg functionality, as previously noted in IBD [34,55]. Indeed, these studies and development of modalities to boost CD39 expression have implications for the development of novel therapeutic strategies in Crohn's disease.

Supporting Information

Figure S1   Experimental protocol for T-cell activation. CD4^{mem} and CD4^{naive} T-cells, purified as CD4$^+$CD45RO$^+$ and CD4$^+$CD45RA$^+$ cells, were initially activated under Th17 polarizing conditions. This comprised of IL-6+IL-1β+rTGF-β+ anti-CD3/anti-CD28 T-cell expander (bead/cell ratio: 1:50) for 3 days. Cells were then exposed to iT-reg skewing conditions with high concentration IL-2 and anti-CD3/anti-CD28 T-cell expander (bead/cell ratio: 1:2) for 4 days, and then were re-activated under Th17 polarizing conditions for 3 days.

Figure S2   Frequency of IL-17$^+$, CD25$^+$ and FOXP3$^+$ cells in Th17, iT-reg and supTh17. Frequency of (A) IL-17$^+$, (B) CD25$^+$ and (C) FOXP3$^+$ cells in CD4^{mem} at baseline, Th17, iT-reg and supTh17 cells was determined in 12 healthy subjects; ***$P<0.001$.

Figure S3   iT-reg phenotype. Flow cytometry plots of FOXP3 (*X* axis) and IFNγ or IL-2 (*Y* axis) fluorescence. Frequency of cells is shown in each quadrant. A representative of two independent experiments is shown.

Figure S4   T-cell suppressive ability. (A) Mean (+SEM) CD4 effector cell proliferation, expressed as mean count per minute (cpm) in the absence or presence of Th17, iT-reg and supTh17 cells. Proliferation of Th17, iT-reg and supTh17 on their own is also shown. (B) Mean (+SEM) CD4 effector cell IL-17 and IFNγ production in the absence or presence of Th17, iT-reg and supTh17 cells. Production of IL-17 and IFNγ by Th17, iT-reg and supTh17, in isolation, are also shown. Results are obtained from 10 healthy subjects. *$P≤0.05$; **$P≤0.01$; ***$P<0.001$. (C)

Representative flow cytometry plots of CD4 (*X* axis) and IL-17 or IFNγ (*Y* axis) fluorescence in CD4 effectors alone and in the presence of Th17, iT-reg or supTh17 cells.

Figure S5   Frequency of CD39$^+$ and CD73$^+$ cells within Th17, iT-reg and supTh17. (A) Frequency of CD39$^+$ cells was determined after exposing CD4^{mem} cells to different Th17 polarizing conditions, i.e. 1) IL-6+IL-1β+rTGF-β; 2) IL-6+IL-1β+IL-23; and 3) IL-6+IL-1β+rTGF-β+IL-23. Flow cytometry plots of CD4 (*X* axis) and CD39 (*Y* axis) fluorescence. A representative of 5 independent experiments is shown. (B) Flow cytometry plots of CD4 (*X* axis) and CD73 (*Y* axis) fluorescence. Cells were gated on CD39$^+$ lymphocytes.

Figure S6   Phenotype of Th1, iT-reg and supTh17 cells. Mean (+SEM) frequency of lymphocytes positive for (A) FOXP3, (B) IL-10 and (C) RORC within CD39$^+$ cells in CD4^{mem} at baseline, Th17, iT-reg and supTh17. Results are obtained from 12 healthy subjects. *$P≤0.05$; **$P≤0.01$. Representative flow cytometry plots of CD4 (*X* axis) and (A) FOXP3, (B) IL-10 and (C) RORC (*Y* axis) fluorescence in CD4^{mem} at baseline, Th17, iT-reg and supTh17 are shown. Cells are gated on CD39$^+$ lymphocytes.

Figure S7   Effect of adenosine on CD39 expression. Flow cytometry plots of CD4 (*X* axis) and CD39 (*Y* axis) fluorescence in Th17, iT-reg and supTh17 cells in the absence and presence of adenosine in a representative individual of 12 healthy subjects tested.

Figure S8   Frequency of supTh17 in PBMCs and LPMCs. supTh17 were identified by initially gating CD4$^+$CD45RO$^+$ cells within PBMCs or LPMCs and then by determining the proportion of cells positive for CD39 and IL-17 and expressing FOXP3 within this population. Flow cytometry plots of CD4 (*X* axis) and IL-17 (*Y* axis) fluorescence in PBMCs and LPMCs from one healthy subject and one patient with Crohn's disease. Cells were gated on CD39$^+$ lymphocytes. Histograms of FOXP3 fluorescence in CD4$^+$IL-17$^+$ cells within CD39$^+$ lymphocytes are also shown.

Acknowledgments

The authors are deeply grateful to Professor Terry B Strom for very helpful suggestions on the overall project and for critical review of the manuscript draft.

Author Contributions

Conceived and designed the experiments: AC SCR. Performed the experiments: MSL HH. Analyzed the data: MSL AM AB YW. Wrote the paper: MSL FJQ SCR.

References

1. Shevach EM, DiPaolo RA, Andersson J, Zhao DM, Stephens GL, et al. (2006) The lifestyle of naturally occurring CD4+ CD25+ Foxp3+ regulatory T cells. Immunol Rev 212: 60–73.

2. Sakaguchi S, Yamaguchi T, Nomura T, Ono M (2008) Regulatory T cells and immune tolerance. Cell 133: 775–787.

3. Josefowicz SZ, Lu LF, Rudensky AY (2012) Regulatory T cells: mechanisms of differentiation and function. Annu Rev Immunol 30: 531–564.

4. Deaglio S, Robson SC (2011) Ectonucleotidases as regulators of purinergic signaling in thrombosis, inflammation, and immunity. Adv Pharmacol 61: 301–332.

5. Hawrylowicz CM, O'Garra A (2005) Potential role of interleukin-10-secreting regulatory T cells in allergy and asthma. Nat Rev Immunol 5: 271–283.

6. Asseman C, Mauze S, Leach MW, Coffman RL, Powrie F (1999) An essential role for interleukin 10 in the function of regulatory T cells that inhibit intestinal inflammation. J Exp Med 190: 995–1004.

7. Nakamura K, Kitani A, Strober W (2001) Cell contact-dependent immunosuppression by CD4(+)CD25(+) regulatory T cells is mediated by cell surface-bound transforming growth factor beta. J Exp Med 194: 629–644.

8. Green EA, Gorelik L, McGregor CM, Tran EH, Flavell RA (2003) CD4+ CD25+ T regulatory cells control anti-islet CD8+ T cells through TGF-beta-

TGF-beta receptor interactions in type 1 diabetes. Proc Natl Acad Sci U S A 100: 10878–10883.

9. Collison LW, Workman CJ, Kuo TT, Boyd K, Wang Y, et al. (2007) The inhibitory cytokine IL-35 contributes to regulatory T-cell function. Nature 450: 566–569.

10. Vignali DA, Collison LW, Workman CJ (2008) How regulatory T cells work. Nat Rev Immunol 8: 523–532.

11. Cederbom L, Hall H, Ivars F (2000) CD4+CD25+ regulatory T cells down-regulate co-stimulatory molecules on antigen-presenting cells. Eur J Immunol 30: 1538–1543.

12. Thornton AM, Shevach EM (1998) CD4+CD25+ immunoregulatory T cells suppress polyclonal T cell activation in vitro by inhibiting interleukin 2 production. J Exp Med 188: 287–296.

13. Deaglio S, Dwyer KM, Gao W, Friedman D, Usheva A, et al. (2007) Adenosine generation catalyzed by CD39 and CD73 expressed on regulatory T cells mediates immune suppression. J Exp Med 204: 1257–1265.

14. Gandhi R, Kumar D, Burns EJ, Nadeau M, Dake B, et al. (2010) Activation of the aryl hydrocarbon receptor induces human type 1 regulatory T cell-like and Foxp3(+) regulatory T cells. Nat Immunol 11: 846–853.

15. Miossec P, Korn T, Kuchroo VK (2009) Interleukin-17 and type 17 helper T cells. N Engl J Med 361: 888–898.

16. Korn T, Bettelli E, Oukka M, Kuchroo VK (2009) IL-17 and Th17 Cells. Annu Rev Immunol 27: 485–517.

17. Chen W, Jin W, Hardegen N, Lei KJ, Li L, et al. (2003) Conversion of peripheral CD4+CD25- naive T cells to CD4+CD25+ regulatory T cells by TGF-beta induction of transcription factor Foxp3. J Exp Med 198: 1875–1886.

18. Davidson TS, DiPaolo RJ, Andersson J, Shevach EM (2007) Cutting Edge: IL-2 is essential for TGF-beta-mediated induction of Foxp3+ T regulatory cells. J Immunol 178: 4022–4026.

19. Zhang P, Tey SK, Koyama M, Kuns RD, Olver SD, et al. (2013) Induced Regulatory T Cells Promote Tolerance When Stabilized by Rapamycin and IL-2 In Vivo. J Immunol 191: 5291–5303.

20. Huber S, Gagliani N, Flavell RA (2012) Life, death, and miracles: Th17 cells in the intestine. Eur J Immunol 42: 2238–2245.

21. Zhou X, Bailey-Bucktrout SL, Jeker LT, Penaranda C, Martinez-Llordella M, et al. (2009) Instability of the transcription factor Foxp3 leads to the generation of pathogenic memory T cells in vivo. Nat Immunol 10: 1000–1007.

22. Xu L, Kitani A, Fuss I, Strober W (2007) Cutting edge: regulatory T cells induce CD4+CD25-Foxp3- T cells or are self-induced to become Th17 cells in the absence of exogenous TGF-beta. J Immunol 178: 6725–6729.

23. Dominguez-Villar M, Baecher-Allan CM, Hafler DA (2011) Identification of T helper type 1-like, Foxp3+ regulatory T cells in human autoimmune disease. Nat Med 17: 673–675.

24. McGeachy MJ, Bak-Jensen KS, Chen Y, Tato CM, Blumenschein W, et al. (2007) TGF-beta and IL-6 drive the production of IL-17 and IL-10 by T cells and restrain T(H)-17 cell-mediated pathology. Nat Immunol 8: 1390–1397.

25. O'Connor W, Jr., Zenewicz LA, Flavell RA (2010) The dual nature of T(H)17 cells: shifting the focus to function. Nat Immunol 11: 471–476.

26. Schnyder-Candrian S, Togbe D, Couillin I, Mercier I, Brombacher F, et al. (2006) Interleukin-17 is a negative regulator of established allergic asthma. J Exp Med 203: 2715–2725.

27. Chalmin F, Mignot G, Bruchard M, Chevriaux A, Vegran F, et al. (2012) Stat3 and Gfi-1 transcription factors control Th17 cell immunosuppressive activity via the regulation of ectonucleotidase expression. Immunity 36: 362–373.

28. Enjyoji K, Sevigny J, Lin Y, Frenette PS, Christie PD, et al. (1999) Targeted disruption of cd39/ATP diphosphohydrolase results in disordered hemostasis and thromboregulation. Nat Med 5: 1010–1017.

29. Enjyoji K, Kotani K, Thukral C, Blumel B, Sun X, et al. (2008) Deletion of cd39/entpd1 results in hepatic insulin resistance. Diabetes 57: 2311–2320.

30. Borsellino G, Kleinewietfeld M, Di Mitri D, Sternjak A, Diamantini A, et al. (2007) Expression of ectonucleotidase CD39 by Foxp3+ Treg cells: hydrolysis of extracellular ATP and immune suppression. Blood 110: 1225–1232.

31. Dwyer KM, Hanidziar D, Putheti P, Hill PA, Pommey S, et al. (2010) Expression of CD39 by human peripheral blood CD4+ CD25+ T cells denotes a regulatory memory phenotype. Am J Transplant 10: 2410–2420.

32. Fletcher JM, Lonergan R, Costelloe L, Kinsella K, Moran B, et al. (2009) CD39+Foxp3+ regulatory T Cells suppress pathogenic Th17 cells and are impaired in multiple sclerosis. J Immunol 183: 7602–7610.

33. Grant CR, Liberal R, Holder BS, Cardone J, Ma Y, et al. (2013) Dysfunctional CD39 regulatory T cells and aberrant control of T helper type 17 cells in autoimmune hepatitis. Hepatology.

34. Friedman DJ, Kunzli BM, YI AR, Sevigny J, Berberat PO, et al. (2009) From the Cover: CD39 deletion exacerbates experimental murine colitis and human polymorphisms increase susceptibility to inflammatory bowel disease. Proc Natl Acad Sci U S A 106: 16788–16793.

35. Zhou Q, Yan J, Putheti P, Wu Y, Sun X, et al. (2009) Isolated CD39 expression on CD4+ T cells denotes both regulatory and memory populations. Am J Transplant 9: 2303–2311.

36. Acosta-Rodriguez EV, Napolitani G, Lanzavecchia A, Sallusto F (2007) Interleukins 1beta and 6 but not transforming growth factor-beta are essential for the differentiation of interleukin 17-producing human T helper cells. Nat Immunol 8: 942–949.

37. Manel N, Unutmaz D, Littman DR (2008) The differentiation of human T(H)-17 cells requires transforming growth factor-beta and induction of the nuclear receptor RORgammat. Nat Immunol 9: 641–649.

38. Longhi MS, Liberal R, Holder B, Robson SC, Ma Y, et al. (2012) Inhibition of interleukin-17 promotes differentiation of CD25(−) cells into stable T regulatory cells in patients with autoimmune hepatitis. Gastroenterology 142: 1526–1535 e1526.

39. Walker MR, Kasprowicz DJ, Gersuk VH, Benard A, Van Landeghen M, et al. (2003) Induction of FoxP3 and acquisition of T regulatory activity by stimulated human CD4+CD25- T cells. J Clin Invest 112: 1437–1443.

40. Hoffmann P, Eder R, Kunz-Schughart LA, Andreesen R, Edinger M (2004) Large-scale in vitro expansion of polyclonal human CD4(+)CD25high regulatory T cells. Blood 104: 895–903.

41. Chen Y, Corriden R, Inoue Y, Yip L, Hashiguchi N, et al. (2006) ATP release guides neutrophil chemotaxis via P2Y2 and A3 receptors. Science 314: 1792–1795.

42. Sun X, Wu Y, Gao W, Enjyoji K, Csizmadia E, et al. (2010) CD39/ENTPD1 expression by CD4+Foxp3+ regulatory T cells promotes hepatic metastatic tumor growth in mice. Gastroenterology 139: 1030–1040.

43. Beldi G, Wu Y, Banz Y, Nowak M, Miller L, et al. (2008) Natural killer T cell dysfunction in CD39-null mice protects against concanavalin A-induced hepatitis. Hepatology 48: 841–852.

44. Longhi MS, Meda F, Wang P, Samyn M, Mieli-Vergani G, et al. (2008) Expansion and de novo generation of potentially therapeutic regulatory T cells in patients with autoimmune hepatitis. Hepatology 47: 581–591.

45. Ohta A, Sitkovsky M (2001) Role of G-protein-coupled adenosine receptors in downregulation of inflammation and protection from tissue damage. Nature 414: 916–920.

46. Bengsch B, Seigel B, Flecken T, Wolanski J, Blum HE, et al. (2012) Human Th17 cells express high levels of enzymatically active dipeptidylpeptidase IV (CD26). J Immunol 188: 5438–5447.

47. Esplugues E, Huber S, Gagliani N, Hauser AE, Town T, et al. (2011) Control of TH17 cells occurs in the small intestine. Nature 475: 514–518.

48. Lee Y, Awasthi A, Yosef N, Quintana FJ, Xiao S, et al. (2012) Induction and molecular signature of pathogenic TH17 cells. Nat Immunol 13: 991–999.

49. Acosta-Rodriguez EV, Rivino L, Geginat J, Jarrossay D, Gattorno M, et al. (2007) Surface phenotype and antigenic specificity of human interleukin 17-producing T helper memory cells. Nat Immunol 8: 639–646.

50. Mills JH, Kim DG, Krenz A, Chen JF, Bynoe MS (2012) A2A adenosine receptor signaling in lymphocytes and the central nervous system regulates inflammation during experimental autoimmune encephalomyelitis. J Immunol 188: 5713–5722.

51. Zarek PE, Huang CT, Lutz ER, Kowalski J, Horton MR, et al. (2008) A2A receptor signaling promotes peripheral tolerance by inducing T-cell anergy and the generation of adaptive regulatory T cells. Blood 111: 251–259.

52. Moriyama K, Sitkovsky MV (2010) Adenosine A2A receptor is involved in cell surface expression of A2B receptor. J Biol Chem 285: 39271–39288.

53. Chamouard P, Monneaux F, Richert Z, Voegeli AC, Lavaux T, et al. (2009) Diminution of Circulating CD4+CD25 high T cells in naive Crohn's disease. Dig Dis Sci 54: 2084–2093.

54. Ishikawa D, Okazawa A, Corridoni D, Jia LG, Wang XM, et al. (2012) Tregs are dysfunctional in vivo in a spontaneous murine model of Crohn's disease. Mucosal Immunol.

18

Serological Investigation of Food Specific Immunoglobulin G Antibodies in Patients with Inflammatory Bowel Diseases

Chenwen Cai, Jun Shen, Di Zhao, Yuqi Qiao, Antao Xu, Shuang Jin, Zhihua Ran, Qing Zheng*

Key Laboratory of Gastroenterology & Hepatology, Ministry of Health, Division of Gastroenterology and Hepatology, Ren Ji Hospital, School of Medicine, Shanghai Jiao Tong University, Shanghai Institute of Digestive Diseases, 145 Middle Shandong Road, Shanghai 200001, China

Abstract

Objective: Dietary factors have been indicated to influence the pathogenesis and nature course of inflammatory bowel diseases (IBD) with their wide variances. The aim of the study was to assess the prevalence and clinical significance of 14 serum food specific immunoglobulin G (sIgG) antibodies in patients with IBD.

Methods: This retrospective study comprised a total of 112 patients with IBD, including 79 with Crohn's disease (CD) and 33 with ulcerative colitis (UC). Medical records, clinical data and laboratory results were collected for analysis. Serum IgG antibodies against 14 unique food allergens were detected by semi-quantitative enzyme linked immunosorbent assay (ELISA).

Results: Food sIgG antibodies were detected in 75.9% (60/79) of CD patients, 63.6% (21/33) of UC patients and 33.1% (88/266) of healthy controls (HC). IBD patients showed the significantly higher antibodies prevalence than healthy controls (CD vs. HC, $P=0.000$; UC vs. HC, $P=0.001$). However no marked difference was observed between CD and UC groups ($P=0.184$). More subjects were found with sensitivity to multiple antigens ($\geq$3) in IBD than in HC group (33.9% vs.0.8%, $P=0.000$). Egg was the most prevalent food allergen. There was a remarkable difference in the levels of general serum IgM ($P=0.045$) and IgG ($P=0.041$) between patients with positive and negative sIgG antibodies. Patients with multiple positive allergens ($\geq$3) were especially found with significant higher total IgG levels compared with sIgG-negative patients ($P=0.003$). Age was suggested as a protective factor against the occurrence of sIgG antibodies ($P=0.002$).

Conclusions: The study demonstrates a high prevalence of serum IgG antibodies to specific food allergens in patients with IBD. sIgG antibodies may potentially indicate disease status in clinical and be utilized to guide diets for patients.

Editor: David L Boone, University of Chicago, United States of America

Funding: The work was supported by grants from the National Key Technology R&D Program of China (No. 2012BAI06B03), http://kjzc.jhgl.org/and National Natural Science Foundations of China (No. 81170362, 81200280 and 81370508), http://isisn.nsfc.gov.cn. The funders had no role in study design, data collection and analysis, decision to publish, or preparation of the manuscript.

Competing Interests: The authors have declared that no competing interests exist.

* Email: qingzheng101@163.com

Introduction

Inflammatory bowel diseases (IBD) include two main types, Crohn's disease (CD) and ulcerative colitis (UC), both characterized by mucosal ulceration in gut. Patients with IBD suffer from abdominal pain, diarrhea, weight loss and fatigue. As diseases progress, they can cause perianal lesion, abdominal abscess, intestinal perforation or even canceration as diverse complications. Extraintestinal manifestations including oral ulcer, arthritis, iritis and cholangitis may also occur simultaneously [1]. The tendentiousness of the constant alternation of relapses and remissions seriously affects the quality of life in IBD patients [2]. For the moment the mechanisms involved in the pathogenesis can be summarized that the influence of environmental factors to genetically susceptible individuals triggers abnormal mucosal immune reaction in gut with the involvement of intestinal flora and eventually leads to the bowel inflammation and ulceration [3].

IBD has long been regarded as a problem threatening public health in the Western world. However in recent decades the rising incidence of it in developing nations has made IBD a global issue. In Asia, according to an epidemiological survey, the rapid westernization and modernization may attribute to the condition [4]. Among various environmental factors, diet has been implicated to play a considerable role in the course of IBD [5–8]. A Japanese study suggested the intake of a high fat diet and sweets may associate with CD and UC [9]. Another research also pointed an increased consumption of alcohol and red meat might cause higher incidence of relapse in UC patients [10]. Meanwhile food intolerance, which is defined as a reproducible adverse reaction to specific food or food ingredients, has become more common in recent years [11–12]. Banai J. considered all kinds of

Table 1. Demographic data of all subjects.

Clinicopathological features	CD (N = 79)	UC (N = 33)	HC (N = 266)
Male (n, %)	47(59.5)	18(54.5)	146(54.9)
Female (n, %)	32(40.5)	15(45.5)	120(45.1)
Age (yr) (mean, 95% CI)	36.5(33.6–39.4)	40.7 (35.9–45.7)	46.4(45.2–47.6)
Age range (yr)	18–68	17–73	24–71
Duration of disease (yr) (n, %)			
<1	21 (26.6)	13 (39.4)	/
1–5	38 (48.1)	11 (33.3)	/
5–10	16 (20.3)	7 (21.2)	/
>10	4 (5.1)	2 (6.1)	/
Disease activity (n, %)			
Remission	7 (8.9)	0 (0)	/
Mild	16 (20.3)	12 (36.4)	/
Moderate	33 (41.8)	14 (42.4)	/
Severe	23 (29.1)	7 (21.2)	/
Localization of disease (n, %)			
L1 (terminal ileum)	40 (50.6)	/	/
L2 (colon)	10 (12.7)	/	/
L3 (ileocolon)	29 (36.7)	/	/
E1 (rectum)	/	1 (3.0)	/
E2 (left-sided colon)	/	14 (42.4)	/
E3 (entire colon)	/	18 (54.5)	/
Complications of disease (n, %)			
None	32 (40.5)	31 (93.9)	/
1 item	42 (53.2)	2 (6.1)	/
2 items	5 (6.3)	/	/
Extraintestinal manifestations (n, %)			
None	60 (75.9)	26 (78.8)	/
1 item	18 (22.8)	7 (21.2))	/
2 items	1 (1.3)	/	/
Intestinal surgery	15 (19.0)	0 (0.0)	/

CD: Crohn's disease; UC: ulcerative colitis; HC: healthy controls; yr: year; 95% CI: 95% confidence interval; L1,L2,L3: disease localization of Crohn's disease by Montreal Classification; E1,E2,E3: disease localization of ulcerative colitis by Montreal Classification.

food could be antigenic properties to cause chronic mild inflammation in gut and eventually lead to ulcerative colitis [13]. For example, intolerance to milk has long been believed involving in the pathogenesis of IBD [14,15]. Glassman *et al* reported during infancy stage the frequency of symptoms compatible with milk protein sensitivity was greater in UC compared with control population (P<0.03) [16]. Furthermore patients who underwent milk intolerance were found to develop UC at an earlier age compared to those without a history of hypersensitivity to milk (P<0.02) [16]. The statistics suggested the early antigenic stimuli might play a role in development of IBD at a later age [17]. However the causality of food intolerance and IBD still remains controversial and needs further researches to figure out.

Studies on food adverse reactions mediated by immunoglobulin G (IgG) in certain intestinal diseases, such as irritable bowel syndrome (IBS), have been increasingly reported [18–19]. Researchers used to mainly focus on food intolerance classically by the presence of serous IgE antibodies but it seemed that the characteristically immediate allergic reactions were quite rare in

some conditions [20–21]. By contrast, the circulating IgG antibodies provide a more delayed or even asymptomatic response after the exposure to a unique food antigen [22]. Considering that IBD patients mostly suffer a long course of the chronic disease, we hypothesize IgG may have a stronger relevance with IBD than IgE.

Food is a complicated field to study because of its enormous varieties. In another way this feature also makes it a resource palace for us researchers to explore. In this study we aimed to identify the prevalence and significance of 14 food specific IgG antibodies in IBD patients through serological investigation. We expected the results may provide a more clear and detailed connection between food intolerance and IBD in our patient population as well as a supporting evidence for the antibody test to serve the clinical.

Subjects and Methods

Ethics Statement

This study was approved by Medical Ethics Committee of Ren Ji Hospital of Shanghai Jiao Tong University School of Medicine.

Table 2. Prevalence of food specific IgG antibodies in patients with Crohn's disease (CD), ulcerative colitis (UC) and healthy controls (HC).

Group	N	Seropositive Degree (n)				Antibodies (−)	Antibodies (+)
		0	+1	+2	+3	(n, %)	(n, %)
CD	79	19	10	14	36	19 (24.1)	60 (75.9)
UC	33	12	9	4	8	12 (36.4)	21 (63.6)
HC	266	178	41	24	23	178 (66.9)	88 (33.1)

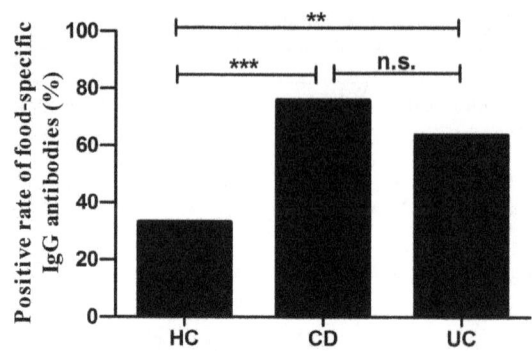

Figure 1. Positive rate of food-specific IgG antibodies in Crohn's disease (CD), ulcerative colitis (UC) and healthy control (HC) groups. Chi-square test, *** $P<0.001$, **$P<0.005$, n.s. not significant.

Informed consent wasn't applied as the medical records and private information of all the subjects were anonymized and de-identified prior to analysis.

Subjects

The study included a total of 112 patients with CD (n = 79) or UC (n = 33) in Ren Ji Hospital from June 2011 to December 2013. All patients met the diagnostic criteria for CD or UC according to the consensus on the diagnosis of IBD drawn up by European Crohn's and Colitis Organization (ECCO) [23,24] and were serologically tested of the food sIgG antibodies during their visit in hospital. In addition another 266 people, who came to our Health Care Centre to do checkups which contained the test as a routine item, were randomly chosen to represent the general population as healthy controls (HC).

Data Collection

Medical records and clinical data of all the IBD patients were comprehensively reviewed and the general demographic data were summarized. The disease severity of CD or UC was based on Harvey-Bradshaw Index [25] or Modified Truelove-Witts Classi-

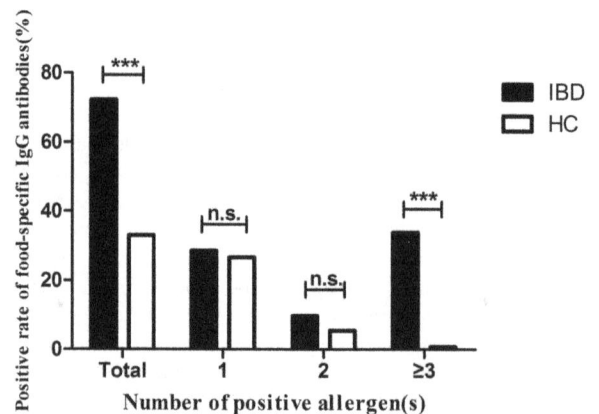

Figure 2. Distribution of the number of positive allergen(s) with positive rate of food-specific IgG antibodies in patients with inflammatory bowel diseases (IBD) and healthy controls (HC). Chi-square test, *** $P<0.001$, n.s. not significant.

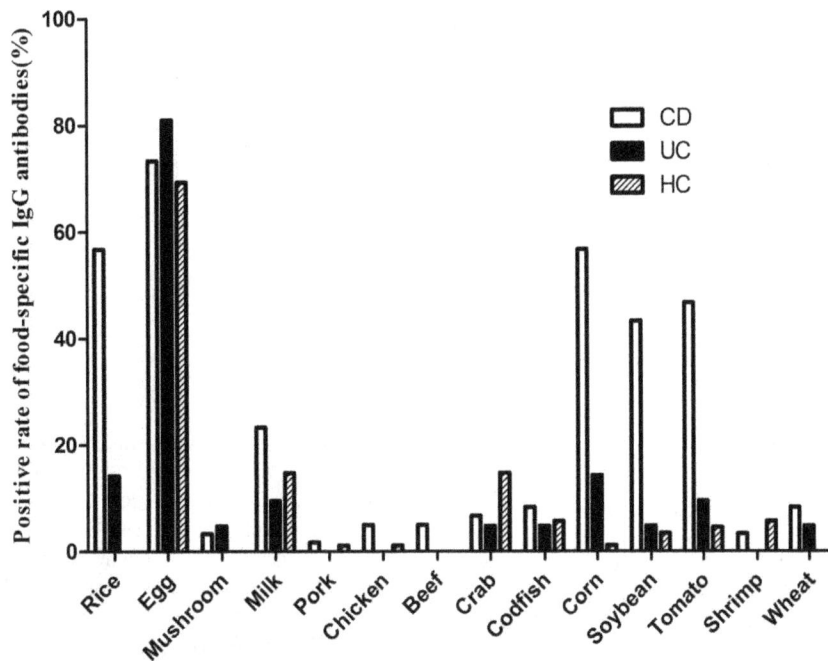

Figure 3. Distribution of positive food allergens in Crohn's disease (CD), ulcerative colitis (UC) and healthy control (HC) groups.

fication [26], respectively. The disease localization of both CD and UC was determined by Montreal Classification [27]. The complications that patients carried consisted of fistula, abdominal abscess, intestinal obstruction, perianal disease, hemorrhage of gastrointestinal tract and acute perforation. The simultaneous extraintestinal manifestations included oral ulcer, sacro-iliitis, rheumatoid arthritis, iritis, primary sclerotic cholangitis, hepatic adipose infiltration and cholelithiasis. Relevant laboratory findings contained peripheral white blood cell (WBC) counts, eosinophile granulocyte (EOS) counts, lymphocyte (LYM) counts, haemoglobin (Hb), serum albumin, erythrocyte sedimentation rate (ESR), high-sensitivity C-reactive protein (hs-CRP), serum total immunoglobulin (IgM, IgA and IgG) and anti double-stranded DNA antibodies (anti-dsDNA).

Enzyme Linked Immunosorbent Assay (ELISA)

ELISA tests for the semi-quantitative analysis of serum IgG antibodies to 14 unique food allergens, including rice, egg, mushroom, milk, pork, chicken, beef, crab, codfish, corn, soybean, tomato, shrimp and wheat, were performed by the detection kit according to the operation manual (Biomerica, Inc. USA). The IgG concentration less than 50U/ml was considered negative

(Grade 0). The values between 50–100U/ml, 100–200U/ml and more than 200U/ml were represented mild sensitivity (Grade +1), moderate sensitivity (Grade +2) and high sensitivity (Grade +3), respectively.

Data Analysis

Statistics were performed with SPSS 19.0 (SPSS Inc. USA). Enumeration data were analyzed using chi-squared test, in which rates of multiple samples were compared by R×C contingency table analysis. Continuous numerical variables were expressed in the form of mean with 95% confidence interval (95% CI) and analyzed by Student's t test. Regression analysis was utilized to identify the correlation/risk factors among variables. Two-tailed P-value < 0.05 was regarded statistically significant.

Results

Demographic data of all subjects

The characteristic information of IBD patients and healthy controls were summarized in **Table 1**.

Table 3. Distribution of food specific IgG antibodies in different disease localizations.

Localization	sIgG antibodies (+)	sIgG antibodies (−)
	(n, %)	(n, %)
Only small intestine (N = 40)	33 (82.5)	3 (17.5)
Only large intestine (N = 43)	26 (60.5)	17 (39.5)
Both small & large intestine (N = 29)	22 (75.9)	7 (24.1)
P-value	0.072△	

△ Chi-square test (R×C contingency table analysis), not statistically significant (P>0.05).

Table 4. Distribution of food specific IgG antibodies at different IBD activity status.

Disease status	sIgG antibodies (+)	Multiple positive (≥2)	High sensitivity
	n (%)	n (%)	n (%)
Remission (N = 7)	6 (85.7)	5 (71.4)	3 (42.9)
Mild (N = 28)	18 (64.3)	7 (25)	9 (32.1)
Moderate (N = 47)	35 (74.5)	23 (48.9)	18 (38.3)
Severe (N = 30)	22 (73.3)	14 (46.7)	14 (46.7)
P-value	0.647△	0.079△	0.719△

△Chi-square test (R×C contingency table analysis), not statistically significant (P>0.05).

Prevalence of serum IgG antibodies to 14 unique food allergens

Food specific IgG antibodies were detected positive in 75.9% (60/79) of CD patients, 63.6% (21/33) of UC patients and 33.1% (88/266) of HC (**Table 2**). The antibodies showed a significantly higher frequency in both CD and UC groups than in healthy controls (CD vs HC, P = 0.000; UC vs HC, P = 0.001) (**Figure 1**). However, there was no significant difference between CD and UC groups (P = 0.184). In general the total positive rate of all IBD patients was 72.3% (81/112), higher than the control group (P = 0.000). Among them 28.6% (32/112), 9.8% (11/112) and 33.9% (38/112) of subjects were respectively sensitive to one, two and more than two food allergens while the corresponding ratios of healthy controls were 26.7% (71/266), 5.6% (15/266) and 0.8% (2/266). There were more subjects who got intolerant to 3 or more antigens in IBD group than in HC group (P = 0.000) (**Figure 2**).

In the present study, the top five prevalent food allergens which caused positive sIgG antibodies in CD patients were egg (44/60, 73.3%), rice (34/60, 56.7%), corn (34/60, 56.7%), tomato (28/60, 46.7%) and soybean (26/60, 43.3%). Besides, the top five prevalent food allergens in UC group were egg (17/21, 81.0%), rice (3/21, 14.3%), corn (3/21, 14.3%), tomato (2/21, 9.5%) and

milk (2/21, 9.5%). And healthy controls demonstrated the compositions of egg (61/88, 69.3%), milk (13/88, 14.8%), crab (13/88, 14.8%), codfish (5/88, 5.7%) and shrimp (5/88, 5.7%), which were similar to the results of a reported epidemiological survey in general population [28]. **Figure 3** showed the distribution of positive food allergens in CD, UC and HC groups.

Association of food specific IgG antibodies with inflammatory segments

To analyze the association between food sIgG antibodies status and disease extent in gut, all 112 patients were divided into three subgroups according to endoscopic results (**Table 3**). The positive rate was found higher (82.5%) in patients with only small intestine involved but the statistical difference wasn't remarkable (P = 0.072).

Relevance of food specific IgG antibodies with disease activity

We divided all 112 IBD patients into four subgroups according to clinical disease activity and compared the ratios of patients with positive IgG antibodies, multiple positive antibodies (≥2) and high sensitivity to at least one food allergen (**Table 4**). Although the

Table 5. Comparison of laboratory results in IBD patients with positive and negative food specific IgG antibodies.

Laboratory results	sIgG antibodies (+)	sIgG antibodies (−)	P-value
	(N = 81)	(N = 31)	
WBC (×10⁹/L)	7.15(6.50–7.86)	6.66(5.79–7.56)	0.437
EOS (×10⁹/L)	0.16(0.12–0.23)	0.15(0.10–0.21)	0.833
LYM (×10⁹/L)	1.44(1.31–1.59)	1.54(1.32–1.81)	0.501
Hb (g/L)	114.31(109.52–119.06)	114.23(104.84–122.58)	0.986
Albumin (g/L)	36.19(34.82–37.72)	35.98(33.67–38.28)	0.889
ESR (mm/h)	28.07(23.01–33.58)	21.35(15.65–27.61)	0.160
hs-CRP (mg/L)	18.84(13.78–23.89)	11.75(6.51–18.51)	0.083
IgM (g/L)	1.22(0.99–1.49)	0.79(0.60–1.03)	0.045*
IgA (g/L)	2.80(2.37–3.27)	2.60(2.13–3.05)	0.597
IgG (g/L)	12.90(11.94–13.94)	10.92(9.50–12.48)	0.041*
anti-dsDNA (IU/mL)	3.31(2.85–3.75)	3.56(2.72–4.61)	0.609

Statistics were expressed as mean with 95% confidence interval.
Normal range: white blood cell (WBC), 3.69–9.16×10⁹/L; eosinophile granulocyte (EOS), 0.02–0.50×10⁹/L; lymphocyte (LYM), 0.8–4.0×10⁹/L; haemoglobin (Hb), 113–172 g/L; albumin, 35–55 g/L; erythrocyte sedimentation rate (ESR) 0–20 mm/h; high-sensitivity C-reactive protein (hs-CRP), 0–3 mg/L; immunoglobulin M (IgM) 0.4–2.3 g/L; IgA, 0.7–4.0 g/L; IgG, 7–16 g/L; anti double-stranded DNA antibodies (anti-dsDNA), 0–7.0 IU/mL
Student's t test, *P<0.05.

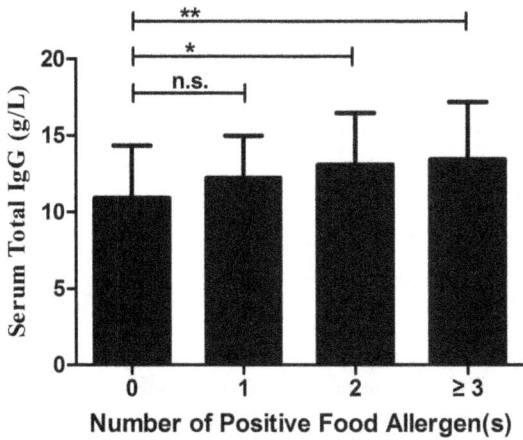

Figure 4. Serum total IgG values in inflammatory bowel disease patients with multiple positive food allergens. Statistics were shown as mean ± standard deviation. Chi-square test, * $P<0.05$; ** $P<0.005$, n.s. not significant.

general antibodies and multi-antibodies were found more common in remission group (85.7% and 71.4%) while the patients who were highly sensitive to specific food allergens seemed to be severer (46.7%), there was no significant differences among the four subgroups.

To further analyze the possible association with several laboratory values related to disease activity, IBD patients were classified into positive and negative IgG antibodies subgroups (**Table 5**). We did find a notable difference in general serum IgM ($P = 0.045$) and IgG ($P = 0.041$) levels between the two groups. Mean values of WBC, ESR and hs-CRP in the positive patients were recognized higher compared with the other group although no marked differences were found. The rest lab findings of the two groups were resembled.

Considering the relative levels of total IgG in relation to antigen specific IgG, we then divided all the IBD patients into 4 groups according to the number of positive allergen(s) (0, 1, 2, ≥3) and compared the difference of serum general IgG values among the groups (**Figure 4**). The mean values of each group were 10.92 (9.50–12.48) g/L, 12.24 (11.31–13.32) g/L, 13.08 (11.31–14.97) g/L and 13.42 (12.24–14.58) g/L, respectively. Patients with multiple positive allergens (≥2) were found with significant higher total IgG levels than sIgG-negative patients ($P = 0.044$, $P = 0.003$, respectively).

Predictors for the occurrence of food specific IgG antibodies

To further identify the predictive factors, we utilized binary logistic regression analyses of several demographic and clinical parameters. The independent variables contained disease type (CD/UC), gender, age, complication, extraintestinal manifestation and intestinal surgery (**Table 6**). Only age was found as a predisposing as well as protective factor against the development of serum food-related IgG antibodies ($P = 0.002$).

Discussion

In the present study, we have demonstrated that IgG antibodies against food specific allergens are distinctly elevated in IBD patients compared with healthy controls. This serologic antibody investigation is served as an aid in the diagnosis and management of food intolerance in clinical activities [29]. Food intolerance can be defined as a series of unpleasant symptoms including eructation, abdominal pain, diarrhea, fatigue, headache and palpitation after the intake of particular food products [29]. It is usually caused by enzyme deficiency as well as pharmacological effects of vasoactive amines present in foods. When certain food can't be fully digested, bodies may produce specific IgG antibodies which would form immune complexes with food particles and lead to excessive protective immune responses [30]. Food intolerance is not so similar to food allergy as the latter mainly occurs through the classically immediate IgE-mediated antibody responses and the obvious symptoms can be detected by most patients [31]. Meanwhile, IgG-mediated reaction characteristically acts as a particular delayed-type hypersensitivity response after the exposure to antigens and sometimes the symptoms are too occult for patients to recognize [22]. Some investigators considered them to be physiological since that the food sIgG antibodies can appear in healthy individuals [32], which was also proved in our data. However, several studies including our results have shown the higher prevalence of sIgG antibodies to food in IBD patients or animal models in contrast to normal controls [19,33], which arouse the attention to the relevance between IBD and food intolerance. Van Den Bogaerde *et al.* used colonoscopic allergen provocation test to determine the gut mucosal response to food antigens in Crohn's disease [34]. This intuitionistic study provided both *in vivo* and *in vitro* evidence that CD patients were more sensitive to exogenous food antigens than healthy people and the reactions were gut specific.

Food sIgG antibodies were discovered frequent in IBD patients with small intestine involved in the present research, which resembled the result of a study on the correlation of lactose malabsorption and disease segments [35]. Mishkin *et al.* demon-

Table 6. Correlation of food specific IgG antibodies with demographic and clinical parameters.

Parameters	Odds ratio	95% CI	P-value
Disease type (CD vs. UC)	1.167	0.389–3.498	0.783
Gender	0.758	0.306–1.879	0.549
Age	0.945	0.912–0.979	0.002**
Complication	2.269	0.719–7.157	0.162
Extraintestinal manifestation	1.302	0.438–3.868	0.635
Intestinal surgery	1.613	0.329–7.905	0.556

95% CI: 95% confidence interval; CD: Crohn's disease; UC: ulcerative colitis.
Binary logistic regression, **$P<0.005$.

strated that CD of the proximal small bowel (duodenum, jejunum), terminal ileum, terminal ileum plus colon and colon alone were related with lactose malabsorption of 100%, 68.1%, 54.5% and 43.5%, respectively. Regression analysis of our data indicated age as a protective factor of food intolerance in IBD patients, which is opposite to the result of a cross sectional epidemiological study in other area of China [28]. We assume the difference might be associated with age structure of onset as inflammatory bowel diseases, especially Crohn's disease, tend to occur in younger people based on our clinical observation.

A survey demonstrated that 15.6% IBD patients believed diet could initiate the disease while 57.8% were convinced certain foods could play a role in causing relapses [36]. In our study, we found food sIgG antibodies were more frequent in patients who were during remission. Meanwhile, the patients who were highly sensitive to food allergens tended to be serious in disease activity and mean levels of ESR and hs-CRP were detected higher in sIgG-positive patients. Although the results didn't show statistical significance, they did provide us with a tendency. We consider the few remission cases (only 7) contributed to the above conflicting results.

The increased serum IgM values tested in sIgG-positive patients may indicate recent infection. Besides, we also found a higher level of serum total IgG antibodies in patients with positive allergens, especially with multiple ones in the study. The general increase on IgG levels may be an important reason for the increased amount of sIgG antibodies against food epitopes. It has been reported that mast cells can respond not only to IgE antibodies but also to IgG antibodies [37]. In addition IgG antibodies in food allergy may even influence allergen-IgE complex formation and bind to B cells, which is quite opposite the traditional concept that IgG antibodies are supposed to inhibit these processes [38]. Therefore IgG antibodies probably serve as mediation effects rather than inhibition in hypersensitivity reaction caused by food intolerance. Serum sIgG antibodies to non-food related antigens are mostly studied within inhaled antigens in respiratory allergic disorders such as asthma. Wang et al. investigated the relevance between asthma morbidity and sIgE/sIgG levels to inhaled allergen exposure [39]. They concluded that sIgE levels could serve as markers of asthma however sIgG was not that important as predictor or modifier. Due to the rich diversity of food and non-food allergens, we believe that the immune reactions can be very distinct for different allergens and the mechanisms of how sIgG functions may be complicated and needs further study.

How IBD and food intolerance interact with each other remains controversial. Disruption of epithelial tight junctions causes hyperpermeability in the gut of IBD patients and allows the antigen presenting cells (dendritic cells) to directly encounter food antigens in lamina propria to activate Th/B cells, thus resulting in high levels of sIgG antibodies [40]. Simultaneously this defect may also exacerbate inflammatory conditions. In another respect, lack of certain enzyme may lead to incomplete digestion of food and the remaining polypeptides then stimulate the secretion of sIgG antibodies as well as inflammatory cytokines, thereby bringing impairments to normal intestines [41]. The definite mechanism still remains unclear.

Although we used several methods to improve our study, there were still some limitations to the present results. The small quantity of cases may bring about the first shortcoming. The sample size needs to be enlarged to see the exact trend. We didn't contain the follow-up data of whether or not the IBD patients eliminated the food based on the presence of sIgG antibodies and whether the subsequent diet elimination had an effect on the diseases, which is also a limitation of our research. However, promising results have been reported in a randomized controlled trial [19]. Bentz et al. designed a double-blind, cross-over nutritional diet intervention according to circulating food sIgG antibodies with 40 CD patients and it did show therapeutic effects with regard to abdominal pain, stool frequency and general well-being. However, the investigators could not elucidate the exact mechanisms of the contribution of sIgG antibodies to disease activity. Anyway, we still consider serologic investigation of IgG antibodies to food antigens may bring benefits to dietary modification for IBD patients.

In conclusion, the prevalence of food specific IgG antibodies is remarkably higher in patients with inflammatory bowel diseases than healthy controls, and age may acts as a protective factor for their occurrence. Although the mechanisms of the interaction between food intolerance and IBD remain obscure, the sIgG antibodies may potentially show the clinical significance to indicate disease status and to ameliorate symptoms by guiding diets for patients.

Acknowledgments

The authors would like to thank the Department of Clinical Laboratory at Ren Ji Hospital for assisting us to conduct the study.

Author Contributions

Conceived and designed the experiments: CC QZ ZR. Performed the experiments: CC QZ. Analyzed the data: CC DZ AX SJ. Contributed reagents/materials/analysis tools: JS YQ DZ SJ. Wrote the paper: CC JS DZ ZR QZ.

References

1. Bernstein CN (2001) Extraintestinal manifestations of inflammatory bowel disease. Curr Gastroenterol Rep 3: 477–483.

2. Vidal A, Gomez-Gil E, Sans M, Portella MJ, Salamero M, et al. (2008) Health-related quality of life in inflammatory bowel disease patients: the role of psychopathology and personality. Inflamm Bowel Dis 14: 977–983.

3. Macdonald TT, Monteleone G (2005) Immunity, inflammation, and allergy in the gut. Science 307: 1920–1925.

4. Goh K, Xiao SD (2009) Inflammatory bowel disease: a survey of the epidemiology in Asia. J Dig Dis 10: 1–6.

5. Magee EA, Edmond LM, Tasker SM, Kong SC, Curno R, et al. (2005) Associations between diet and disease activity in ulcerative colitis patients using a novel method of data analysis. Nutr J 4: 7.

6. Hou JK, Abraham B, El-Serag H (2011) Dietary intake and risk of developing inflammatory bowel disease: a systematic review of the literature. Am J Gastroenterol 106: 563–573.

7. Brunner B, Scheurer U, Seibold F (2007) Differences in yeast intolerance between patients with Crohn's disease and ulcerative colitis. Dis Colon Rectum 50: 83–88.

8. Haboubi NY, Jones S (2005) Influence of dietary factors on the clinical course of inflammatory bowel disease. Gut 54: 567.

9. Sakamoto N, Kono S, Wakai K, Fukuda Y, Satomi M, et al. (2005) Dietary risk factors for inflammatory bowel disease: a multicenter case-control study in Japan. Inflamm Bowel Dis 11: 154–163.

10. Jowett SL, Seal CJ, Pearce MS, Phillips E, Gregory W, et al. (2004) Influence of dietary factors on the clinical course of ulcerative colitis: a prospective cohort study. Gut 53: 1479–1484.

11. Sampson HA (2004) Update on food allergy. J Allergy Clin Immunol 113: 805–819; quiz 820.

12. David TJ (2000) Adverse reactions and intolerance to foods. Br Med Bull 56: 34–50.

13. Banai J (2009) Nutrition in inflammatory bowel disease. Orv Hetil 150: 839–845.

14. Binder JH, Gryboski JD, Thayer WR Jr, Spiro HM (1966) Intolerance to milk in ulcerative colitis. A preliminary report. Am J Dig Dis 11: 858–864.

15. Truelove SC (1961) Ulcerative colitis provoked by milk. Br Med J 1: 154–160.

16. Glassman MS, Newman LJ, Berezin S, Gryboski JD (1990) Cow's milk protein sensitivity during infancy in patients with inflammatory bowel disease. Am J Gastroenterol 85: 838–840.

17. Cashman KD, Shanahan F (2003) Is nutrition an aetiological factor for inflammatory bowel disease? Eur J Gastroenterol Hepatol 15: 607–613.

18. Atkinson W, Sheldon TA, Shaath N, Whorwell PJ (2004) Food elimination based on IgG antibodies in irritable bowel syndrome: a randomised controlled trial. Gut 53: 1459–1464.

19. Bentz S, Hausmann M, Piberger H, Kellermeier S, Paul S, et al. (2010) Clinical relevance of IgG antibodies against food antigens in Crohn's disease: a double-blind cross-over diet intervention study. Digestion 81: 252–264.

20. Zar S, Kumar D, Benson MJ (2001) Food hypersensitivity and irritable bowel syndrome. Aliment Pharmacol Ther 15: 439–449.

21. Mekkel G, Barta Z, Ress Z, Gyimesi E, Sipka S, et al. (2005) Increased IgE-type antibody response to food allergens in irritable bowel syndrome and inflammatory bowel diseases. Orv Hetil 146: 797–802.

22. Crowe SE, Perdue MH (1992) Gastrointestinal food hypersensitivity: basic mechanisms of pathophysiology. Gastroenterology 103: 1075–1095.

23. Stange EF, Travis SP, Vermeire S, Reinisch W, Geboes K, et al. (2008) European evidence-based Consensus on the diagnosis and management of ulcerative colitis: Definitions and diagnosis. J Crohns Colitis 2: 1–23.

24. Van Assche G, Dignass A, Panes J, Beaugerie L, Karagiannis J, et al. (2010) The second European evidence-based Consensus on the diagnosis and management of Crohn's disease: Definitions and diagnosis. J Crohns Colitis 4: 7–27.

25. Harvey RF, Bradshaw JM (1980) A simple index of Crohn's-disease activity. Lancet 1: 514.

26. Truelove SC, Witts LJ (1955) Cortisone in ulcerative colitis; final report on a therapeutic trial. Br Med J 2: 1041–1048.

27. Satsangi J, Silverberg MS, Vermeire S, Colombel JF (2006) The Montreal classification of inflammatory bowel disease: controversies, consensus, and implications. Gut 55: 749–753.

28. Sai XY, Zheng YS, Zhao JM, Zhao W (2011) A cross sectional survey on the prevalence of food intolerance and its determinants in Beijing, China. Chin J Epidemiol 32(3):302–05 (in Chinese).

29. Palmieri B, Esposito A, Capone S, Fistetto G, Iannitti T (2011) Food intolerance: reliability and characteristics of different diagnostic alternative tests. Minerva Gastroenterol Dietol 57: 1–10.

30. Ortolani C, Pastorello EA (2006) Food allergies and food intolerances. Best Pract Res Clin Gastroenterol 20: 467–483.

31. Wuthrich B (2009) Food allergy, food intolerance or functional disorder. Praxis (Bern 1994) 98: 375–387.

32. Husby S, Oxelius VA, Teisner B, Jensenius JC, Svehag SE (1985) Humoral immunity to dietary antigens in healthy adults. Occurrence, isotype and IgG subclass distribution of serum antibodies to protein antigens. Int Arch Allergy Appl Immunol 77: 416–422.

33. Foster AP, Knowles TG, Moore AH, Cousins PD, Day MJ, et al. (2003) Serum IgE and IgG responses to food antigens in normal and atopic dogs, and dogs with gastrointestinal disease. Vet Immunol Immunopathol 92: 113–124.

34. Van Den Bogaerde J, Cahill J, Emmanuel AV, Vaizey CJ, Talbot IC, et al. (2002) Gut mucosal response to food antigens in Crohn's disease. Aliment Pharmacol Ther 16: 1903–1915.

35. Mishkin B, Yalovsky M, Mishkin S (1997) Increased prevalence of lactose malabsorption in Crohn's disease patients at low risk for lactose malabsorption based on ethnic origin. Am J Gastroenterol 92: 1148–1153.

36. Zallot C, Quilliot D, Chevaux JB, Peyrin-Biroulet C, Gueant-Rodriguez RM, et al. (2013) Dietary beliefs and behavior among inflammatory bowel disease patients. Inflamm Bowel Dis 19: 66–72.

37. Malbec O, Daeron M (2007) The mast cell IgG receptors and their roles in tissue inflammation. Immunol Rev 217: 206–221.

38. Meulenbroek LA, de Jong RJ, den Hartog Jager CF, Monsuur HN, Wouters D, et al. (2013) IgG antibodies in food allergy influence allergen-antibody complex formation and binding to B cells: a role for complement receptors. J Immunol 191: 3526–3533.

39. Wang J, Visness CM, Calatroni A, Gergen PJ, Mitchell HE, et al. (2009) Effect of environmental allergen sensitization on asthma morbidity in inner-city asthmatic children. Clin Exp Allergy 39: 1381–1389.

40. Chahine BG, Bahna SL (2010) The role of the gut mucosal immunity in the development of tolerance against allergy to food. Curr Opin Allergy Clin Immunol 10: 220–225.

41. Isolauri E, Rautava S, Kalliomaki M (2004) Food allergy in irritable bowel syndrome: new facts and old fallacies. Gut 53: 1391–1393.

19

Comparison of Microbiological, Histological, and Immunomodulatory Parameters in Response to Treatment with Either Combination Therapy with Prednisone and Metronidazole or Probiotic VSL#3 Strains in Dogs with Idiopathic Inflammatory Bowel Disease

Giacomo Rossi[1], Graziano Pengo[2], Marco Caldin[3], Angela Palumbo Piccionello[1], Jörg M. Steiner[4], Noah D. Cohen[5], Albert E. Jergens[6], Jan S. Suchodolski[4]*

1 School of Veterinary Medical Sciences, University of Camerino, Camerino, Italy, 2 Clinic "St. Antonio", Cremona, Italy, 3 San Marco Laboratories, Padova, Italy, 4 Gastrointestinal Laboratory, Department of Small Animal Clinical Sciences, College of Veterinary Medicine and Biomedical Sciences, Texas A&M University, College Station, Texas, United States of America, 5 Department of Large Animal Clinical Sciences, College of Veterinary Medicine and Biomedical Sciences, Texas A&M University, College Station, Texas, United States of America, 6 Department of Veterinary Clinical Sciences, College of Veterinary Medicine, Iowa State University, Ames, Iowa, United States of America

Abstract

Background: Idiopathic inflammatory bowel disease (IBD) is a common chronic enteropathy in dogs. There are no published studies regarding the use of probiotics in the treatment of canine IBD. The objectives were to compare responses to treatment with either combination therapy (prednisone and metronidazole) or probiotic strains (VSL#3) in dogs with IBD.

Methodology and Principal Findings: Twenty pet dogs with a diagnosis of IBD, ten healthy pet dogs, and archived control intestinal tissues from three euthanized dogs were used in this open label study. Dogs with IBD were randomized to receive either probiotic (D-VSL#3, n = 10) or combination drug therapy (D-CT, n = 10). Dogs were monitored for 60 days (during treatment) and re-evaluated 30 days after completing treatment. The CIBDAI (P<0.001), duodenal histology scores (P< 0.001), and CD3+ cells decreased post-treatment in both treatment groups. FoxP3+ cells (p<0.002) increased in the D-VSL#3 group after treatment but not in the D-CT group. TGF-β+ cells increased in both groups after treatment (P = 0.0043) with the magnitude of this increase being significantly greater for dogs in the D-VSL#3 group compared to the D-CT group. Changes in apical junction complex molecules occludin and claudin-2 differed depending on treatment. *Faecalibacterium* and *Turicibacter* were significantly decreased in dogs with IBD at T0, with a significant increase in *Faecalibacterium* abundance observed in the animals treated with VSL#3 strains.

Conclusions: A protective effect of VSL#3 strains was observed in dogs with IBD, with a significant decrease in clinical and histological scores and a decrease in CD3+ T-cell infiltration. Protection was associated with an enhancement of regulatory T-cell markers (FoxP3+ and TGF-β+), specifically observed in the probiotic-treated group and not in animals receiving combination therapy. A normalization of dysbiosis after long-term therapy was observed in the probiotic group. Larger scale studies are warranted to evaluate the clinical efficacy of VSL#3 in canine IBD.

Editor: Mathias Chamaillard, INSERM, France

Funding: There was no external funding support for this research. VSL Pharmaceuticals supplied the probiotic strains used in this study, but otherwise did not provide any financial support and had no role in study design, data collection, analysis, interpretation or preparation of the manuscript.

Competing Interests: VSL Pharmaceuticals supplied the probiotic strains used in this study. Graziano Pengo is employed by Clinic "St. Antonio" and Marco Caldin by San Marco Laboratories. There are no further patents, products in development or marketed products to declare.

* E-mail: jsuchodolski@cvm.tamu.edu

Introduction

Similar to human inflammatory bowel disease (IBD), three main factors are considered to be fundamental in the pathogenesis of canine idiopathic IBD: the interactions between the mucosal immune system, host genetic susceptibility, and environmental factors (e.g., microbiota, nutrition) [1–3]. Experimental evidence supports a role for commensal bacteria in the pathogenesis of IBD;

for example, spontaneous colitis develops in mice deficient in interleukin (IL)-2 [4] and IL-10 [5] when colonized with a complex microbiota, but not in mice raised under germ-free conditions. Recent studies suggest involvement of the intestinal microbiota in the pathogenesis of canine and feline IBD [2,6–9]. Also, antibiotics such as metronidazole are useful in the treatment of IBD in humans [10] and dogs [11], and there is evidence that children with IBD respond to probiotic administration [12]. Collectively, these findings suggest that the intestinal microbiota plays a crucial role in the pathogenesis of IBD and modulation of intestinal microbiota may be beneficial in the treatment of mucosal inflammation. While probiotics are used frequently in small animal practice, there are only few published studies regarding their efficacy in dogs with chronic enteropathies. In one investigation, a probiotic cocktail was shown to reduce clinical severity in a prospective, placebo-controlled trial in dogs with food-responsive diarrhea treated with an elimination diet [13], but studies evaluating idiopathic IBD have not been reported.

VSL#3 is a high-dose, multi-strain probiotic product containing viable lyophilized bacteria consisting of 4 strains of *Lactobacillus* (*L. casei, L. plantarum. L. acidophilus*, and *L. delbrueckii* subsp. *bulgaricus*), 3 strains of *Bifidobacterium* (*B. longum, B. breve*, and *B. infantis*), and 1 strain of *Streptococcus sulivarius* subsp *thermophilus*. The VSL#3 strains have shown efficacy in humans for the prevention, treatment, and maintenance of remission of both pouchitis and ulcerative colitis in adults and children [12,14,15].

The purpose of the present study was to perform a randomized open-label trial to compare the microbiological, histological, and immunomodulatory effects between the commercial multi-strain probiotic SIVOY, a probiotic product formulated with VSL#3 strains for pets (VSL Pharmaceuticals, Inc., Gaithersburg, MD, USA) and combination therapy with prednisone and metronidazole in canine IBD.

Our results suggest a protective effect of the probiotic mixture in dogs with IBD, with a significant decrease in clinical and histological scores, and a decrease in CD3+ T-cell infiltration. Protection was associated with an enhancement of regulatory T-cell markers (FoxP3+ and TGF-β+), specifically observed in the probiotic-treated group and not in animals receiving combination therapy. The protective effect of the probiotic VSL#3 strains was also associated with normalization of dysbiosis, specifically increases in *Faecalibacterium* spp.

Materials and Methods

Animals

The study was approved by the Camerino University Institutional Animal Care and Use Committee protocol and all owners of the IBD dogs gave informed written consent before enrollment. Twenty pet dogs (Table 1) with a long-time diagnosis of IBD according to published criteria [16] were evaluated at the Veterinary Teaching Hospital, Camerino University, for chronic gastroenteritis. Inclusion criteria included recurrence of clinical signs and absence of any immunomodulating drug therapy (e.g., corticosteroids, metronidazole, and sulfasalazine) within a month before referral. Diagnostic criteria for IBD included: persistent (>3 weeks) gastrointestinal signs, failed responses to dietary (hydrolysate or commercial intact protein elimination diet) or symptomatic therapies (anthelminthics, antibiotics, anticholinergics, gastrointestinal protectants) alone, a thorough diagnostic evaluation with failure to document other causes for gastroenteritis, and histopathologic evidence of intestinal inflammation. The minimum diagnostic evaluation in all dogs included a complete blood count, serum biochemistry, urinalysis, direct (wet mount) and

indirect (flotation) examination of feces for endoparasites, and survey abdominal radiographs. In some instances, additional tests including contrast radiography, abdominal ultrasound (performed in 16 of the 20 dogs) and measurement of serum concentrations of trypsin-like immunoreactivity and/or folate and cobalamin were performed. Additional inclusion criteria were the absence of extra-alimentary tract inflammation based on results obtained from initial diagnostic testing. Dogs with hypoproteinemia or a suspicion of intestinal lymphangiectasia were excluded from the study.

Ten pet dogs (Table 1), living in home environments and free of gastrointestinal signs for at least four months, were enrolled as control group (D–H) for comparison of fecal microbiota between healthy dogs and dogs with IBD. Control dogs were judged to be healthy based on normal results on physical examination, complete blood count, serum biochemistry, urinalysis, repeated fecal examinations, and dirofilarial antigen assay.

Study design

The trial was a 90 day open-label evaluation to compare the effects of VSL#3 strains versus combination drug therapy on histological, microbiological, and immunological markers. Dogs were randomized into two groups using a computer-generated randomization list. The VSL#3 group (D-VSL#3; n = 10) received between 112 and 225 billion (112 to 225×10^9) lyophilized bacteria per 10 kg daily for 60 consecutive days; the D-CT group (n = 10) received a combination protocol of metronidazole at 20 mg/Kg q12 h and prednisone at 1 mg/kg body weight/day. The clinical disease activity (CIBDAI score) was assessed at baseline (T0) and after 90 days (T1) of enrollment, which was 30 days following completion of either treatment. The CIBDAI is based on 6 criteria, each scored on a scale from 0–3: attitude/activity, appetite, vomiting, stool consistency, stool frequency, and weight loss. After summation, the total composite score is determined to be clinically insignificant (score 0–3), mild (score 4–5), moderate (score 6–8) or severe (score 9 or greater) [17].

Fecal samples were also collected at each visit then immediately stored at −80°C, until microbiota analysis. The evaluation time point 30 days post-treatment was chosen to determine whether individual dogs would relapse within 30 days following completion of either treatment regimen.

Tissue sampling

After enrollment (time point T0) and after 90 days (T1), multiple (10–15 specimens) mucosal biopsy specimens were procured endoscopically from the small and/or large intestine of all dogs with IBD (n = 20, 10 dogs per treatment group). Fifteen dogs having predominantly upper gastrointestinal signs (i.e., vomiting, small bowel diarrhea, anorexia, and/or weight loss) underwent esophagogastroduodenoscopy, whereas upper and lower endoscopic examinations were performed in 5 dogs having mixed signs of enterocolitis (i.e., GI signs associated with tenesmus, hematochezia, mucoid feces, and/or frequent defecation). Biopsy specimens were obtained directly from mucosal lesions of increased granularity, friability, or erosions as well as areas of normal-appearing mucosa. Tissues for histopathology were placed in 10% neutral buffered formalin, then paraffin embedded and serial 3 μm thick sections were prepared. For ethical considerations, no endoscopic examinations were performed in healthy dogs. Histopathology was performed by a single pathologist, who was blinded regarding history, clinical signs, or endoscopic observations. A severity score was assigned for each dog, by using a standardized and previously described histologic grading system, based on the extent of architectural disruption and mucosal

Table 1. Summary characteristics of enrolled dogs.

| | Treatment groups | | |
	VSL#3 (n = 10)	CT (n = 10)	Healthy Control (n = 10)
Breed	Golden Retriever, Husky, Boxer, Rottweiler, Jack Russell Terrier, WHW Terrier, German shepherd (2), Shih Tzu, Yorkshire Terrier	Golden retriever (2), Cocker Spaniel, Boxer, Bull Terrier, Carlino, WHW Terrier, German shepherd, Shar Pei, Yorkshire Terrier	Golden Retriever, Epagneul Breton, Chow Chow, Rottweiler, Border collie, German shepherd, Bolognese, Miniature Schnauzer, Yorkshire Terrier (2)
Sex	m = 5, mn = 1, f = 1, fs = 3	m = 5, f = 2,fs = 3	m = 5, f = 5
Median age (range) in years	5.8 (2.5–11)	5.5 (1.5–9)	6.5 (1–12)
Body weight (range) in kg	18.9 (2–36)	18.7 (1.5–30)	20.6 (2.8–45)
Median (range) time to remission (days)	10.6 (5–15)	4.8 (2.5–7)	n/a

m = male, mn = neutered male, f = female, fs = spayed female; CT = combination therapy; n/a-not applicable.

Immunohistochemical evaluation

epithelial changes [17,18], as recently been proposed by the WSAVA for diagnosis of gastrointestinal inflammation [19].

Tissues were also evaluated for expression patterns of apical junction complex (AJC) molecules in both dog groups after end of the therapy. To obtain control tissue from healthy dogs for this analysis, archived formalin-fixed and paraffin–embedded colonic tissues from three male dogs with no clinical signs of intestinal disease were retrieved from the University of Camerino Veterinary Pathology Unit archives. These samples had been obtained immediately post-mortem from dogs that were presented for euthanasia (euthanized dogs, ED) for old age (n = 1), nasal carcinoma (n = 1), or splenic haemangiosarcoma (n = 1). Ages ranged from 7 years to 14 years and histopathological examination of full-thickness intestinal biopsies was normal in all these ED cases.

Immunohistochemical evaluation

Paraffin sections were rehydrated and neutralized for endogenous peroxidases with 3% hydrogen peroxide for 5 minutes followed by rinsing for 5 minutes in distilled water. For antigen retrieval, slides were incubated in three antigen retrieval solutions: citrate buffer (pH 6.0) for TGF-β, EDTA (pH 8.0) for CD3 and FoxP3, and 0.01 M Tris-EDTA buffer (pH 9.0) for claudin 2, occludin and E-cadherin in a steamer (Black & Decker, Towson, MD, USA) for 20 minutes. Non-specific binding was blocked by incubation of slides for 10 minutes with a protein-blocking agent (Protein-blocking agent, Dako, Carpinteria, CA, USA) before application of the primary antibody. Slides were incubated overnight in a moist-chamber with the following primary antibodies: monoclonal (mAb) rat anti-human CD3 (Monoclonal rat anti-human CD3 clone MCA1477, Serotec abD, Biorad Laboratories, Hercules, CA, USA) diluted 1:50, mAb anti-mouse/ rat FoxP3 antibodies (Monoclonal anti-mouse/rat FoxP3 antibodies clone FJK-16s, eBioscience, San Diego, CA, USA) diluted 1:400, and mAb mouse anti-TGF-β (Monoclonal mouse anti-TGF-β, clone 1D11, Serotec abD, Biorad Laboratories, Hercules, CA, USA) diluted 1:25 [19,20]. Polyclonal rabbit anti-claudin-2 (Polyclonal rabbit anti-claudin-2 (PAD: MH44), Invitrogen Ltd.,

Paisley, UK) and anti-occludin (anti-occludin PAD: Z-T22, Invitrogen Ltd., Paisley, UK) antibodies and monoclonal mouse anti-E-cadherin IgG2α (Monoclonal mouse anti-E-cadherin IgG2α (clone: 36), BD Biosciences, Oxford, UK) were used as described previously [21].

The immunoreaction with streptavidin–immunoperoxidase (Streptavidin–immunoperoxidase, Black & Decker, Towson, MD, USA) was visualized with 3,3′-diaminobenzidine substrate (3,3′-diaminobenzidine substrate, Vector, Burlingame, UK). Tissues were counterstained with Mayer's hematoxylin. For negative immunohistochemical controls the primary antibodies were omitted. Sections of canine spleen and tonsil served as positive control tissues for CD3 and FoxP3 cell staining and sections of canine placenta for that of TGF-β expression. Positive control tissues for claudin/occludin and E-cadherin staining consisted of canine lung and kidney sections, respectively.

For scoring of intestinal CD3+ T-lymphocytes, FoxP3+ cells, and TGF-β+ cells, these cells were quantified in select compartments of the GI tract (small intestine: villi, basal crypt area, villus-crypt junction; large intestine: apical crypt area, basal crypt area). All cellular types were evaluated using a light microscope (Carl Zeiss, Jena, Germany), a ×40 objective, a ×10 eyepiece, and a square eyepiece graticule (10×10 squares, having a total area of 62,500 μm^2). Ten appropriate fields were chosen for each compartment and arithmetic means were calculated for each intestinal region. Results were expressed as IHC positive cells per 62,500 μm^2. For all parameters, cells on the margins of the tissue sections were not considered for evaluation to avoid inflation of positive cell numbers.

For the evaluation of different lymphocytes subsets in the same histological sections, consecutive 3-μm-thick bioptic cross sections were cut. Sections were placed consecutively on each of eight separate slides, after which the ninth section was placed on the first slide, next to the first section, continuing for 48 sections. A single slide, upon which were six bioptic cross sections from each dog, was analyzed for any given immunostain. Numbers of CD3+ T-lymphocytes, FoxP3+ cells, and TGF-β+ cells, were quantified by using an image-analysis system consisting of a light microscope

Table 2. Oligonucleotides primers/probes used in this study.

qPCR primers/probe	Sequence (5'-3')	Target	Annealing (°C)	Reference
Forward	CCGGAWTYATTGGGTTTAAAGGG	Bacteroidetes	60	[45]
Reverse	GGTAAGGTTCCTCGCGTA			
Forward	GAAGGCGGCCTACTGGGCAC	*Faecalibacterium*	60	[47]
Reverse	GTGCAGGCGAGTTGCAGCCT			
Forward	ACTGAGAGGTTGAACGGCCA	Family Ruminococcaceae	59	[47]
Reverse	CCTTTACACCCAGTAAWTCCGGA			
Forward	CGCATAACGTTGAAAGATGG			
Reverse	CCTTGGTAGGCCGTTACCC	*C. perfringens* 16S	58	[48]
Probe	TCATCATTCAACCAAAGGAGCAATCC			
Forward	KGGGCTCAACMCMGTATTGCGT	Fusobacteria	51	[9]
Reverse	TCGCGTTAGCTTGGGCGCTG			
Forward	TCTGATGTGAAAGGCTGGGGCTTA	*Blautia*	56	[9]
Reverse	GGCTTAGCCACCCGACACCTA			
Forward	CCTACGGGAGGCAGCAGT	Universal Bacteria	59	[49]
Reverse	ATTACCGCGGCTGCTGG			
Forward	CAGACGGGGACAACGATTGGA	*Turicibacter*	63	[9]
Reverse	TACGCATCGTCGCCTTGGTA			
Forward	TCGCGTCCGGTGTGAAAG	*Bifidobacterium*	60	[50]
Reverse	CCACATCCAGCATCCAC			
Forward	CCCTTATTGTTAGTTGCCATCATT	*Enterococcus*	61	[46]
Reverse	ACTCGTTGTACTTCCCATTGT			
Forward	AGCAGTAGGGAATCTTCCA[a]	*Lactobacillus*	58	[46]
Reverse	CACCGCTACACATGGAG[b]			
Forward	TTATTTGAAAGGGGCAATTGCT	*Streptococcus*	54	[51]
Reverse	GTGAACTTTCCACTCTCACAC			

[a]Originally described by [52].
[b]Originally described by [53].

(Carl Zeiss, Jena, Germany) attached to a Javelin JE3462 high-resolution camera and a personal computer equipped with a Coreco-Oculus OC-TCX frame grabber and high-resolution monitor. Computerized color-image analysis was performed by using Image-Pro Plus software (Media Cybernetics). The area of each biopsy in all six cross sections in every dog was recorded, as was the total number of T-lymphocytes determined by immunostaining as previously described. For each dog, the total bioptic area was calculated as the sum of the areas of all fields in all six bioptic cross sections on one slide. CD3+ T-lymphocytes, FoxP3+ cells, and TGF-β+ cells were counted per section, and stained cell densities were expressed as the number of lymphocytes/cells per square millimeter of analyzed bioptic area [22].

To assess AJC expression (claudin-2, occludin, and E-cadherin) in biopsies sampled after treatment in both groups (at T1 for D-VSL#3 and D-CT), and to compare data to the AJC expression in non-IBD control dogs (ED group), stained tissue sections were evaluated at ×200 and ×630 (oil immersion) magnification to identify areas of consistent staining and acceptable orientation. Immunostaining was evaluated along the length of multiple enteric/colonic crypts and in areas of intact luminal epithelium. Stain intensity was subjectively graded as absent (−), weak (+), moderate (++), or strong (+++), and the localization and distribution of chromogen were noted. For evaluation, intestinal epithelium was divided into luminal, proximal, and distal gland/crypt regions, and the intercellular junction was divided into apical and basolateral compartments. Finally, the scoring of intestinal AJC molecules expression was calculated as previously described for CD3+ T-cells, FoxP3+ cells, and TGF-β+ cells. The AJC molecules were assessd only at T1 (following treatment intervention), because at T0 all dogs had endoscopically visible lesions of intestinal inflammation including erosions, friability, and increased mucosal granularity. Also, dogs had histopathologic lesions of intestinal inflammation of varying severity. Intestinal inflammation was associated with different degrees of epithelial infiltration by lymphocytes (i.e., intraepithelial lymphocytes) in all dogs of both groups. In these instances, it was not considered useful to evaluate AJCs as they were assumed to be altered, but instead AJC molecules were evaluated at T1 when the previously observed endoscopic lesions of inflammation had resolved.

Plasma citrulline

Plasma concentrations of citrulline were measured in the D-VSL#3 treated group only. Plasma samples were taken at baseline (T0) and after 90 days (T1) and stored at −80°C until evaluation. Samples were precipitated with organic solvents and quantified by MS/MS mass spectrometer equipped with electrospray ionization (ESI) interface in positive ion mode (Waters TQ Detector, Water Corp., Milford, MA, USA). All assays were performed in duplicate fashion. All data collected in centroid mode were processed using commercial software (MassLynx 4.1 software, Water Corp., Milford, Ma, USA).

Microbiota analysis

Fresh naturally voided samples were collected from all 20 diseased dogs (at T0 and T1) and 10 healthy dogs (one time point), flash-frozen in liquid nitrogen and stored at −80°C. DNA was extracted using a bead-beating method (PowerSoil DNA Isolation Kit, MoBio Laboratories, Carlsbad, CA) according to the manufacturer's protocol. Selected bacterial groups within the fecal microbiota were analyzed by quantitative PCR (qPCR) assays as described previously for canine fecal samples (Table 2) [9,23]. Amplified DNA from each bacterial group was normalized for total amplified bacterial DNA (log_{10} amplified DNA for each bacterial group divided by log_{10} of amplified bacterial DNA) as described previously [23].

Data analysis (statistics)

To evaluate differences at baseline as well as post-treatment between both treatment groups, a combined statistical analysis model was used. This model takes into account differences between the treatment groups at T0 as well as post-treatment at T1. The effects of time (i.e., T0 or T1), treatment, and their 2-way interaction on the various outcome parameters were measured (viz., histology, CIBDAI, TGF-β+, CD3+, and FoxP3+ cells). Dog was modeled as a random effect to account for repeated measures (before and after treatment) for individual dogs; time, treatment, and their 2-way interaction were modeled as fixed, categorical variables. Datasets for TGF-β and FoxP3+ were log_{10}-transformed to meet distributional assumptions underlying the statistical modeling. Confidence intervals (CIs) were estimated using maximum likelihood methods. The correlation structure for mixed-effects modeling was that of compound symmetry. Model fit was assessed visually by examining plots of standardized residuals versus fitted values, and by examining the AIC and BIC values for models. A significance level of P<0.05 was used for all analyses (S-PLUS, Version 8.2, TIBCO, Inc., Palo Alto, CA, USA). Changes in plasma citrulline concentrations were compared in the D-VSL#3 group between T0 and T1 using a Wilcoxon matched pairs test. The expression of AJC molecules expression (claudin-2, occludin, and E-cadherin) were compared at T1 between the dogs in the D-VSL#3, the D-CT, and the ED group using a Kruskal-Wallis-Test. The microbiota data obtained by qPCR were compared between healthy dogs and both treatment groups at T0 using an ANOVA or Kruskal-Wallis test where appropriate after evaluating for normal distribution using the Kolmogorov–Smirnov test. Changes in bacterial groups between T0 and T1 were compared using Wilcoxon matched pairs tests. Resulting P-values were corrected for multiple comparisons using the false discovery rate as described by Benjamini & Hochberg, and a P<0.05 was considered significant [9].

Results

Table 1 summarizes the signalment of the dogs enrolled into the study. No significant differences for age, sex, or body weights were identified (P>0.05 for each) between the dog groups. Table 3 and Figure 1 summarize the changes in histology scores, CIBDAI, and TGF-β+, FoxP3+, and CD3+ T-cell expression in both treatment groups.

Histology scores

Although there was a residual inflammatory infiltrate present (Figure 2), histology scores were significantly (P<0.0001) reduced at T1 relative to T0 in both treatment groups (Table 3 and Figure 1). There were no significant differences in the magnitude of this reduction between treatments (P = 0.1452).

CIBDAI

Despite computer randomization, the severity of clinical signs, as judged by the CIBDAI score, was significantly higher at baseline in the D-CT group (median 9, range 7–13) compared to the D-VSL#3 group (median 7, range 5–10; P<0.0001). This was, in part, related to the fact that the all 3 dogs with severe disease were randomly allocated to the D-CT group. Another explanation was the presence of active (versus quiescent) clinical disease at presentation in some dogs. Both groups, however, had overall moderate-to-severe median disease activity at presentation. Clinical scores decreased significantly in both treatment groups over time (P<0.0001). As reported by the owners, recovery was more rapid in the D-CT group compared to the D-VSL#3 group (P = 0.0011). The median time of clinical remission of the main clinical sign (i.e., diarrhea or vomiting) of the dogs in the D-CT group was 4.8 days (range, 2.5 to 7.0 days); while in D-VSL#3 group an improvement was observed in a median of 10.6 days (range, 5.0 to 15.0 days).

TGF-β+

While the TGF-β expression increased significantly in both treatment groups between T0 and T1 (P = 0.0043), the magnitude of this increase was significantly greater for dogs in the D-VSL#3 group than those for the dogs in the D-CT group at Time T1 (P = 0.0008) without any obvious preferential localization throughout the small or large intestine (Figure 1).

CD3+ T-cells

The number of CD3+ lymphocytes was increased in dogs with IBD in both treatment groups at T0 (before treatment), with small or large intestinal involvement depending of intestinal tract involved in the inflammatory process. CD3+ T-cells were significantly (P<0.0001) reduced at T1 relative to T0 in both treatment groups (Figure 1 and 2), and there were no significant differences in the magnitude of this reduction between both treatments (P = 0.7527).

FoxP3+ cells

At T0, there were no significant differences in the number of cells between the two treatment groups (Figure 1). No significant increase in FoxP3+ cells was observed in the D-CT group (P = 0.3296). However, a significant increase in FoxP3+ cells between T0 and T1 (P = 0.0001) was observed in the D-VSL#3 group.

Expression of AJC proteins

Mucosal biopsies were evaluated in both treatment groups at T1 (Figure 3 and 4). Additionally, samples from 3 ED dogs were utilized as controls. Occludin was significantly lower in the D-CT group (P<0.0001) compared to the D-VSL#3 and ED groups. In contrast, Claudin-2 in the large intestine was significantly higher in the D-CT group (P<0.0001; Table 3, Figure 4) compared to the D-VSL#3 and ED groups. No significant differences were observed for the other AJC proteins.

Stain intensity was subjectively graded as absent (−), weak (+), moderate (++), or strong (+++), and the localization and distribution of chromogen was noted. Occludin-specific labeling was most intense at the epithelial cell AJC (Fig. 3), with fainter labeling observed along the basolateral membranes. This staining

Table 3. Summary statistics for evaluated markers.

	VSL#3		CT		ED	
	T0	T1	T0	T1	-	
Histology score	11.5 (7–14)	4 (3–7)	9 (3–14)	3 (0–9)	—	P<0.0001*
CIBDAI score	7 (5–10)	0 (0–2)	9 (7–13)	0 (0–3)	—	P<0.0001*
CD3+ cells[†]	3318 (±447.1)	1204 (±240.4)	3427 (±1813)	845 (±849)	—	P<0.0001*
FoxP3+ cells[†]	26.9 (±26.9)	353.6 (±175.1)	11.1 (±9.5)	51.5 (±32.2)	—	P = 0.0001**
TGF-β+ cells[†]	35.4 (±30.3)	791.8 (±771.9)	32.6 (±21.8)	136.7 (±122)	—	P = 0.0043*
Citrulline (μg/ml)	3.46 (±1.82)	4.66 (±2.34)	—	—	—	P = 0.0113
E-caderin[†]	—	4767 (±2288)	—	4735 (±1319)	4877 (±971)	P = 0.9467
Occludin[†]	—	4523 (±1366)	—	814 (±387)	6511 (±1239)	P<0.0001
Claudin-2 (SI) [†]	—	4274 (±1201)	—	4421 (±1293)	4994 (±1183)	P = 0.7944
Claudin-2 (LI) [†]	—	525 (±264)	—	5771 (±1588)	680 (±305)	P<0.0001

Numerical data are expressed as median (range) for histology and CIBDAI and as mean (± SD) for remaining data.
*significant differences between T0 and T1 in both treatment groups.
**significant differences between T0 and T1 for the VSL#3 group only.
[†]cells per 62,500 μm².

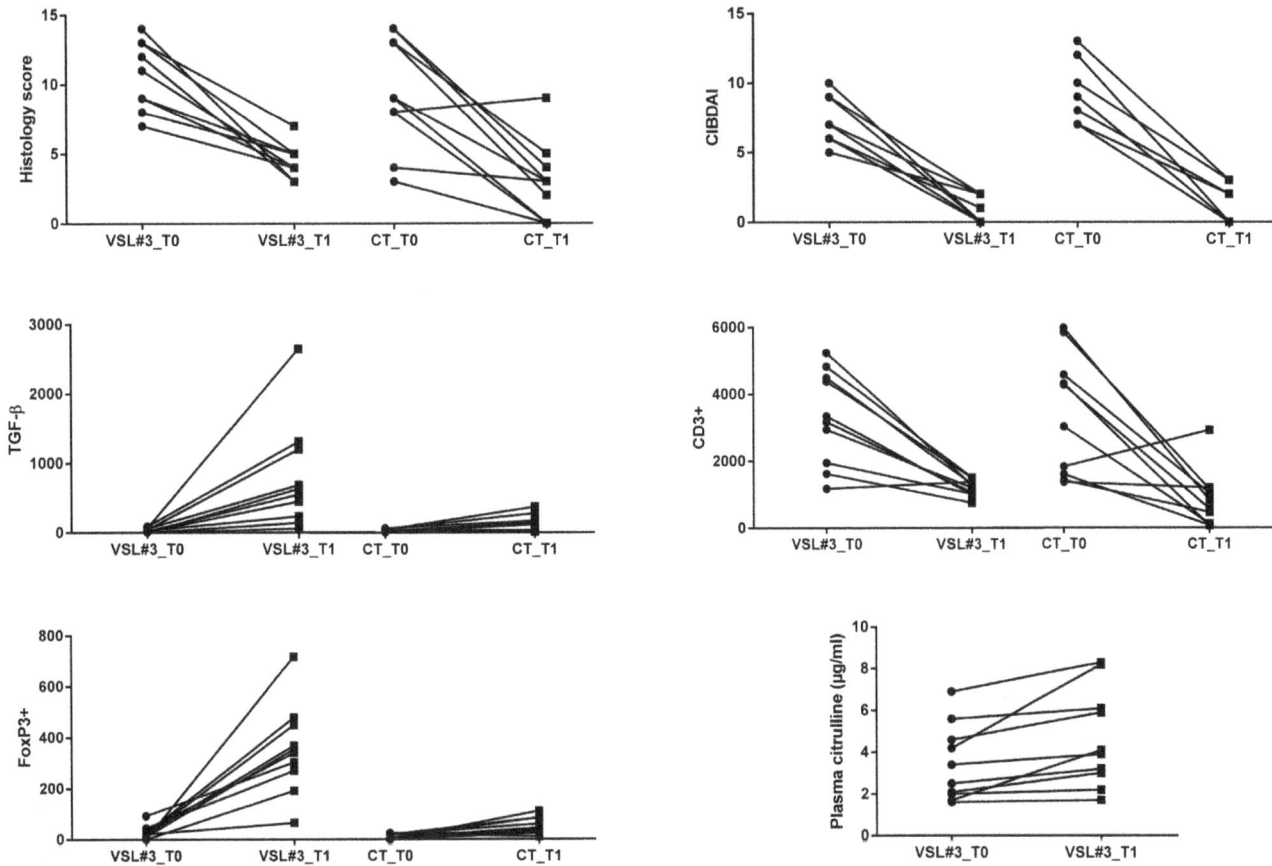

Figure 1. Results for histology scores, CIBDAI, CD3+ cells, FoxP3+ cells, TGF-β cells, and plasma citrulline concentrations. Significant differences between baseline (T0) and 30 days after the end of therapy (T1) were observed for all parameters in both treatment groups except the expression of FoxP3+ T-cells in the CT group (P = 0.3296). While TGF-β increased significantly in both treatment groups, the magnitude of the increase was significantly higher in dogs treated with VSL#3 (P = 0.0008). Data for CD3+ cells, FoxP3+ cells, TGF-β cells expressed as cells per 62,500 μm².

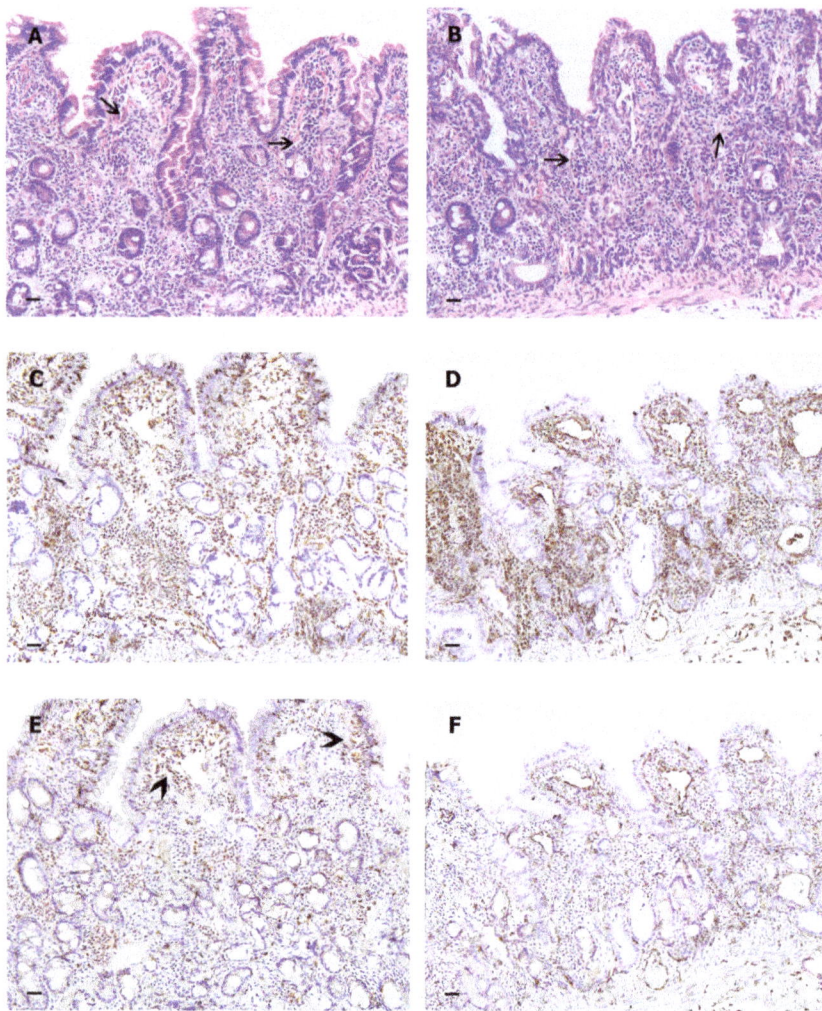

Figure 2. Histology of intestinal mucosa of dogs with IBD after treatment with VSL#3 (A, C, E) and CT (B, D, F). A residual inflammatory infiltrate with lymphocytic-plasmacytic cells (arrows) is evident after the therapy in both samples (H&E, 40X). In both treatment groups ssimilar patterns of mucosal infiltrations with CD3+ T-lymphocytes are evident (C and D). Infiltration with Fox-P3+ cells are proportionally increased in a sample belonging to a VSL#3 treated dog (E) compared to the sample from CT treated dog (F). Note the particular Fox-P3+ T-cells concentrations at the apical portion of villi in the VSL#3 treated dog (E) (arrow-heads) (IHC, ABC method, Harris haematoxylin nuclear counterstain, 40X).

appeared to be uniformly expressed throughout the epithelium of both ED and D-VSL#3 groups. On the contrary, weak to absent expression was observed in the luminal epithelium and in the small intestinal glands of some dogs in the D-CT group. No discernible difference in the distribution or staining intensity of E-cadherin was observed between normal and affected dogs; as, the overall intensity of E-cadherin expression decreased from the luminal epithelium to the distal crypts. At the luminal epithelium, labeling was uniform along the length of the intercellular junction, while the expression was becoming polarized toward the AJC in the distal glands/crypts. E-cadherin-specific labeling was restricted to the AJC and basolateral membranes of intestinal epithelial cells. Moreover, there was little evidence of specific labeling outside the epithelium. In ED and D-VSL#3 groups, claudin-2 was readily detectable in the duodenal epithelium and glands and in colonic crypt epithelium. Immunostaining decreased in intensity from the distal to the proximal crypt and was minimally detectable at the luminal surface of the colon. Claudin-2-specific labeling was largely restricted to the epithelial cell AJC, with some punctate basolateral labeling noted. However, claudin-2 expression was increased in the proximal crypt and luminal epithelium in all CT dogs.

Citrulline

Plasma citrulline concentrations increased significantly in dogs in the D-VSL#3 group between T0 and T1 (P = 0.0113; Figure 1 and Table 3).

Microbiota analysis

The qPCR results (Figure 5) showed that at T0 dogs with IBD (in both treatment groups) had significantly decreased abundance of *Faecalibacterium* spp. (p = 0.008) and *Turicibacter* spp. (p = 0.0078) when compared to healthy dogs. No other bacterial groups evaluated were significantly different compared to the healthy dogs. The qPCR analysis, revealed that the abundance of *Faecalibacterium* spp. increased significantly in the D-VSL#3 group (T1 vs T0; p = 0.03) but not in the D-CT group (T1. vs. T0; p = 0.46). No significant changes were observed for any other bacterial groups in response to treatment.

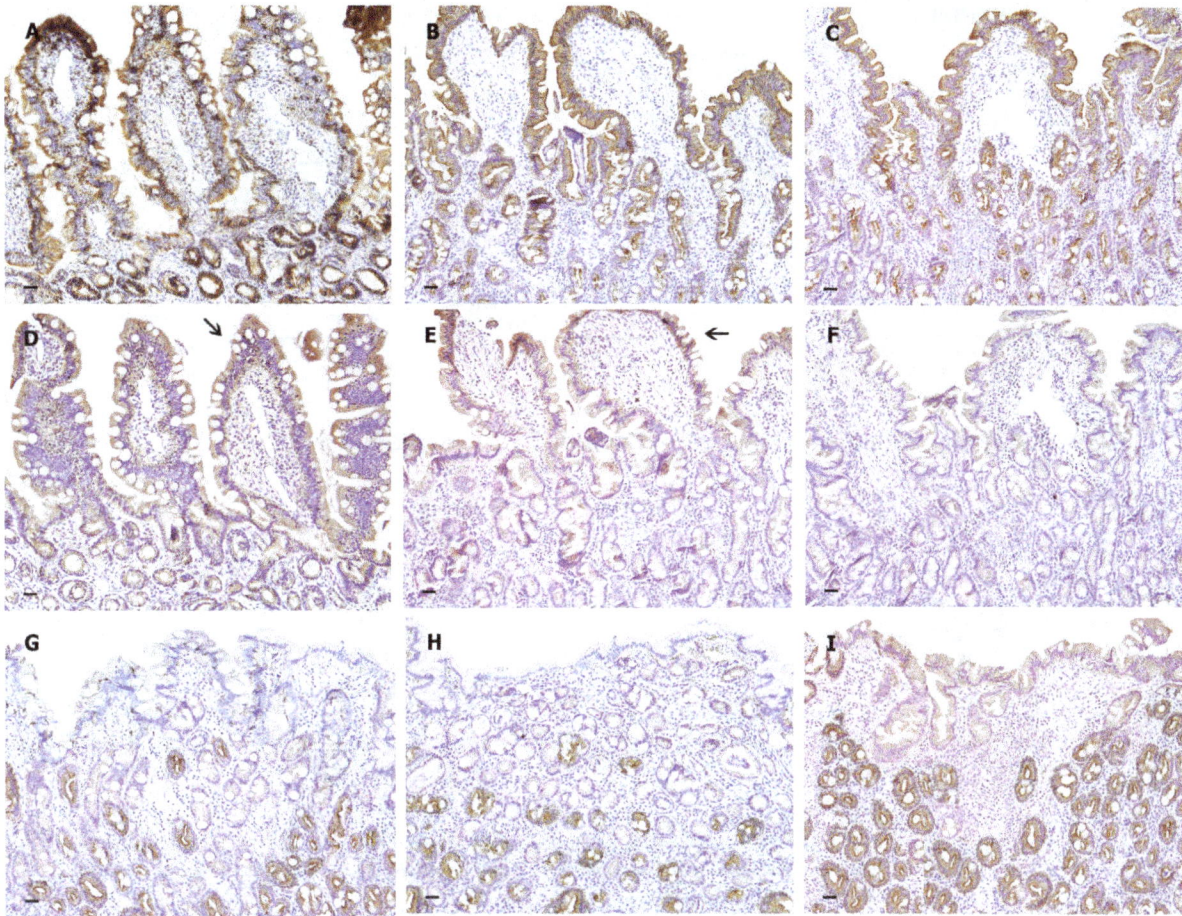

Figure 3. Expression of AJC proteins in the intestinal mucosa of control dogs (ED group) (A, D, G) and dogs treated with VSL#3 (B, E, H) or CT (C, F, I). No discernible differences in the distribution or staining intensity of E-cadherin are observed between normal mucosa (A) and IBD samples (B and C); the overall intensity of E-cadherin staining decreased from the luminal epithelium to the distal crypts. Occludin-specific labelling is most intense at the epithelial cell AJC (arrows) of the luminal epithelium covering the apical portion of villi in ED (D) and VSL#3 (E); a weak to absent expression is observed in the luminal epithelium and in some intestinal glands of the small intestine of the CT sample (F). In colonic samples belonging to ED (G) and VSL#3 (H) groups, claudin-2 is readily detectable only in the colonic crypt epithelium, decreasing in intensity from the distal to the proximal crypt and becoming barely detectable at the luminal surface of the colon. In contrast, claudin-2 expression is increased in the proximal crypt and luminal epithelium of all samples from CT dogs (I).

Discussion

In this study, 20 dogs with long standing IBD were randomized to receive either a probiotic containing VSL#3 strains (SIVOY) or a combination therapy of prednisone and metronidazole. Using a statistical analysis that takes into account differences between the treatment groups at enrollment (T0) as well as post-treatment (T1), we observed differences in some of the evaluated variables depending on the treatment regimen. Histology scores, CIBDAI, and infiltration with mucosal CD3+ T-cells decreased significantly in both treatment groups, and there was no significant effect between the two treatments. FoxP3+ T-cells increased in dogs treated with VSL#3 but not in the D-CT group. While TGF-β+ cells increased significantly in both treatment groups, the magnitude of the increase was significantly greater in dogs treated with VSL#3. The expression of occludin and claudin-2 was also significantly different between dogs treated with probiotic VSL#3 compared to combination therapy.

Although the etiology of canine IBD is poorly understood, there is evidence from clinical observations, studies in humans, and animal models to incriminate the intestinal microbiota as one

factor influencing aberrant host responses. Evidence for the role of enteric microbiota in the pathogenesis of IBD in humans is supported by clinical responses to fecal stream diversion in patients with Crohn's disease (CD) and antimicrobial therapy in both CD and ulcerative colitis (UC) patients [3,10]. Furthermore, genetic mutations in NOD2/CARD15 and TLR-4 (Toll-like-receptor-4) in IBD patients make them less able to respond to bacterial components, resulting in defective innate immune responses to enteric microbiota [24]. Dietary factors also appear to play a role in mediating mucosal inflammation in dogs based on the beneficial clinical response to elimination or "hypoallergenic" diets in many of these animals [16]. All 20 patients enrolled in this study were diagnosed as having long-standing idiopathic IBD, and in the past had undergone unsuccessful dietary trials (e.g., elimination diets to exclude adverse food events). During the study period, all dogs remained on their pre-trial diets, and no dietary changes were performed as part of the here presented study. These diets were similar in nutritional composition across both treatment groups. In the D-VSL#3 group, 4 dogs were on an Adult Dry Maintenance Diet, 4 dogs were on a novel protein diet, and 2 dogs were on an elimination diet. The dogs in the D-CT group had a similar diet

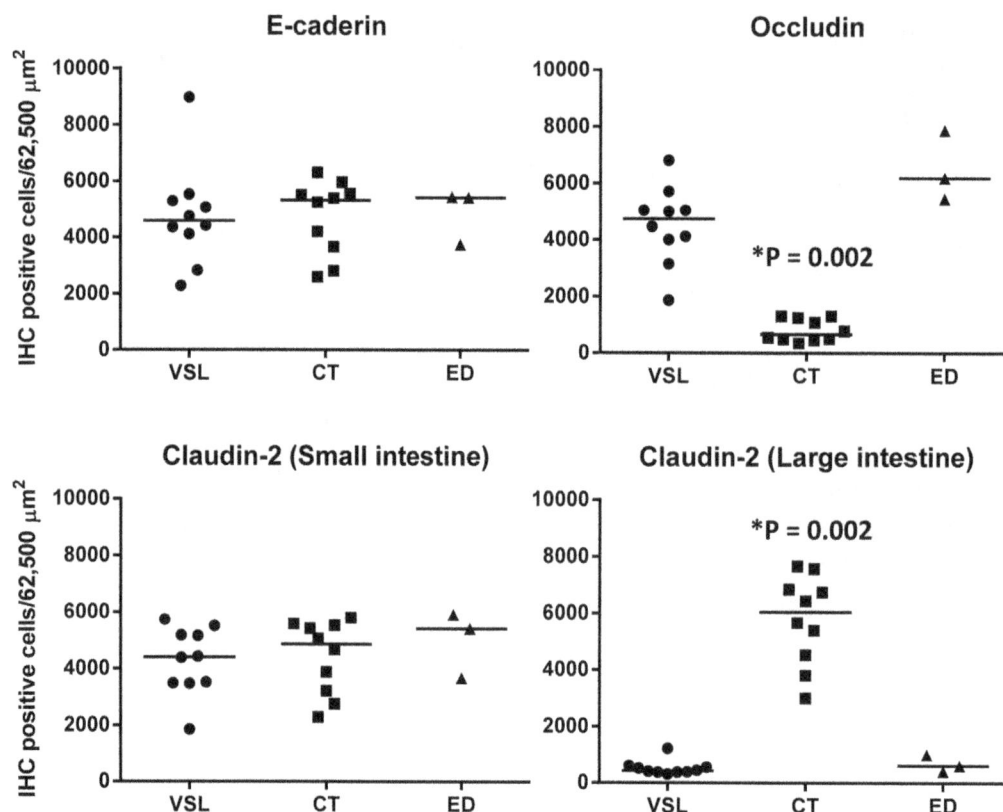

Figure 4. Expression of AJC proteins. Mucosal biopsies were evaluated after the end of treatment (T1) either with the probiotic (VSL) or combination drug therapy (CT), and compared to archived mucosal samples from dogs euthanized for non-gastrointestinal disorders (ED). (*significantly different to the other 2 groups; line denotes median).

distribution, with 4 dogs receiving an Adult Dry Maintenance Diet, 5 dogs receiving a novel protein diet, and 1 dog receiving an elimination diet. Therefore, it is unlikely that the diets were a significant confounding factor in this study since they were broadly similar in both treatment groups.

Probiotic therapy is becoming increasingly popular in veterinary medicine, and has been recommended for the treatment or prevention of a variety of gastrointestinal disorders. However, few objective studies attesting clinical efficacy of probiotics for gastroenteritis are available. The administration of probiotics to dogs with IBD represents warrants further investigation. It has been demonstrated that colitis in both humans and mice is associated with increased levels of cytokines such as TNF-α, IL-6, IL-12p70 and IL-23 [25,26]. Thus, a proper selection of probiotic strains for the treatment of IBD is crucial and should be based on their potential ability to induce an anti-inflammatory pattern of cytokines (IL- 10^{high}, TGF-β^{high}, IL-12p70^{low}, IL-23^{low}, TNF-α^{low}) and attenuate intestinal inflammation. Apart from their immunomodulatory effects, it has been suggested that probiotics have an effect on the gut microbiome by their antimicrobial activities directed toward intestinal pathogens [3]. In humans, VSL#3 showed efficacy for maintenance of remission of ulcerative colitis [14]. To our knowledge, this is the first study to investigate the microbiological, histological, and immunomodulatory effects of VSL#3 in dogs with IBD and to compare these effects to a commonly used combination therapy with prednisone and metronidazole.

Based on qPCR analysis, only the bacterial genera *Faecalibacterium* and *Turicibacter* were found to be significantly decreased in dogs

with IBD at baseline relative to healthy dogs. These results are consistent with recent findings [9], where *Faecalibacterium* was also the predominant bacterial group decreased in fecal samples of dogs with IBD. *Faecalibacterium prausnitzii* is also consistently decreased in human IBD patients and considered an important bacterial group for maintaining microbial homeostasis [27]. A suggested direct immunomodulatory mechanism of action of *F. prausnitzii* is the secretion of metabolites with anti-inflammatory effects, due to blocking NF-κB activation and IL-8 production [27]. In contrast to previous findings, Fusobacteria were not significantly different in dogs with IBD relative to healthy dogs in the current study [9]. Neither treatment with VSL#3 nor with conventional therapy led to major changes in the overall microbial abundance of bacterial phyla (Bacteroidetes, Firmicutes, Fusobacteria) as assessed 30 days following discontinuation of treatment (at T1). Figure 5 illustrates that there were no significant luminal increases in the administered probiotic genera (i.e., *Bifidobacterium*, *Lactobacillus*, and *Streptococcus*) in dogs receiving VSL#3. This is in line with some studies demonstrating that the administration of probiotics do appear to have only minor and transient detectable effects on fecal microbial communities as assessed by qPCR assays or sequencing of 16S rRNA genes [23,28,29]. In the VSL#3 group, however, *Faecalibacterium* spp. increased significantly after treatment, although a trend for an increase in this bacterial group was also observed in the CT group. These results are in line with a previous study, in which *Faecalibacterium* increased after 4 months of conventional treatment in dogs with IBD and this increase correlated with the improvement in clinical disease activity [9]. This would suggest that the significant increase in fecal

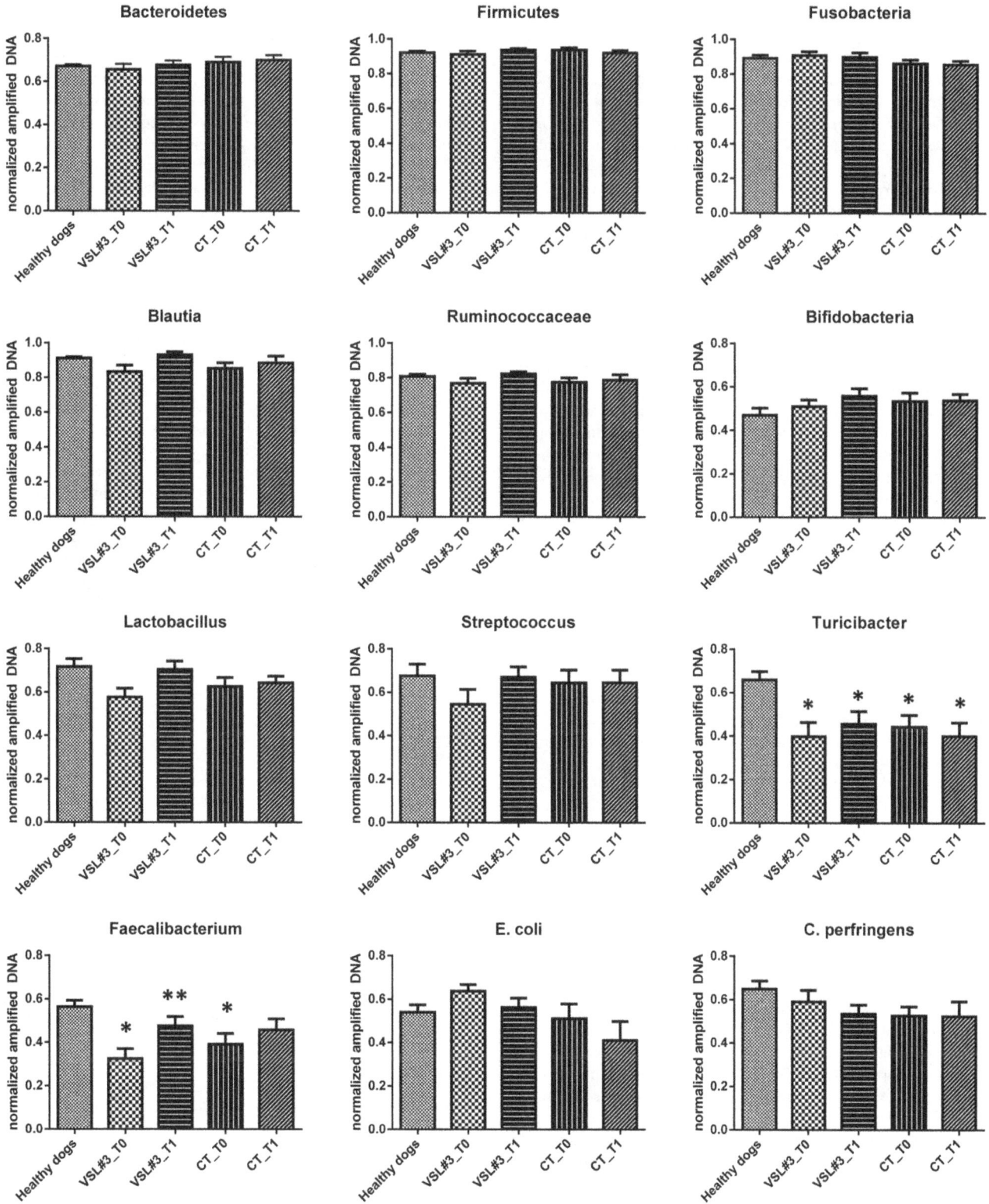

Figure 5. Results of quantitative PCR assays for selected bacterial groups. Dogs with IBD (in both treatment groups) had significantly decreased abundance of *Faecalibacterium* spp. (p = 0.008) and *Turicibacter* spp. (p = 0.0078) compared to the healthy dogs. *Faecalibacterium* spp. increased significantly in the VSL#3 treated dogs at T1 but not in the CT group. (*significantly different compared to healthy dogs; **significantly different after treatment compared to pre-treatment).

Faecalibacterium is not necessarily specific for the probiotic treatment, but may be a general indicator for normalization of fecal dysbiosis after long-term therapy. The *Faecalibacterium–Subdoligranulum* group is a major bacterial group in the canine gastrointestinal tract, comprising 16% of total bacterial counts in feces of healthy dogs and is believed to be of importance in canine gastrointestinal health [30]. Therefore, more-in depth studies evaluating the functional properties of canine *Faecalibacterium* strains are warranted. Some limitation of the microbiota analysis performed in this study need to be noted. Analyzing the fecal microbiota using sequencing of 16S rRNA genes may have revealed potential changes either in microbial diversity indices or in bacterial groups that were not covered by our qPCR assays. For technical reasons, a sequencing approach was not possible in this study. However, we have utilized qPCR assays targeting the microbiota on various phylogenetic levels and also targeting bacterial groups that are major bacterial groups in the canine intestine and that have been shown to be important in canine IBD [9]. Furthermore, in the current study, only fecal samples were analyzed, and the potential impact of treatment on the composition of the small intestinal mucosa-associated microbiota may have been missed. Previous studies have revealed that dogs with IBD have significant differences in small intestinal microbiota compared to controls, and future studies should evaluate the effect of probiotics on the small intestinal microbiota of these dogs [8]. Also, in this study we assessed the fecal microbiota 30 days after the discontinuation of therapy, and it is possible that a transient change in the fecal microbiota during the administration period may have remained undetected and/or changed during the 30 days post-treatment.

It has been speculated that IBD is associated with a loss of intestinal barrier function, as multiple genes encoding for proteins responsible for maintenance of intestinal barrier function (i.e., those encoding for claudin-8, metallothionein, and matrix metalloproteinases) were down-regulated in dogs with IBD in a previous study [31]. The observation that the expression and distribution of occludin and claudin-2 in the large intestine were not significantly different between dogs treated with VSL#3 and the non-IBD control dogs (ED group), but were significantly different compared to the D-CT group, suggests potential effects of VSL#3 on intestinal barrier function, warranting further studies [32]. Similar changes in the distribution of claudin-2 expression have been observed in humans with active UC, where claudin-2 was detected at the surface epithelium [33]. Similarly, down regulation of occludin has been observed in the intestinal mucosa of patients with both UC and CD [34]. Here we compared the expression patterns of AJC proteins between healthy dogs (euthanized dogs; group ED) and dogs with IBD after the two different types of treatment (VSL # 3 or CT treated dogs). The expression pattern of AJC proteins in the ED group was similar to that described by Ohta *et al.* in healthy dogs [35]. In contrast, based on our results it seems that dogs in the CT-group had a greater deviation from the physiological conditions in expression of Claudin-2 in the colon. This particular expression pattern resembles that observed in samples from the colon of dogs with colitis [21]. While we cannot conclusively state that there was an improvement in the expression pattern after probiotic treatment, as samples were not evaluated at T0, we speculate that the expression pattern of AJC proteins in dogs treated with VSL#3 appears to resembles more the physiological state as observed in healthy dogs [35]. Future studies are warranted to confirm this observation. At this point it remains also unclear why claudin-2 is increased in the large intestine of dogs treated with drug therapy,

and further work is needed to elucidate the mechanism behind this increased expression of claudin-2.

Dogs treated with VSL#3 showed significantly increased plasma citrulline concentrations 30 days after end of administration, suggesting restitution of the mucosal barrier. Plasma citrulline concentrations are a marker of global enterocyte mass in humans, rodents, and pigs [36], and have recently been shown to reflect intestinal mucosal recovery in response to severe injury in dogs [37]. Unfortunately, we were able to statistically evaluate the blood levels of citrulline only in the D-VSL#3 group, as plasma citrulline concentrations were not available for all dogs in the D-CT group. Because of the small samples size in the D-CT group, we decided not to perform any statistical analysis to compare plasma citrulline concentrations between treatments. Therefore, it is currently unknown whether the observed increase in plasma citrulline concentrations was specific for the treatment with VSL#3 strains, or would also be present in dogs treated with conventional therapy.

The immunohistochemical results showed cross-reactivity for canine tissues of all antibodies used in this study. This is in line with results from previous studies which have shown that these antibodies are useful for immunohistochemical assessment of canine tissues. In particular, cross-reactivity of the rat anti-human CD3 antigen, clone MCA1477, for canine CD3 positive T-lymphocytes has been shown previously on gastric tissue of dogs [20]. Cross-reactivity of the clone FJK-16s used to stain canine FoxP3-lymphocytes has been reported in another study [38]. Similarly, other authors have successfully used the monoclonal antibody against TGF-β positive dog lymphocytes (clone 1D11) [39]. Finally, the specificities of the antibodies used for canine AJC proteins (i.e., pAb anti-claudin-2 (PAD: MH44), anti-occludin (PAD: Z-T22), and mAb anti-E-cadherin (IgG2α, clone: 36) were, similarly to our study, also reported on sections of intestinal tissue in dogs with IBD [21].

The evaluation of immunomorphological variables suggests a potential anti-inflammatory effect of VSL#3 strains, as decreased mucosal CD3+ T-lymphocytes, and increased FoxP3+ and TGF-β+ positive cells were observed 30 days after the end of administration. Immunohistochemistry results showed a difference in the predominant immunophenotype of infiltrating cells in intestinal lamina propria of biopsies from VSL#3 treated dogs. More specifically, the VSL#3 treated dogs showed increases in CD3+/FoxP3+ cells (Figure 2) in the intestinal mucosa, while dogs treated with prednisone and metronidazole displayed an overall decrease in all inflammatory cell populations that was accompanied by a decrease of FoxP3+ lymphocytes and TGF-β expressing cells (Figure 2). These findings are consistent with a previous study in a mouse model, where VSL#3 also led to increased FoxP3+ expressing T-cells in intestinal lymphoid follicles [40]. In clinical studies with human IBD patients as well as studies on rodent models of IBD, VSL#3 has shown various other anti-inflammatory mechanisms. For example, VSL#3 was shown to induce heat-shock-proteins in intestinal epithelial cells (IEC) [41] or enhance proliferation of IL-10-dependent TGF-β-bearing regulatory T-cells in Th1-dependent murine colitis [42]. These variables have not been examined in the current study, and it would be useful to evaluate these markers in future clinical studies. Furthermore, qPCR quantification of both pro-inflammatory (i.e., TNF-α, IL1-β, IL-8) as well as regulatory genes (FoxP3, IL-10) would have been useful to perform since canine probes have already been published [43] and these studies showed increases in IL-8 in colorectal inflammation [44].

As limitations to this study it should be noted that only a small number of dogs was evaluated, and the power to detect differences in some of the evaluated variables may have been insufficient to detect differences between treatment groups. Furthermore, this was an open-label study and no placebo group was included. Ideally, the clinical effect of the treatment with probiotic strains should be evaluated in a double-blinded placebo controlled trial and compared to a non-treated group. However, in the case of chronic IBD, it is difficult to enroll a non-treated group as these dogs show chronic signs of disease, and therefore we chose in this study to compare the effects of VSL#3 strains to the commonly used combination therapy with prednisone and metronidazole. Our study results suggest that probiotic treatment induces differential anti-inflammatory immune responses when compared

to routine combination therapy as evidenced by significant increases in FoxP3+ cells and a significantly larger increase in TGF-β. The findings lay the foundation for future larger scale placebo controlled clinical studies to evaluate clinical benefits of probiotic VSL#3 strains in the treatment of dogs with IBD.

Author Contributions

Conceived and designed the experiments: GR GP AEJ JSS. Performed the experiments: GR GP MC APP JSS. Analyzed the data: GR NDC AEJ JMS JSS. Contributed reagents/materials/analysis tools: GR GP MC APP. Wrote the paper: GR JMS NDC AEJ JSS.

References

1. Suchodolski JS (2011) Companion animals symposium: Microbes and gastrointestinal health of dogs and cats. J Anim Sci 89: 1520–1530.
2. Allenspach K, House A, Smith K, McNeill FM, Hendricks A, et al. (2010) Evaluation of mucosal bacteria and histopathology, clinical disease activity and expression of Toll-like receptors in German shepherd dogs with chronic enteropathies. Vet Microbiol 146: 326–335.
3. Rioux KP, Madsen KL, Fedorak RN (2005) The role of enteric microflora in inflammatory bowel disease: Human and animal studies with probiotics and prebiotics. Gastroenterol Clin North Am 34: 465–482.
4. Contractor NV, Bassiri H, Reya T, Park AY, Baumgart DC, et al. (1998) Lymphoid hyperplasia, autoimmunity, and compromised intestinal intraepithelial lymphocyte development in colitis-free gnotobiotic IL-2-deficient mice. J Immunol 160: 385–394.
5. Sellon RK, Tonkonogy S, Schultz M, Dieleman LA, Grenther W, et al. (1998) Resident enteric bacteria are necessary for development of spontaneous colitis and immune system activation in interleukin-10-deficient mice. Infect Immun 66: 5224–5231.
6. Xenoulis PG, Palculict B, Allenspach K, Steiner JM, Van House AM, et al. (2008) Molecular-phylogenetic characterization of microbial communities imbalances in the small intestine of dogs with inflammatory bowel disease. FEMS Microbiol Ecol 66: 579–589.
7. Suchodolski JS, Xenoulis PG, Paddock CG, Steiner JM, Jergens AE (2010) Molecular analysis of the bacterial microbiota in duodenal biopsies from dogs with idiopathic inflammatory bowel disease. Vet Microbiol 142: 394–400.
8. Suchodolski JS, Dowd SE, Wilke V, Steiner JM, Jergens AE (2012) 16S rRNA Gene Pyrosequencing Reveals Bacterial Dysbiosis in the Duodenum of Dogs with Idiopathic Inflammatory Bowel Disease. Plos ONE 7: e39333.
9. Suchodolski JS, Markel ME, Garcia-Mazcorro JF, Unterer S, Heilmann RM, et al. (2012) The fecal microbiome in dogs with acute diarrhea and idiopathic inflammatory bowel disease. Plos ONE 7: e51907.
10. Sutherland L, Singleton J, Sessions J, Hanauer S, Krawitt E, et al. (1991) Double-Blind, Placebo Controlled Trial of Metronidazole in Crohns-Disease. Gut 32: 1071–1075.
11. Jergens AE, Crandell J, Morrison JA, Deitz K, Pressel M, et al. (2010) Comparison of oral prednisone and prednisone combined with metronidazole for induction therapy of canine inflammatory bowel disease: a randomized-controlled trial. J Vet Intern Med 24: 269–277.
12. Turner D, Levine A, Escher JC, Griffiths AM, Russell RK, et al. (2012) Management of pediatric ulcerative colitis: joint ECCO and ESPGHAN evidence-based consensus guidelines. J Pediatr Gastroenterol Nutr 55: 340–361.
13. Sauter SN, Benyacoub J, Allenspach K, Gaschen F, Ontsouka E, et al. (2006) Effects of probiotic bacteria in dogs with food responsive diarrhoea treated with an elimination diet. J Anim Physiol Anim Nutr (Berl) 90: 269–277.
14. Bibiloni R, Fedorak RN, Tannock GW, Madsen KL, Gionchetti P, et al. (2005) VSL#3 probiotic-mixture induces remission in patients with active ulcerative colitis. Am J Gastroenterol 100: 1539–1546.
15. Tursi A, Brandimarte G, Papa A, Giglio A, Elisei W, et al. (2010) Treatment of Relapsing Mild-to-Moderate Ulcerative Colitis With the Probiotic VSL#3 as Adjunctive to a Standard Pharmaceutical Treatment: A Double-Blind, Randomized, Placebo-Controlled Study. Am J Gastroenterol: 2218–2227.
16. Simpson KW, Jergens AE (2011) Pitfalls and progress in the diagnosis and management of canine inflammatory bowel disease. Vet Clin North Am Small Anim Pract 41: 381–398.
17. Jergens AE, Schreiner CA, Frank DE, Niyo Y, Ahrens FE, et al. (2003) A scoring index for disease activity in canine inflammatory bowel disease. J Vet Intern Med 17: 291–297.
18. German AJ, Helps CR, Hall EJ, Day MJ (2000) Cytokine mRNA expression in mucosal biopsies from German Shepherd dogs with small intestinal enteropathies. Dig Dis Sci 45: 7–17.
19. Day MJ, Bilzer T, Mansell J, Wilcock B, Hall EJ, et al. (2008) Histopathological Standards for the Diagnosis of Gastrointestinal Inflammation in Endoscopic Biopsy Samples from the Dog and Cat: A Report from the World Small Animal Veterinary Association Gastrointestinal Standardization Group. J Comp Pathol 138 S1–S43.
20. Rossi G, Fortuna D, Pancotto L, Renzoni G, Taccini E, et al. (2000) Immunohistochemical study of lymphocyte populations infiltrating the gastric mucosa of beagle dogs experimentally infected with Helicobacter pylori. Infect Immun 68: 4769–4772.
21. Ridyard AE, Brown JK, Rhind SM, Else RW, Simpson JW, et al. (2007) Apical junction complex protein expression in the canine colon: differential expression of claudin-2 in the colonic mucosa of dogs with idiopathic colitis. J Histochem Cytochem 55: 1049–1058.
22. Engel AG, Arahata K (1986) Mononuclear cells in myopathies: quantitation of functionally distinct subsets, recognition of antigen-specific cell-mediated cytotoxicity in some diseases, and implications for the pathogenesis of the different inflammatory myopathies. Hum Pathol 17: 704–721.
23. Garcia-Mazcorro JF, Lanerie DJ, Dowd SE, Paddock CG, Grutzner N, et al. (2011) Effect of a multi-species synbiotic formulation on fecal bacterial microbiota of healthy cats and dogs as evaluated by pyrosequencing. FEMS Microbiol Ecol 78: 542–554.
24. Franchimont D, Vermeire S, El Housni H, Pierik M, Van Steen K, et al. (2004) Deficient host-bacteria interactions in inflammatory bowel disease? The toll-like receptor (TLR)-4 Asp299gly polymorphism is associated with Crohn's disease and ulcerative colitis. Gut 53: 987–992.
25. Becker C, Dornhoff H, Neufert C, Fantini MC, Wirtz S, et al. (2006) Cutting edge: IL-23 cross-regulates IL-12 production in T cell-dependent experimental colitis. J Immunol 177: 2760–2764.
26. Fuss IJ, Becker C, Yang Z, Groden C, Hornung RL, et al. (2006) Both IL-12p70 and IL-23 are synthesized during active Crohn's disease and are down-regulated by treatment with anti-IL-12 p40 monoclonal antibody. Inflamm Bowel Dis 12: 9–15.
27. Sokol H, Pigneur B, Watterlot L, Lakhdari O, Bermudez-Humaran LG, et al. (2008) Faecalibacterium prausnitzii is an anti-inflammatory commensal bacterium identified by gut microbiota analysis of Crohn disease patients. PNAS 105: 16731–16736.
28. Vitali B, Ndagijimana M, Cruciani F, Carnevali P, Candela M, et al. (2010) Impact of a synbiotic food on the gut microbial ecology and metabolic profiles. BMC Microbiol 10: 4.
29. Larsen N, Vogensen FK, Gobel R, Michaelsen KF, Abu Al-Soud W, et al. (2011) Predominant genera of fecal microbiota in children with atopic dermatitis are not altered by intake of probiotic bacteria Lactobacillus acidophilus NCFM and Bifidobacterium animalis subsp. lactis Bi-07. FEMS Microbiol Ecol 75: 482–496.
30. Garcia-Mazcorro JF, Dowd SE, Poulsen J, Steiner JM, Suchodolski JS (2012) Abundance and short-term temporal variability of fecal microbiota in healthy dogs. MicrobiologyOpen 1: 340–347.
31. Wilke VL, Nettleton D, Wymore MJ, Gallup JM, Demirkale CY, et al. (2012) Gene expression in intestinal mucosal biopsy specimens obtained from dogs with chronic enteropathy. Am J Vet Res 73: 1219–1229.
32. Madsen K, Cornish A, Soper P, McKaigney C, Jijon H, et al. (2001) Probiotic bacteria enhance murine and human intestinal epithelial barrier function. Gastroenterol 121: 580–591.
33. Prasad S, Mingrino R, Kaukinen K, Hayes KL, Powell RM, et al. (2005) Inflammatory processes have differential effects on claudins 2, 3 and 4 in colonic epithelial cells. Lab Invest 85: 1139–1162.
34. Gassler N, Rohr C, Schneider A, Kartenbeck J, Bach A, et al. (2001) Inflammatory bowel disease is associated with changes of enterocytic junctions. Am J Physiol Gastrointest Liver Physiol 281: G216–228.
35. Ohta H, Yamaguchi T, Rajapakshage BK, Murakami M, Sasaki N, et al. (2011) Expression and subcellular localization of apical junction proteins in canine duodenal and colonic mucosa. Am J Vet Res 72: 1046–1051.
36. Curis E, Nicolis I, Osowska S, Zerrouk N, Benazeth S, et al. (2005) Almost all about citrulline in mammals. Amino Acids 29: 177–205.
37. Dossin O, Rupassara SI, Weng HY, Williams DA, Garlick PJ, et al. (2011) Effect of Parvoviral Enteritis on Plasma Citrulline Concentration in Dogs. J Vet Intern Med 25: 215–221.
38. Pinheiro D, Singh Y, Grant CR, Appleton RC, Sacchini F, et al. (2011) Phenotypic and functional characterization of a CD4(+) CD25(high) FOX-P3(high) regulatory T-cell population in the dog. Immunol 132: 111–122.

39. Colitz CM, Malarkey D, Dykstra MJ, McGahan MC, Davidson MG (2000) Histologic and immunohistochemical characterization of lens capsular plaques in dogs with cataracts. Am J Vet Res 61: 139–143.

40. Bassaganya-Riera J, Viladomiu M, Pedragosa M, De Simone C, Carbo A, et al. (2012) Probiotic bacteria produce conjugated linoleic acid locally in the gut that targets macrophage PPAR gamma to suppress colitis. Plos ONE 7: e31238.

41. Petrof EO, Kojima K, Ropeleski MJ, Musch MW, Tao Y, et al. (2004) Probiotics inhibit nuclear factor-kappaB and induce heat shock proteins in colonic epithelial cells through proteasome inhibition. Gastroenterol 127: 1474–1487.

42. Di Giacinto C, Marinaro M, Sanchez M, Strober W, Boirivant M (2005) Probiotics ameliorate recurrent Th1-mediated murine colitis by inducing IL-10 and IL-10-dependent TGF-beta-bearing regulatory cells. J Immunol 174: 3237–3246.

43. Ohta H, Takada K, Torisu S, Yuki M, Tamura Y, et al. (2013) Expression of CD4+ T cell cytokine genes in the colorectal mucosa of inflammatory colorectal polyps in miniature dachshunds. Vet Immunol Immunopathol 155: 259–263.

44. Tamura Y, Ohta H, Torisu S, Yuki M, Yokoyama N, et al. (2013) Markedly increased expression of interleukin-8 in the colorectal mucosa of inflammatory colorectal polyps in miniature dachshunds. Vet Immunol Immunopathol 156: 32–42.

45. Muhling M, Woolven-Allen J, Murrell JC, Joint I (2008) Improved group-specific PCR primers for denaturing gradient gel electrophoresis analysis of the genetic diversity of complex microbial communities. ISME J 2: 379–392.

46. Malinen E, Rinttila T, Kajander K, Matto J, Kassinen A, et al. (2005) Analysis of the fecal microbiota of irritable bowel syndrome patients and healthy controls with real-time PCR. Am J Gastroenterol 100: 373–382.

47. Garcia-Mazcorro JF, Suchodolski JS, Jones KR, Clark-Price SC, Dowd SE, et al. (2012) Effect of the proton pump inhibitor omeprazole on the gastrointestinal bacterial microbiota of healthy dogs. FEMS Microbiol Ecol 80: 624–636.

48. Wise MG, Siragusa GR (2005) Quantitative detection of Clostridium perfringens in the broiler fowl gastrointestinal tract by real-time PCR. Appl Environ Microbiol 71: 3911–3916.

49. Lubbs DC, Vester BM, Fastinger ND, Swanson KS (2009) Dietary protein concentration affects intestinal microbiota of adult cats: a study using DGGE and qPCR to evaluate differences in microbial populations in the feline gastrointestinal tract. J Anim Physiol Anim Nutr (Berl) 93: 113–121.

50. Rinttila T, Kassinen A, Malinen E, Krogius L, Palva A (2004) Development of an extensive set of 16S rDNA-targeted primers for quantification of pathogenic and indigenous bacteria in faecal samples by real-time PCR. J Appl Microbiol 97: 1166–1177.

51. Furet JP, Quenee P, Tailliez P (2004) Molecular quantification of lactic acid bacteria in fermented milk products using real-time quantitative PCR. Int J Food Microbiol 97: 197–207.

52. Walter J, Hertel C, Tannock GW, Lis CM, Munro K, et al. (2001) Detection of Lactobacillus, Pediococcus, Leuconostoc, and Weissella species in human feces by using group-specific PCR primers and denaturing gradient gel electrophoresis. Appl Environ Microbiol 67: 2578–2585.

53. Heilig HG, Zoetendal EG, Vaughan EE, Marteau P, Akkermans AD, et al. (2002) Molecular diversity of Lactobacillus spp. and other lactic acid bacteria in the human intestine as determined by specific amplification of 16S ribosomal DNA. Appl Environ Microbiol 68: 114–123.

20

Mucosal Healing did not Predict Sustained Clinical Remission in Patients with IBD after Discontinuation of One-Year Infliximab Therapy

Cong Dai, Wei-Xin Liu, Min Jiang, Ming-Jun Sun*

Department of Gastroenterology, First Affiliated Hospital, China Medical University, Shenyang City, Liaoning Province, China

Abstract

Aim: To assess the endoscopic activity and Clinical activity after a one-year period of infliximab therapy and to evaluate the association between mucosal healing and need for retreatment after stopping infliximab in patients with Inflammatory bowel disease (IBD).

Methods: The data from 109 patients with Crohn's disease (CD) and 107 patients with Ulcerative colitis (UC) received one-year infliximab were assessed. The primary endpoint of the study was the proportion of clinical remission, mucosal healing and full remission in IBD after the one-year period of maintenance infliximab therapy. The secondary endpoint was the frequency of relapses in the next year.

Results: A total of 84.4% (92/109) CD patients and 81.3% (87/107) UC patients achieved clinical remission, 71.56% (78/109) of CD patients and 69.16% (74/107) of UC patients achieved mucosal healing, 56.88% (62/109) of CD patients and 54.21% (58/107) of UC patients achieved full remission at the end of the year of infliximab therapy. Infliximab therapy was restarted in the 10.19% (22/216) patients (13 CD, 9 UC) who achieved mucosal healing, and 13.89% (30/216) patients (18 CD, 12 UC) who achieved clinical remission and 6.48% (14/216) patients (8 CD, 6 UC) who achieved full remission had to be retreated within the next year. Neither clinical remission nor mucosal healing was associated with the time to restarting Infliximab therapy in IBD.

Conclusion: Mucosal healing did not predict sustained clinical remission in patients with IBD in whom the infliximab therapies had been stopped. And stopping or continuing infliximab therapy may be determined by assessing the IBD patient's general condition and the clinical activity.

Editor: Mathias Chamaillard, INSERM, France

Funding: The authors have no support or funding to report.

Competing Interests: The authors have declared that no competing interests exist.

* Email: 273159833@qq.com

Introduction

Inflammatory bowel disease (IBD) is a chronic recurrent disease, which mainly consists of ulcerative colitis (UC) and Crohn's disease (CD) [1]. And it is a growing worldwide health burden especially in many developing countries. Although not completely defined, the aetiopathology of IBD is thought to be a consequence of immune dysregulation, impaired mucosal integrity, enteric bacterial dysbiosis and genetic susceptibility factors [2,3,4]. The aims of treatment in IBD are to induce and maintain remission, to improve quality of life and to prevent the development of complications and the need for surgery. Now the pharmaceutical therapies have included corticosteroids, 5-aminosalicylic acids (5-ASAs), immunomodulators such as azathioprine, 6-mercaptopurine (6-MP), methotrexate, and biological therapy such as infliximab, adalimumab [5,6].

Colonoscopies play an important role in the diagnosis, management and monitoring of IBD. Now the most important goals in the treatment of IBD is mucosal healing, because some studies have demonstrated that mucosal healing can alter the course of IBD due to its association with sustained clinical remission and reduced rates of hospitalization and surgery [7]. And mucosal healing at the time of treatment withdrawal may predict better outcomes in IBD [8].

The endoscopy provides a direct evaluation of the mucosal lesions in IBD and intestinal activity may be quantified by indices of endoscopic activity, but a clear definition of mucosal healing is still lacking. Most of the clinical trials define mucosal healing as the total disappearance of mucosal ulcerations. The Simplified Endoscopic Activity Score for Crohn's Disease (SES-CD) is a relatively easy tool to evaluate the endoscopic activity in CD [9], and the Mayo endoscopic score is common indices to evaluate the endoscopic activity in UC [10,11]. The weaknesses of these endoscopic activity indices include the absence of a clear definition and the lack of validation of mucosal healing [12]. At the same time, routine endoscopic follow-up is recommended for all IBD patients who have achieved clinical remission with medical therapy; for those with persistent complaints, in order to rule out post-inflammatory irritable bowel syndrome; for those still within their first year after surgery; and for those who are stopping biological therapies but continuing immunosuppressants [13,14].

The introduction of monoclonal anti-TNF-α drugs revolutionised the management of IBD. Although the precise mechanism of action is unknown, it is thought that anti-TNF-α drugs cause apoptosis of inflammatory cells carrying membrane-bound TNF-α, an important cytokine in the pathogenesis of IBD. And anti-TNF-α drugs have proven their efficacy in inducing and maintaining clinical and endoscopic remission in both CD and UC. For example, Good data exist demonstrating the efficacy of anti-TNF-α drugs for inducing and sustaining remission for patients with moderate to severely CD, with approximately 60% of patients showing overall clinical improvement [15,16]. Long-term data have shown infliximab to be beneficial, in initial responders, over a median follow-up period of 4.6 years [17]. The efficacy of anti-TNF-α drugs in the treatment of UC is less impressive than their effect in CD. The ACT UC Trials were large, multicentre RCTs that compared infliximab with placebo in the treatment of moderate to severe active UC [13]. There was a modest, but significant benefit in clinical improvement over placebo.

According to the Consensus Statement on Diagnoses and Treatment of IBD in China, biological therapies (infliximab approved for the treatment of CD and UC) have to be discontinued after a one-year maintaining clinical remission treatment period. The endoscopic healing of the mucosa is commonly evaluated at the end of the one-year treatment period with biological therapies. In the present study, we want to assess the endoscopic activity and the rate of mucosal healing after a one-year period of infliximab therapy and to evaluate how the endoscopic findings of the mucosa predict the frequency of relapses and the need for restarting infliximab therapy.

Materials and Methods

Study design

This was a prospective observational study conducted in the Department of Gastroenterology, First Affiliated Hospital, China Medical University between January 2010 and December 2013. The study was approved by China Medical University Regional and Institutional Committee of Science and Research Ethics and by the Regional and Institutional Human Medical Biological Research Ethics Committee of China Medical University. All participants have provided their written informed consent to participate in our study. The ethics committees have approved this consent procedure. We have also obtained informed consent from the next of kin, caretakers, or guardians on behalf of the minors/children enrolled in our study.

The analysis focused on patients who underwent an ileocolonoscopy before and after the one-year maintenance infliximab therapy and in whom infliximab therapy were discontinued at the end of the year. Endoscopies were performed by two experienced gastroenterologists after stopping the one-year infliximab therapy.

One hundred and nine CD patients (59 females, 41 males, mean disease duration at the beginning of biological therapy: 6.2 years) and 107 UC patients (59 females, 48 males, mean disease duration at the beginning of biological therapy: 11.4 years) were prospectively followed up in this study. Twelve CD patients (8 females, 4 males, mean disease duration at the beginning of biological therapy: 5.8 years) and 8 UC patients (5 females, 3 males, mean disease duration at the beginning of biological

therapy: 9.9 years) were lost in the follow-up. There was no significant difference about the basic clinical characteristics of patients between included and not included in the study. All patients received maintenance infliximab therapy for one year in accordance with the Consensus Statement on Diagnoses and Treatment of IBD in China. CD disease phenotypes were determined according to the Montreal Classification [18]. These patients received the last dose of infliximab therapy at least 3 month before the repeated one-year therapy. Seventy-three patients were naive to biological therapy (did not receive biological therapy before the one-year treatment period analyzed in the study) in the CD group, and 68 patients in the UC group. The concomitant immunosuppression during the induction therapy was corticosteroids in 100 (CD: 66, UC: 34) and azathioprine in 66 (CD: 45, UC: 21) patients. The clinical characteristics of the patients are presented in Table 1. Patients' data regarding smoking status, previous appendectomy, perianal involvement, presence of extraintestinal manifestation, outcome of induction therapy, previous surgical procedures, and previous biological therapy were collected.

Assessment of clinical and endoscopic remission

Clinical activities, as determined by the Crohn's Disease Activity Index (CDAI) [19] in CD and by the Mayo score [10] in UC, were calculated at the end of infliximab therapy when the endoscopic assessment was performed, while partial Mayo scores were calculated when infliximab therapy needed to be restarted. Clinical remission was defined as a CDAI of <150 points and a Mayo score of <2 points. Sustained clinical remission was defined as a stable, steroid-free clinical remission during the 1-year follow-up period. The definition of relapse and indication for restarting biologicals were an increase of >100 points in CDAI and a CDAI of >150 points and a partial Mayo score of >3 points.

The endoscopic severity of CD was quantified with SES-CD in CD [8] and with Mayo endoscopic subscore in UC [10]. The endoscopic scores were prospectively assessed by two investigators (Min Jiang and Ming-Jun Sun). Mucosal healing was defined using the endoscopic indices as SES-CD between 0 and 3 and Mayo endoscopic subscore as 0.

Endpoints

Data collection and analysis were performed at the Department of Gastroenterology, First Affiliated Hospital, China Medical University. The primary endpoint of the study was the proportion of mucosal healing in IBD after the one-year period of maintenance infliximab therapy. The secondary endpoint was the frequency of relapses in the next year.

Statistical analysis

Variables were tested for normality using Shapiro-Wilk's W test. The χ^2-test and logistic regression analysis were used to assess the association between categorical clinical variables and clinical/endoscopic outcomes. The variables analyzed were gender, disease duration, active smoking, appendectomy, location/extent, behavior, associated perineal disease, extraintestinal manifestations, previous surgery, previous biological therapy, clinical activities, CRP levels, and outcomes of induction therapy. The difference between patients with mucosal healing and those who failed to achieve endoscopic remission was assessed by chi-square or Fisher's exact tests. Kaplan-Meier survival curves were plotted for analysis with the Log-Rank and Breslow tests. For the statistical analysis, SPSS 11.5 was used. And P<0.05 was considered significant.

Mucosal Healing did not Predict Sustained Clinical Remission in Patients with IBD after Discontinuation...

195

Table 1. Demographic and clinical characteristics of patients.

	CD patients (*n*= 109)	UC patients (*n*= 107)
Female/male	68/41	59/48
Mean age at diagnosis (yr)	26 (14–63)	31 (12–57)
Mean age at the beginning of infliximab therapy (yr)	32 (19–64)	42 (15–65)
Age at diagnosis		
<20 years (A1)	15	17
20–40 years (A2)	73	68
>40 years (A3)	21	22
Location		
Ileal (L1)	20	-
Colonic (L2)	31	-
Ileocolonic (L3)	56	-
Upper GI (L4)	2	-
Proctitis	-	0
Left-sided colitis	-	64
Extensive colitis	-	43
Behaviour		
Inflammatory (B1)	53	-
Stricturing (B2)	17	-
Penetrating (B3)	35	-
Perianal manifestation	41	-
Extraintestinal manifestation	39	12
Surgery before infliximab therapy	23	5
Previous biological therapy	17	3
Median CDAI/pMayo at the start of infliximab therapy	328	9.8
Median CRP level at the start of infliximab therapy (mg/l)	13.8	11.2
Current smokers	74	21
Appendectomy	13	1

Results

Clinical activity of IBD after the one-year period of infliximab therapy

The median CDAI was 72 (interquartile range: 36.8–97.5) ($P<$ 0.01) and the partial Mayo score was 1.4 (interquartile range: 0–5.2) ($P<0.01$) at the end of the treatment period. A total of 92/109 patients with CD (84.4%) and 87/107 with UC (81.3%) achieved clinical remission at the end of the year of infliximab therapy.

Endoscopic activity of IBD before and after the one year period of infliximab therapy

Colonoscopies reached the terminal ileum in each patient. The median values of the SES-CD and the Mayo endoscopic subscores significantly improved after infliximab therapy [18 (interquartile range: 11–25) vs 6 (interquartile range: 2–11), $P<0.01$, and 3 (interquartile range: 2–4) vs 1 (interquartile range: 0–3), $P<0.01$]. Mucosal healing was achieved in 71.56% (78/109) of CD patients and 69.16% (74/107) of UC patients. Full remission – both mucosal healing and clinical remission - was achieved in 56.88% (62/109) of CD patients and 54.21% (58/107) of UC patients.

The frequency of relapses in the next year

During the next year follow up period, 13.89% (30/216) of patients (18 CD, 12 UC) in the clinical remission group and 6.48% (14/216) patients (8 CD, 6 UC) in the full remission group had to be retreated. In CD, infliximab therapy was restarted due to clinical relapse in 21.1% (23/109) of patients after a median 4.8 month (interquartile range: 3.2–6.3 month). The median CDAI was 327 (interquartile range: 115–369) at the time of relapse. In UC, infliximab therapy needed to be restarted in 14.02% (15/107) patients after a median 6.7 month (interquartile range: 2.8–9.7 month). The median partial Mayo score was 5.9 (interquartile range: 4.5–7.2) at the time of retreatment. Of note, infliximab therapy was restarted in the 10.19% (22/216) patients (13 CD, 9 UC) who achieved mucosal healing, and 13.89% (30/216) patients (18 CD, 12 UC) who achieved clinical remission and 6.48% (14/216) patients (8 CD, 6 UC) who achieved full remission had to be retreated within the next year. Endoscopic activity was not assessed in each patient when the infliximab therapy was restarted. The response rates for retreatment were 78.26% (18/23) in CD and 66.67% (10/15) in UC within an average of three months after the reintroduction of infliximab therapy.

In a univariate or Kaplan-Meier analysis using the Log-Rank and Breslow tests, neither clinical remission nor mucosal healing was associated with the time to restarting infliximab therapy in either CD (Figure 1) or UC (Figure 2). In univariate analysis or logistic regression analysis, none of the investigated parameters (e.g., gender, disease duration, smoking status, history of appendectomy, location/extent, behavior, extraintestinal manifestations, previous surgery, previous biological therapy, CRP level, or the effect of induction therapy) was associated with the need to restart infliximab therapy in either CD or UC (Table 2).

Discussion

In this prospective observational study conducted in patients with CD and UC receiving infliximab therapy for one year, mucosal healing was observed in 71.56% and 69.16% of the patients, respectively. Full remission, including both clinical and endoscopic remission, was detected in 56.88% and 54.21% of patients with CD and UC. Retreatment with infliximab therapy was necessary in 16.67% (13/78) of CD patients and in 12.16% (9/74) of UC patients, despite their achieving mucosal healing at the end of the year of infliximab therapy. Our results showed that mucosal healing after one year of infliximab treatment was not associated with sustained clinical remission.

Regarding the therapeutic approach of IBD, anti-TNF-α drugs proved to be the most effective in inducing mucosal healing. For example, The ACT trials confirmed the efficacy of infliximab in inducing and maintaining mucosal healing in active UC [20]. And The ACCENT I study confirmed that scheduled infliximab therapy is more effective in achieving mucosal healing than episodic treatment [21] for CD. In our study, infliximab therapy proved to be more effective in achieving mucosal healing in CD than in UC. This result may be due to the difference in the sizes of the inflamed area and the proportion of patients with previous biological therapy in the CD and UC groups. Now mucosal healing is very important for patients with IBD, because it seems to

be associated with better outcomes (reduced rate of complications, surgery and hospitalization) in CD [21,22]. In a Norwegian study, mucosal healing was associated with lower colectomy rate in UC and decreased need for steroid treatment in CD [23]. The STORI trial suggested that one of the most important predictors of relapse was the absence of mucosal healing at the time of drug withdrawal [14]. The study of Baert et al [24] confirmed that complete mucosal healing in patients with early stage CD predicted sustained steroid-free remission 3 and more years. At the same time, Ananthakrishnan have found that mucosal healing as an endpoint is cost effective in CD patients [25].

Now an important question is when mucosal healing should be established. International guidelines recommend assessing endoscopic mucosal healing before stopping the therapy with anti-TNF agents. But our results do not support the guidelines because more than 13.82% of the patients with mucosal healing relapsed and needed retreatment after one-year infliximab therapy. At the same time, there is no established guideline on when anti-TNF agents can be discontinued. Different studies have concluded different views. For example, In the STORI study, infliximab therapy was terminated in 115 CD patients in clinical remission after treatment with scheduled infliximab for at least one year [14]. But Forty-five percent of patients relapsed following withdrawal from infliximab. In a Danish single-center study, 24% of CD patients and 30% of UC patients discontinued infliximab while in clinical steroid-free remission [26]. The proportion of patients in remission declined steadily, with 61% of CD patients and 75% of UC patients remaining in remission after 1 year. Half of these patients maintained their remission after a median of 2 years. In total, 96% of CD patients and 71% of UC patients experienced complete clinical remission when retreated with infliximab after their relapses. In our study, the relapsed rate of the full remission patients was 11.67%, and the response rates for retreatment were

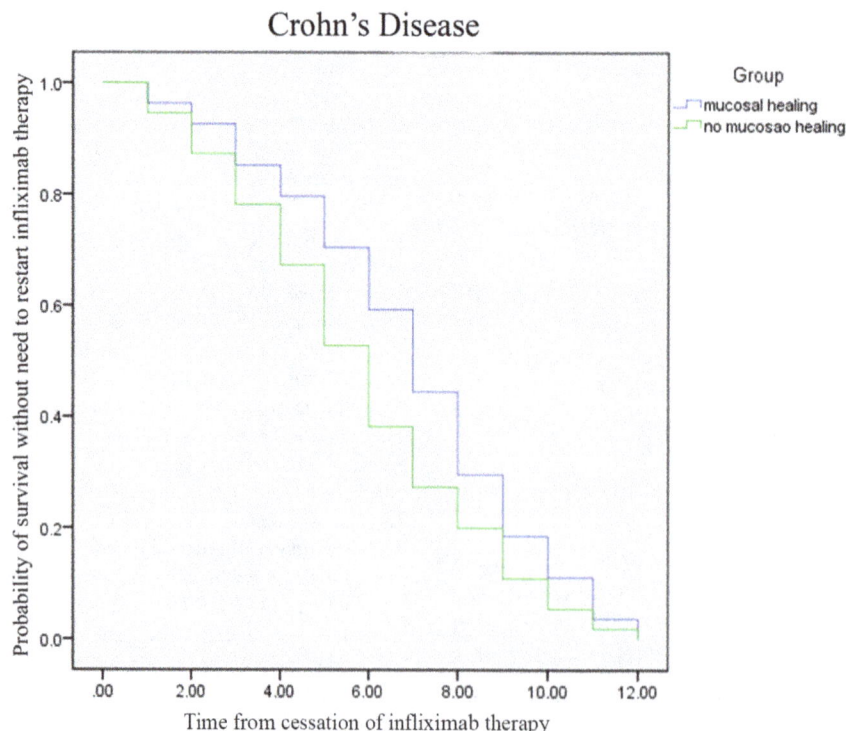

Figure 1. Kaplan-Meier analysis using Log-Rank and Breslow tests (clinical remission or mucosal healing was not associated with the time to restarting infliximab therapy in Crohn's disease).

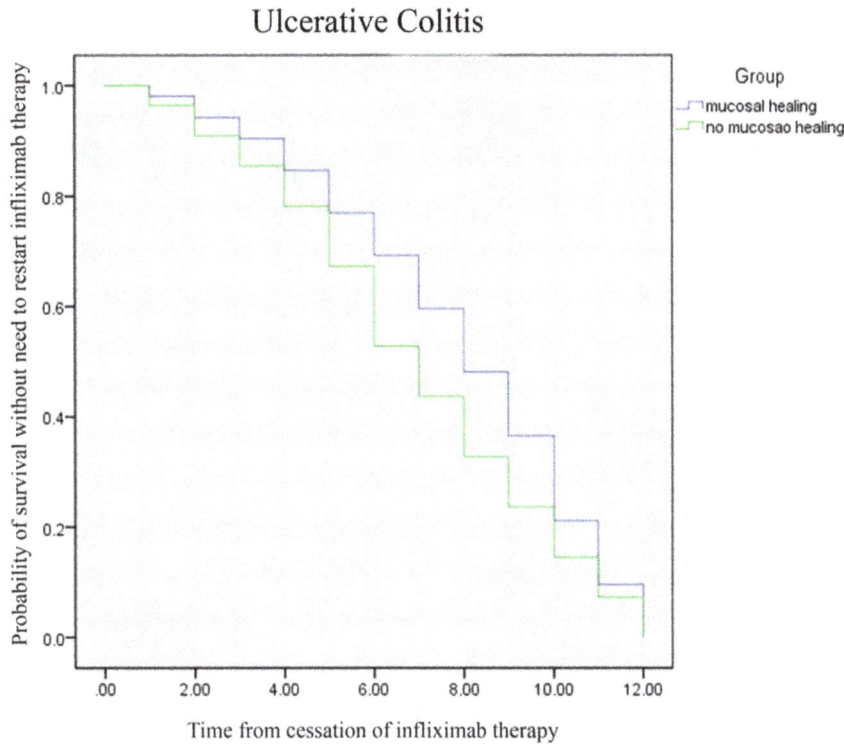

Figure 2. Kaplan-Meier analysis using Log-Rank and Breslow tests (clinical remission or mucosal healing was not associated with the time to restarting infliximab therapy in Ulcerative colitis).

78.26% in CD and 66.67% in UC at the end of the year of infliximab therapy.

There are some limitations in our study. Firstly, biopsy samples were not taken routinely to assess microscopic activity of patients with IBD. Theoretically, the microscopic evaluation of the mucosa reflects the therapeutic response more accurately than an endoscopy, but it should be noted that the histological assessment of biopsy samples demonstrates only mucosal abnormalities. For example, the transmural pattern of CD is difficult to evaluate [27] by biopsy. And Laharie *et al* [28] did not find any correlation between histologically confirmed microscopic inflammation and

endoscopic activity indices in patients with IBD. Therefore, the necessity for microscopic evaluation in the assessment of mucosal healing in IBD may be worthy of further consideration. Secondly, there is no widespread agreement regarding an acceptable definition of mucosal healing. The disappearance of mucosal ulcers and erosions may be used for mucosal healing more frequently in clinical practice. In our study, mucosal healing was evaluated on the basis of endoscopic activity indices. Finally, the sample size of our study is not particularly large, but we think that the tendency of our results is worth considering.

Table 2. Univariate regression analysis of need for retreatment with infliximab therapy.

Factor	CD-P value	UC-P value
Gender	0.87	0.63
Disease duration	0.12	0.15
Smoking status	0.96	0.53
Appendectomy	0.98	-
Location/extent	0.92	0.87
Behaviour	0.98	-
Extraintestinal manifestations	0.37	-
Steroid therapy at inclusion	0.19	0.13
Previous surgery	0.98	-
Previous biological therapy	0.42	-
Elevated CRP level	0.51	0.86
Outcome of induction therapy	0.29	0.23

Now the primary goals of treatment in IBD are not only the induction and maintenance of clinical remission but also the induction of mucosal healing in an attempt to alter the course of IBD. And mucosal healing represents a more reliable and objective marker in the assessment of therapeutic response than clinical activity indices. Macroscopic findings of the mucosa represent its real alterations of patients with IBD, so endoscopy is the gold standard method of assessing mucosa lesions of patients with IBD.

But none of the studies support that mucosal healing correlates with clinical activity of IBD. Our results have revealed a high proportion of patients who relapsed even after mucosal healing. The higher relapse rates in patients with IBD who achieved mucosal healing may be explained by the shorter duration of their infliximab therapy. Therefore, the necessity of the routine endoscopic examinations at the end of the one-year period of infliximab therapy is worth considering. In conclusion, we think that stopping or continuing infliximab therapy may be determined by assessing the IBD patient's general condition and the clinical activity. At the same time, we have concluded that the long-term advantages of mucosal healing can be achieved only if we continue previous effective therapies, even after mucosal healing by the endoscopic examination. In future, large controlled clinical trials are required to confirm these results.

Author Contributions

Conceived and designed the experiments: CD MS. Performed the experiments: CD WL. Analyzed the data: MJ. Contributed reagents/materials/analysis tools: CD MJ. Contributed to the writing of the manuscript: CD MS.

References

1. Baumgart DC, Sandborn WJ (2007) Inflammatory bowel disease: clinical aspects and established and evolving therapies. Lancet 369: 1641–1657.
2. Wardle RA, Mayberry JF (2014) Patient knowledge in inflammatory bowel disease: the Crohn's and Colitis Knowledge Score. Eur J Gastroenterol Hepatol 26: 1–5.
3. Ye L, Cao Q, Cheng J (2013) Review of Inflammatory Bowel Disease in China. ScientificWorldJournal 2013: 296470.
4. Mulder DJ, Noble AJ, Justinich CJ, Duffin JM (2013) A tale of two diseases: The history of inflammatory bowel disease. J Crohns Colitis.
5. Speight RA, Mansfield JC (2013) Drug advances in inflammatory bowel disease. Clin Med 13: 378–382.
6. Danese S (2012) New therapies for inflammatory bowel disease: from the bench to the bedside. Gut 61: 918–932.
7. Pineton de Chambrun G, Peyrin-Biroulet L, Lemann M, Colombel JF (2010) Clinical implications of mucosal healing for the management of IBD. Nat Rev Gastroenterol Hepatol 7: 15–29.
8. Armuzzi A, Van Assche G, Reinisch W, Pineton de Chambrun G, Griffiths A, et al. (2012) Results of the 2nd scientific workshop of the ECCO (IV): therapeutic strategies to enhance intestinal healing in inflammatory bowel disease. J Crohns Colitis 6: 492–502.
9. Daperno M, D'Haens G, Van Assche G, Baert F, Bulois P, et al. (2004) Development and validation of a new, simplified endoscopic activity score for Crohn's disease: the SES-CD. Gastrointest Endosc 60: 505–512.
10. Dave M, Loftus EV Jr (2012) Mucosal healing in inflammatory bowel disease-a true paradigm of success? Gastroenterol Hepatol (N Y) 8: 29–38.
11. Schroeder KW, Tremaine WJ, Ilstrup DM (1987) Coated oral 5-aminosalicylic acid therapy for mildly to moderately active ulcerative colitis. A randomized study. N Engl J Med 317: 1625–1629.
12. Rutgeerts P, Vermeire S, Van Assche G (2007) Mucosal healing in inflammatory bowel disease: impossible ideal or therapeutic target? Gut 56: 453–455.
13. Rutgeerts P, Sandborn WJ, Feagan BG, Reinisch W, Olson A, et al. (2005) Infliximab for induction and maintenance therapy for ulcerative colitis. N Engl J Med 353: 2462–2476.
14. Louis E, Mary JY, Vernier-Massouille G, Grimaud JC, Bouhnik Y, et al. (2012) Maintenance of remission among patients with Crohn's disease on antimetabolite therapy after infliximab therapy is stopped. Gastroenterology 142: 63–70 e65; quiz e31.
15. Hanauer SB, Feagan BG, Lichtenstein GR, Mayer LF, Schreiber S, et al. (2002) Maintenance infliximab for Crohn's disease: the ACCENT I randomised trial. Lancet 359: 1541–1549.
16. Hanauer SB, Sandborn WJ, Rutgeerts P, Fedorak RN, Lukas M, et al. (2006) Human anti-tumor necrosis factor monoclonal antibody (adalimumab) in Crohn's disease: the CLASSIC-I trial. Gastroenterology 130: 323–333; quiz 591.
17. Schnitzler F, Fidder H, Ferrante M, Noman M, Arijs I, et al. (2009) Long-term outcome of treatment with infliximab in 614 patients with Crohn's disease: results from a single-centre cohort. Gut 58: 492–500.
18. Silverberg MS, Satsangi J, Ahmad T, Arnott ID, Bernstein CN, et al. (2005) Toward an integrated clinical, molecular and serological classification of inflammatory bowel disease: report of a Working Party of the 2005 Montreal World Congress of Gastroenterology. Can J Gastroenterol 19 Suppl A: 5A–36A.
19. Best WR, Becktel JM, Singleton JW, Kern F Jr (1976) Development of a Crohn's disease activity index. National Cooperative Crohn's Disease Study. Gastroenterology 70: 439–444.
20. Rutgeerts P, Feagan BG, Lichtenstein GR, Mayer LF, Schreiber S, et al. (2004) Comparison of scheduled and episodic treatment strategies of infliximab in Crohn's disease. Gastroenterology 126: 402–413.
21. Rutgeerts P, Diamond RH, Bala M, Olson A, Lichtenstein GR, et al. (2006) Scheduled maintenance treatment with infliximab is superior to episodic treatment for the healing of mucosal ulceration associated with Crohn's disease. Gastrointest Endosc 63: 433–442; quiz 464.
22. Schnitzler F, Fidder H, Ferrante M, Noman M, Arijs I, et al. (2009) Mucosal healing predicts long-term outcome of maintenance therapy with infliximab in Crohn's disease. Inflamm Bowel Dis 15: 1295–1301.
23. Froslie KF, Jahnsen J, Moum BA, Vatn MH (2007) Mucosal healing in inflammatory bowel disease: results from a Norwegian population-based cohort. Gastroenterology 133: 412–422.
24. Baert F, Moortgat L, Van Assche G, Caenepeel P, Vergauwe P, et al. (2010) Mucosal healing predicts sustained clinical remission in patients with early-stage Crohn's disease. Gastroenterology 138: 463–468; quiz e410–461.
25. Ananthakrishnan AN, Korzenik JR, Hur C (2013) Can Mucosal Healing Be a Cost-effective Endpoint for Biologic Therapy in Crohn's Disease? A Decision Analysis. Inflamm Bowel Dis 19: 37–44.
26. Steenholdt C, Molazahi A, Ainsworth MA, Brynskov J, Ostergaard Thomsen O, et al. (2012) Outcome after discontinuation of infliximab in patients with inflammatory bowel disease in clinical remission: an observational Danish single center study. Scand J Gastroenterol 47: 518–527.
27. Freeman HJ (2010) Limitations in assessment of mucosal healing in inflammatory bowel disease. World J Gastroenterol 16: 15–20.
28. Laharie D, Filippi J, Roblin X, Nancey S, Chevaux JB, et al. (2013) Impact of mucosal healing on long-term outcomes in ulcerative colitis treated with infliximab: a multicenter experience. Aliment Pharmacol Ther 37: 998–1004.

21

Cytomegalovirus Infection in Inflammatory Bowel Disease is not Associated with Worsening of Intestinal Inflammatory Activity

Alexandre Medeiros do Carmo[1]*, Fabiana Maria Santos[1], Carmen Lucia Ortiz-Agostinho[1], Iêda Nishitokukado[1], Cintia S. Frota[1], Flavia Ubeda Gomes[1], André Zonetti de Arruda Leite[1], Claudio Sérgio Pannuti[2], Lucy Santos Vilas Boas[3], Magaly Gemio Teixeira[4], Aytan Miranda Sipahi[1]

1 Departamento de Gastroenterologia, Hospital das Clínicas da Faculdade de Medicina da Universidade de São Paulo – LIM 07, São Paulo, São Paulo, Brazil, **2** Instituto de Medicina Tropical e Departamento de Doenças Infecciosas e Parasitarias (LIM-HC) da Faculdade de Medicina da Universidade de São Paulo, São Paulo, São Paulo, Brazil, **3** Instituto de Medicina Tropical e Hospital das Clínicas da Faculdade de Medicina (LIM-HC), Universidade de São Paulo, São Paulo, São Paulo, Brazil, **4** Departamento de Cirurgia do Serviço de Cirurgia do Cólon Reto e Ânus, Hospital das Clínicas da Faculdade de Medicina da Universidade de São Paulo, São Paulo, São Paulo, Brazil

Abstract

Background: Cytomegalovirus is highly prevalent virus and usually occurs in immunocompromised patients. The pathophysiology and treatment of inflammatory bowel disease often induce a state of immunosuppression. Because this, there are still doubts and controversies about the relationship between inflammatory bowel disease and cytomegalovirus.

Aim: Evaluate the frequency of cytomegalovirus in patients with inflammatory bowel disease and identify correlations.

Methods: Patients with inflammatory bowel disease underwent an interview, review of records and collection of blood and fecal samples. The search for cytomegalovirus was performed by IgG and IgM blood serology, by real-time PCR in the blood and by qualitative PCR in feces. Results were correlated with red blood cell levels, C-reactive protein levels, erythrocyte sedimentation rates and fecal calprotectin levels for each patient.

Results: Among the 400 eligible patients, 249 had Crohn's disease, and 151 had ulcerative colitis. In the group of Crohn's disease, 67 of the patients had moderate or severe disease, but 126 patients presented with active disease, based on the evaluation of the fecal calprotectin. In patients with ulcerative colitis, only 21 patients had moderate disease, but 76 patients presented with active disease, based on the evaluation of the fecal calprotectin. A large majority of patients had positive CMV IgG. Overall, 10 patients had positive CMV IgM, and 9 patients had a positive qualitative detection of CMV DNA by PCR in the feces. All 400 patients returned negative results after the quantitative detection of CMV DNA in blood by real-time PCR. Analyzing the 19 patients with active infections, we only found that such an association occurred with the use of combined therapy (anti-TNF-alpha + azathioprine)

Conclusion: The findings show that latent cytomegalovirus infections are frequent and active cytomegalovirus infection is rare. We did not find any association between an active infection of CMV and inflammatory bowel disease activity.

Editor: Juliet Spencer, University of San Francisco, United States of America

Funding: This project received funding from FAPESP helping to buy products to experiments (project 2010/18275-8, http://www.fapesp.br/). The funders had no role in study design, data collection and analysis, decision to publish, or preparation of the manuscript.

Competing Interests: The authors have declared that no competing interests exist.

* Email: amccirurgia@gmail.com

Introduction

Cytomegalovirus (CMV) is a ß herpes-virus with double-stranded DNA and represents a common viral infection in humans, with infection levels ranging from 40% in developed countries to 100% in developing countries [1]. Primary CMV infection is subclinical in most patients and is often followed by CMV disease or latent CMV infection. CMV disease is rare in immunocompetent patients but not among the immunocompromised population. The organs affected by CMV disease include the eyes, lungs, liver, urinary tract, pancreas, central nervous system, heart and gastrointestinal tract [2].

The different grades of CMV infection can be defined as not infected, latent infection, active infection and disease [3] (Table 1)

Inflammatory Bowel diseases (IBD), which include ulcerative colitis (UC) and Crohn's disease (CD), consist of chronic, non-specific inflammatory diseases of unknown etiology that affect the digestive tract and can be differentiated mainly due to the depth and extent of disease involvement. To determine the degree of

Table 1. The different grades of CMV infection.

CMV infection status	Description
Not infected	Not infected with the virus; negative IgG and IgM antibodies against CMV
Latent infection	Carrier of the CMV genome without active replication
Active infection	Detectable viral replication in peripheral blood or organs or a significant rise in IgM antibodies against CMV
Disease	Clinical expression of active infection, that is, active CMV infection with end-organ involvement

inflammation, it is necessary to use a combination of parameter settings, covering clinical, endoscopic, laboratory, endoscopic and radiological values. The CDAI (Crohn's disease activity index) and the TrueLove-Witts are clinical indices that are widely used as a means to quantify the inflammatory activity of CD and UC, respectively [4,5,6]. In addition, Fecal Calprotectin (FC) is a very good marker of intestinal inflammation that has a close correlation with endoscopic and histological findings, as well as good sensitivity and specificity [7,8].

A clinical treatment is not curative and often relies on the use of immunosuppressive drugs. The pathophysiology of a disease may compromise the immune system. This observation, in combination with the fact that CMV presents a tropism for sites of inflammation, prompted us to hypothesize whether patients with IBD are more susceptible to CMV infection and disease [9,10].

Several authors have tried to correlate CMV and IBD, hypothesizing the following: possible triggering of CMV infection at the onset of IBD [11,12]; a worsening of the infection [13,14,15,16]; an association between the use of anti TNF-alpha and a higher risk of CMV disease [17,18]; or the higher prevalence of CMV disease in UC patients, compared with CD [19,20]. On the other hand, other authors have advocated that CMV is only a bystander or surrogate marker of severe colitis [21,22,23,24,25] or that the anti TNF-alpha therapies may reduce the risk of CMV reactivation in UC patients [26].

The prevalence of CMV infection in patients with IBD is highly variable. One reason for this wide variation is the difficulty and lack of standardization among indices for diagnosing the different grades of CMV infection [13,27]. The prevalence of CMV infection and its clinical significance in IBD, especially in outpatients, have yet to be determined.

In this context, the aim of this study was to explore the prevalence of CMV infection in 400 outpatients with IBD, using serology, a real-time quantitative PCR assay on blood samples, and a qualitative PCR assay on fecal samples. Another objective was to correlate CMV viral replication with various demographic, therapeutic and inflammatory activities in IBD patients.

Patients and Methods

Patients and Samples

The study was carried out from June 2011 to August 2012 with IBD outpatients from the *Hospital das Clínicas*, School of Medicine, University of São Paulo (HC-FMUSP). The authors followed the Resolution number 196/96, the National Health Council/MS, respecting the basic principles of bioethics, autonomy, non-maleficence, beneficence and justice. The study was submitted to the Ethics Committee of the *Hospital das Clínicas*, Faculty of Medicine, University of São Paulo (USP-HC) (Research Protocol: 0144/11) and accepted in session on 11/05/2011, before it starts. All patients or guardians, after reading, filled in and signed the consent form and agreed to participate in the study.

The diagnosis of inflammatory bowel disease, UC or CD, had been previously established by clinical, laboratory, endoscopic, radiological and histological findings, according to standard criteria.

Patients were asked to bring a fecal sample and were submitted to an interview on the day of consultation. Patients were evaluated to verify the levels of their disease activity, according to the pathology: CD (CDAI- Crohn's disease activity index) [5] and UC (Truelove-Witts index) [6]. After data collection, all patients were referred to the laboratory for collection of venous blood samples.

All of the data collected were analyzed and compared with data collected from these patients medical records. Those who did not meet the established criteria, did not sign the consent form, or failed to collect or deliver laboratory fecal materials were automatically excluded from the study.

Definition of active CMV infection

Active CMV infection was defined by a positive IgM test and/or detection of CMV DNA in peripheral blood or fecal samples by qualitative or real time PCR

Laboratory Analysis

Peripheral blood samples were collected, and the tests performed included the following: complete blood count, erythrocyte sedimentation rate, C-reactive protein(CRP), and IgG and IgM antibodies against CMV.

Real Time Quantitative PCR (qPCR)

Extraction of viral DNA was performed by processing whole bloodusing a QIAamp DNA Mini-kit (Qiagen, Valencia, Calif.) according to the manufacturer's instructions.

For Amplification and detection of viral DNA, the sequences of the PCR primers and probe were selected from the US17 region of CMV AD169, as previously described [28]. Summarizing, forward and reverse primers were 5'-GCGTGCT-TTTTAGCCTCTGCA-3' and 5'-AAAAGTTTGTGCCC-CAACGGTA-3', respectively, and the probe FAM -TG-ATCGGCGTTATCGCGTTCTTGATC - BHQ. PCR was performed using TaqMan Universal PCR master mix (Applied Biosystems), prepared as follows: 20μL of DNA from whole blood was mixed with 25 μl of PCR master mix, 15 pmol of each of the primers, 10 pmol of the TaqMan probe, and DPOC water were added to final volume of 50 μl.

Reactions were performed using the ABI PRISM 7300 Real Time PCR System (Applied Biosystems, Foster City, Calif.) with the following cycling conditions: 1 cycle at 50°C for 2 min and 95°C for 10 min to activate the Taq-Polymerase followed by 45 cycles at 95°C for 15 s and 61°C for 1 min.

To determine the sensitivity of the method, standard DNA at a concentration of 15.000 copies/ml (DNA from ADN169, Sellex,

Table 2. Demographic and clinical profile of the inflammatory bowel disease patients.

Characteristics	Crohn's disease	Ulcerative Colitis
Number of cases	249	151
Gender M:F	113:136	64:87
Age variation (mean)	15–82 (45,5)	23–80 (49,92)
Duration of disease, months (mean)	12–456 (132,5)	6–576 (118,77)
BMI, kg/m² (mean)	15,42–48,05 (24,3)	16,9–37,32 (25,51)
Disease location		
	ileal 64 (25,7%)	**distal** 50 (33,1%)
	colonic 65 (26,1%)	**left colonic** 41 (27,1%)
	ileocolonic 108 (43,3%)	**pancolonic** 60 (39,4%)
	upper GI 12 (4,8%)	
Clinical Index (CDAI/Truelove)		
Remission	126 (50,8%)	
Mild	55 (22,18%)	129 (86%)
Moderate	57 (22,98%)	21 (14%)
Severe	10 (4%)	0
FC≥150, number (%)	126 (50,6%)	76 (50,8%)
Anemia, number (%)	56 (22,5%)	28 (18,5%)
C-reactive protein≥5, number (%)	92 (37,7%)	56 (37,6%)
Previous surgery	100/247 (40,5%)	15/151 (9,9%)

Washington, DC, USA) was serially diluted until the concentration of 150 copies/ml and tested in triplicate.

For specificity, DNAs of the following pathogens: Epstein-Barr virus, Adenovirus, *Mycoplasma pneumoniae*, Herpes Simplex Virus Type 1, Herpes Simplex Virus Type 2, Varicella-Zoster Virus, *Pneumocystis jiroveci*, *Toxoplasma gondii*), obtained from commercial crops, acquired from SellexInc (Washington DC, USA), were subjected to PCR.

After performing the RT-PCR, DNA samples extracted from 300 of the 400 randomly selected patients) were analyzed by conventional qualitative PCR. The same qualitative technique was used for stool samples[29].

Qualitative PCR

The fecal DNA was extracted using a Qiagen (QIAamp DNA stool Mini Kit) kit, and the detection of the cytomegalovirus genome was performed using the qualitative PCR technique (conventional) to amplify a specific segment of the CMV gB, with specific primers gB 1319 and gB 1604 of the glycoprotein B gene [29,30].

Table 3. Medications used by the patients enrolled in the study.

Drug	Crohn's disease	Ulcerative colitis
Sulfasalazine	39 (15,7%)	70 (46,7%)
Mesalazine	55 (22,2%)	68 (45,3%)
Azathioprine	143 (57,7%)	41 (27,3%)
Steroids	23 (9,3%)	9 (6,0%)
Methotrexat	1 (0,4%)	0
Infliximab	66 (26,6%)	15 (10,0%)
Adalimumab	19 (7,7%)	2 (1,3%)
Ciprofloxacin	37 (14,9%)	10 (6,7%)
Metronidazole	23 (9,3%)	7 (4,7%)
Cyclosporine	0	1 (0,7%)
No medication	22 (8,9%)	13 (8,7%)
Combo therapy	48 (19.3%)	7 (4,7%)
Total	**248**	**150**

Table 4. Serologic distribution for CMV in patients with CD and UC.

Serologic	CD	UC	Total
IgG (-) IgM (-)	16 (7%)	8 (5,6%)	24 (6,5%)
IgG (+) IgM (-)	207 (90,4%)	131 (91,6%)	338 (90,9%)
IgG (+) IgM (+)	6 (2,6%)	4 (2,8%)	10 (2,6%)
IgG (-) IgM (+)	0	0	0
Not performed	20	8	28

The result was revealed by the presence or absence of a band at the expected segment of DNA electrophoresis on an agarose gel marked with ethidium bromide. Internal, negative and positive controls were performed in parallel to assess the proper operation of the reaction.

Fecal Calprotectin

Stool samples were stored at $-20°C$ to be thawed later, and a survey of fecal calprotectin using ELISA, PhiCal (Caprotectin Elisa Kit) was conducted [8,31].

Statistical Analysis

A statistical analysis to determine the characteristics associated with CMV and IBDs patients was conducted. Descriptive analyses were performed first, and the Fisher's exact test and Mann-Whitney test were used for categorical variables, with Student's t test being used for continuous variables. In a more detailed study, a simple and multiple logistic regression was considered. A P value <0.05 was considered significant.

Results

Clinical Characteristics

The clinical and demographic characteristics of the 400 patients involved in the study are shown in Table 2. Using clinical indices, including the Crohn's disease activity index (CDAI) for CD and the Truelove, for UC, only 67 CD patients and 21 UC patients presented with moderate or severe disease. However, using fecal calprotectin (FC), over half of the patients had an FC above 149 ng/ml, suggesting active inflammatory bowel disease. Analyzing these data, we found associations among FC≥150, CRP≥5 and anemia. The association between FC≥150 and the clinical indices (CDAI and Truelove) did not achieve statistical significance.

The medications used are shown in Table 3. Immunosuppressive agents were widely used among these patients. Analyzing the combined therapy (anti TNF-α plus azathioprine), 37 patients with CD used infliximab and azathioprine, and 11 patients used adalimumab and azathioprine. Among UC patients, six used

infliximab and azathioprine, and one used adalimumab and azathioprine.

CMV Status

The serologic status of CMV in the blood of patients is shown in Table 4. Only 24 patients were not infected with CMV, and 90,9% of patients exhibited IgG antibodies against CMV in the blood, indicating previous CMV infection. Ten patients were IgG positive, whereas 28 patients did not complete the tests. The analysis of fecal samples from 394 study patients by a qualitative PCR revealed that nine of them exhibited CMV DNA (Table 5). The detection of CMV DNA by RT-PCR in the blood produced values under the inferior limit (150 copies/mL) in all 400 patients. As a result of these overall negative results, we randomly selected 300 patients and repeated the detection of CMV by PCR in blood using qualitative PCR, the same technique used on the feces. Again, all of the samples were negative.

The detection of CMV DNA by real time PCR in the blood produced values under the inferior limit (150 copies/mL) in all 400 patients. In order to double-check these overall negative results, we randomly selected 300 patients and repeated the detection of CMV in blood by using the same qualitative technique used on the feces. Again, all blood samples were negative.

Using serology and the results from the CMV DNA PCR, it is possible to conclude that 24 patients were not infected with CMV, 332 patients were infected without viral replication, and 19 were infected with viral replication. (Table 6)

Clinical-Virological Correlations

After dividing the patients into three different groups, the not infected, the latent infection and the active infection groups, we looked for associations between these groups and the variables of interest.

Analyzing exclusively CD patients, we found an association between the use of infliximab and CMV viral replication (p = 0.0045) and between the use of combined therapy and viral replication (p = 0.005). In UC patients, no variable was significantly associated with the three different groups of CMV infection.

Table 5. Analysis of CMV DNA by qualitative PCR on the feces of study patients.

Feces PCR	CD	UC	Total
(+)	5 (2,01%)	4 (2,65%)	9 (2,25%)
(-)	239 (95,98%)	146 (96,69%)	385 (96,25%)
Not performed	5 (2,01%)	1 (0,66%)	6 (1,5%)

Table 6. Patients distribution regarding CMV infection.

	CD	UC	Total
Not infected	16 (6.42%)	8 (5.3%)	24 (6%)
Infected without viral replication (latent infection)	204 (81.93%)	128 (84.77%)	332 (83%)
Infected with viral replication (active infection)	11 (4.42%)	8 (5.3%)	19 (4.75%)
CMV IgM or feces PCR not performed	18 (7.23%)	7 (4.63%)	25 (6.25%)

Considering all patients with inflammatory bowel disease, the likelihood ratio test demonstrated a statistically significant association between the use of combined therapy and the CMV infection group (Table 7).

Utilizing the variables in univariate tests with descriptive levels below 0.2 (p<0.2), we verified whether the infection's characteristics as whole could influence replication. We found that a patient using combined therapy had a chance of replication that was 3.63 times greater than that of patients not using this treatment (p = 0.014) (Table 8).

Discussion

This study examined patients with IBD. Without any previous selection, 400 outpatients were randomly selected in order to evaluate a group that would best represent the general population of patients with IBD from the HCFMUSP.

More than half of these patients had intestinal disease activity, as confirmed by fecal calprotectin. Based on the clinical index, most patients were categorized with quiescent/mild disease (50.8%/22.18%CD and 0/86% of UC). However, such clinical indices have been criticized due to their highly variable sensitivity and specificity, and we believe that fecal calprotectin is the better parameter to demonstrate that half of the patients had active IBD. These results corroborate the literature, which is quite critical of these indices but reports a good sensitivity and specificity of fecal calprotectin in relation to endoscopic findings [8,31,32].

The very high percentage of patients infected with CMV, as evidenced by the presence of IgG antibodies to CMV, can be justified by the socioeconomic status of the study group [19,33,34]. Using Fischer's test and simple logistic regression, we did not find significant differences between the group of uninfected patients and the group with latent infections in relation to the activity index of IBD, CRP levels or fecal calprotectin. This contradicts the original hypothesis, which held that the latent CMV infection could worsen the IBD activity compared to the uninfected CMV patients [14,15,16,35]. It is worth noting that only 24 patients (6.45%) were not infected, instead having negative antibodies IgG and IgM for CMV.

Despite the large number of patients undergoing immunosuppressive therapy, comprising more than half of patients with active IBD, viral replication was not detected by PCR in their blood in any case. These null results may have been obtained because our sample was composed of IBD outpatients, rather than a specifically selected population. Our study corroborates other studies arguing that the frequency of viral replication and CMV disease in patients with IBD is not as high as sometimes reported, questioning the virulence of CMV in patients with IBD [21,24,25,26,27]. The detection of CMV DNA in the fecal specimens by a qualitative PCR assay employing primers to the gB region, a highly variable region of HCMV, could underestimate the number of patients shedding CMV in feces. However, as this assay was performed blindly in all samples regardless of the clinical category or activity index of inflammatory bowel disease, we believe that our result concerning the lack of association between CMV and worsening of intestinal inflammatory activity was not affected.

When we began our study, the association between IBD and CMV was controversial, with the literature pointing to the risk that the rates of CMV infection, replication and disease might be higher in IBD patients. As the present project has progressed, new studies have emerged to challenge these ideas, suggesting that CMV is an occasional finding, a bystander in IBD enterocolitis [21,24,25,26,27].

In our series of ulcerative colitis patients, we did not find any patients with a severe form of the disease, according to the Truelove-Witts classification, which affects the assessment of the role of CMV in this particular group of patients. CD patients were found in all categories of CMV infection, but we did not find any correlation between CMV and the severity of IBD. We found that, in patients with mild and moderate forms of CD and UC, there was no association between the severity of IBD and CMV viral replication in the blood or stool specimens.

Pillet et al. [26] suggest that immunosuppressive therapy does not appear to have an impact on CMV reactivation in CD patients. They state that TNF alpha enhances CMV viral replication and that anti-TNF drugs may reduce the risk of CMV reactivation. However, we detected CMV viral replication in UC and CD patients, indicating that anti-TNF alpha does not protect against viral replication. In CD patients, an association was found between the viral replication of CMV and anti-TNF alpha, contradicting the hypothesis put forth by Pillet et al.

In the present study, we found a statistically significant association between CMV viral replication and the use of combined therapy, consisting of biological therapy (infliximab or adalimumab) plus an immunosuppressive drug (azathioprine or methotrexat). We believe that higher immunosuppression favors viral replication. However, the increase in CMV replication was not accompanied by a greater intestinal inflammatory activity, as evidenced by fecal the calprotectin levels. The present findings further support the hypothesis that CMV is a spectator of the inflammatory process in IBD. The higher the degree of immunosuppressive state caused by the therapy and/or disease is, the greater the chance for CMV replication; however, this finding did not seem to worsen the IBD activity.

The methodological difficulties in achieving a clear categorization of the CMV infections in uninfected, infected non-replicating, and infected with replication and with CMV disease patients might jeopardize the critical evaluation of each work. This effect can be seen in the large variation among the rates of CMV disease that have been published in previous works, suggesting that many cases of the disease were most likely misdiagnosed as CMV infection or CMV replication.

Table 7. Description of the cytomegalovirus groups, according to characteristics of interest in all patients and the results of the tests of association.

Variable	Not infected		Infected without replication		Infected with replication		Total	p
	N	%	N	%	N	%		
Hemoglobin								0.195#
No anemia	17	5.8	264	90.1	12	4.1	293	
Anemia	7	8.5	68	82.9	7	8.5	82	
CRP								0.395
<5	14	6.1	207	90.0	9	3.9	230	
≥5	9	6.4	122	86.5	10	7.1	141	
Fecal calprotectin								0.464
<150	10	5.6	163	90.6	7	3.9	180	
≥150	14	7.2	168	86.6	12	6.2	194	
Sulfasalazine								0.587
No	19	7.0	237	87.5	15	5.5	271	
Yes	5	4.9	94	91.3	4	3.9	103	
Mesalazine								0.704
No	18	6.9	230	88.5	12	4.6	260	
Yes	6	5.3	101	88.6	7	6.1	114	
Azathioprine								0.165
No	10	5.1	181	91.4	7	3.5	198	
Yes	14	8.0	150	85.2	12	6.8	176	
Steroids								0.433#
No	21	6.1	305	89.2	16	4.7	342	
Yes	3	9.4	26	81.3	3	9.4	32	
Ifx								0.068#
No	22	7.3	266	88.7	12	4.0	300	
Yes	2	2.7	65	87.8	7	9.5	74	
Ada								0.066#
No	24	6.8	314	88.7	16	4.5	354	
Yes	0	0.0	17	85.0	3	15.0	20	
Combo therapy								**0.001#**
No	24	7.4	287	88.9	12	3.7	323	
Yes	0	0.0	44	86.3	7	13.7	51	

Result of the chi-square.
Result of the likelihood ratio

Table 8. Results of the multiple logistic regression model to explain the replication of cytomegalovirus.

Variable	OR	IC (95%)		P
		Inferior	Superior	
Hemoglobin				
No anemia	1.00			
Anemia	1.38	0.45	4.28	0.576
CRP				
<5	1.00			
≥5	1.54	0.54	4.38	0.419
Combo therapy				
No	1.00			
Yes	3.63	1.30	10.12	**0.014**
Results of the logistic regression				

Based on the improved standardization of diagnostic methods and increasing understanding of the pathophysiology of CMV, studies should soon converge on lower rates of diagnosis for CMV disease in the IBD population.

In summary, our study has shown that latent infection by CMV was quite prevalent in a study group of patients with inflammatory bowel disease. We found no association between IBD activity and CMV infection in IBD patients, even among patients with viral replication using immunosuppressive therapy. Finally, although the use of combined therapies in patients with IBD was associated with the viral replication of CMV, such therapies bore no relation to inflammatory activity of IBD.

Author Contributions

Conceived and designed the experiments: AMC AZAL CSP MGT AMS. Performed the experiments: AMC FMS CLOA IN CSF FUG LSVB. Analyzed the data: AMC AZAL CSP MGT AMS. Wrote the paper: AMC FMS CLOA AZAL CSP MGT AMS.

References

1. Staras SA, Dollard SC, Radford KW, Flanders WD, Pass RF, et al. (2006) Seroprevalence of cytomegalovirus infection in the United States, 1988–1994. Clin Infect Dis 43: 1143–1151.
2. Goodgame RW (1993) Gastrointestinal cytomegalovirus disease. Ann Intern Med 119: 924–935.
3. Rowshani AT, Bemelman FJ, van Leeuwen EM, van Lier RA, ten Berge IJ (2005) Clinical and immunologic aspects of cytomegalovirus infection in solid organ transplant recipients. Transplantation 79: 381–386.
4. Vilela EG, Torres HO, Martins FP, Ferrari Mde L, Andrade MM, et al. (2012) Evaluation of inflammatory activity in Crohn's disease and ulcerative colitis. World J Gastroenterol 18: 872–881.
5. Best WR, Becktel JM, Singleton JW, Kern F Jr (1976) Development of a Crohn's disease activity index. National Cooperative Crohn's Disease Study. Gastroenterology 70: 439–444.
6. Truelove SC, Witts LJ (1955) Cortisone in ulcerative colitis; final report on a therapeutic trial. Br Med J 2: 1041–1048.
7. Konikoff MR, Denson LA (2006) Role of fecal calprotectin as a biomarker of intestinal inflammation in inflammatory bowel disease. Inflamm Bowel Dis 12: 524–534.
8. Vieira A, Fang CB, Rolim EG, Klug WA, Steinwurz F, et al. (2009) Inflammatory bowel disease activity assessed by fecal calprotectin and lactoferrin: correlation with laboratory parameters, clinical, endoscopic and histological indexes. BMC Res Notes 2: 221.
9. Papadakis KA, Tung JK, Binder SW, Kam LY, Abreu MT, et al. (2001) Outcome of cytomegalovirus infections in patients with inflammatory bowel disease. Am J Gastroenterol 96: 2137–2142.
10. Maher MM, Nassar MI (2009) Acute cytomegalovirus infection is a risk factor in refractory and complicated inflammatory bowel disease. Dig Dis Sci 54: 2456–2462.
11. Orvar K, Murray J, Carmen G, Conklin J (1993) Cytomegalovirus infection associated with onset of inflammatory bowel disease. Dig Dis Sci 38: 2307–2310.
12. Lakatos PL (2009) Environmental factors affecting inflammatory bowel disease: have we made progress? Dig Dis 27: 215–225.
13. Criscuoli V, Rizzuto MR, Cottone M (2006) Cytomegalovirus and inflammatory bowel disease: is there a link? World J Gastroenterol 12: 4813–4818.
14. Kambham N, Vij R, Cartwright CA, Longacre T (2004) Cytomegalovirus infection in steroid-refractory ulcerative colitis: a case-control study. Am J Surg Pathol 28: 365–373.
15. Kishore J, Ghoshal U, Ghoshal UC, Krishnani N, Kumar S, et al. (2004) Infection with cytomegalovirus in patients with inflammatory bowel disease: prevalence, clinical significance and outcome. J Med Microbiol 53: 1155–1160.
16. Onyeagocha C, Hossain MS, Kumar A, Jones RM, Roback J, et al. (2009) Latent cytomegalovirus infection exacerbates experimental colitis. Am J Pathol 175: 2034–2042.
17. Helbling D, Breitbach TH, Krause M (2002) Disseminated cytomegalovirus infection in Crohn's disease following anti-tumour necrosis factor therapy. Eur J Gastroenterol Hepatol 14: 1393–1395.
18. Pickering O, Weinstein T, Rubin LG (2009) Fatal disseminated cytomegalovirus infection associated with infliximab and 6-mercaptopurine therapy in a child with Crohn disease. Pediatr Infect Dis J 28: 556.
19. Domenech E, Vega R, Ojanguren I, Hernandez A, Garcia-Planella E, et al. (2008) Cytomegalovirus infection in ulcerative colitis: a prospective, comparative study on prevalence and diagnostic strategy. Inflamm Bowel Dis 14: 1373–1379.
20. Dimitroulia E, Spanakis N, Konstantinidou AE, Legakis NJ, Tsakris A (2006) Frequent detection of cytomegalovirus in the intestine of patients with inflammatory bowel disease. Inflamm Bowel Dis 12: 879–884.
21. Matsuoka K, Iwao Y, Mori T, Sakuraba A, Yajima T, et al. (2007) Cytomegalovirus is frequently reactivated and disappears without antiviral agents in ulcerative colitis patients. Am J Gastroenterol 102: 331–337.
22. Criscuoli V, Casa A, Orlando A, Pecoraro G, Oliva L, et al. (2004) Severe acute colitis associated with CMV: a prevalence study. Dig Liver Dis 36: 818–820.
23. Maconi G, Colombo E, Zerbi P, Sampietro GM, Fociani P, et al. (2005) Prevalence, detection rate and outcome of cytomegalovirus infection in ulcerative colitis patients requiring colonic resection. Dig Liver Dis 37: 418–423.
24. Lawlor G, Moss AC (2010) Cytomegalovirus in inflammatory bowel disease: Pathogen or innocent bystander? Inflamm Bowel Dis.
25. Leveque N, Brixi-Benmansour H, Reig T, Renois F, Talmud D, et al (2010) Low frequency of cytomegalovirus infection during exacerbations of inflammatory bowel diseases. J Med Virol 82: 1694–1700.
26. Pillet S, Pozzetto B, Jarlot C, Paul S, Roblin X (2012) Management of cytomegalovirus infection in inflammatory bowel diseases. Dig Liver Dis 44: 541–548.
27. Kim JJ, Simpson N, Klipfel N, Debose R, Barr N, et al. (2010) Cytomegalovirus infection in patients with active inflammatory bowel disease. Dig Dis Sci 55: 1059–1065.

28. Bankier AT, Beck S, Bohni R, Brown CM, Cerny R, et al. (1991) The DNA sequence of the human cytomegalovirus genome. DNA Seq 2: 1–12.

29. Chou SW, Dennison KM (1991) Analysis of interstrain variation in cytomegalovirus glycoprotein B sequences encoding neutralization-related epitopes. J Infect Dis 163: 1229–1234.

30. Boom R, Sol C, Weel J, Lettinga K, Gerrits Y, et al. (2000) Detection and quantitation of human cytomegalovirus DNA in faeces. J Virol Methods 84: 1–14.

31. Gisbert JP, McNicholl AG (2009) Questions and answers on the role of faecal calprotectin as a biological marker in inflammatory bowel disease. Dig Liver Dis 41: 56–66.

32. Denis MA, Reenaers C, Fontaine F, Belaiche J, Louis E (2007) Assessment of endoscopic activity index and biological inflammatory markers in clinically active Crohn's disease with normal C-reactive protein serum level. Inflamm Bowel Dis 13: 1100–1105.

33. Pannuti CS, Vilas-Boas LS, Angelo MJ, Carvalho RP, Segre CM (1985) Congenital cytomegalovirus infection. Occurrence in two socioeconomically distinct populations of a developing country. Rev Inst Med Trop Sao Paulo 27: 105–107.

34. Suassuna JH, Leite LL, Villela LH (1995) Prevalence of cytomegalovirus infection in different patient groups of an urban university in Brazil. Rev Soc Bras Med Trop 28: 105–108.

35. Kandiel A, Lashner B (2006) Cytomegalovirus colitis complicating inflammatory bowel disease. Am J Gastroenterol 101: 2857–2865.

22

Job Strain and the Risk of Inflammatory Bowel Diseases: Individual-Participant Meta-Analysis of 95,000 Men and Women

Katriina Heikkilä[1]*, Ida E. H. Madsen[2], Solja T. Nyberg[1], Eleonor I. Fransson[3,4,5], Kirsi Ahola[1], Lars Alfredsson[3], Jakob B. Bjorner[2], Marianne Borritz[6], Hermann Burr[7], Nico Dragano[8], Jane E. Ferrie[9,10], Anders Knutsson[11], Markku Koskenvuo[12], Aki Koskinen[1], Martin L. Nielsen[6], Maria Nordin[13], Jan H. Pejtersen[14], Jaana Pentti[15], Reiner Rugulies[2,16], Tuula Oksanen[15], Martin J. Shipley[10], Sakari B. Suominen[17,18,19], Töres Theorell[5], Ari Väänänen[1], Jussi Vahtera[15,18], Marianna Virtanen[1], Hugo Westerlund[5], Peter J. M. Westerholm[20], G. David Batty[10,21], Archana Singh-Manoux[10,22], Mika Kivimäki[1,10], for the IPD-Work Consortium

1 Finnish Institute of Occupational Health, Helsinki, Finland, 2 National Research Centre for the Working Environment, Copenhagen, Denmark, 3 Institute of Environmental Medicine, Karolinska Institutet, Stockholm, Sweden, 4 School of Health Sciences, Jönköping University, Jönköping, Sweden, 5 Stress Research Institute, Stockholm University, Stockholm, Sweden, 6 Department of Occupational and Environmental Medicine, Bispebjerg University Hospital, Copenhagen, Denmark, 7 Federal Institute for Occupational Safety and Health (BAuA), Berlin, Germany, 8 Institute for Medical Sociology, Medical Faculty, University of Düsseldorf, Düsseldorf, Germany,, 9 School of Community and Social Medicine, University of Bristol, Bristol, United Kingdom, 10 Department of Epidemiology and Public Health, University College London, London, United Kingdom, 11 Department of Health Sciences, Mid Sweden University, Sundsvall, Sweden, 12 Department of Public Health, University of Helsinki, Helsinki, Finland, 13 Department of Psychology, Umeå University, Umeå, Sweden, 14 The Danish National Centre for Social Research, Copenhagen, Denmark, 15 Finnish Institute of Occupational Health, Helsinki, Tampere and Turku, Finland, 16 Department of Public Health and Department of Psychology, University of Copenhagen, Copenhagen, Denmark, 17 Folkhälsan Research Center, Helsinki, Finland, 18 Department of Public Health, University of Turku, Turku, Finland, 19 Nordic School of Public Health, Göteborg, Sweden, 20 Occupational and Environmental Medicine, Uppsala University, Uppsala, Sweden, 21 Centre for Cognitive Ageing and Cognitive Epidemiology, University of Edinburgh, Edingurgh, United Kingdom, 22 Inserm U1018, Centre for Research in Epidemiology and Population Health, Villejuif, France

Abstract

Background and Aims: Many clinicians, patients and patient advocacy groups believe stress to have a causal role in inflammatory bowel diseases, such as Crohn's disease and ulcerative colitis. However, this is not corroborated by clear epidemiological research evidence. We investigated the association between work-related stress and incident Crohn's disease and ulcerative colitis using individual-level data from 95 000 European adults.

Methods: We conducted individual-participant data meta-analyses in a set of pooled data from 11 prospective European studies. All studies are a part of the IPD-Work Consortium. Work-related psychosocial stress was operationalised as job strain (a combination of high demands and low control at work) and was self-reported at baseline. Crohn's disease and ulcerative colitis were ascertained from national hospitalisation and drug reimbursement registers. The associations between job strain and inflammatory bowel disease outcomes were modelled using Cox proportional hazards regression. The study-specific results were combined in random effects meta-analyses.

Results: Of the 95 379 participants who were free of inflammatory bowel disease at baseline, 111 men and women developed Crohn's disease and 414 developed ulcerative colitis during follow-up. Job strain at baseline was not associated with incident Crohn's disease (multivariable-adjusted random effects hazard ratio: 0.83, 95% confidence interval: 0.48, 1.43) or ulcerative colitis (hazard ratio: 1.06, 95% CI: 0.76, 1.48). There was negligible heterogeneity among the study-specific associations.

Conclusions: Our findings suggest that job strain, an indicator of work-related stress, is not a major risk factor for Crohn's disease or ulcerative colitis.

Editor: Yvette Tache, University of California, Los Angeles, United States of America

Funding: IPD-Work Consortium is supported by the EU New OSH ERA research programme (funded by the Finnish Work Environment Fund, Finland, the Swedish Research Council for Working Life and Social Research, Sweden and the Danish National Research Centre for the Working Environment, Denmark), the Academy of Finland (grant no. 132944), the BUPA Foundation (grant 22094477), and the British Heart Foundation. Mika Kivimäki is supported by the Medical Research Council, UK (grant no. K013351), the US National Institutes of Health (grant nos. R01HL036310, R01AG034454), and a professorial fellowship from the Economic and Social Research Council, UK. Funding bodies for the individual studies are listed on the study websites. The funding bodies had no role in the study design, data collection and analysis, decision to publish the findings or preparation of the manuscript.

Competing Interests: Töres Theorell receives royalties for books written on various topics, including psychosocial factors; music and health; and Sweden's working life in the 1990s. Hugo Westerlund's institution has received a research grant from Saint-Gobain Ecophon AB, a manufacturer of soundabsorbing materials, to study the effect of such materials on stress, job satisfaction and productivity in open-plan offices. Other authors declare no conflicts of interest.

* E-mail: katriina.heikkila@ttl.fi

Introduction

Inflammatory bowel diseases, Crohn's disease and ulcerative colitis, are incurable abnormalities of the adaptive mucosal immune response in the small and large intestines. Crohn's disease is perpetual inflammation of the small intestine, mainly driven by a sub-population of mucosal CD4+ T cells and T-helper type 1 (Th-1) cells, and marked by superficial and deep ulceration of the small intestine, with intestinal and perianal abscesses and fistulae [1]. Ulcerative colitis is mucosal inflammation of the rectum and colon, and is characterised by an abnormal T-helper type 2 (Th-2) response, which leads to epithelial cell cytotoxicity, increased apoptosis and epithelial barrier dysfunction in the colorectal area [2]. Typical symptoms of both inflammatory bowel diseases are abdominal pain, recurring diarrhoea, blood in faeces, fatigue and weight loss. Differential diagnosis between these diseases is usually made based on endoscopies or various types of imaging and scans.

Crohn's disease and ulcerative colitis are often diagnosed in individuals aged between 20 and 40 and whilst Crohn's disease is 20–30% more common in women, colitis occurs 60% more often in men [1]. Both diseases are rare at population level, as the prevalence of Crohn's disease in the Western countries is approximately 50 to 200 per 100 000 and of colitis about 120 to 200 per 100 000 [1]. Both also have a genetic background [3] and family history is indeed the most important predictor of developing either of them [4,5]. Risk factors for Crohn's disease and ulcerative colitis include dietary factors (such as low fruit, vegetable and fibre intake), appendectomy, and medications [4,6,7]. Evidence from observational studies suggest that tobacco smoking is associated with an increased risk of Crohn's disease but a decreased risk of ulcerative colitis [4], which highlights the importance of investigating these diseases separately in risk factor studies. A further less well understood risk factor implicated in inflammatory bowel diseases is stress. It has been suggested that stress could initiate or reactivate gastrointestinal inflammation that causes the symptoms of inflammatory bowel diseases. [8–10] Stress activates neural pathways from the hypothalamus to the sympathetic and parasympathetic nervous systems, which in turn link to the enteric nervous system that controls gut motility and endocrine and exocrine functions in the gastrointestinal tract. [9,11]

Many patients with Crohn's disease or ulcerative colitis believe stress to have caused or triggered their disease [10]. Epidemiological evidence from clinic-based studies, along with a recent systematic review pooling together findings from animal studies and observational studies in humans, indicated that stress can indeed worsen the symptoms and is associated with exacerbations in both diseases. [8,12–14] Preclinical data also suggest that stress has a role in experimental colitis. [14] However, the observational epidemiological evidence for the associations between stress and the onset of Crohn's disease and ulcerative colitis is based on a small number of retrospective studies, which have had conflicting findings, with positive as well as null-results reported [9,15,16]. Findings from studies based on retrospectively collected data are prone to recall and other biases and cannot provide reliable evidence for an association between stress and the risk of disease.

We examined the hypothesis that stress is associated with risk of developing Crohn's disease and ulcerative colitis using prospectively collected data from 11 European studies with over 95 000 participants. As these diseases are most often diagnosed in working-age individuals, we focused on stress at work, operationalised as job strain, and the incidence of these diseases and conducted individual-participant data meta-analyses of job strain and the risk of Crohn's disease and ulcerative colitis.

Methods

Studies and participants

Individual-level data were obtained from the following 11 prospective cohort studies: Copenhagen Psychosocial Questionnaire I and II (COPSOQ-I and COPSOQ-II), Danish Work Environment Cohort Study (DWECS), Finnish Public Sector study (FPS), Health and Social Support (HeSSup), Intervention Project on Absence and Well-being (IPAW), Burnout, Motivation and Job Satisfaction study (Danish acronym PUMA), Still Working, Whitehall II and Work Lipids and Fibrinogen (WOLF) Norrland and Stockholm studies). These studies, begun between 1986 and 2005 in Finland, Sweden, Denmark and the UK, are a part of the "Individual-participant-data Meta-analysis in Working Populations" (IPD-Work) Consortium [17]. Each study in the IPD-Work consortium was approved by the relevant local or national ethics committees and all participants gave informed consent to take part. Details of the ethical approval are provided in Appendix S1. Details of the design and participants in all the studies have been published previously and are described, with references to previous publications, in Appendix S1. Our analyses were based on men and women who were employed at study baseline and had complete data on job strain, inflammatory bowel disease outcomes and potential confounders. Participants with a diagnosis of Crohn's disease (n = 108) or colitis (n = 271) before the study baseline or within the first month of follow-up were excluded from the analyses.

Job strain exposure

Job strain, which is the most extensively used operationalisation of work stress, was ascertained from the baseline self-report questionnaire [18,19]. Detailed descriptions of the job strain instrument and its harmonisation have been published previously [20]. Briefly, participants were asked to rate various psychosocial aspects of their job (statements such as "my job requires working very fast") and mean response scores were calculated for job demands items and job control items for each participant. A job demands score higher than the study-specific median score was defined as "high demands" and a job control score lower than the study-specific median score as "low control". Job strain was defined as high demands and low control at work.

Inflammatory bowel disease outcomes

In each study, the participants' records were linked to national hospitalisation registries (including in-patient and out-patient appointments) and incident Crohn's disease and ulcerative colitis events during the study follow-up and the dates for these events were ascertained from these registers. In the Finnish studies (FPS, HeSSup and Still Working), we also used information from the Medical Reimbursement Register, kept by the Social Insurance Institution of Finland, to identify Crohn's disease and colitis events. All permanent residents in Finland are eligible for special reimbursement for the cost of medication for certain diseases, including Crohn's disease or colitis (75% of the cost during the study follow-up). A condition for eligibility is a diagnosis of Crohn's disease or ulcerative colitis made in specialised health care or by a specialist physician in gastroenterology, internal medicine, paediatrics or surgery, which are further reviewed by the expert board of the Social Insurance Institute. [21] The dates for the disease events ascertained from the Medical Reimbursement

Register were the dates when the right to special reimbursement was granted.

Crohn's disease events were defined as diagnoses that were registered as International Classification of Diseases (ICD) version 10 code K50 and ICD-9 and earlier versions codes beginning with 555. Ulcerative colitis events were defined correspondingly as K51 and codes beginning with 556.

Potential confounders

Potential confounders were identified based on a priori knowledge of their associations with job strain and Crohn's disease or ulcerative colitis. Potentially confounding factors were age and sex [1,22,23], socioeconomic position [6,24], tobacco smoking [4,25] and body mass index [7,26]. There are a number of recognised as well as proposed risk factors to Crohn's disease and ulcerative colitis, including appendectomy, infections, dietary factors and medications [6], but there is currently no evidence of these being associated with job strain and our analyses were not adjusted for these.

Baseline data on all potential confounders were harmonised to be consistent across the studies. Participants' sex and age were ascertained from population registries or interview (in COPSOQ-I, COPSOQ-II, DWECS, FPS, IPAW, PUMA, Still Working, WOLF Norrland and WOLF Stockholm) or were self-reported (in HeSSup and Whitehall II). Socioeconomic position was defined based on occupational title, which was register-based (in COPSOQ-I, COPSOQ-II, DWECS, FPS, IPAW, PUMA and Still Working) or self-reported (in Whitehall II, WOLF Norrland and WOLF Stockholm). In HeSSup, socioeconomic position was based on self-reported highest educational qualification. Socioeconomic position was categorised into low, intermediate, high

and other [26]. Tobacco smoking was ascertained from self-report and categorised into never, ex- and current smoking. Body mass index (BMI: weight in kilograms divided by height in meters squared) was calculated using height and weight, which were measured by baseline assessors (in Whitehall II, WOLF Norrland and WOLF Stockholm) or self-reported (in COPSOQ-II, DWECS, FPS, HeSSup, IPAW and PUMA). BMI data were not collected in COPSOQ-I and Still Working. BMI was categorised according to the World Health Organization recommendations into <18.5 kg/m^2 (underweight), 18.5–24.9 kg/m^2 (normal weight), 25–29.9 kg/m^2 (overweight) and $> = 30$ kg/m^2 (obese). Extreme BMI values (<15 or >50), which were probably due to measurement error, were excluded from the analysis.

Statistical analyses

Job strain was modelled as a binary variable, job strain (high demands and low control) versus no strain (all other combinations of demands and control). Incident Crohn's disease and ulcerative colitis were binary outcomes. The associations between job strain and incident Crohn's disease or ulcerative colitis were modelled using Cox proportional hazards regression. Time at risk was defined as beginning at birth and observation time as starting at study baseline. The inflammatory bowel disease cases' follow-up ended at the date of their first disease event (Crohn's disease or ulcerative colitis). Participants who were free of these diseases were followed-up until their date of death or end of the hospital registry follow-up. The proportional hazards assumption was checked visually, by comparing the plots of log hazards against time in the exposed and the unexposed, and by using the Schoenfeld-test, and found valid. We ran age and sex-adjusted and multivariable- (age, sex, socioeconomic position, smoking and BMI)-adjusted models

Table 1. Job strain at baseline and inflammatory bowel diseases during the follow-up, by study.

Study, country	Baseline	Median (range) follow-up time (years)	N (%) free of Crohn's disease or ulcerative colitis	N (%) incident Crohn's disease	N (%) incident ulcerative colitis	N (%) job strain
Copenhagen Psychosocial Questionnaire I (COPSOQ-I), Denmark	1997	12.1 (0.02, 12.1)	1 706 (99.3)	4 (0.2)	8 (0.5)	354 (20.6)
Copenhagen Psychosocial Questionnaire II (COPSOQ-II), Denmark	2004–2005	5.0 (0.4, 5.3)	3 314 (99.79	1[1] (0.03)	9 (0.3)	470 (14.1)
Danish Work Environment Cohort Study (DWECS), Denmark	2000	9.1 (0.1, 10.0)	5 394 (99.5)	5 (0.1)	20 (0.4)	1 203 (22.2)
Finnish Public Sector (FPS), Finland	2000	9.2 (0.06, 11.0)	43 683 (99.5)	52 (0.1)	158 (0.4)	7 044 (16.1)
Health and Social Support (HeSSup), Finland	1998	7.0 (0.04, 7.7)	14 909 (99.6)	14 (0.1)	41 (0.3)	2 642 (17.7)
Intervention Project on Absence and Well-being (IPAW), Denmark	1996–1997	13.0 (0.6, 13.79	2[1] (0.1)	3 (0.2)	338 (17.3)	
Burnout, Motivation and Job Satisfaction study (Danish acronym PUMA), Denmark	1999–2000	10.1 (0.5, 10.9)	1 747 (99.3)	5[1] (0.3)	8 (0.5)	266 (15.1)
Still Working, Finland	1986	22.8 (0.03, 23.4)	8 979 (99.1)	15 (0.2)	66 (0.7)	1 412 (15.6)
Whitehall II, UK	2003–2004	6.5 (0.08, 7.3)	2 959 (98.4)	4 (0.1)	43 (1.4)	499 (16.6)
Work Lipids and Fibrinogen (WOLF) Norrland, Sweden	1996–1998	11.8 (0.1, 11.6)	4 637 (99.2)	7[1] (0.1)	31 (0.7)	597 (12.8)
Work Lipids and Fibrinogen (WOLF) Stockholm, Sweden	1992–1995	14.8 (0.04, 18.2)	5 562 (99.3)	17 (0.3)	27 (0.5)	903 (16.1)
All	**1986–2005**	**10.5 (0.02, 23.4)**	**94 839 (99.4)**	**126 (0.1)**	**414 (0.4)**	**15 728 (16.5)**
				111 (0.1)[2]		

[1]COPSOQ-II, IPAW, PUMA and WOLF Norrland were excluded from the analyses of job strain and Crohn's disease risk because in these studies no-one with job strain developed Crohn's disease.
[2]After exclusions NB: Inflammatory bowel diseases here refer to Crohn's disease and ulcerative colitis

Study, disease outcome, n incident cases

HR (95% CI)   Weight

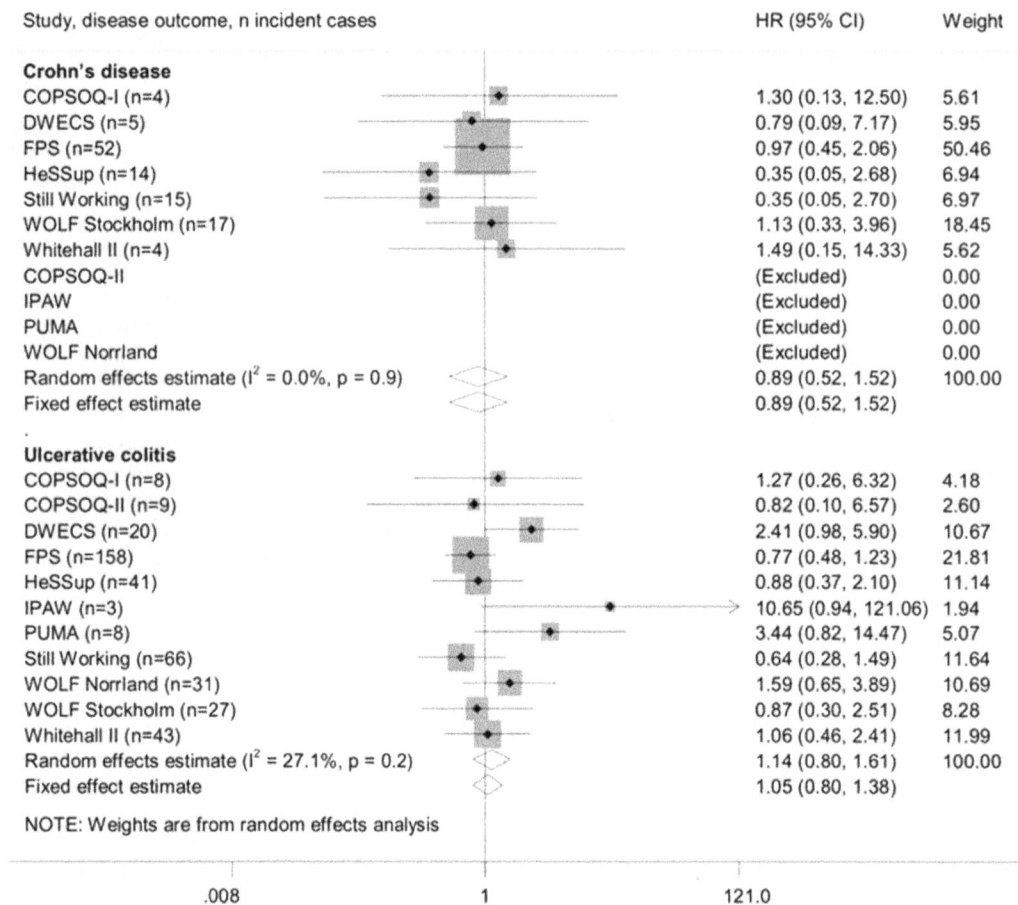

Study, disease outcome, n incident cases	HR (95% CI)	Weight
Crohn's disease		
COPSOQ-I (n=4)	1.30 (0.13, 12.50)	5.61
DWECS (n=5)	0.79 (0.09, 7.17)	5.95
FPS (n=52)	0.97 (0.45, 2.06)	50.46
HeSSup (n=14)	0.35 (0.05, 2.68)	6.94
Still Working (n=15)	0.35 (0.05, 2.70)	6.97
WOLF Stockholm (n=17)	1.13 (0.33, 3.96)	18.45
Whitehall II (n=4)	1.49 (0.15, 14.33)	5.62
COPSOQ-II	(Excluded)	0.00
IPAW	(Excluded)	0.00
PUMA	(Excluded)	0.00
WOLF Norrland	(Excluded)	0.00
Random effects estimate (I^2 = 0.0%, p = 0.9)	0.89 (0.52, 1.52)	100.00
Fixed effect estimate	0.89 (0.52, 1.52)	
Ulcerative colitis		
COPSOQ-I (n=8)	1.27 (0.26, 6.32)	4.18
COPSOQ-II (n=9)	0.82 (0.10, 6.57)	2.60
DWECS (n=20)	2.41 (0.98, 5.90)	10.67
FPS (n=158)	0.77 (0.48, 1.23)	21.81
HeSSup (n=41)	0.88 (0.37, 2.10)	11.14
IPAW (n=3)	10.65 (0.94, 121.06)	1.94
PUMA (n=8)	3.44 (0.82, 14.47)	5.07
Still Working (n=66)	0.64 (0.28, 1.49)	11.64
WOLF Norrland (n=31)	1.59 (0.65, 3.89)	10.69
WOLF Stockholm (n=27)	0.87 (0.30, 2.51)	8.28
Whitehall II (n=43)	1.06 (0.46, 2.41)	11.99
Random effects estimate (I^2 = 27.1%, p = 0.2)	1.14 (0.80, 1.61)	100.00
Fixed effect estimate	1.05 (0.80, 1.38)	

NOTE: Weights are from random effects analysis

.008   1   121.0

Figure 1. Age and sex-adjusted associations of job strain with Crohn's disease or ulcerative colitis.

in each study in turn. As BMI was not measured in COPSOQ-I and Still Working, the multivariable-adjusted models in these studies were not adjusted for it. The study-specific effect estimates were pooled using fixed effect and random effects meta-analyses [27] and heterogeneity in the effect estimates was assessed using the I^2 statistic. All statistical analyses were conducted using Stata 11 (Stata Corporation Ltd., College Station, Texas, US) apart from study-specific analyses in COPSOQ-I, COPSOQ-II, DWECS, IPAW and PUMA, which were conducted using SAS 9.2 (SAS Institute Inc., Cary, North Carolina, US).

Results

Of the 95 379 participants who were free of Crohn's disease or ulcerative colitis at baseline, 126 men and women developed Crohn's disease and 414 developed ulcerative colitis during the follow-up. 94 839 participants remained free of these diseases throughout follow-up. COPSOQ-II, IPAW, PUMA, Still Working and WOLF Norrland were excluded from the analyses of job strain and Crohn's disease risk as no-one with job strain went on to develop Crohn's disease and these analyses were thus based on 111 incident cases of Crohn's disease (Table 1). Median follow-up was 10.5 years. Participant characteristics are provided in Appendix S2, Table S1. A sensitivity analysis showed that the exclusion of COPSOQ-II, IPAW, PUMA, Still Working and WOLF Norrland had not influenced our analyses of job strain and Crohn's disease risk (Appendix S2, Table S2).

The age and sex-adjusted associations between job strain and incident Crohn's disease and ulcerative colitis are shown in Figure 1 and multivariable-adjusted associations in Figure 2. Job strain was not associated with the risk of developing Crohn's disease in the age and sex-adjusted analyses (random effects hazard ratio (HR): 0.89, 95% CI: 0.52, 1.52) Further adjustment (in addition to age and sex) for socioeconomic position, BMI and smoking did not markedly change this estimate (random effects HR: 0.83, 95% CI: 0.48, 1.43). There was little heterogeneity in the estimated associations between job strain and incident Crohn's disease (I^2: 0%).

The association estimates for ulcerative colitis were more heterogeneous than the estimates for Crohn's disease (with approximately 20–30% heterogeneity in minimum- and multivariable-adjusted analyses). Job strain was not associated with the risk of ulcerative colitis in the age and sex-adjusted analyses (random effects HR: 1.14, 95% CI: 0.80, 1.61). Further adjustment for socioeconomic position, BMI and smoking attenuated this estimate even closer to the null-value (random effects HR: 1.06, 95% CI: 0.76, 1.48).

Discussion

Summary of findings in the context of previous research

Better understanding the association between work-related stress and the risk of inflammatory bowel diseases is important because both Crohn's disease and ulcerative colitis are often diagnosed in working-age individuals [1]. Our meta-analyses

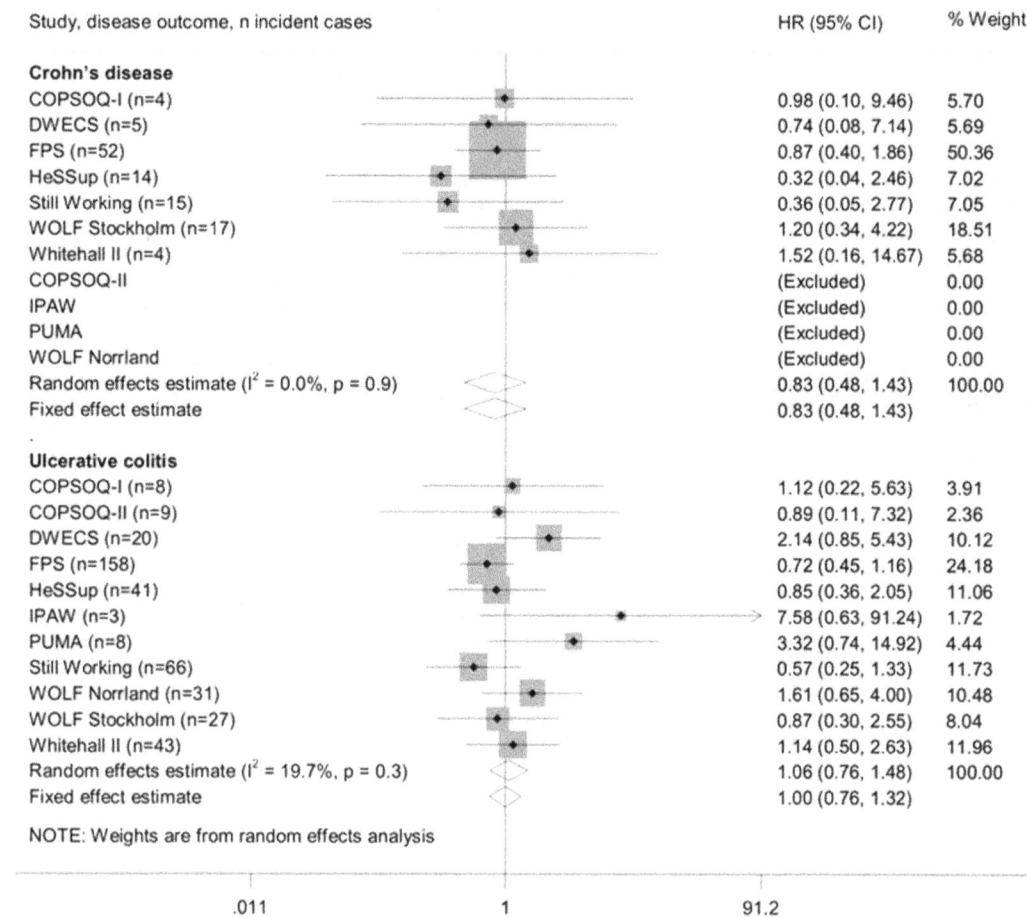

Figure 2. Multivariable-adjusted associations of job strain with Crohn's disease or ulcerative colitis (adjusted for age, sex, socioeconomic position, smoking and BMI).

suggest that job strain, the most extensively studied operationalisation of work-related psychosocial stress, is not associated with the risk of Crohn's disease or ulcerative colitis after adjustment for age, sex, socioeconomic position, smoking and BMI, thus providing evidence against the belief shared by many patients that work-related stress might have a causal role in their disease [10]. These findings do not, of course, take away from the evidence from cross-sectional studies that inflammatory bowel disease patients often experience stress [28,29], or that stress can trigger symptoms and exacerbations in these diseases [8]. The trigger-effect is evident in studies in which the time from the stressful event or experience to the onset of symptoms or diagnosis of inflammatory bowel disease is relatively short. Our analyses, however, were based on several years of follow-up, which is ideal for disentangling the possible impact of job strain on the disease process. Also, our findings are not necessarily generalisable to other indicators of work-related stress or sources of stress outside work. Further large, prospective, population-based studies would help to determine whether other operationalisations of work-related stress or stress in other areas of life have a role in the aetiology of inflammatory bowel diseases

Strengths and limitations

The main strength of the IPD-Work Consortium is its size, which allowed us to investigate relatively rare diseases, such as Crohn's disease and colitis, in a prospective cohort design. Thus far the evidence for an association between stress and the risk of

inflammatory bowel diseases has been based on small, retrospective studies, with findings prone to recall and other biases [9,15,16]. The lack of large, prospective, population-based studies may relate, at least partly, to inflammatory bowel diseases being rare at population-level (the incidence of Crohn's disease in the Western countries is about 6 to 17 per 100 000 and of colitis about 8 to 17 per 100 000).[1] The need to recruit large numbers of participants to ensure sufficient statistical power for the analyses is evident in our investigation which, as far as we are aware, is the largest study of this topic thus far yet still includes just over 100 incident cases of Crohn's disease and 400 incident cases of colitis. The incidence of both inflammatory bowel diseases was lower among the men and women included in our analyses than in the general population, which we suspect is because one eligibility criterion for our analyses was that the participants had to work at study baseline and the working population tends to be healthier than those who do not work.

A further strength in our analyses is that incident Crohn's disease and colitis cases were ascertained from hospitalisation and drug reimbursement registries, which generally have good coverage and are not prone to recall bias. Inflammatory bowel disease diagnoses are made by specialist clinicians using endoscopies or imaging. These techniques allow differential diagnosis of Crohn's and colitis, which is a further strength of our study. The diagnostic tests can be done in primary health care where facilities exist, or at out-patient hospital appointments, but even those initially diagnosed in primary care attend hospital early on in the disease process, for confirmation of their diagnosis or planning and monitoring of their treatment. The hospitalisation data in the studies analysed here covered outpatient appointments onwards from the mid-1990s in the Danish and Finnish studies [30] and from 2003 in the UK study [31]. The Swedish data on specialised outpatient care were available from 2001 and have been shown to have good coverage from 2005-06 onwards [32]. Although there have been some concerns about its previous coverage, the validity of the diagnoses is likely to be good. Thus, as we used registers to ascertain incident cases, it is possible that a small number of individuals who had an inflammatory bowel disease before the study baseline were misclassified as disease-free at the start of the follow-up and defined as incident cases according to a later hospitalisation or drug reimbursement record. Also, misdiagnoses can occur and it is possible that as a result, some healthy individuals have been misclassified as having Crohn's disease or ulcerative colitis, or individuals with either of these diseases misclassified as healthy or having the incorrect disease. Such misclassification is unlikely to be related to any job strain exposure and thus it may have diluted our association estimates, though probably not substantially.

Generally, our analyses of prospectively collected data are unlikely to have been influenced by reverse causality. However, as the symptoms of inflammatory bowel diseases can be vague and differential diagnosis, with the various tests required, can take time. It is therefore possible that the symptoms of an underlying disease have contributed to some individuals reporting high job demands and (though less likely) low control at baseline. If anything, this should artificially inflate the estimated associations between job strain and inflammatory bowel diseases, a result that was not seen in the present analyses Also, the follow-up in the studies included in our analyses span two decades, during which the diagnostic methods for inflammatory bowel disease have changed and improved. It is possible that some outcome misclassification (e.g. irritable bowel syndrome misdiagnosed as inflammatory bowel disease) may have occurred, especially during the early years of follow-up in the older studies. Due to the rarity of inflammatory bowel diseases and the relatively small numbers of cases in our analyses, we were unable to conduct sensitivity analyses excluding cases diagnosed during the early follow-up, though individuals with an inflammatory bowel disease diagnosis within the very first month of follow-up were left out of the analyses. We used a well-recognised, validated and harmonised exposure measure, job strain [18,20]. However, we did not have

data on biological markers of stress, such as dysregulation of the hypothalamic-pituitary-adrenal axis or the activation of the autonomous nervous system, and were thus unable to explore the potential biological pathways linking stress and inflammatory bowel diseases.

Conclusions

Our findings suggest that job strain is unlikely to be an important risk factor for developing Crohn's disease or ulcerative colitis. Whilst these findings would not change the current clinical practice, they provide information to alleviate concerns by patients that work-related stress, as indicated by job strain, would lead to either disease. Further large, prospective, population-based studies would help to determine whether other types of work-related stress or stress in other areas of life have a role in the aetiology of inflammatory bowel diseases.

Supporting Information

Appendix S1   Individual-participant Data Meta-analysis of Working Populations (IPD-Work) Consortium, studies and participants.

Appendix S2   Participant characteristics and a sensitivity analysis.

Checklist S1   STROBE Checklist.

Checklist S2   MOOSE Checklist.

Author Contributions

Conceived and designed the experiments: KH IEHM STN EIF KA LA JBB MB HB ND JEF A. Knutsson M. Koskenvuo A. Koskinen MLN MN JHP JP RR TO MJS SBS TT AV JV MV HW PJMW GDB ASM M. KivimÃ¤ki. Analyzed the data: KH IEHM. Contributed reagents/materials/analysis tools: KH IEHM STN EIF KA LA JBB MB HB ND JEF A. Knutsson M. Koskenvuo A. Koskinen MLN MN JHP JP RR TO MJS SBS TT AV JV MV HW PJMW GDB ASM M. KivimÃ¤ki. Wrote the paper: KH IEHM STN EIF KA LA JBB MB HB ND JEF A. Knutsson M. Koskenvuo A. Koskinen MLN MN JHP JP RR TO MJS SBS TT AV JV MV HW PJMW GDB ASM M. KivimÃ¤ki.

References

1. Cosnes J, Gower-Rousseau C, Seksik P, Cortot A (2011) Epidemiology and natural history of inflammatory bowel diseases. Gastroenterology 140: 1785–1794.
2. Danese S, Fiocchi C (2011) Ulcerative colitis. N Engl J Med 365: 1713–1725.
3. Anderson CA, Boucher G, Lees CW, Franke A, D'Amato M, et al. (2011) Meta-analysis identifies 29 additional ulcerative colitis risk loci, increasing the number of confirmed associations to 47. Nat Genet 43: 246–252.
4. Cabre E, Domenech E (2012) Impact of environmental and dietary factors on the course of inflammatory bowel disease. World J Gastroenterol 18: 3814–3822.
5. Han DY, Fraser AG, Dryland P, Ferguson LR (2010) Environmental factors in the development of chronic inflammation: a case-control study on risk factors for Crohn's disease within New Zealand. Mutat Res 690: 116–122.
6. Carbonnel F, Jantchou P, Monnet E, Cosnes J (2009) Environmental risk factors in Crohn's disease and ulcerative colitis: an update. Gastroenterol Clin Biol 33 Suppl 3: S145–157.
7. Mendall MA, Gunasekera AV, John BJ, Kumar D (2011) Is obesity a risk factor for Crohn's disease? Dig Dis Sci 56: 837–844.
8. Maunder RG, Levenstein S (2008) The role of stress in the development and clinical course of inflammatory bowel disease: epidemiological evidence. Curr Mol Med 8: 247–252.
9. Mawdsley JE, Rampton DS (2005) Psychological stress in IBD: new insights into pathogenic and therapeutic implications. Gut 54: 1481–1491.

10. Sajadinejad MS, Asgari K, Molavi H, Kalantari M, Adibi P (2012) Psychological Issues in Inflammatory Bowel Disease: An Overview. Gastroenterol Res Pract 2012: 106502.
11. Goyal RK, Hirano I (1996) The enteric nervous system. N Engl J Med 334: 1106–1115.
12. Bitton A, Dobkin PL, Edwardes MD, Sewitch MJ, Meddings JB, et al. (2008) Predicting relapse in Crohn's disease: a biopsychosocial model. Gut 57: 1386–1392.
13. Bernstein CN, Singh S, Graff LA, Walker JR, Miller N, et al. (2010) A prospective population-based study of triggers of symptomatic flares in IBD. Am J Gastroenterol 105: 1994–2002.
14. Bonaz BL, Bernstein CN (2013) Brain-gut interactions in inflammatory bowel disease. Gastroenterology 144: 36–49.
15. Lerebours E, Gower-Rousseau C, Merle V, Brazier F, Debeugny S, et al. (2007) Stressful life events as a risk factor for inflammatory bowel disease onset: A population-based case-control study. Am J Gastroenterol 102: 122–131.
16. Li J, Norgard B, Precht DH, Olsen J (2004) Psychological stress and inflammatory bowel disease: a follow-up study in parents who lost a child in Denmark. Am J Gastroenterol 99: 1129–1133.
17. Kivimaki M, Nyberg ST, Batty GD, Fransson E, Heikkila K, et al. (2012) Job strain as a risk factor for future coronary heart disease: Collaborative meta-analysis of 2358 events in 197,473 men and women. Lancet 380: 1491–1497.

18. Karasek R, Brisson C, Kawakami N, Houtman I, Bongers P, et al. (1998) The Job Content Questionnaire (JCQ): an instrument for internationally comparative assessments of psychosocial job characteristics. J Occup Health Psychol 3: 322–355.

19. Karasek R, Theorell T (1990) Healthy work: Stress, productivity, and the reconstruction of working life. New York: Basic Books.

20. Fransson EI, Nyberg ST, Heikkila K, Alfredsson L, Bacquer de D, et al. (2012) Comparison of alternative versions of the job demand-control scales in 17 European cohort studies: the IPD-Work consortium. BMC Public Health 12: 62. doi:10.1186/1471-2458-12-62.

21. Martikainen J, Rajaniemi S (2002) Drug Reimbursement System in EU Member States, Iceland and Norway. Helsinki.

22. Gadinger MC, Fischer JE, Schneider S, Terris DD, Kruckeberg K, et al. (2010) Gender moderates the health-effects of job strain in managers. Int Arch Occup Environ Health 83: 531–541.

23. Lidwall U, Marklund S (2006) What is healthy work for women and men? - A case-control study of gender- and sector-specific effects of psycho-social working conditions on long-term sickness absence. Work 27: 153–163.

24. Elovainio M, Kivimaki M, Ek E, Vahtera J, Honkonen T, et al. (2007) The effect of pre-employment factors on job control, job strain and psychological distress: a 31-year longitudinal study. Soc Sci Med 65: 187–199.

25. Heikkilä K, Nyberg ST, Fransson EI, Alfredsson L, De Bacquer D, et al. (2012) Job Strain and Tobacco Smoking: An Individual-participant Data Meta-analysis of 166 130 Adults in 15 European Studies. PLoS ONE 7: e35463.

26. Nyberg ST, Heikkila K, Fransson EI, Alfredsson L, De Bacquer D, et al. (2012) Job strain in relation to body mass index: pooled analysis of 160 000 adults from 13 cohort studies. Journal of Internal Medicine 272: 65–73.

27. Higgins JP, Thompson SG, Deeks JJ, Altman DG (2003) Measuring inconsistency in meta-analyses. British Medical Journal 327: 557–560.

28. Pellissier S, Dantzer C, Canini F, Mathieu N, Bonaz B (2010) Psychological adjustment and autonomic disturbances in inflammatory bowel diseases and irritable bowel syndrome. Psychoneuroendocrinology 35: 653–662.

29. Singh S, Blanchard A, Walker JR, Graff LA, Miller N, et al. (2011) Common symptoms and stressors among individuals with inflammatory bowel diseases. Clin Gastroenterol Hepatol 9: 769–775.

30. Lynge E, Sandegaard JL, Rebolj M (2011) The Danish National Patient Register. Scand J Public Health 39: 30–33.

31. HESonline Hospital Episode Statistics. The Health and Social Care Information Centre, the National Health Service, United Kingdom. Accessed October 2013.

32. Jacobsson A, Serden L (2013) Kodningskvalitet i patientregistret – Ett nytt verktyg för att mäta kvalitet. Socialstyrelsen, Stockholm, Sweden.

23

PR3-ANCA: A Promising Biomarker in Primary Sclerosing Cholangitis (PSC)

Laura M. Stinton[1]*, **Chelsea Bentow**[2], **Michael Mahler**[2], **Gary L. Norman**[2], **Bertus Eksteen**[1], **Andrew L. Mason**[3], **Gilaad G. Kaplan**[1], **Bjorn Lindkvist**[4], **Gideon M. Hirschfield**[5], **Piotr Milkiewicz**[6,8], **Angela Cheung**[7], **Harry L. A. Janssen**[7], **Marvin J. Fritzler**[1]

1 Department of Medicine, University of Calgary, Calgary, Alberta, Canada, **2** Inova Diagnostics, Inc., San Diego, California, United States of America, **3** Department of Medicine, University of Alberta, Edmonton, Alberta, Canada, **4** Institute of Medicine, Sahlgrenska Academy, University of Gothenburg, Gothenburg, Sweden, **5** Centre for Liver Research, NIHR Biomedical Research Unit, University of Birmingham, Birmingham, United Kingdom, **6** Department of General, Transplant and Liver Surgery, Warsaw Medical University, Warsaw, Poland, **7** University Health Network, Division of Gastroenterology, Toronto Western Hospital, Toronto, Ontario, Canada, **8** Liver Research Laboratories, Pomeranian Medical University, Szczecin, Poland

Abstract

Background and Aims: The only recognized biomarker for primary sclerosing cholangitis (PSC) is atypical anti-neutrophil cytoplasmic antibodies (aANCA), which, in addition to having low sensitivity and specificity, is an indirect immunofluorescence (IIF) test lacking the advantages of high throughput and objectivity. Recent reports have shown that antibodies to proteinase-3 (PR3-ANCA) might add diagnostic value in inflammatory bowel disease (IBD), specifically in ulcerative colitis (UC). As PSC is associated with IBD, the objective of this study was to evaluate the frequency and clinical significance of PR3-ANCA in a large cohort of patients.

Methods: A total of 244 PSC and 254 control [autoimmune hepatitis (AIH), primary biliary cirrhosis (PBC), hepatitis C viral infection (HCV), hepatitis B viral infection (HBV), and healthy controls] sera and their clinical correlations were retrospectively analyzed for PR3-ANCA determined by ELISA and a new chemiluminescence immunoassay (CIA). Testing was also performed for aANCA by IIF.

Results: When measured by CIA, PR3-ANCA was detected in 38.5% (94/244) of PSC patients compared to 10.6% (27/254) controls ($p < 0.0001$). By ELISA, PR3-ANCA was detected in 23.4% (57/244) of PSC patients compared to 2.7% (6/254) controls ($p < 0.0001$). PR3-ANCA in PSC patients was not associated with the presence or type of underlying IBD, and, in fact, it was more frequent in Crohn's disease (CD) patients with PSC than previously reported in CD alone. PR3-ANCA in PSC measured by CIA correlated with higher liver enzymes.

Conclusion: PR3-ANCA is detected in a significant proportion of PSC patients compared to other liver diseases including PBC and AIH. PR3-ANCA is associated with higher liver enzyme levels in PSC, and is not solely related to underlying IBD.

Editor: Niklas K. Björkström, Karolinska Institutet, Sweden

Funding: L. Stinton received funding from the 2013 Clinical Research Award from the American College of Gastroenterology. Part of it was used for this project. A. Mason is supported by Alberta Heritage Foundation for Medical Research (AHFMR) as a Senior Scholar. B. Lindkvist is supported by the medical research council of Västra Götaland in Sweden (ALF-22101) and the Rolf Olsson memorial scholarship fund. G. Hirschfield is supported as a co-investigator by the Medical Research Council as part of a stratified medicine team grant; www.ukpbc.com. P. Milkiewicz is supported by the grant no. 2011/01/B/NZ5/04216 from National Science Centre in Poland. The funders had no role in study design, data collection and analysis, decision to publish, or preparation of the manuscript. M. Mahler, C. Bentow and G. Norman are employees of Inova Diagnostics Inc. (San Diego). Inova Diagnostics Inc. provided support in the form of salaries for authors MM, CB and GLN, but did not have any additional role in the study design, data collection and analysis, decision to publish, or preparation of the manuscript. The specific roles of these authors are articulated in the 'author contributions' section.

Competing Interests: M. Fritzler is a paid consultant, has received honoraria or has received gifts in kind from ImmunoConcepts Inc. (Sacramento, CA), Bio-Rad (Hercules, CA) and INOVA Diagnostics (San Diego, CA), Mikrogen GmbH (Neuried, Germany), Euroimmun GmbH (Lubeck, Germany) and Dr. Fooke Laboratorien GmbH (Neuss, Germany). M. Mahler, C. Bentow and G. Norman are employees of Inova Diagnostics Inc. (San Diego) a manufacturer of autoantibody diagnostic kits. There are no patents, products in development or marketed products to declare.

* Email: laura.stinton@ucalgary.ca

Introduction

Primary sclerosing cholangitis (PSC) is a chronic, cholestatic syndrome characterized by inflammation and fibrosis of the intra- and extra-hepatic bile ducts, leading to multifocal bile duct strictures. The clinical course and complications of PSC vary considerably, but usually follows a progressive course, ultimately leading to cirrhosis, hepatic failure, and in 10–20% of patients, cholangiocarcinoma. PSC is associated with inflammatory bowel disease (IBD) in 70–80% of cases, most commonly ulcerative colitis (UC) [1,2].

The diagnosis of large duct PSC is based on a cholestatic elevation of liver enzymes and typical cholangiographic findings including bile duct irregularities with multiple strictures and segmental dilatations. A variety of autoantibodies have been observed in the sera of PSC patients, but none are disease-specific [3]. Anti-neutrophil cytoplasmic antibodies (ANCA), directed against various subcellular constituents of neutrophil or myeloid cells, have been reported in 65–95% of PSC patients [4–6]. ANCA are routinely detected by indirect immunofluorescence (IIF) assays using ethanol and formalin-fixed neutrophils [7]. The IIF ANCA staining pattern in PSC has been characterized as broad, non-homogeneous enhancement of the nuclear periphery combined with multiple intranuclear foci. This has been referred to as atypical ANCA (aANCA), anti-neutrophil nuclear antibodies (p-ANNA), or xANCA [7]. aANCA have been reported in the context of UC and PSC, but also in other liver diseases including autoimmune hepatitis (AIH), primary biliary cirrhosis (PBC), and viral and alcoholic hepatitis [2] [5,6,8,9]. The other well known IIF ANCA patterns are cytoplasmic (cANCA) and perinuclear (pANCA). cANCA is largely attributed to the presence of autoantibodies targeting the serine protease proteinase-3 (PR3-ANCA), while pANCA is associated with antibodies directed against a number of antigens, including myeloperoxidase (MPO-ANCA), lactoferrin, lysozyme, azurocidin, elastase, cathepsin G, and bactericidal/permeability-increasing enzyme (BPI)[10,11]. PR3-ANCA are an established marker for the diagnosis of small vessel vasculitis including granulomatosis with polyangiitis (GPA) (formerly Wegener's granulomatosus); MPO is the most frequently identified antigen in pANCA and is associated with crescentic glomerulonephritis, microscopic polyaangitis (MPA), and eosinophilic granulomatosis with polyangiitis (EGPA) (formerly Churg-Strauss syndrome) [7,12]. aANCA has been widely investigated and putative targets include high mobility group non-histone, high mobility group chromosomal proteins HMG1/2 [13], beta-tubulin isotype 5 [14,15], and DNA-bound lactoferrin[16].

In contrast to previously reported data [17], more recent studies indicate that PR3-ANCA are detected in a significant proportion of patients with IBD, specifically UC [18,19]. This is particularly true when PR3-ANCA are detected by capture or anchor immunoassays, possibly because they bind conformational epitopes that are not available for binding in conventional enzyme-linked immunosorbent assays (ELISA) [18,20]. PR3-ANCA measured by conventional ELISA has previously been reported in PSC, however the prevalence has ranged from 4–44% [3,21]. The goal of this multi-centre international study was to evaluate the frequency of PR3-ANCA in PSC patients as measured by ELISA and a new chemiluminescence immunoassay (CIA) and to determine clinical correlations with PR3-ANCA. The utility of PR3-ANCA to aid in the diagnosis of PSC was compared to aANCA detected by IIF, while the diagnostic specificity of these assays was assessed in PSC and compared to other liver diseases including those of autoimmune etiology [primary biliary cirrhosis (PBC), autoimmune hepatitis (AIH) and overlap syndromes of AIH-PBC, AIH-PSC]. Finally, the use of PR3-ANCA and aANCA IIF in PSC and IBD was assessed.

Materials and Methods

Patient Samples

A total of 498 patient biobanked sera were analysed in this study. Serum samples from 222 PSC patients and 22 AIH-PSC originating from 5 clinical centres (Center I: Sahlgrenska University Hospital, Gothenburg, Sweden, n = 114; Center II: University Health Network, Toronto Western Hospital, Toronto, Ontario, Canada, n = 59; Center III: University of Calgary, Calgary, Alberta, Canada (Including the Alberta IBD Consortium), n = 27); Center IV: University of Alberta Hospital, Edmonton, Alberta, Canada, n = 26; Center V: Pomeranian Medical University, Szczecin, Poland, n = 18). A diagnosis of PSC was confirmed by clinical experts in the field based on the following criteria: chronically elevated liver enzymes; standard cholangiographic (magnetic resonance cholangiography [MRCP] or endoscopic retrograde cholangiography [ERCP]) bile duct changes with multifocal strictures and segmental dilatations and/or liver biopsy consistent with PSC, and exclusion of secondary cause of cholangitis. Small duct PSC was defined as a liver biopsy with histopathology consistent with PSC and a normal ERCP or MRCP. Clinical data from the PSC patients was collected when available and included age, sex, disease duration, type of PSC including small-duct PSC, presence of cholangiocarcinoma, cirrhosis, ascites, hepatic encephalopathy, esophageal varices, use of ursodeoxycholic acid (UDCA), and laboratory measurements (alanine aminotransferase (ALT), aspartate aminotransferase (AST), alkaline phosphatase (ALP), total bilirubin, international normalized ratio (INR), hemoglobin, platelet count, and creatinine). All clinical information correlated with the date of serum collection. Each site also provided the IBD status of the PSC patients. The diagnosis of IBD was made by experts in the field based on established diagnostic criteria including a combination of clinical, endoscopic, histological and serological results. Patients with PSC who were not evaluated for IBD were excluded. 254 serum samples from patients with various hepatic diseases were also included as pathological controls (65 AIH, 81 PBC, 10 AIH-PBC, 18 hepatitis C viral infection (HCV), 32 hepatitis B viral infection (HBV), 48 healthy controls) (Inova Diagnostics Inc., San Diego, CA, in-house control cohorts). Written consent was obtained from all patients in accordance with the project approved by the local ethical committees including the Conjoint Health Ethics Review Board at the University of Calgary and fulfilled the ethical guidelines established in the Declaration of Helsinki.

Autoantibody Assays

PR3-ANCA positivity was determined by a novel CIA (QUANTA Flash PR3 on BIO-FLASH CIA, Inova Diagnostics Inc.) which uses native PR3 antigen coupled to paramagnetic beads. The PR3 CIA is designed around the BIO-FLASH instrument, containing a luminometer, as well as all the hardware and liquid handling accessories necessary to perform the assay. Native purified human PR3 is coated onto paramagnetic beads and assayed on the BIO-FLASH system as previously described [22]. The PR3 CIA utilizes a predefined lot specific Master Curve that is uploaded into the instrument through the reagent pack barcode. Based on the results of running two calibrators, an instrument specific Working Curve is created, which is used to calculate chemiluminescent units (CUs) for each serum. For the PR3 CIA IgA version, the isoluminol conjugated anti-human IgG was replaced by isoluminol conjugated anti-human IgA. All samples were tested by PR3 ELISA and by the PR3 CIA. The suggested cut-off value of 20 chemiluminescent units (CU) for the CIA as suggested by the manufacturer was utilized. Anti-PR3 was also determined by traditional ELISA (QUANTA Lite PR3, Inova Diagnostics, Inc.), which uses the same native antigen as the CIA system. ANCA was tested by IIF on formalin and ethanol-fixed neutrophil substrates (ANCA: Inova Diagnostics Inc.) and read on an Olympus CX31 microscope (Olympus America Inc., Melville, NY) by an experienced technologist.

Statistical Methods

Statistical evaluation was performed using Analyse-it software (Version 2.03; Analyse-it Software, Ltd., Leeds, UK). Sensitivities, specificities and likelihood ratios were calculated where appropriate. Descriptive statistics and Fisher's exact test were used to compare groups where applicable. Mann-Whitney test and ANOVA were used for the comparison of continuous data. Receiver operator characteristic (ROC) curves were calculated to determine the ability of PR3-ANCA to discriminate PSC from the control groups. Mean titers of both the CIA and ELISA tests were used. Where appropriate, 95% confidence intervals (CI) were provided. For all statistical methods, p values <0.05 were considered significant.

Results

Prevalence of PR3-ANCA in PSC and liver disease controls

By CIA, 94/244 (38.5%) of PSC patients [82/222 (36.9%) PSC, 12/22 (54.5%) AIH-PSC] were positive for PR3-ANCA compared to 27/254 (10.6%) of controls (p<0.0001). By comparison the control sera had a remarkably lower frequency of PR3-ANCA: AIH 14/65 (21.5%), AIH-PBC 3/10 (30%), PBC 9/81 (11.1%), HBV 1/32 (3.1%), HCV 0/18, healthy controls 0/48. By ELISA, 57/244 (23.4%) of PSC patients [51/222 (23.0%) PSC, 6/22 (27.3%) AIH-PSC] were positive for PR3-ANCA compared to 6/254 (2.7%) of controls (p<0.0001) [AIH 5/65 (7.7%), AIH-PBC 0/10, PBC 0/81, HCV 0/18, HBV 0/32, healthy controls 1/48 (2.1%)]. aANCA by IIF were detected in 101/244 (41.4%) of PSC patients [89/222 (40.1%) PSC, 12/22 (54.5%) AIH-PSC] compared to 51/254 (20.1%) of controls (p<0.0001) [AIH 26/65 (40%), AIH-PBC 2/10 (20%), PBC 8/81 (9.9%), HCV 0/18, HBV 3/32 (9.4%), healthy controls 2/48 (4.2%)] (Table 1).

Comparison of PR3-ANCA and Established Assays

The sensitivity and specificity for PSC were 38.5% and 89.4%, respectively when compared to all controls by CIA. When compared to AIH the specificity was 78.5% and to PBC was 86.8%. The likelihood ratios (LR+/LR-) were 3.62/0.69 for PSC vs. all controls, 1.79/0.78 for PSC vs. AIH, and 2.92/0.71 for PSC vs. PBC. By ELISA, the sensitivity and specificity in PSC were 23.4% and 97.6%, respectively when compared to all controls. When compared to AIH the specificity was 92.3% and to PBC was 100%. The LR+/LR- were 9.89/0.78 for PSC vs. all controls, 3.04/083 for PSC vs. AIH, and +∞/0.77 for PSC vs. PBC.

Measurement of aANCA by IIF had a sensitivity and specificity of 41.4% and 83.9% respectively when PSC was compared to all controls. When compared to AIH the specificity was 60.0% and to PBC was 89.0%. The LR+/LR- were 2.56/0.70 for PSC vs. all controls and 1.03/0.98 for PSC vs. AIH, and 3.77/0.66 for PSC vs. PBC (Table 2).

ROC curves were used to test the ability of the serological tests to discriminate PSC from other liver controls (Figure 1). When PSC was compared to all controls the area under the curve (AUC) values were 0.67 (CIA), 0.78 (ELISA), and 0.69 (IIF), respectively. When PSC was compared to AIH the area under the curve (AUC) values were 0.56 (CIA), 0.68 (ELISA), and 0.52 (IIF), respectively. When PSC was compared to PBC the area under the curve (AUC) values were 0.60 (CIA), 0.81 (ELISA), and 0.75 (IIF), respectively.

Mean titers of PR3-ANCA CIA were significantly higher in PSC (PSC 39.9CU, AIH-PSC 58.7CU) compared to other liver cohorts (p<0.0001): AIH 17.3 CU, AIH-PBC 15.6 CU, PBC 9.8 CU, HCV 4.7 CU, HBV 4.2 CU, healthy controls 2.5 CU. Mean titers of PR3-ANCA ELISA were significantly higher in PSC (PSC 14.9 CU, AIH-PSC 22.3) compared to controls (p<0.0001): AIH

Table 1. Frequency of PR3-ANCA by CIA, ELISA, and aANCA in PSC vs. all controls, vs. AIH and vs. PBC.

| | PSC | | | Controls | | | Relevance |
	All PSC, n (%)	PSC, n (%)	AIH-PSC, n (%)	All Controls, n (%)	AIH, n (%)	PBC, (%)	p value
PR3-ANCA CIA	94/244 (38.5%)	82/222 (36.9%)	12/22 (54.5%)	27/254 (10.6%)	14/65 (21.5%)	12/91 (13.2%)	<0.0001[a] 0.014[b] <0.0001[c]
PR3-ANCA ELISA	57/244 (23.4%)	51/222 (23.0%)	6/22 (27.3%)	6/254 (2.7%)	5/65 (7.7%)	0/91 (0%)	<0.0001[a] 0.005[b] <0.0001[c]
aANCA IIF (Titer 1-20)	101/244 (41.4%)	89/222 (40.1%)	12/22 (54.5%)	51/254 (20.1%)	26/65 (40%)	10/91 (11%)	<0.0001[a] 0.955[b] <0.0001[c]

[a] p value for PSC vs. all controls.
[b] p value for PSC vs. AIH.
[c] p value for PSC vs. PBC.

Table 2. Sensitivity, specificity and likelihood ratios (LR+/LR-) in PSC when compared to controls.

	Sensitivity (95% CI)	Specificity PSC vs. All controls (95% CI)	Specificity PSC vs. AIH (95% CI)	Specificity PSC vs. PBC (95% CI)	LR+/LR- PSC vs. All Controls	LR+/LR- PSC vs. AIH	LR+/LR- PSC vs. PBC
PR3 CIA	38.50% (32.4-44.9)	89.40% (84.9-92.9)	78.50% (66.5-87.7)	86.80% (78.1-93.0)	3.62/0.69	1.79/0.78	2.92/0.71
PR3 ELISA	23.40% (18.2-29.2)	97.60% (94.9-99.1)	92.30% (83.0-97.5)	100% (96.0-100)	9.89/0.78	3.04/0.83	+∞/0.77
aANCA IIF	41.40% (35.1-47.9)	83.90% (78.7-88.2)	60.00% (47.1-72.0)	89.00% (80.7-94.6)	2.56/0.70	1.03/0.98	3.77/0.66

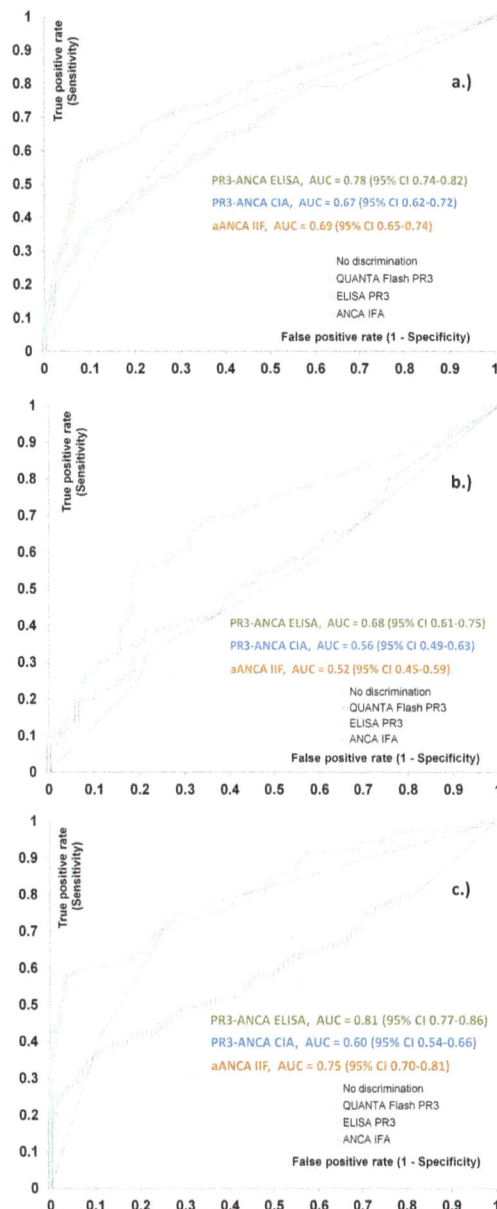

Figure 1. Comparative receiver operating characteristic (ROC) curves analysis. Comparative ROC analysis is shown for PR3-ANCA by ELISA, chemiluminescence immunoassay (CIA) and ANCA by indirect immunofluorescence (pANCA). Primary sclerosing cholangitis (PSC) vs. all liver controls (a) and vs. autoimmune hepatitis (AIH) (b), and vs. primary biliary cirrhosis (PBC) (c). Area under the curve (AUC) and 95% Confidence Intervals (CI) values for the individual assays are presented in the figure.

6.4 CU, AIH-PBC 3.7 CU, PBC 2.7 CU, HCV 2.1 CU, HBV 2.7 CU, healthy controls 4.4 CU (Figure 2).

Clinical parameters of PSC patients

The available clinical and biochemical parameters of the PSC patients are reported in Table 3. PR3-ANCA positivity by CIA was associated with younger age (p<0000.1), higher ALT (p = 0.0002), AST (p<0.0001), ALP (p<0.0001), and platelet levels (p = 0.0076). PR3-ANCA did not significantly distinguish between sex, disease duration, small duct PSC, cholangiocarcinoma, cirrhosis, esophageal varices, ascites, hepatic encephalop-

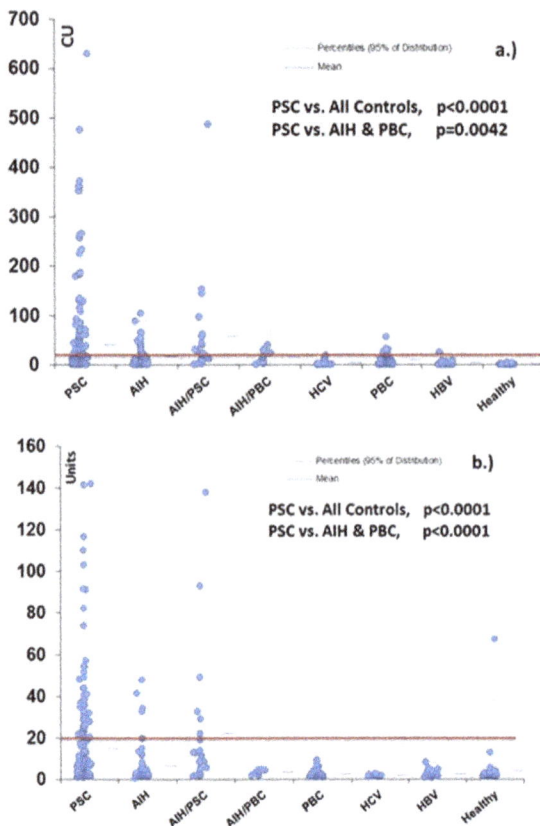

Figure 2. Comparative descriptive analysis. PR3-ANCA in primary sclerosing cholangitis (PSC) and various pathological and healthy controls (a. PR3-ANCA chemiluminescence immunoassay (CIA), b. PR3-ANCA ELISA). The recommended cut-off by the manufacturer is 20 chemiluminescent units (CU). Groups are as follows: autoimmune hepatitis (AIH); primary biliary cirrhosis (PBC); AIH-PSC overlap; AIH-PBC overlap; hepatitis C virus (HCV) infection; hepatitis B virus (HBV) infection; healthy controls.

Discussion

PR3-ANCA is an extensively described diagnostic and prognostic serological biomarker for primary systemic vasculitis [23]. More recently, PR3-ANCA, when measured by a novel CIA platform, has been described in a significant proportion of IBD patients, specifically UC, where it was related to disease severity [18,24]. Because PSC is commonly associated with IBD [25], we were interested to determine if PR3-ANCA is also a biomarker of this condition. In this study we found that the frequency of PR3-ANCA when measured by CIA is 38.5% in PSC patient sera and only 10.6% in liver disease controls ($p<0.0001$). When measured by ELISA, the prevalence of PR3-ANCA in PSC is lower at 23.3%; however, it had a higher specificity compared to CIA (97.6% vs. 89.4%). PR3-ANCA measured by both CIA and ELISA were more specific than the IIF aANCA (83.9%), which is a traditional serological marker of PSC [26]. These results are clinically and diagnostically important as the IIF testing for aANCA is associated with a number of limitations. For example, IIF assays are time consuming, observer-dependent, low throughput, and require highly trained personnel. In addition, the standardization of ELISA has proven challenging largely because of inter-manufacturer variation of ANCA detection kits [27–29]. Taken together, despite international consensus and guidelines for ANCA testing [7,30], these factors still generate significant inter-laboratory variation of results [31,32]. Although aANCA is currently used as a biomarker for PSC, it also has significant overlap with other disorders including AIH and UC. Our study has shown that PR3-ANCA performs better than aANCA for the diagnosis of PSC and avoids the challenges associated with IIF testing.

Patients presenting with elevated liver enzymes require a full diagnostic workup and the differential diagnosis of potential hepatopathies is wide. The present data suggest that the measurement of PR3-ANCA are a useful biomarker to aid in the differentiation of PSC and other liver diseases including AIH, PBC. Other serological biomarkers are used for the diagnosis of AIH (ANA, F-actin, ASMA [33]) and PBC (i.e. AMA, gp210, sp100) [34,35], however, apart from aANCA by IIF, which can also be seen in AIH, no simple serological test is currently available to alert the clinician to possible PSC. With multiplex assays becoming more common [36,37], perhaps the addition of PR3-ANCA to a liver panel should be considered: given that PSC is rare and not encountered frequently by many clinicians, such a blood result could initiate further investigation, such as a MRCP, in a more prompt way outside of specialist centers.

In our study, PR3-ANCA in PSC was associated with higher levels of hepatocellular (ALT, AST) and cholestatic (ALP) liver enzymes. Although there was no statistically significant difference between PR3-ANCA in disease severity or progression as measured by the presence of cirrhosis, esophageal varices, hepatic encephalopathy, or ascites, the relative number of these patients in the cohort was low. Additionally, the ability of PR3-ANCA to predict small duct PSC or the development of cholangiocarcinoma was limited by small sample numbers. However, the finding that PR3-ANCA is associated with patients with higher liver enzymes may represent a subgroup of patients with a more inflammatory phenotype who potentially may respond to future anti-inflammatory compounds. Larger prospective studies will be needed to further identify the clinical association of PR3-ANCA in PSC, including identifying subgroups of patients and response to medications.

Our data also demonstrate that PR3-ANCA in PSC is not exclusively related to underlying IBD. Due to differences in data

athy, or UDCA use. Due to the lower frequency of PR3-ANCA measured by ELISA, only CIA results were analyzed for clinical parameters.

Clinical associations of PR3-ANCA in PSC and IBD

The clinical association of IBD in the PSC patients was available in 204/244 (83.6%) of the cohort. 62/244 (25.4%) had no associated IBD, 27/242 (11.1%) had Crohn's disease (PSC-CD), 111/244 (45.5%) had UC (PSC-UC) and 4/244 (1.6%) had IBD-unclassified (PSC-IBD-U). By CIA, 58/142 (40.8%) of the PSC & IBD patients [PSC-CD 13/27 (48.1%), PSC-UC 45/111 (40.5%), PSC-IBD-U 0/4] were positive for PR3-ANCA compared to 19/62 (30.6%) of the PSC with no associated IBD patients ($p=0.22$). By ELISA, 38/142 (26.8%) of the PSC & IBD patients [PSC-CD 6/27 (22.2%), PSC-UC 32/111 (28.8%), PSC-IBD-U 0/4] were positive for PR3-ANCA compared to 10/62 (16.1%) of the PSC & no associated IBD patients ($p=0.14$). aANCA by IIF were detected in 58/142 (40.8%) of the PSC & IBD patients [PSC-CD 7/27 (25.9%), PSC-UC 47/111 (25.9%), PSC-IBD-U 4/4 (100%)] compared to 26/62 (41.9%) of the PSC & no associated IBD patients ($p=1$) (Table 4). There was no significant difference between any of the tests when PSC-CD was compared to PSC-UC.

Table 3. Comparison of the clinical parameters of PSC patients at the time of serum testing according to the PR3-ANCA status as measured by chemiluminescence immunoassay (CIA).

	PSC patients	PR3-ANCA positive	PR3-ANCA negative	p value
Age, years (range) (n)	45.3 (18–86) (n = 218)	39.4 (19–78) (n = 78)	48.6 (18–86) (n = 140)	<0.0001[a]
Sex, male (%)/female (%)	133 (61%)/85 (39%)	55 (71%)/23 (29%)	78 (56%)/62 (44%)	0.067[b]
ALT, U/L (range) (n)	91 (8–576) (n = 201)	133 (8–576) (n = 74)	66 (12–294) (n = 127)	<0.0001[a]
AST, U/L (range) (n)	74 (17–730) (n = 198)	109 (17–730) (n = 73)	55 (18–247) (n = 125)	<0.0001[a]
ALP, U/L (range) (n)	273 (41–1959) (n = 202)	352 (52–1959) (n = 74)	228 (41–1349) (n = 128)	<0.0001[a]
Total bilirubin, mg/dL (range) (n)	22 (3–445) (n = 202)	25 (5–340) (n = 74)	20 (3–445) (n = 128)	0.12[a]
INR (range) (n)	1.1 (0.9–2.4) (n = 194)	1.1 (0.9–2.0) (n = 71)	1.1 (0.9–2.4) (n = 123)	0.08[a]
Albumin, g/L (range) (n)	41 (21–54) (n = 78)	41 (28–50) (n = 31)	41 (21–54) (n = 47)	0.98[a]
Hemoglobin g/L (range) (n)	135 (79–167) (n = 204)	133 (89–167) (n = 75)	137 (79–167) (n = 129)	0.18[a]
Platelet count ×10⁹/L (range) (n)	266 (37–608) (n = 185)	288 (98–608) (n = 64)	253 (37–589) (n = 121)	0.0076[a]
Creatinine μmol/L (range) (n)	78 (50–127) (n = 29)	76 (60–102) (n = 9)	79 (50–127) (n = 20)	0.91[a]
Disease duration, years (range) (n)	7.8 (0–27) (n = 201)	7.4 (0–25) (n = 72)	8.0 (0–27) (n = 129)	0.73[a]
Small duct PSC, n (%)	28/202 (14%)	11/28 (39%)	17/28 (61%)	0.9[b]
Cholangiocarcinoma, n (%)	5/167 (3%)	3/5 (60%)	2/5 (40%)	0.3[b]
Cirrhosis, n (%)	34/74 (46%)	16/34 (47%)	18/34 (53%)	0.21[b]
Ursodeoxycholic Acid (UDCA) use, n (%)	64/87 (74%)	27/64 (42%)	37/64 (58%)	0.82[b]
Varices, n (%)	15/52 (29%)	7/15 (47%)	8/15 (53%)	0.51[b]
Ascites, n (%)	12/55 (22%)	7/12 (58%)	5/12 (42%)	0.15[b]
Hepatic encephalopathy, n (%)	5/54 (9%)	3/5 (60%)	2/5 (40%)	0.58[b]

ALP, alkaline phosphatase; ALT, alanine aminotransferase; AST, aspartate aminotransferase, INR, international normalized ratio; UDCA, ursodeoxycholic acid.
[a]Mann-Whitney test was used for continuous variables.
[b]Student's t-test was used for qualitative measurements.

collection between the clinical sites, the IBD status was only known in 83.6%. Despite this, there was no significant difference between PR3-ANCA in PSC-CD, PSC-UC, PSC-IBD-U, or PSC without associated IBD. However, PR3-ANCA may be a marker of PSC in CD. Previous studies have shown that the frequency of PR3-ANCA in CD is low (i.e. <2%) [18,38], however these studies did not include patients with PSC. Our study found that 48.1% of PSC-CD patients had PR3-ANCA when measured by CIA. Although larger studies are needed to confirm this association, if PR3-ANCA is seen in CD, it may predict and/or prompt the clinician to evaluate the patient for associated PSC.

We acknowledge limitations of our study including the fact that it is retrospective and lacks the serial measurements of PR3-ANCA during the disease course. Although the diagnosis of PSC was made by experts in the field, due to the multi-centre nature of the study, a lack of a standardized diagnostic approach, is a limitation. Although the specificity of PR3-ANCA in PSC is high, we acknowledge that the sensitivity of the test is very low. At this point we are not recommending the use of this test to solely rule out the diagnosis of PSC. Additional studies are warranted to investigate if PR3-ANCA in PSC is associated with disease prognosis or response to medications and if PR3-ANCA in CD may indicate an increased likelihood of the presence of PSC in these patients.

Table 4. Frequency of PR3-ANCA in PSC & IBD subgroups.

	PSC & IBD	PSC-CD	PSC-UC	PSC-IBD-U	PSC & no IBD	p value
PR3-ANCA CIA	58/142 (40.8%)	13/27 (48.1%)	45/111 (40.5%)	0/4	19/62	0.22[a]
				0%	-30.60%	1.00[b]
PR3-ANCA ELISA	38/142 (26.7%)	6/27 (22.2%)	32/111 (28.8%)	0/4	Oct-62	0.14[a]
				0%	−16.10%	0.41[b]
aANCA IIF	58/142 (40.8%)	7/27 (25.9%)	47/111 (42.3%)	4-Apr	26/62	1.00[a]
				−100%	−41.90%	0.64[b]

[a] P value calculated between PSC & IBD and PSC & no IBD.
[b] P value calculated between PSC-CD and PSC-UC.

Conclusions

Our data demonstrate that PR3-ANCA can be detected in a significant proportion of PSC patients and are a specific biomarker in the context of other liver disorders including autoimmune liver diseases. PR3-ANCA in PSC was found to be associated with higher liver enzymes and may represent a more inflammatory subtype of disease. PR3-ANCA in PSC do not seem to be related to a co-diagnosis of IBD and more studies are needed to determine if it may be a biomarker of PSC in CD.

Acknowledgments

We acknowledge the help of Andrea Seaman, Zakera Shums, Jay Milo, Shay Middleton and Cassandra Bryant from Inova Diagnostics, Meifeng Zhang and Haiyan Hou from Mitogen Laboratory, and Mark Fritzler from Eve Technologies.

Author Contributions

Conceived and designed the experiments: LMS CB MM GLN MJF. Performed the experiments: LMS CB. Analyzed the data: LMS CB MM GLN MJF. Contributed reagents/materials/analysis tools: LMS BE ALM GGK BL GMH PM AC HLAJ MJF. Wrote the paper: LMS CB MM GLN BE ALM GGK BL GMH PM AC HLAJ MJF.

References

1. Wiesner RH, Grambsch PM, Dickson ER, Ludwig J, MacCarty RL, et al. (1989) Primary sclerosing cholangitis: natural history, prognostic factors and survival analysis. Hepatology 10: 430–436. S0270913989001837 [pii].
2. Hirschfield GM, Karlsen TH, Lindor KD, Adams DH (2013) Primary sclerosing cholangitis. Lancet 382: 1587–1599. S0140-6736(13)60096-3 [pii];10.1016/S0140-6736(13)60096-3 [doi].
3. Angulo P, Peter JB, Gershwin ME, DeSotel CK, Shoenfeld Y, et al. (2000) Serum autoantibodies in patients with primary sclerosing cholangitis. J Hepatol 32: 182–187. S0168-8278(00)80061-6 [pii].
4. Roozendaal C, de Jong MA, van den Berg AP, van Wijk RT, Limburg PC, et al. (2000) Clinical significance of anti-neutrophil cytoplasmic antibodies (ANCA) in autoimmune liver diseases. J Hepatol 32: 734–741. S016882780080241X [pii].
5. Duerr RH, Targan SR, Landers CJ, LaRusso NF, Lindsay KL, et al. (1991) Neutrophil cytoplasmic antibodies: a link between primary sclerosing cholangitis and ulcerative colitis. Gastroenterology 100: 1385–1391. S0016508591001798 [pii].
6. Deniziaut G, Ballot E, Johanet C (2013) Antineutrophil cytoplasmic auto-antibodies (ANCA) in autoimmune hepatitis and primary sclerosing cholangitis. Clin Res Hepatol Gastroenterol 37: 105–107. S2210-7401(12)00212-4 [pii];10.1016/j.clinre.2012.07.008 [doi].
7. Savige J, Gillis D, Benson E, Davies D, Esnault V, et al. (1999) International Consensus Statement on Testing and Reporting of Antineutrophil Cytoplasmic Antibodies (ANCA). Am J Clin Pathol 111: 507–513.
8. De Riva V, Celadin M, Pittoni M, Plebani M, Angeli P (2009) What is behind the presence of anti-neutrophil cytoplasmatic antibodies in chronic liver disease? Liver Int 29: 865–870. LIV1989 [pii];10.1111/j.1478-3231.2009.01989.x [doi].
9. Fulcher DA (2000) Anti-neutrophil cytoplasmic antibodies in hepatobiliary disease. J Gastroenterol Hepatol 15: 344–345.
10. Savige JA, Davies DJ, Gatenby PA (1994) Anti-neutrophil cytoplasmic antibodies (ANCA): their detection and significance: report from workshops. Pathology 26: 186–193.
11. Talor MV, Stone JH, Stebbing J, Barin J, Rose NR, et al. (2007) Antibodies to selected minor target antigens in patients with anti-neutrophil cytoplasmic antibodies (ANCA). Clin Exp Immunol 150: 42–48. CEI3453 [pii];10.1111/j.1365-2249.2007.03453.x [doi].
12. Fabbri C, Jaboli MF, Giovanelli S, Azzaroli F, Pezzoli A, et al. (2003) Gastric autoimmune disorders in patients with chronic hepatitis C before, during and after interferon-alpha therapy. World J Gastroenterol 9: 1487–1490.
13. Sobajima J, Ozaki S, Uesugi H, Osakada F, Inoue M, et al. (1999) High mobility group (HMG) non-histone chromosomal proteins HMG1 and HMG2 are significant target antigens of perinuclear anti-neutrophil cytoplasmic antibodies in autoimmune hepatitis. Gut 44: 867–873.
14. Terjung B, Spengler U, Sauerbruch T, Worman HJ (2000) "Atypical p-ANCA" in IBD and hepatobiliary disorders react with a 50-kilodalton nuclear envelope protein of neutrophils and myeloid cell lines. Gastroenterology 119: 310–322. S0016508500010738 [pii].
15. Terjung B, Sohne J, Lechtenberg B, Gottwein J, Muennich M, et al. (2010) p-ANCAs in autoimmune liver disorders recognise human beta-tubulin isotype 5 and cross-react with microbial protein FtsZ. Gut 59: 808–816. gut.2008.157818 [pii];10.1136/gut.2008.157818 [doi].
16. Teegen B, Niemann S, Probst C, Schlumberger W, Stocker W, et al. (2009) DNA-bound lactoferrin is the major target for antineutrophil perinuclear cytoplasmic antibodies in ulcerative colitis. Ann N Y Acad Sci 1173: 161–165. NYAS4752 [pii];10.1111/j.1749-6632.2009.04752.x [doi].
17. Ooi CJ, Lim BL, Cheong WK, Ling AE, Ng HS (2000) Antineutrophil cytoplasmic antibodies (ANCAs) in patients with inflammatory bowel disease show no correlation with proteinase 3, lactoferrin, myeloperoxidase, elastase, cathepsin G and lysozyme: a Singapore study. Ann Acad Med Singapore 29: 704–707.
18. Mahler M, Bogdanos DP, Pavlidis P, Fritzler MJ, Csernok E, et al. (2013) PR3-ANCA: A promising biomarker for ulcerative colitis with extensive disease. Clin Chim Acta 424C: 267–273. S0009-8981(13)00246-5 [pii];10.1016/j.cca.2013.06.005 [doi].
19. Arias-Loste MT, Bonilla G, Moraleja I, Mahler M, Mieses MA, et al. (2013) Presence of Anti-proteinase 3 Antineutrophil Cytoplasmic Antibodies (Anti-PR3 ANCA) as Serologic Markers in Inflammatory Bowel Disease. Clin Rev Allergy Immunol 45: 109–116. 10.1007/s12016-012-8349-4 [doi].
20. Holle JU, Csernok E, Fredenhagen G, Backes M, Bremer JP, et al. (2010) Clinical evaluation of hsPR3-ANCA ELISA for detection of antineutrophil cytoplasmatic antibodies directed against proteinase 3. Ann Rheum Dis 69: 468–469. 69/2/468 [pii];10.1136/ard.2009.109868 [doi].
21. Roozendaal C, Van Milligen de Wit AW, Haagsma EB, Horst G, Schwarze C, et al. (1998) Antineutrophil cytoplasmic antibodies in primary sclerosing cholangitis: defined specificities may be associated with distinct clinical features. Am J Med 105: 393–399. S0002934398002940 [pii].
22. Mahler M, Radice A, Yang W, Bentow C, Seaman A, et al. (2012) Development and performance evaluation of novel chemiluminescence assays for detection of anti-PR3 and anti-MPO antibodies. Clin Chim Acta 413: 719–726. S0009-8981(12)00010-1 [pii];10.1016/j.cca.2012.01.004 [doi].
23. Long SA, Van de Water J, Gershwin ME (2002) Antimitochondrial antibodies in primary biliary cirrhosis: the role of xenobiotics. Autoimmun Rev 1: 37–42. S1568997201000209 [pii].
24. Arias-Loste MT, Bonilla G, Moraleja I, Mahler M, Mieses MA, et al. (2013) Presence of Anti-proteinase 3 Antineutrophil Cytoplasmic Antibodies (Anti-PR3 ANCA) as Serologic Markers in Inflammatory Bowel Disease. Clin Rev Allergy Immunol. 10.1007/s12016-012-8349-4 [doi].
25. Bambha K, Kim WR, Talwalkar J, Torgerson H, Benson JT, et al. (2003) Incidence, clinical spectrum, and outcomes of primary sclerosing cholangitis in a United States community. Gastroenterology 125: 1364–1369. S0016508503013568 [pii].
26. Terjung B, Worman HJ (2001) Anti-neutrophil antibodies in primary sclerosing cholangitis. Best Pract Res Clin Gastroenterol 15: 629–642. 10.1053/bega.2001.0209 [doi];S1521691801902094 [pii].
27. Trevisin M, Pollock W, Dimech W, Melny J, Paspaliaris B, et al. (2008) Antigen-specific ANCA ELISAs have different sensitivities for active and treated vasculitis and for nonvasculitic disease. Am J Clin Pathol 129: 42–53. W32U6598233K2436 [pii];10.1309/F6L4C48RHFMT4AAU [doi].
28. Pollock W, Clarke K, Gallagher K, Hall J, Luckhurst E, et al. (2002) Immunofluorescent patterns produced by antineutrophil cytoplasmic antibodies (ANCA) vary depending on neutrophil substrate and conjugate. J Clin Pathol 55: 680–683.
29. Trevisin M, Neeson P, Savige J (2004) The binding of proteinase 3 antineutrophil cytoplasmic antibodies (PR3-ANCA) varies in different ELISAs. J Clin Pathol 57: 303–308.
30. Savige J, Dimech W, Fritzler M, Goeken J, Hagen EC, et al. (2003) Addendum to the International Consensus Statement on testing and reporting of antineutrophil cytoplasmic antibodies. Quality control guidelines, comments, and recommendations for testing in other autoimmune diseases. Am J Clin Pathol 120: 312–318. 10.1309/WAEP-ADW0-K4LP-UHFN [doi].
31. Pollock W, Jovanovich S, Savige J (2009) Antineutrophil cytoplasmic antibody (ANCA) testing of routine sera varies in different laboratories but concordance is greater for cytoplasmic fluorescence (C-ANCA) and myeloperoxidase specificity (MPO-ANCA). J Immunol Methods 347: 19–23. S0022-1759(09)00171-9 [pii];10.1016/j.jim.2009.05.008 [doi].
32. Joossens S, Daperno M, Shums Z, Van SK, Goeken JA, et al. (2004) Interassay and interobserver variability in the detection of anti-neutrophil cytoplasmic antibodies in patients with ulcerative colitis. Clin Chem 50: 1422–1425. 10.1373/clinchem.2004.032318 [doi];50/8/1422 [pii].
33. Czaja AJ, Freese DK (2002) Diagnosis and treatment of autoimmune hepatitis. Hepatology 36: 479–497. S0270913902000563 [pii];10.1053/jhep.2002.34944 [doi].
34. Czaja AJ (2009) Autoimmune liver disease. Curr Opin Gastroenterol 25: 215–222. 10.1097/MOG.0b013e328324ed06 [doi];00001574-200905000-00009 [pii].
35. Czaja AJ, Norman GL (2003) Autoantibodies in the diagnosis and management of liver disease. J Clin Gastroenterol 37: 315–329.

36. Trevisin M, Pollock W, Dimech W, Savige J (2008) Evaluation of a multiplex flow cytometric immunoassay to detect PR3- and MPO-ANCA in active and treated vasculitis, and in inflammatory bowel disease (IBD). J Immunol Methods 336: 104–112. S0022-1759(08)00115-4 [pii];10.1016/j.jim.2008.03.012 [doi].

37. Fritzler MJ, Fritzler ML (2009) Microbead-based technologies in diagnostic autoantibody detection. Expert Opin Med Diagn 3: 81–89. 10.1517/17530050802651561 [doi].

38. Vidali M, Stewart SF, Rolla R, Daly AK, Chen Y, et al. (2003) Genetic and epigenetic factors in autoimmune reactions toward cytochrome P4502E1 in alcoholic liver disease. Hepatology 37: 410–419. 10.1053/jhep.2003.50049 [doi];S0270913902141632 [pii].

Permissions

All chapters in this book were first published in PLOS ONE, by The Public Library of Science; hereby published with permission under the Creative Commons Attribution License or equivalent. Every chapter published in this book has been scrutinized by our experts. Their significance has been extensively debated. The topics covered herein carry significant findings which will fuel the growth of the discipline. They may even be implemented as practical applications or may be referred to as a beginning point for another development.

The contributors of this book come from diverse backgrounds, making this book a truly international effort. This book will bring forth new frontiers with its revolutionizing research information and detailed analysis of the nascent developments around the world.

We would like to thank all the contributing authors for lending their expertise to make the book truly unique. They have played a crucial role in the development of this book. Without their invaluable contributions this book wouldn't have been possible. They have made vital efforts to compile up to date information on the varied aspects of this subject to make this book a valuable addition to the collection of many professionals and students.

This book was conceptualized with the vision of imparting up-to-date information and advanced data in this field. To ensure the same, a matchless editorial board was set up. Every individual on the board went through rigorous rounds of assessment to prove their worth. After which they invested a large part of their time researching and compiling the most relevant data for our readers.

The editorial board has been involved in producing this book since its inception. They have spent rigorous hours researching and exploring the diverse topics which have resulted in the successful publishing of this book. They have passed on their knowledge of decades through this book. To expedite this challenging task, the publisher supported the team at every step. A small team of assistant editors was also appointed to further simplify the editing procedure and attain best results for the readers.

Apart from the editorial board, the designing team has also invested a significant amount of their time in understanding the subject and creating the most relevant covers. They scrutinized every image to scout for the most suitable representation of the subject and create an appropriate cover for the book.

The publishing team has been an ardent support to the editorial, designing and production team. Their endless efforts to recruit the best for this project, has resulted in the accomplishment of this book. They are a veteran in the field of academics and their pool of knowledge is as vast as their experience in printing. Their expertise and guidance has proved useful at every step. Their uncompromising quality standards have made this book an exceptional effort. Their encouragement from time to time has been an inspiration for everyone.

The publisher and the editorial board hope that this book will prove to be a valuable piece of knowledge for researchers, students, practitioners and scholars across the globe.

List of Contributors

Lauren Elizabeth Veit, Jay Fong and Benjamin Udoka Nwosu
Department of Pediatrics, University of Massachusetts Medical School, Worcester, Massachusetts, United States of America

Louise Maranda
Department of Quantitative Health Sciences, University of Massachusetts Medical School, Worcester, Massachusetts, United States of America

Jan S. Suchodolski, Melissa E. Markel, Romy M. Heilmann, Yasushi Minamoto and Jörg M. Steiner
Gastrointestinal Laboratory, Small Animal Clinical Sciences, College of Veterinary Medicine and Biomedical Sciences, Texas A&M University, College Station, Texas, United States of America

Jose F. Garcia-Mazcorro
Facultad de Medicina Veterinaria, Universidad Autónoma de Nuevo León. Gral. Escobedo, Nuevo León, México

Stefan Unterer
Clinic of Small Animal Medicine, Ludwig-Maximillians-University, Munich, Germany

Scot E. Dowd
Molecular Research DNA Laboratory, Shallowater, Texas, United States of America

Priyanka Kachroo, Ivan Ivanov, Enricka M. Dillman and Audrey K. Cook
College of Veterinary Medicine and Biomedical Sciences, Texas A&M University, College Station, Texas, United States of America

Linda Toresson
Helsingborg Referral Animal Hospital, Helsingborg, Sweden

Jacilene S. Mesquita and Daniel F. Feijó
Departamento de Imunologia, Instituto de Microbiologia Professor Paulo de Góes, Universidade Federal do Rio de Janeiro (UFRJ), Rio de Janeiro, Brazil

Marcelo T. Bozza
Departamento de Imunologia, Instituto de Microbiologia Professor Paulo de Góes, Universidade Federal do Rio de Janeiro (UFRJ), Rio de Janeiro, Brazil
Departamento de Clínica Médica, Laboratório Multidisciplinar de Pesquisa, Universidade Federal do Rio de Janeiro (UFRJ), Rio de Janeiro, Brazil

Iranaia Assuncão-Miranda
Departamento de Virologia, Instituto de Microbiologia Professor Paulo de Góes, Universidade Federal do Rio de Janeiro (UFRJ), Rio de Janeiro, Brazil

Marta G. Cavalcanti
Departamento de Imunologia, Instituto de Microbiologia Professor Paulo de Góes, Universidade Federal do Rio de Janeiro (UFRJ), Rio de Janeiro, Brazil
Serviço de Doenças Infecciosas e Parasitárias, Universidade Federal do Rio de Janeiro (UFRJ), Rio de Janeiro, Brazil

Heitor S. P. Souza
Departamento de Clínica Médica, Laboratório Multidisciplinar de Pesquisa, Universidade Federal do Rio de Janeiro (UFRJ), Rio de Janeiro, Brazil

Kalil Madi
Departamento de Patologia, Hospital Universitário Clementino Fraga Filho, Universidade Federal do Rio de Janeiro (UFRJ), Rio de Janeiro, Brazil
Laboratório Sérgio Franco, Rio de Janeiro, Brazil

Eliseo Papa
Harvard/MIT Health Science and Technology Institute, Cambridge, Massachusetts, United States of America

Michael Docktor, Sarah Weber, Jay Ingram and Athos Bousvaros
Inflammatory Bowel Disease Center, Children's Hospital Boston, Boston, Massachusetts, United States of America

Christopher Smillie
Computational and Systems Biology Initiative, Massachusetts Institute of Technology, Cambridge, Massachusetts, United States of America

Sarah P. Preheim
Department of Civil and Environmental Engineering, Massachusetts Institute of Technology, Cambridge, Massachusetts, United States of America

Eric J. Alm
Department of Civil and Environmental Engineering, Massachusetts Institute of Technology, Cambridge, Massachusetts, United States of America
The Broad Institute, 7 Cambridge Center, Cambridge, Massachusetts, United States of America
Department of Biological Engineering, Massachusetts Institute of Technology, Cambridge, Massachusetts, United States of America

Dirk Gevers, Georgia Giannoukos, Dawn Ciulla, Diana Tabbaa and Doyle V. Ward
The Broad Institute, 7 Cambridge Center, Cambridge, Massachusetts, United States of America

David B. Schauer
Department of Biological Engineering, Massachusetts Institute of Technology, Cambridge, Massachusetts, United States of America
Division of Comparative Medicine, Massachusetts Institute of Technology, Cambridge, Massachusetts, United States of America

Joshua R. Korzenik
Gastrointestinal Unit, Center for Inflammatory Bowel Disease, Massachusetts General Hospital, Harvard Medical School, Boston, Massachusetts, United States of America

Ramnik J. Xavier
The Broad Institute, 7 Cambridge Center, Cambridge, Massachusetts, United States of America
Gastrointestinal Unit, Center for Inflammatory Bowel Disease, Massachusetts General Hospital, Harvard Medical School, Boston, Massachusetts, United States of America
Center for Computational and Integrative Biology, Harvard Medical School, Massachusetts General Hospital, Boston, Massachusetts, United States of America

Zhengting Wang, Rong Fan, Jie Zhou and Jie Zhong
Department of Gastroenterology, Ruijin Hospital, Shanghai Jiaotong University School of Medicine, Shanghai, China

Jiajia Hu
Department of Nuclear Medicine, Ruijin Hospital, Shanghai Jiaotong University School of Medicine, Shanghai, China

Magali Fasseu, Cécile Guichard, Eric Pedruzzi, Christophe Richard, Fanny Daniel, Richard Moreau, Marc Laburthe, André Groyer and Eric Ogier-Denis
INSERM U773, Centre de Recherche Biomédicale Bichat Beaujon, Paris, France
Université Paris 7 Denis Diderot, Paris, France

Xavier Tréton and Yoram Bouhnik
INSERM U773, Centre de Recherche Biomédicale Bichat Beaujon, Paris, France
Université Paris 7 Denis Diderot, Paris, France
Service de Gastroentérologie et d'Assistance Nutritive, Hôpital Beaujon, Clichy, France

Dominique Cazals-Hatem
INSERM U773, Centre de Recherche Biomédicale Bichat Beaujon, Paris, France

Université Paris 7 Denis Diderot, Paris, France
Service d'Anatomo-Pathologie, Hôpital Beaujon, Clichy, France

Thomas Aparicio and Jean-Claude Soulé
INSERM U773, Centre de Recherche Biomédicale Bichat Beaujon, Paris, France,
Université Paris 7 Denis Diderot, Paris, France
Service de Gastroentérologie, Hôpital Xavier Bichat, Paris, France

Yazan Ismail, Hoyul Lee and Li Zhang
School of Biotechnology and Biomolecular Sciences, University of New South Wales, Sydney, New South Whales, Australia

Stephen M. Riordan
Gastrointestinal and Liver Unit, The Prince of Wales Hospital, Sydney, New South Whales, Australia
Faculty of Medicine, University of New South Wales, Sydney, New South Whales, Australia

Michael C. Grimm
St George Clinical School, University of New South Wales, Sydney, New South Whales, Australia

Jane J. Sohn, Aaron J. Schetter, Izumi Horikawa, Mohammed A. Khan, Ana I. Robles, S. Perwez Hussain, Akiteru Goto, Elise D. Bowman and Curtis C. Harris
Laboratory of Human Carcinogenesis, Center for Cancer Research, National Cancer Institute, Bethesda, Maryland, United States of America

Harris G. Yfantis
Pathology and Laboratory Medicine, Baltimore Veterans Affairs Medical Center, and Department of Pathology, University of Maryland School of Medicine, Baltimore, Maryland, United States of America

Lisa A. Ridnour and David A. Wink
Radiation Biology Branch, National Cancer Institute, Bethesda, Maryland, United States of America

Lorne J. Hofseth
Department of Pharmaceutical and Biomedical Sciences, South Carolina College of Pharmacy, University of South Carolina, Columbia, South Carolina, United States of America

Jirina Bartkova
Cancer Society Research Center, Copenhagen, Denmark

Jiri Bartek
Cancer Society Research Center, Copenhagen, Denmark
Institute of Molecular and Translational Medicine, Faculty of Medicine and Dentistry, Palacky University, Olomouc, Czech Republic

Gerald N. Wogan
Department of Biological Engineering, Center for Environmental Health Sciences, Massachusetts Institute of Technology, Cambridge, Massachusetts, United States of America

Jesper Lindhardsen, Christian Torp-Pedersen, Gunnar Hilmar Gislason and Peter Riis Hansen
Department of Cardiology, Copenhagen University Hospital Gentofte, Hellerup, Denmark

Søren Lund Kristensen and Ole Ahlehoff
Department of Cardiology, Copenhagen University Hospital Gentofte, Hellerup, Denmark
Department of Cardiology, Copenhagen University Hospital Roskilde, Roskilde, Denmark

Gunnar Vagn Jensen
Department of Cardiology, Copenhagen University Hospital Roskilde, Roskilde, Denmark

Rune Erichsen
Department of Clinical Epidemiology, Aarhus University Hospital, Denmark

Ole Haagen Nielsen
Department of Gastroenterology, Copenhagen University Hospital Herlev, Herlev, Denmark

Indrani Mukhopadhya, Charlotte E. Nicholl, Yazeid A. Alhaidan, John M. Thomson, Susan H. Berry, Emad M. El-Omar and Georgina L. Hold
Gastrointestinal Research Group, Division of Applied Medicine, University of Aberdeen, Foresterhill, Aberdeen, United Kingdom

Richard Hansen
Gastrointestinal Research Group, Division of Applied Medicine, University of Aberdeen, Foresterhill, Aberdeen, United Kingdom
Child Health, University of Aberdeen, Royal Aberdeen Children's Hospital, Foresterhill, Aberdeen, United Kingdom

Craig Pattinson and David A. Stead
Aberdeen Proteomics Group, Institute of Medical Sciences, University of Aberdeen, Foresterhill, Aberdeen, United Kingdom

Richard K. Russell
Department of Paediatric Gastroenterology, Royal Hospital for Sick Children, Glasgow, United Kingdom

Maciej Chichlowski and Greg S. Westwood
Department of Pathology, Duke University Medical Center, Durham, North Carolina, United States of America

Soman N. Abraham
Department of Pathology, Duke University Medical Center, Durham, North Carolina, United States of America
Department of Molecular Genetics and Microbiology, Duke University Medical Center, Durham, North Carolina, United States of America
Department of Immunology, Duke University Medical Center, Durham, North Carolina, United States of America

Laura P. Hale
Department of Pathology, Duke University Medical Center, Durham, North Carolina, United States of America
The Human Vaccine Institute, Duke University Medical Center, Durham, North Carolina, United States of America

Anna Latiano, Orazio Palmieri, Fabrizio Bossa, Tiziana Latiano, Giuseppe Corritore, Maria Rosa Valvano and Angelo Andriulli
Division of Gastroenterology, IRCCS 'Casa Sollievo della Sofferenza', San Giovanni Rotondo, Italy

Luca Pastorelli and Maurizio Vecchi
Gastroenterology and Gastrointestinal Endoscopy Unit, IRCCS Policlinico San Donato, San Donato Milanese, Italy
Department of Medical and Surgical Sciences, University of Milan, Milan, Italy

Theresa T. Pizarro
Department of Pathology, Case Western Reserve University School of Medicine, Cleveland, Ohio, United States of America

Giuseppe Merla and Bartolomeo Augello
Medical Genetic Unit, IRCCS 'Casa Sollievo della Sofferenza', San Giovanni Rotondo, Italy

Alessia Settesoldi and Vito Annese
Gastroenterology Unit, AOU Careggi Hospital, Florence, Italy

Renata D'Inca
Department of Surgical and Gastroenterological Sciences, University of Padua, Padua, Italy

Laura Stronati
Department of Radiobiology and Human Health, Italian National Agency for New Technologies, Energy and Sustainable Economic Development (ENEA), Rome, Italy

Julia Seiderer, Cornelia Tillack, Florian Beigel, Johannes Stallhofer, Christian Steib, Burkhard Göke, Thomas Ochsenkühn and Stephan Brand
Department of Medicine II - Grosshadern, Ludwig-Maximilians-University (LMU), Munich, Germany

Johanna Wagner, Christoph Fries, Matthias Friedrich and Julia Diegelmann
Department of Medicine II - Grosshadern, Ludwig-Maximilians-University (LMU), Munich, Germany
Department of Preventive Dentistry and Periodontology, LMU, Munich, Germany

Jürgen Glas
Department of Medicine II - Grosshadern, Ludwig-Maximilians-University (LMU), Munich, Germany
Department of Preventive Dentistry and Periodontology, LMU, Munich, Germany
Department of Human Genetics, Rheinisch-Westfälische Technische Hochschule (RWTH), Aachen, Germany

Torsten Olszak
Department of Medicine II - Grosshadern, Ludwig-Maximilians-University (LMU), Munich, Germany
Division of Gastroenterology, Brigham & Women's Hospital, Harvard Medical School, Boston, United States of America

Martin Wetzke
Department of Medicine II - Grosshadern, Ludwig-Maximilians-University (LMU), Munich, Germany
Department of Preventive Dentistry and Periodontology, LMU, Munich, Germany
Department of Pediatrics, Hannover Medical School, Hannover, Germany

Darina Czamara
Max-Planck-Institute of Psychiatry, Munich, Germany

Valérie Bézirard, Christel Salvador-Cartier, Valérie Bacquié, Corinne Lencina, Mathilde Lévêque, Viorica Braniste, Sandrine Ménard, Vassilia Théodorou and Eric Houdeau
Neuro-Gastroenterology and Nutrition, Institut National de la Recherche Agronomique, UMR1331 Toxalim, INRA/INPT/UPS, Toulouse, France

Lara Moussa
Neuro-Gastroenterology and Nutrition, Institut National de la Recherche Agronomique, UMR1331 Toxalim, INRA/INPT/UPS, Toulouse, France
GENIBIO, Lorp-Sentaraille, France

Anna Latiano, Orazio Palmieri, Tiziana Latiano, Giuseppe Corritore, Fabrizio Bossa, Giuseppina Martino, Giuseppe Biscaglia, Daniela Scimeca, Maria Rosa Valvano and Angelo Andriulli
Gastroenterology Unit, IRCCS "Casa Sollievo della Sofferenza," San Giovanni Rotondo, Italy

Maria Pastore and Antonio Marseglia
Division of Paediatrics, IRCCS "Casa Sollievo della Sofferenza," San Giovanni Rotondo, Italy

Renata D'Incá
Department of Surgical and Gastroenterological Sciences, University of Padua, Padua, Italy,

Vito Annese
Division of Gastroenterology, University Hospital Careggi, Florence, Italy

Alan Moss, Aiping Bai, Yan Wu, Huang Huang, Adam Cheifetz and Simon C. Robson
Division of Gastroenterology, Department of Medicine, Beth Israel Deaconess Medical Center, Harvard University, Boston, United States of America

Maria Serena Longhi
Division of Gastroenterology, Department of Medicine, Beth Israel Deaconess Medical Center, Harvard University, Boston, United States of America
Institute of Liver Studies, King's College London School of Medicine at King's College Hospital, London, United Kingdom

Francisco J. Quintana
Center for Neurologic Diseases, Brigham and Women's Hospital, Harvard Medical School, Boston, United States of America

Chenwen Cai, Jun Shen, Di Zhao, Yuqi Qiao, Antao Xu, Shuang Jin, Zhihua Ran and Qing Zheng
Key Laboratory of Gastroenterology & Hepatology, Ministry of Health, Division of Gastroenterology and Hepatology, Ren Ji Hospital, School of Medicine, Shanghai Jiao Tong University, Shanghai Institute of Digestive Diseases, 145 Middle Shandong Road, Shanghai 200001, China

Giacomo Rossi and Angela Palumbo Piccionello
School of Veterinary Medical Sciences, University of Camerino, Camerino, Italy

Graziano Pengo
Clinic "St. Antonio", Cremona, Italy

Marco Caldin
San Marco Laboratories, Padova, Italy

Jörg M. Steiner and Jan S. Suchodolski
Gastrointestinal Laboratory, Department of Small Animal Clinical Sciences, College of Veterinary Medicine and Biomedical Sciences, Texas A&M University, College Station, Texas, United States of America

Noah D. Cohen
Department of Large Animal Clinical Sciences, College of Veterinary Medicine and Biomedical Sciences, Texas A&M University, College Station, Texas, United States of America

Albert E. Jergens
Department of Veterinary Clinical Sciences, College of Veterinary Medicine, Iowa State University, Ames, Iowa, United States of America

Cong Dai, Wei-Xin Liu, Min Jiang and Ming-Jun Sun
Department of Gastroenterology, First Affiliated Hospital, China Medical University, Shenyang City, Liaoning Province, China

Alexandre Medeiros do Carmo, Fabiana Maria Santos, Carmen Lucia Ortiz-Agostinho, Iêda Nishitokukado, Cintia S. Frota, Flavia Ubeda Gomes, André Zonetti de Arruda Leite and Aytan Miranda Sipahi
Departamento de Gastroenterologia, Hospital das Clínicas da Faculdade de Medicina da Universidade de São Paulo – LIM 07, São Paulo, São Paulo, Brazil

Claudio Sérgio Pannuti
Instituto de Medicina Tropical e Departamento de Doenc,as Infecciosas e Parasitarias (LIM-HC) da Faculdade de Medicina da Universidade de São Paulo, São Paulo, São Paulo, Brazil

Lucy Santos Vilas Boas
Instituto de Medicina Tropical e Hospital das Clínicas da Faculdade de Medicina (LIM-HC), Universidade de São Paulo, São Paulo, São Paulo, Brazil

Magaly Gemio Teixeira
Departamento de Cirurgia do Serviço de Cirurgia do Cólon Reto e Ânus, Hospital das Clínicas da Faculdade de Medicina da Universidade de de São Paulo, São Paulo, São Paulo, Brazil

Katriina Heikkilä, Solja T. Nyberg, Kirsi Ahola, Aki Koskinen, Marianna Virtanen and Ari Väänänen
Finnish Institute of Occupational Health, Helsinki, Finland

Ida E. H. Madsen and Jakob B. Bjorner
National Research Centre for the Working Environment, Copenhagen, Denmark

Lars Alfredsson
Institute of Environmental Medicine, Karolinska Institutet, Stockholm, Sweden

Eleonor I. Fransson
Institute of Environmental Medicine, Karolinska Institutet, Stockholm, Sweden
School of Health Sciences, Jönkö ping University, Jönkö ping, Sweden
Stress Research Institute, Stockholm University, Stockholm, Sweden

Töres Theorell and Hugo Westerlund
Stress Research Institute, Stockholm University, Stockholm, Sweden

Marianne Borritz and Martin L. Nielsen
Department of Occupational and Environmental Medicine, Bispebjerg University Hospital, Copenhagen, Denmark

Hermann Burr
Federal Institute for Occupational Safety and Health (BAuA), Berlin, Germany

Nico Dragano
Institute for Medical Sociology, Medical Faculty, University of Düsseldorf, Düsseldorf, Germany

Jane E. Ferrie
School of Community and Social Medicine, University of Bristol, Bristol, United Kingdom,
Department of Epidemiology and Public Health, University College London, London, United Kingdom

Martin J. Shipley
Department of Epidemiology and Public Health, University College London, London, United Kingdom

Anders Knutsson
Department of Health Sciences, Mid Sweden University, Sundsvall, Sweden

Markku Koskenvuo
Department of Public Health, University of Helsinki, Helsinki, Finland

Maria Nordin
Department of Psychology, Umeå University, Umeå, Sweden,

Jan H. Pejtersen
The Danish National Centre for Social Research, Copenhagen, Denmark

Jaana Pentti and Tuula Oksanen
Finnish Institute of Occupational Health, Helsinki, Tampere and Turku, Finland

Reiner Rugulies
National Research Centre for the Working Environment, Copenhagen, Denmark,
Department of Public Health and Department of Psychology, University of Copenhagen, Copenhagen, Denmark

Jussi Vahtera
Finnish Institute of Occupational Health, Helsinki, Tampere and Turku, Finland
Department of Public Health, University of Turku, Turku, Finland

Sakari B. Suominen
Folkhälsan Research Center, Helsinki, Finland
Department of Public Health, University of Turku, Turku, Finland
Nordic School of Public Health, Göteborg, Sweden

Peter J. M. Westerholm
Occupational and Environmental Medicine, Uppsala University, Uppsala, Sweden

G. David Batty
Department of Epidemiology and Public Health, University College London, London United Kingdom
Centre for Cognitive Ageing and Cognitive Epidemiology, University of Edinburgh, Edingurgh, United Kingdom

Archana Singh-Manoux
Department of Epidemiology and Public Health, University College London, London, United Kingdom
Inserm U1018, Centre for Research in Epidemiology and Population Health, Villejuif, France

Laura M. Stinton, Bertus Eksteen, Gilaad G. Kaplan and Marvin J. Fritzler
Department of Medicine, University of Calgary, Calgary, Alberta, Canada

Chelsea Bentow, Michael Mahler and Gary L. Norman
Inova Diagnostics, Inc., San Diego, California, United States of America

Andrew L. Mason
Department of Medicine, University of Alberta, Edmonton, Alberta, Canada

Bjorn Lindkvist
Institute of Medicine, Sahlgrenska Academy, University of Gothenburg, Gothenburg, Sweden

Gideon M. Hirschfield
Centre for Liver Research, NIHR Biomedical Research Unit, University of Birmingham, Birmingham, United Kingdom

Piotr Milkiewicz
Department of General, Transplant and Liver Surgery, Warsaw Medical University, Warsaw, Poland
Liver Research Laboratories, Pomeranian Medical University, Szczecin, Poland

Angela Cheung and Harry L. A. Janssen
University Health Network, Division of Gastroenterology, Toronto Western Hospital, Toronto, Ontario, Canada

Index